Handbook of Clinical Dietetics

# HANDBOOK OF CLINICAL DIETETICS

The American Dietetic Association

New Haven and London : Yale University Press

Designed by Sally Harris
and set in Times Roman type.
Printed in the United States of America by
Halliday Lithograph Corp.
West Hanover, Massachusetts

*Library of Congress Cataloging in Publication Data*

American Dietetic Association
  Handbook of clinical dietetics.

  Includes bibliographical references.
  1. Diet therapy.   I. Title.
RM216.A52     1980      615.8′54      80–11317
ISBN 0–300–02256–5


14   13   12   11   10   9   8

# Contents

# Preface

This handbook has been developed in response to a need for a manual, which was expressed in a resolution to the House of Delegates of the American Dietetic Association in 1971. The resolution stated in part, "*Whereas*, There is a great national and regional diversity in defining required dietetic diet content and terminology; *be it therefore resolved*, that The American Dietetic Association develop definitions of diet contents and terminology and accompanying scientific documentation" [1].

A committee of the Diet Therapy Section was appointed with Doris Johnson, Ph.D., R.D., as chairman of the project. Juliette Signore, M.S., R.D., was the principal researcher and writer.

The material compiled has been reviewed, in whole or in part, by a number of people with expertise in particular areas. A consensus was then arrived at for the final manuscript. We are most grateful to all those physicians, medical nutritionists, pharmacists, and dietitians who have in one way or another contributed to this handbook.

One of the unique aspects of the handbook is that it delineates what not to do as well as what to do and lists those practices in diet therapy that are obsolete and should be discarded. This handbook, with its many references, should serve as a guide for the current practice of diet therapy and as a basis for the preparation of diet manuals. If used as it is intended, it should do much to bring about some degree of uniformity and improvement in the practice of diet therapy.

References    1. Annual Report and Proceedings, 1971. Chicago: The American Dietetic Association.

# Introduction

## Purpose and Scope of the Handbook

As the charge to the committee to develop a handbook of dietetic diet content and terminology was carried out, the scope of the project of necessity was broadened in order to establish as precise terminology as possible, based on sound, well-documented principles that govern the modification of each diet being defined. It has been stated that, "When the rationale for a diet is not firmly established, the terminology is likely to be less exact" [1]. Thus the handbook has developed into a manual with definitions of each diet, as well as documentation for the formulation of the diet prescription and guidelines for making appropriate food choices within its confines. The material presented is intended as a reference for prescribing and implementing appropriate diet prescriptions for a projected audience of dietitians, nutritionists, physicians, physicians' assistants, nurse practitioners, nurses, and dietetic technicians. Sample menus for each diet have been evaluated, using the Recommended Dietary Allowances [2] and selected tables of food composition as guides [3,4].

**Modified Diet Prescription**    The format of the handbook is based on the concept of the therapeutic diet as a modification of the normal diet in which altered nutritional components should be prescribed in the same precise manner that governs the prescription of any other mode of therapy. Basic considerations affecting the formulation and use of the diet prescription have been incorporated into the following general headings, which provide the format for each section:

*Definition*    A standardization of the nomenclature in use in describing quantitative and qualitative aspects of the diet.

*Characteristics of the diet*    Description of pertinent aspects of the diet.

*Rationale*    The purpose and the expected effects of the diet and the supportive data.

*Indications for use*    Clinical applications either in the area of preventive nutrition or in the treatment of some preexisting disorder. If known, the ranges in clinical chemistry that may be useful as an index in making the appropriate prescription are included here.

*Possible adverse reactions*    Unwarranted side effects that may result from the use of the diet and suggested mechanisms for minimizing these effects. Nutritional deficits of any diet are also noted here.

*Contraindications*    Specific instances of accompanying conditions in which the consequences of possible adverse reactions would outweigh the beneficial effects of the diet.

*Suggestions for dietitians*     Guidelines for further modification of the diet where indicated, hints for the successful institution and implementation of the diet, and priorities for patient education.

*Guidelines for making appropriate food choices*     Where applicable, lists of foods to be permitted or excluded from the diet or a list of recommendations that will facilitate achievement of the goals of the diet.

*References*     Statements on the basis for the diet or lack of such basis are documented with appropriate references from the medical literature.

Detailed statements about the purpose, effects, indications, and contraindications for use of the diet are not provided if the rationale is highly controversial. Some sections of the manual, such as those on the bland and the purine restricted diets, contain only general statements or recommendations as to the status of the diet or simple guidelines where applicable.

## Limitations of the Handbook

Limitations in currently available tables of food composition have been a handicap in the development of the book, e.g., the lack of values for dietary fiber content of foods. A sound scientific basis for diet therapy principles cannot be documented in the absence of well-controlled clinical trials or where controversy exists over the efficacy of a particular form of nutritional management. Library research for the handbook probably uncovered as many questions as it did answers. It is hoped, however, that the handbook will stimulate a great deal of discussion and interest in clarifying gaps in diet therapy; that it will focus attention on the fact that reliance on subjective clinical impressions leads to empiricism in diet therapy, which cannot be used as the basis for the formulation of therapeutic diet prescriptions; and, finally, that careful consideration of any possible adverse consequences from alterations in the nutritional components of the normal diet should be a prerequisite to the prescription of any modified diet.

## Terms Used to Describe Diets

Diets should be prescribed in qualitative and quantitative terms that leave no room for misinterpretation. When a limitation must be set on the amount of any particular nutrient, the diet contents should be defined in terms of the specific amount to be provided, e.g., 40 g protein, 1 g sodium diet, etc. Additional terminology may also be used to define further the relationship of a specific diet prescription to the normal diet.

*Diet, modified*     A diet based on the normal diet and designed to meet the requirements of a given situation. It may be modified in individual nutrients, caloric value, consistency, flavor, techniques of service or preparation, content of specific foods, or a combination of these factors.

Levels of specific nutrients provided by any modified diet may also be described as being:

**Increased** Providing more of any nutrient than is usually provided by the normal diet.

**Decreased** Providing less of any nutrient than is usually provided by the normal diet.

**Restricted** Limited to a prescribed level in the amount and/or type of one or more nutrients provided. For example, the intake of any one nutrient may be limited to a particular type, as in the gluten restricted diet, or the amount ingested may be limited to a prescribed level, as with the fat restricted diet.

**High** The amount provided of a specific nutrient is increased to a substantial degree above that which is provided by the normal diet.

**Low** The amount provided of a specific nutrient is decreased to a substantial degree below that which is provided by the normal diet.

**Controlled** Implying careful regulation or adjustment of levels of one or more nutrients from day to day as needed according to biochemical changes; also used to refer to a diet in which *both* the amount and the type of one or more nutrients are regulated.

References
1. Robinson, C. H.: Updating clinical dietetics terminology. J. Am. Diet. Assoc. 62: 645, 1973.
2. Food and Nutrition Board, National Research Council: Recommended Dietary Allowances. 9th ed. Washington, DC: National Academy of Sciences, 1980.
3. Nutritive Value of American Foods in Common Portions. Agricultural Handbook No. 456. Washington, DC: Agriculture Research Service, U.S. Department of Agriculture, 1975.
4. Composition of Foods—Raw, Processed, Prepared. Agricultural Handbook No. 8. Washington, DC: Agriculture Research Service, U.S. Department of Agriculture, 1963.

# PART A     Normal Diet

# Normal Diet

***Definition*** A diet whose aim is to maintain a healthy person in a state of nutritive sufficiency [1]. It should provide amounts of energy, protein, vitamins, minerals, and other nutrients sufficient to meet the needs of the individual in his particular stage of the life cycle.

***Recommended Dietary Allowances*** Levels of intake of essential nutrients considered by the Food and Nutrition Board of the National Academy of Sciences, on the basis of available scientific knowledge, to be adequate to meet the known nutritional needs of practically all healthy persons [2] (see pp. I3–I5.) These allowances do not take into account special needs arising from infection, metabolic disorders, chronic diseases, or other abnormal conditions that necessitate therapeutic modifications of the diet, nor should they be confused with the minimum requirements. Except for kilocalories, the allowances are designed to afford a margin of safety sufficiently above average physiological requirements to cover variations among most individuals and to provide a buffer against increased needs during common everyday stresses [3].

Planning the Normal Diet

In order to be practical and meaningful, a standard such as the Recommended Dietary Allowances must be translated into guidelines for the proper selection of foods. One such guide utilizes basic food groups to provide a foundation for the daily planning of nutritious meals [4]. Foods should be chosen from these groups in such a way as to include as varied a selection of different foods as is possible. More specific information as to the nutrient needs in different stages of the life cycle and the formulation of the diet on the basis of these needs is available in excellent publications, which give more detailed information than can be provided within the scope of this handbook [1–15].

Presented here are menu patterns and sample meal plans for the normal adult, the 4- to 6-year-old, the 15- to 18-year-old male, pregnant and lactating women, and persons 55 years of age and older.

**Description of the Daily Food Plan of Normal Diet For an Adult (70 g protein, 1,415–2,415 kcal)**

| •Daily food plan | Description |
|---|---|
| MILK GROUP | |
| 1 pt* | *One pint whole milk* contains 320 kcal, 16 g protein, and calcium, phosphorous, and the B complex in important amounts. One pint buttermilk made from whole milk or ½ pt evaporated milk is similar. |
| | *One pint skim milk* contains 160 kcal, 18 g protein, and important amounts of calcium, phosphorus, and the B complex. If completely skimmed, no fat will be present, which accounts for the 50% decrease in kilocalories. One pint buttermilk made from skim milk or ½–⅔ cup (depending on brand) of nonfat milk solids is similar. |

## Meat Group†

**4 lean meat equivalents**

*One meat equivalent* is approximately equal to 1 oz (edible portion after cooking) beef, veal, lamb, pork, poultry, fish, or cheese, or 1 egg. The 4 equivalents may be distributed throughout the day as desired. (Liver and other variety meats are exceptional sources of vitamin A, iron, and the B complex.) The kilocalories contained in a 1-oz cooked portion of meat will vary with the type of meat equivalent used, depending upon the fat content. One lean meat, protein rich equivalent will contain 50 kcal and 7 g protein; 1 medium fat meat, protein rich equivalent will contain 75 kcal and 7 g protein; and 1 high fat meat, protein rich equivalent contains 95 kcal and 7 g protein. For the types of equivalents within each group see exchange lists on pp. F23–F24.

## Vegetable and Fruit Group

**5 servings**

*A dark green or deep yellow vegetable* is important each day for its vitamin A value. Asparagus, green beans, broccoli, carrots, green peppers, winter squash, pumpkin, and other greens make up this group. Winter squash and pumpkin may contain about 70 kcal per serving; the others contain about 25 kcal per serving.

*Other vegetables*, such as beets, cabbage, cauliflower, celery, cucumber, eggplant, lettuce, mushrooms, onions, peas, tomatoes, or turnips, contribute varied amounts of all nutrients. Peas contribute about 70 kcal per ½ cup serving. The others contain about 25 kcal.

*Citrus fruit or other fruit rich in vitamin C* is important each day. One orange or ½ cup juice, or ½ grapefruit or ½ cup juice, or ½ cup tomato juice, or ¾ cup strawberries, or ⅔ cup red raspberries, or ¼ cantaloupe, or 1 large tangerine contains about 40 kcal per serving and significant amounts of vitamin C.

*Other fruits*, such as 1 apple, 1 peach, 1 pear, 2 whole apricots, 12 grapes, or ½ banana, contribute varied amounts of most nutrients and contain about 40 kcal per serving. For other fruit see exchange lists on pp. F21–F22. If sugar or syrup is added, additional kilocalories must be calculated.

## Bread–Cereal–Potato–Legume Group

**8 servings**

*One serving provides approximately 70 kcal,* important amounts of the B complex, and iron. One serving is equal to 1 slice enriched or whole wheat bread; ½ cup white potato; ¼ cup sweet potato; ⅓ cup corn; ½ cup cooked macaroni, noodles, spaghetti, rice, cornmeal, cooked dried beans or peas, or cooked cereal; ¾ cup flake-type cereal; or 2 graham crackers. For other equivalents see exchange lists on pp. F22–F23.

## Fats and Sweets

*Without this group* the kilocalories for the day approximate 1,245–1,415 (depending on whether skim milk is used). The 2 oz separated fats and oils and 3 oz sugar available per capita in the United States would add approximately 1,000 kcal. Adjustments to fit individual needs may be made as follows:

*If 1 level tsp fat or oil* is used on bread, in vegetables, or in cooking, about 45 kcal is added. One thin slice crisp bacon, 2 tbsp light cream or 1 tbsp heavy cream, 1 tsp mayonnaise or oil, 1 tbsp cream cheese or French dressing, or 5 small olives or 6 small nuts also contain 45 kcal each.

*One level teaspoon sugar, jelly, or honey* in cooking, on cereal, in fruit, or in coffee adds 20 kcal. One-half cup ice cream, pudding, or gelatin dessert may add between 150 and 300 kcal, and 1 serving of cake or pie between 300 and 700 kcal. One slice of bread or equivalent will add 70 kcal.

## Iodized Salt

Iodized salt should be used in regions where iodine is lacking. Iodized salt is especially important in adolescence and pregnancy.

*Source*: Adapted from Handbook of Diet Therapy [1].
* One quart milk during last trimester of pregnancy; 1½ qt milk during lactation.
† If more meat is desired, 1 additional meat equivalent (edible portion: 1 oz cooked meat) may be substituted for 1 serving of the bread group without a substantial change in kilocalories.

**Menu Pattern and Sample Meals for an Adult**
**(75 g protein, 1,415–2,145 kcal)**

| Daily food plan* | Sample menu pattern | Sample meals |
|---|---|---|
| | | **A.M.** |
| **Milk group** | ½ cup citrus fruit or juice | Orange juice |
| 1 pt† | 1 cup cooked enriched or whole grain cereal or 1½ cups flake-type cereal with milk and sugar§ | Enriched farina with milk and sugar§ |
| **Meat group** | | Toast with fortified margarine§ |
| 4 meat equivalents;‡ 1 equivalent equals 1 oz meat (edible portion) weighed after cooking | 1 slice enriched or whole grain toast with fortified margarine§ | Coffee or tea if desired |
| | Coffee or tea, with sugar§ and milk, if desired | |
| **Vegetable and fruit group** | | **Noon** |
| 5 servings or more | 2 meat equivalents | Vegetable soup |
| **Bread–cereal–potato–legume group** | Vegetable | Sandwich—cheese and ham on 2 slices rye bread with fortified margarine |
| 8 servings‡ | Fruit | Sliced peaches with ice cream§ |
| **Fats and sweets§** | 1 cup milk | Milk |
| (Without this group the diet contains approximately 1,415 kcal) | 2 slices enriched or whole grain bread or alternate* with fortified margarine§ | |
| | Dessert§ | |
| | | **P.M.** |
| | 2 meat equivalents | Broiled chicken breast |
| | ½ cup potato or substitute | Baked potato |
| | Dark green or deep yellow vegetable | Broccoli |
| | Other vegetable | Tomato and lettuce salad with dressing§ |
| | Fruit | Baked apple |
| | 2 slices enriched or whole grain bread or alternate* with fortified margarine§ | Rolls with fortified margarine |
| | 1 cup milk | Milk |

*Source*: Adapted from Handbook of Diet Therapy [1].

\* For alternates within each group on this and other daily food plans for the normal diet, see exchange lists on pp. F20–F25.

† The use of 1 pt skim milk instead of 1 pt whole milk will result in a reduction of 160 kcal. One quart of milk should be used daily during last trimester of pregnancy and 1½ qt during lactation.

‡ If 1 additional meat equivalent (1 oz edible portion) is desired, 1 serving of the bread group may be omitted with no important change in the kilocalories.

§ Without sweets and fats, the diet contains about 1,415 kcal. Daily per capita consumption of separated fats and sugar in the United States averages 1,000 kcal. One teaspoon sugar, jelly, or honey adds 20 kcal; 1 tsp fat or oil, 45 kcal. A dessert such as gelatin, ice cream, or pudding may add 150–300 kcal. A dessert such as cake or pie may add between 300 and 700 kcal. A slice of bread or equivalent will add 70 kcal.

**Menu Pattern and Sample Meals for a Child Between 4 and 6 Years of Age (72 g protein, 1,800 kcal)**

| Daily food plan | Sample menu pattern | Sample meals |
|---|---|---|
| | | **A.M.** |
| MILK GROUP | 1 citrus fruit or ½ cup juice | Orange juice |
| 2–3 cups milk* | ½ cup cereal with milk and sugar‡ | Enriched farina with milk and sugar‡ |
| MEAT GROUP | 1 slice toast with fortified margarine‡ | Toast with fortified margarine |
| 3 equivalents;† 1 equivalent equals 1 oz meat (edible portion weighed after cooking) | 1 cup milk | Milk |
| | | **Noon** |
| VEGETABLE AND FRUIT GROUP | 1 meat equivalent | Sliced turkey |
| 4 servings, including a dark green or deep yellow vegetable for vitamin A and a citrus fruit or other fruit rich in vitamin C daily | Vegetables, raw or cooked | Shredded lettuce |
| | Fruit | Baked apple |
| | 1 slice enriched or whole grain bread with fortified margarine‡ | Bread with fortified margarine‡ |
| | ½ cup milk | Milk |
| BREAD–CEREAL–POTATO–LEGUME GROUP | | **P.M.** |
| 5 servings† | 2 meat equivalents | Broiled ground beef |
| FATS AND SWEETS‡ | ½ cup potato or substitute | Baked potato |
| (Without this group the diet contains 1,355 kcal) | Dark green or deep yellow vegetable | Carrot rings |
| | Dessert‡ | Ice cream |
| | 1 slice enriched or whole grain bread with fortified margarine‡ | Bread with fortified margarine‡ |
| | ½ cup milk | Milk |
| | | **Between meals** |
| | ½ cup milk | Milk |

*Source*: Adapted from Handbook of Diet Therapy [1].

* Vitamin D (400 IU) should be used as a concentrate if not contained in milk.

† If additional meat is desired, 1 serving of bread group (as 1 slice of bread) may be omitted for each 1 oz meat added, without changing the caloric value or reducing nutrient content substantially.

‡ One teaspoon sugar adds 20 kcal; 1 tsp fat or oil adds 45 kcal. Such desserts as ice cream, pudding, and gelatin may add 150–300 kcal.

**Menu Pattern and Sample Meals for an Adolescent Male Between 15 and 18 Years of Age (100 g protein, 2,800 kcal)**

## Daily food plan

MILK GROUP

  1 qt whole milk*

MEAT GROUP

  5 equivalents;† 1 equivalent equals 1 oz meat (edible portion) weighed after cooking

VEGETABLE AND FRUIT GROUP

  4 servings or more, including a dark green or deep yellow vegetable daily for vitamin A value and a citrus fruit or other fruit rich in vitamin C daily

BREAD–CEREAL–POTATO–LEGUME GROUP†

  7 servings†

FATS AND SWEETS‡

  (Without this group the diet contains 1,645 kcal)

## Sample menu pattern

1 citrus fruit or ½ cup juice
½ cup cooked cereal or ¾ cup flake-type with milk and sugar‡
1 slice enriched or whole grain toast with fortified margarine‡
1 cup milk

2 meat equivalents
Vegetable
2 slices enriched or whole grain bread or substitute with fortified margarine‡
1 cup milk

3 meat equivalents
½ cup potato or substitute†
Dark green or deep yellow vegetable
Other vegetable
Fruit
2 slices enriched or whole grain bread with fortified margarine‡
1 cup milk

1 cup milk

## Sample meals

A.M.

Grapefruit
Flakes with milk and sugar‡
Toast with fortified margarine‡
Milk

Noon

Sandwich—turkey on bread with fortified margarine‡
Sliced tomatoes
Milk

P.M.

Meat loaf
Baked potato
Carrots
Cabbage slaw
Apple
Rolls with fortified margarine
Milk

Between meals

Milk

---

*Source*: Adapted from Handbook of Diet Therapy [1].

*Notes*: The Recommended Dietary Allowances during adolescence may be met by this pattern, with the exception of iron; iron rich foods may be used to augment this level.

* The use of skim milk would result in a reduction of 320 kcal. Vitamin D (400 IU) should be used as a concentrate if not contained in milk.

* If additional meat is desired, 1 serving of the bread group (as 1 slice bread) may be omitted for each 1 oz meat added, without changing the caloric value or reducing nutrient content substantially.

‡ One teaspoon sugar adds 20 kcal; 1 tsp fat or oil adds 45 kcal. Desserts such as ice cream, pudding, and gelatin may add 150–300 kcal. Cake or pie may add 300–700 kcal. Adjustments in this group should be made to suit individual caloric needs.

## Menu Pattern and Sample Meals during Pregnancy and Lactation
## (100 g protein, 2,720 kcal)

| Daily food plan | Sample menu pattern | Sample meals |
|---|---|---|
| | | **A.M.** |
| MILK GROUP* | 1 citrus fruit or ½ cup juice | Grapefruit |
| 1 qt whole milk | ½ cup cooked cereal or ¾ cup flake-type with milk and sugar‡ | Flakes with milk and sugar‡ |
| MEAT GROUP | 1 slice enriched or whole grain toast with fortified margarine‡ | Toast with fortified margarine‡ |
| 5 equivalents;† 1 equivalent equals 1 oz of meat (edible portion) weighed after cooking | 1 cup milk | Milk |
| | | **Noon** |
| VEGETABLE AND FRUIT GROUP | 2 meat equivalents | Sandwich—turkey on bread with fortified margarine |
| 4 servings or more, including a dark green or deep yellow vegetable daily for vitamin A value and a citrus fruit or other fruit rich in vitamin C daily | Vegetable | Sliced tomatoes and lettuce |
| | 2 slices enriched or whole grain bread or substitute with fortified margarine | Milk |
| | 1 cup milk | |
| BREAD–CEREAL–POTATO–LEGUME GROUP | | **P.M.** |
| 7 servings† | 3 meat equivalents | Meat loaf |
| FATS AND SWEETS‡ | ½ cup potato or substitute | Baked potato |
| (Without this group the diet contains 1,645 kcal) | Dark green or deep yellow vegetable | Carrots |
| | Other vegetable | Cabbage slaw |
| | Fruit | Apple |
| | 2 slices enriched or whole grain bread or substitute with fortified margarine | Rolls with fortified margarine‡ |
| | | Milk |
| | 1 cup milk | |
| | | **Between meals** |
| | 1 cup milk | Milk |

*Source*: Adapted from Handbook of Diet Therapy [1].

*Notes*: The Recommended Dietary Allowances during pregnancy may be met by this pattern, the exceptions being iron and folic acid. Iron rich foods may be used to augment this level, and daily supplements of 30–60 mg iron in the form of ferrous sulfate and 200–400 μg folic acid should be taken. For information on sodium intake see pp. G3–G16.

* During lactation 1½ qt of milk per day would provide the extra protein and other nutrients required to meet the Recommended Dietary Allowances. The use of skim milk would result in a reduction of 320 kcal in 1 qt of milk. If 400 IU vitamin D is not contained in 1 qt of milk, a concentrate should be prescribed.

† If additional meat is desired, 1 serving of the bread group (as 1 slice bread) may be omitted for each 1 oz meat added, without changing the caloric value or reducing nutrient content substantially.

‡ One teaspoon sugar adds 20 kcal; 1 tsp fat or oil adds 45 kcal. Desserts like ice cream, pudding, and gelatin may add 150–300 kcal. Cake or pie may add 300–700 kcal. Adjustments in this group should be made to suit individual caloric needs.

**Menu Pattern and Sample Meals for a Person 55 Years of Age or Over (75 g protein, 1,800 kcal)**

| Daily food plan | Sample menu pattern | Sample meals |
|---|---|---|

**A.M.**

MILK GROUP

1 pt milk

1 citrus fruit or ½ cup juice
½ cooked cup cereal or ¾ cup flake-type cereal with milk and sugar†
1 slice enriched or whole grain toast with fortified margarine†
Coffee or tea if desired†

Orange juice
Flakes with milk and sugar†
Toast with fortified margarine†
Coffee or tea if desired†

MEAT GROUP

4 equivalents;* 1 equivalent equals 1 oz of meat (edible portion) weighed after cooking

VEGETABLE AND FRUIT GROUP

5 servings or more, including a dark green or deep yellow vegetable for vitamin A value and a citrus fruit or other fruit rich in vitamin C daily

**Noon**

2 meat equivalents
½ cup potato, rice, or substitute‡
2 slices enriched or whole grain bread or substitutes
1 cup milk

Vegetable soup with crackers‡
Tuna casserole
Mixed salad greens with dressing†
Peach custard†
Bread with fortified margarine†
Milk

BREAD–CEREAL–POTATO–LEGUME GROUP‡

8 servings*

FATS AND SWEETS†

(Without this group the diet contains 1,415 kcal)

**P.M.**

3 meat equivalents
½ cup potato or substitute‡
Dark green or deep yellow vegetable
Fruit
1 slice enriched or whole grain bread with fortified margarine†

Browned meat patty
Baked potato
Broccoli
Tossed lettuce and tomato salad with dressing†
Applesauce
Bread with fortified margarine†

**Between meals**

1 cup milk
2 graham crackers‡

Milk
Graham crackers‡

*Source:* Adapted from Handbook of Diet Therapy [1].

*Note:* The nutrient content for this plan corresponds to the Recommended Dietary Allowances for the older person.

† If additional meat is desired, 1 serving of the bread group (as 1 slice bread) may be omitted for each 1 oz meat added, without changing the caloric value or reducing nutrient content substantially.

† One teaspoon sugar adds 20 kcal; 1 tsp fat or oil adds 45 kcal. Desserts like ice cream, pudding, or gelatin may add 150–300 kcal. Cake or pie may add 300–700 kcal.

‡ Soda crackers (2 in. square) or 2 graham crackers may be used as an alternate for 1 slice bread. See exchange lists on pp. F22–F23 for other alternates.

References

1. Turner, D.: Handbook of Diet Therapy. 5th ed. Chicago: University of Chicago Press, 1970.
2. Food and Nutrition Board, National Research Council: Recommended Dietary Allowances. 9th ed. Washington, DC: National Academy of Sciences, 1980.
3. Robinson, C. H., and Lawler, M. R.: Normal and Therapeutic Nutrition. 15th ed. New York, Macmillian, 1977.
4. Hill, M.: Foods to satisfy. U.S. Department of Agriculture: Consumers All-Yearbook of Agriculture, 1965, Washington, DC: U.S. Government Printing Office, 1965.
5. Williams, S. R.: Nutrition and Diet Therapy. 3d ed. St. Louis: C. V. Mosby, 1977.
6. Fomon, S. J.: Infant Nutrition. 2d ed. Philadelphia: W. B. Saunders, 1974.
7. Fomon, S. J., Filer, L. J., Jr., Anderson, T. A., and Ziegler, E. E.: Recommendations For Feeding Normal Infants. Pediatrics 63: 52, 1979.
8. Goodhart, R. S., and Shils, M. E., eds.: Modern Nutrition in Health and Disease. 5th ed. Philadelphia: Lea & Febiger, 1973.
9. Carlson, L., editor: Nutrition and Old Age. Stockholm: Almquist & Wikksell, 1972.
10. Raiha, N. C. R.: Biochemical basis for nutritional management of preterm infants. Pediatrics 53: 146, 1974.
11. Fitzgerald, J. F.: Infant feeding. Postgrad. Med. 56: 47, July 1974.
12. Davies, D. P.: Plasma osmolality and feeding practices of healthy infants in first three months of life. Br. Med. J. 2: 340, 1973.
13. Krehl, W. A.: The influence of nutritional environment on aging. Geriatrics 29: 65, May 1974.
14. Deutsch, R. M.: The Family Guide to Better Food and Better Health. Des Moines: Creative Home Library, 1974.
15. Composition of Foods—Raw, Processed, Prepared. Agricultural Handbook No. 8, Washington, DC: Agriculture Research Service, U.S. Department of Agriculture, 1963.

# Nutritional Analysis of Diets

Tables 1 and 2 give the nutritional analysis of the basic food groups in the amounts used in the normal diet. These tables may be used also to evaluate the nutritional intake of an individual. They are of especial value in the monitoring of food intake of individuals on either normal or modified diets and for the assessment of their nutritional status.

Table 3 gives the average nutritional value of normal diets for different age groups and of the modified diets included in the handbook, based on a 3-day menu plan. These menus include the principles set forth in the prudent diet concept. The basic menus were planned to include three eggs per week, lean meat or equivalent, skim milk, polyunsaturated fortified margarine and cooking fats, and enriched or whole grain cereals and breads. The Recommended Dietary Allowances for the normal male and female adult are given in table 3 for comparison of the diets for nutritional adequacy. The Recommended Dietary Allowances (pp. I3–I5) should be consulted for other recommended allowances, such as those for children and pregnant or lactating women, for comparison. The figures given in table 3 for the normal diets will vary from the Recommended Dietary Allowances, since the menu plans contain such foods as pie, cake, and puddings in addition to the basic food groups. Agricultural Handbook No. 8, Composition of Foods, Raw, Processed, Prepared Washington, DC: Agriculture Research Service, U.S. Department of Agriculture, 1963 was used as the source of the nutrient content of the food. Calculations were done by computer.

**Table 1. Nutritive Value of a Basic Diet Plan for an Adult in Health**

| Food | Measure | Weight (g) | Energy (kcal) | Protein (g) | Fat (g) | Carbohydrate (g) | Crude fiber (g) | Calcium (mg) | Phosphorous (mg) | Iron (mg) | Sodium (mg) | Potassium (mg) | Vitamin A value (IU) | Thiamine (mg) | Riboflavin (mg) | Niacin (mg) | Ascorbic acid (mg) | Saturated fat (g) | Oleic acid (g) | Linoleic acid (g) | Cholesterol (mg) |
|---|---|---|---|---|---|---|---|---|---|---|---|---|---|---|---|---|---|---|---|---|---|
| Milk, 2% skim | 2 cups | 488 | 288 | 20 | 10 | 29 | 0 | 698 | 547 | 0.5 | 298 | 854 | 390 | 0.2 | 1.0 | 0.5 | 5 | 4.9 | 4.9 | 0 | 44 |
| *Meat group*†  | | | | | | | | | | | | | | | | | | | | | |
| Egg | 1 | 50 | 70 | 6 | 5 | 0 | 0 | 24 | 90 | 1.1 | 54 | 57 | 520 | 0.1 | 0.1 | 0.1 | 0 | 1.6 | 2.2 | 0.4 | 203 |
| Meat, fish, poultry | 4 oz | 120 | 285 | 31 | 18 | 0 | 0 | 14 | 274 | 3.1 | 88 | 430 | 88 | 0.3 | 0.2 | 7.3 | 0 | 7.7 | 6.9 | 0.9 | 99 |
| *Vegetable group* | | | | | | | | | | | | | | | | | | | | | |
| Leafy green or deep yellow‡ | ¼–⅓ cup | 50 | 12 | 1 | 0 | 2 | 0.5 | 34 | 22 | 0.6 | 12 | 127 | 2,537 | 0 | 0.1 | 0.3 | 20 | 0 | 0 | 0 | 0 |
| Other vegetables§ | ¼–⅓ cup | 50 | 19 | 1 | 0 | 4 | 0.5 | 19 | 22 | 0.5 | 30 | 105 | 347 | 0 | 0 | 0.4 | 7 | 0 | 0 | 0 | 0 |
| *Fruit group* | | | | | | | | | | | | | | | | | | | | | |
| Citrus fruit⊥ | 1 serving | 100 | 44 | 1 | 0 | 10 | 0.2 | 19 | 17 | 0.3 | 1 | 174 | 123 | 0.1 | 0 | 0.3 | 44 | 0 | 0 | 0 | 0 |
| Other fruit° | 1 serving | 100 | 92 | 1 | 0 | 22 | 0.7 | 10 | 16 | 0.6 | 2 | 176 | 496 | 0 | 0 | 0.4 | 5 | 0 | 0 | 0 | 0 |
| *Bread–cereal group*** | | | | | | | | | | | | | | | | | | | | | |
| Cereal, enriched or whole grain | ¾ cup | 30 (dry) | 135 | 4 | 1 | 29 | 3.0 | 13 | 75 | 1.1 | 303 | 73 | 0 | 0.1 | 0 | 1.3 | 0 | 0.1 | 0.1 | 0.1 | 0 |
| Bread, enriched or whole grain | 3 slices | 75 | 205 | 7 | 2 | 39 | 0.7 | 68 | 126 | 1.9 | 414 | 143 | 0 | 0.2 | 0.1 | 2.0 | 0 | 0.8 | 1.6 | 0 | 2 |
| Fortified margarine | 4 tsp | 20 | 144 | 0 | 16 | 0 | 0 | 4 | 12 | 0 | 200 | 4 | 660 | 0 | 0 | 0 | 0 | 3.2 | 6.0 | 6.0 | 0 |
| Sugars | 2 tsp | 10 | 46 | 0 | 0 | 12 | 0 | 0 | 0 | 0 | 0 | 1 | 0 | 0 | 0 | 0 | 0 | 0 | 0 | 0 | 0 |
| Totals | | | 1,337 | 72 | 52 | 147 | 5.6 | 903 | 1,201 | 9.7 | 1,402 | 2,144 | 5,161 | 1.0 | 1.5 | 12.6†† | 81 | 18.3 | 21.7 | 7.4 | 348 |
| *Recommended Dietary Allowances* | | | | | | | | | | | | | | | | | | | | | |
| Female (23–50 yr) | | | 2,000 | 44 | | | | 800 | 800 | 18.0 | | | 4,000 | 1.0 | 1.2 | 13 | 60 | | | | |
| Male (23–50 yr) | | | 2,700 | 56 | | | | 800 | 800 | 10.0 | | | 5,000 | 1.4 | 1.6 | 18 | 60 | | | | |

*Source:* Adapted from Robinson, C. H.; and Lawler, M. R.: Normal and Therapeutic Nutrition. 15th ed. New York: Macmillan 1977.

* Values for foods in the meat, vegetable, fruit, and bread–cereal groups are weighted on the basis of the approximate consumption in the United States.

† Calculations based upon an average weekly intake for meat of 11 oz beef, 7½ oz pork, 6½ oz poultry, 1½ oz lamb and veal, and 1½ oz fish.

‡ Dark green leafy and deep yellow vegetables include carrots, green peppers, broccoli, spinach, endive, escarole, and kale. It is assumed that an average serving of ½ cup is eaten at least every other day.

§ Other vegetables include tomatoes, lettuce, cabbage, snap beans, lima beans, celery, peas, onions, corn, cucumbers, beets, and cauliflower. It is assumed that an average serving of ½ cup is eaten at least every other day.

⊥ Citrus fruit includes fresh, canned, and frozen oranges, orange juice, grapefruit, and grapefruit juice.

° Other fruit includes apples, peaches, pears, apricots, grapes, plums, prunes, berries, and bananas.

** Cereals include corn flakes, wheat flakes, macaroni, oatmeal, shredded wheat, and enriched rice.

†† The protein in this diet contains about 720 mg trytophan, equivalent to 12 mg niacin; thus the niacin equivalent of this diet is 25 mg.

**Table 2. Additional Mineral and Vitamin Values for the Basic Diet Plan**

| Food | Measure | Weight (g) | Magnesium (mg) | Zinc (g) | Vitamin E (mg) | Folacin (µg) | Vitamin B₆ (µg) | Vitamin B₁₂ (µg) | Pantothenic acid (µg) |
|---|---|---|---|---|---|---|---|---|---|
| Milk, 2% skim | 2 cups | 488 | 62 | 1.9 | 0.19 | 5 | 192 | 1.9 | 1,632 |
| *Meat group* | | | | | | | | | |
| Egg | 1 | 50 | 6 | 0.5 | 0.23 | 3 | 55 | 1.0 | 800 |
| Meat, fish, poultry (lean cooked) | 4 oz | 120 | 33 | 5.4 | 0.26 | 9 | 589 | 1.6 | 839 |
| *Vegetable–fruit group* | | | | | | | | | |
| Leafy green or deep yellow | ¼–⅓ cup | 50 | 13 | 0.3 | 0.47 | 22 | 75 | 0 | 133 |
| Other vegetable | ¼–⅓ cup | 50 | 13 | 0.2 | 0.16 | 14 | 50 | 0 | 152 |
| Potato | 1 medium | 122 | 14 | 0.3 | 0.05 | 9 | 212 | 0 | 320 |
| Citrus fruit | 1 serving | 100 | 11 | 0.1 | 0.04 | 3 | 33 | 0 | 206 |
| Other fruit | 1 serving | 100 | 13 | 0.2 | 0.22 | 5 | 100 | 0 | 174 |
| *Bread–cereal group* | | | | | | | | | |
| Cereal, enriched or whole grain* | ¾ cup | 30 (dry) | 21 | 0.5 | 0.22 | 15 | 39 | 0 | 166 |
| Bread, enriched or whole grain* | 3 slices | 75 | 38 | 0.8 | 0.21 | 17 | 78 | 0 | 446 |
| Totals | | | 224 | 10.2 | 2.05 | 102 | 1,423 | 4.5 | 4,868 |
| *Recommended Dietary Allowances* | | | | | | | | | |
| Female (23–50 yr) | | | 300 | 15 | 12 | 400 | 2,000 | 3.0 | |
| Male (23–50 yr) | | | 350 | 15 | 15 | 400 | 2,200 | 3.0 | |

*Source*: Adapted from Robinson and Lawler: Normal and Therapeutic Nutrition.
*Note*: Values are calculated on the basis of the same foods as used for table 1.
* Average of whole grain and enriched cereals.

# Table 3. Nutritional Analysis of Diets (Average of three days' menus)

| Diet | Food energy (kcal) | Protein (g) | Fat (g) | Carbo-hydrate (g) | Fiber (g) | Calcium (mg) | Phos-phorus (mg) | Iron (mg) | Sodium (mg) | Potas-sium (mg) |
|---|---|---|---|---|---|---|---|---|---|---|
| *Recommended Dietary Allowances* | | | | | | | | | | |
| Female (23–50 yr) | 2,000 | 44 | | | | 800 | 800 | 18.0 | | |
| Male (23–50 yr) | 2,700 | 56 | | | | 800 | 800 | 10.0 | | |
| Normal | 2,104 | 76 | 89 | 253 | 3.3 | 1,196 | 1,318 | 13.8 | 2,808 | 3,114 |
| Pregnancy and lactation | 2,704 | 99 | 120 | 310 | 3.9 | 1,736 | 1,841 | 17.7 | 3,706 | 4,151 |
| Toddlers | 1,814 | 72 | 80 | 204 | 2.5 | 1,317 | 1,325 | 10.3 | 2,027 | 2,683 |
| 15–18-year old male | 2,785 | 99 | 131 | 300 | 3.5 | 1,712 | 1,779 | 14.1 | 3,284 | 3,672 |
| 55 years or over | 1,882 | 75 | 68 | 245 | 3.3 | 1,174 | 1,306 | 13.8 | 2,509 | 3,063 |
| Clear liquid | 801 | 10 | 0 | 195 | 0.2 | 42 | 62 | 2.0 | 2,173 | 640 |
| Full liquid | 2,784 | 114 | 114 | 332 | 2.9 | 2,858 | 2,670 | 10.6 | 6,194 | 4,904 |
| Fiber restricted | 2,339 | 86 | 103 | 269 | 3.5 | 1,179 | 1,411 | 18.5 | 3,152 | 3,285 |
| High fiber | 2,478 | 96 | 86 | 362 | 14.8 | 1,423 | 2,129 | 24.4 | 3,314 | 5,207 |
| High calorie, high protein | 3,377 | 172 | 145 | 352 | 5.8 | 2,199 | 2,660 | 23.6 | 3,963 | 5,385 |
| Gluten restricted | 2,548 | 112 | 105 | 296 | 6.0 | 1,550 | 1,941 | 13.9 | 3,304 | 4,341 |
| Tyramine restricted | 2,661 | 114 | 104 | 324 | 6.1 | 1,297 | 1,754 | 20.5 | 3,315 | 4,128 |
| Carbohydrate restricted for management of dumping syndrome | | | | | | | | | | |
| Stage I | 1,463 | 84 | 90 | 84 | 2.4 | 1,041 | 1,472 | 8.6 | 1,932 | 2,172 |
| Stage II | 2,331 | 139 | 129 | 160 | 5.2 | 1,545 | 2,212 | 17.2 | 3,330 | 3,913 |
| Sucrose free | 1,482 | 108 | 90 | 52 | 0 | 1,345 | 1,703 | 6.5 | 1,167 | 2,461 |
| Sucrose restricted | 1,919 | 95 | 104 | 148 | 3.8 | 1,552 | 1,687 | 10.7 | 1,810 | 2,875 |
| Lactose free | 1,857 | 68 | 77 | 225 | 4.0 | 347 | 854 | 17.3 | 2,517 | 2,669 |
| 50 g fat | 2,028 | 98 | 49 | 304 | 6.6 | 1,153 | 1,456 | 19.3 | 2,204 | 4,127 |
| Fat controlled | 2,506 | 106 | 99 | 302 | 7.0 | 1,290 | 1,675 | 21.8 | 2,801 | 4,751 |
| Type I hyperlipoproteinemia 1,700–2,000 kcal | 2,020 | 112 | 24 | 342 | 7.7 | 1,728 | 1,989 | 21.0 | 2,757 | 5,168 |
| Type IIa hyperlipoproteinemia | 1,988 | 97 | 87 | 204 | 4.5 | 1,109 | 1,402 | 17.4 | 2,355 | 3,372 |
| Type IIb + III hyperlipopro-teinemia 1,800 kcal | 1,795 | 105 | 56 | 222 | 6.6 | 1,612 | 1,851 | 18.0 | 2,402 | 4,238 |
| Type IV hyperlipoproteinemia 1,500 kcal | 1,521 | 86 | 62 | 155 | 4.3 | 965 | 1,289 | 14.0 | 1,850 | 3,214 |
| Type V hyperlipoproteinemia 1,500 kcal | 1,581 | 98 | 47 | 192 | 4.4 | 1,301 | 1,566 | 15.2 | 2,117 | 3,623 |
| Fat controlled 1,200 kcal | 1,319 | 73 | 50 | 142 | 4.0 | 996 | 1,155 | 14.4 | 1,448 | 2,881 |
| Fat controlled 1,800 kcal | 1,988 | 97 | 87 | 204 | 4.5 | 1,109 | 1,402 | 17.4 | 2,355 | 3,372 |
| Calorie, carbohydrate, protein, and fat controlled 1,800 kcal | 1,898 | 101 | 67 | 224 | 5.7 | 1,402 | 1,595 | 17.6 | 2,402 | 3,814 |
| Calorie restricted 1,200 kcal | 1,283 | 76 | 44 | 146 | 4.3 | 1,200 | 1,271 | 18.3 | 1,460 | 3,084 |
| *Medium chain triglyceride-based ketogenic (+ MCT) | 577 | 39 | 14 | 74 | 1.6 | 561 | 629 | 5.0 | 750 | 1,565 |
| *Medium chain triglyceride–long chain triglyceride restricted (+ MCT) | 1,617 | 83 | 28 | 261 | 5.6 | 1,086 | 1,364 | 18.6 | 2,021 | 3,842 |
| Vegans | 2,173 | 81 | 83 | 303 | 14.3 | 672 | 1,677 | 24.3 | 3,038 | 4,727 |
| Lactovegetarian | 2,546 | 94 | 121 | 286 | 9.1 | 1,713 | 2,043 | 13.7 | 3,785 | 4,446 |
| Lactoovovegetarian | 2,505 | 104 | 113 | 283 | 8.7 | 1,638 | 2,203 | 15.8 | 3,932 | 4,475 |
| High potassium | 2,695 | 130 | 105 | 324 | 9.8 | 1,782 | 2,534 | 26.0 | 3,675 | 5,992 |
| 500 mg sodium | 1,930 | 82 | 67 | 251 | 5.7 | 1,124 | 1,392 | 18.3 | | 3,501 |
| 1,000 mg sodium | 1,934 | 81 | 70 | 245 | 5.7 | 1,116 | 1,387 | 18.1 | | 3,491 |
| 1,500 mg sodium | 2,030 | 87 | 74 | 255 | 5.6 | 1,105 | 1,439 | 18.4 | | 3,593 |
| 2,000 mg sodium | 2,096 | 95 | 79 | 253 | 5.8 | 1,172 | 1,540 | 19.0 | | 3,802 |
| Controlled protein, sodium and potassium | 2,259 | 46 | 65 | 372 | 4.9 | 450 | 672 | 13.6 | 1,447 | 1,956 |

* Does not include calories and fat from MCT.

# Table 3. (Continued)

| Diet | Vitamin A value (IU) | Thiamine (mg) | Riboflavin (mg) | Niacin (mg N.E.) | Ascorbic acid (mg) | Saturated fat (g) | Oleic acid (g) | Linoleic acid (g) | Cholesterol (mg) |
|---|---|---|---|---|---|---|---|---|---|
| *Recommended Dietary Allowances* | | | | | | | | | |
| Female (23–50 yr) | 4,000 | 1.0 | 1.2 | 13.0 | 60 | | | | |
| Male (23–50 yr) | 5,000 | 1.4 | 1.6 | 18.0 | 60 | | | | |
| Normal | 8,568 | 1.3 | 1.9 | 15.5 | 123 | 28.7 | 36.9 | 16.6 | 248 |
| Pregnancy and lactation | 9,732 | 1.6 | 2.7 | 19.8 | 138 | 45.9 | 44.7 | 16.7 | 363 |
| Toddlers | 7,567 | 0.8 | 1.7 | 11.1 | 89 | 39.4 | 30.1 | 8.9 | 288 |
| 15–18-year old male | 10,302 | 1.5 | 2.7 | 17.0 | 128 | 48.4 | 48.6 | 21.6 | 367 |
| 55 years or over | 7,813 | 1.3 | 1.8 | 15.4 | 122 | 24.5 | 29.1 | 8.2 | 245 |
| Clear liquid | 364 | 0.2 | 0 | 1.4 | 84 | 0.1 | 0.2 | 0 | 6 |
| Full liquid | 11,187 | 1.5 | 4.3 | 7.3 | 113 | 53.2 | 39.4 | 11.0 | 1,203 |
| Fiber restricted | 11,110 | 1.4 | 1.9 | 19.2 | 124 | 36.7 | 37.6 | 18.6 | 312 |
| High fiber | 16,761 | 1.6 | 2.3 | 25.5 | 196 | 29.5 | 30.1 | 15.7 | 284 |
| High calorie, high protein | 20,254 | 2.1 | 3.5 | 30.9 | 180 | 54.9 | 52.0 | 19.1 | 782 |
| Gluten restricted | 18,756 | 1.4 | 2.3 | 19.8 | 178 | 36.2 | 34.3 | 18.7 | 500 |
| Tyramine restricted | 18,627 | 1.6 | 2.2 | 22.8 | 178 | 33.4 | 38.2 | 18.0 | 503 |
| Carbohydrate restricted for management of dumping syndrome | | | | | | | | | |
| Stage I | 4,994 | 0.8 | 1.4 | 16.7 | 105 | 31.7 | 33.1 | 13.6 | 475 |
| Stage II | 15,845 | 1.9 | 2.2 | 32.7 | 153 | 44.4 | 49.5 | 18.9 | 581 |
| Sucrose free | 3,489 | 0.8 | 2.5 | 15.2 | 10 | 39.8 | 31.9 | 6.7 | 765 |
| Sucrose restricted | 6,682 | 1.1 | 2.6 | 14.1 | 89 | 41.3 | 35.7 | 14.5 | 729 |
| Lactose free | 8,036 | 1.3 | 0.9 | 19.8 | 131 | 22.9 | 29.3 | 15.6 | 236 |
| 50 g fat | 16,558 | 1.7 | 2.2 | 22.8 | 206 | 12.7 | 17.4 | 7.1 | 209 |
| Fat controlled | 16,423 | 2.0 | 2.5 | 24.5 | 281 | 22.9 | 34.8 | 29.6 | 269 |
| Type I hyperlipoproteinemia 1,700–2,000 kcal | 15,207 | 2.2 | 3.2 | 24.3 | 288 | 7.4 | 9.5 | 0.8 | 135 |
| Type IIa hyperlipoproteinemia | 13,320 | 1.5 | 2.0 | 21.9 | 153 | 17.9 | 30.0 | 29.7 | 311 |
| Type IIb + III hyperlipoproteinemia 1,800 kcal | 12,556 | 1.8 | 3.0 | 21.2 | 200 | 12.9 | 19.1 | 16.0 | 147 |
| Type IV hyperlipoproteinemia 1,500 kcal | 9,172 | 1.3 | 1.7 | 19.8 | 154 | 14.0 | 20.9 | 21.2 | 139 |
| Type V hyperlipoproteinemia 1,500 kcal | 9,383 | 1.6 | 2.2 | 21.1 | 161 | 12.2 | 17.4 | 11.5 | 145 |
| Fat controlled 1,200 kcal | 12,759 | 1.2 | 1.7 | 15.3 | 150 | 11.4 | 17.4 | 15.8 | 190 |
| Fat controlled 1,800 kcal | 13,320 | 1.5 | 2.0 | 21.9 | 153 | 17.9 | 30.0 | 29.7 | 311 |
| Calorie, carbohydrate, protein, and fat controlled 1,800 kcal | 14,542 | 1.6 | 2.2 | 21.3 | 179 | 26.3 | 28.0 | 6.2 | 437 |
| Calorie restricted 1,200 kcal | 11,772 | 1.2 | 1.9 | 15.7 | 155 | 18.8 | 18.9 | 2.7 | 229 |
| *Medium chain triglyceride-based ketogenic (+ MCT) | 3,703 | 0.5 | 1.0 | 7.8 | 75 | 4.4 | 6.0 | 2.7 | 59 |
| *Medium chain triglyceride–long chain triglyceride restricted (+ MCT) | 10,759 | 1.7 | 2.0 | 20.0 | 186 | 8.4 | 11.6 | 3.6 | 183 |
| Vegans | 13,289 | 2.1 | 1.0 | 24.4 | 181 | 17.4 | 31.2 | 25.9 | 49 |
| Lactovegetarian | 15,996 | 1.6 | 2.3 | 18.5 | 184 | 50.0 | 44.3 | 15.8 | 268 |
| Lactoovovegetarian | 14,486 | 1.7 | 2.5 | 18.9 | 164 | 38.9 | 43.5 | 17.4 | 863 |
| High potassium | 19,463 | 2.0 | 3.0 | 32.4 | 239 | 37.1 | 40.3 | 15.1 | 352 |
| 500 mg sodium | 5,770 | 1.5 | 1.9 | 18.0 | 169 | 22.2 | 27.2 | 10.1 | 222 |
| 1,000 mg sodium | 5,769 | 1.5 | 1.9 | 18.0 | 166 | 23.2 | 28.6 | 10.4 | 225 |
| 1,500 mg sodium | 5,840 | 1.6 | 2.0 | 19.3 | 166 | 24.9 | 30.0 | 10.6 | 246 |
| 2,000 mg sodium | 6,042 | 1.6 | 2.1 | 21.2 | 168 | 27.0 | 31.5 | 10.7 | 266 |
| Controlled protein, sodium and potassium | 7,038 | 0.9 | 0.8 | 10.9 | 137 | 10.7 | 17.6 | 11.0 | 81 |

* Does not include calories and fat from MCT.

# Nutritional Assessment

Evaluation of the nutritional status of a person, i.e., "the condition of health of the individual as influenced by the utilization of nutrients" [1], permits early intervention in both the treatment of established malnutrition and its prevention in individuals at high risk. The assessment of nutritional status implies a surveillance system that encompasses three principal areas:

1. Clinical information
2. Dietary history
3. Biochemical data

The development of a practical, cost-effective method of nutritional assessment that is clinically relevant to the specific population being served is one of the challenges which confronts today's dietitian.

A great deal of information on the methodology of nutritional assessment techniques and their use in nutritional support of patients has been published [2–14]. Prior to the institution of a nutritional assessment program in any facility, dietitians should familiarize themselves with the latest techniques. Some form of self-study should be undertaken in order to tailor the methodology used to the patient population, as well as to resources available, including finances, time, equipment, the number and expertise level of supportive personnel, the nutritional knowledge of the medical staff, etc. Medical care evaluation studies or patient care audits that include an evaluation of the quality of nutritional care provided may help to highlight overlooked or recurrent problems that are not being addressed [8]. A review of dietary records is also helpful.

## Identification of Nutritional Problems

One approach to the development of a nutritional assessment program begins with the formulation of a decision tree or algorithm, a type of flow chart that enables the dietitian to decide which patients need additional care and whether it needs to be in depth. It involves a screening procedure for identifying nutritional problems as well as a methodical way of questioning the benefits of what is to be done. One example of such an alogarithm has been included as table 1. In order to identify individuals who are at nutritional risk or to answer the question "Is there a nutrition problem?" a set of screening criteria should be developed that is consistent with the resources of the dietitian as well as clinically relevant to the population being assessed. Medical and dietetic records should be screened for specific problems, and the initial patient or client dietitian interview should be restructured in order to provide more information [9].

## Preliminary Nutritional Screening Criteria

### INITIAL LABORATORY TESTS

Preliminary nutritional screening criteria will vary from institution to institution. One example is provided in table 2. Among the screening tests routinely performed in most hospitals are a complete blood count (hemoglobin, hematocrit, red blood cell indices, red blood cell count, white blood cell count and differential) and SMA-12. The latter includes nutrition related laboratory tests such as cholesterol, total protein, albumin, alkaline phosphatase, blood urea nitrogen, creatinine, electrolytes, etc., or an SMA-6 (blood urea nitrogen, creatinine, serum sodium, serum potassium and serum chloride determinations) [9].

Table 3 is a summary of differential findings in the anemia of iron deficiency, pernicious anemia, or $B_{12}$ or folate deficiency and the anemia of chronic disease [9]. The anemia of chronic disease does not respond to iron therapy. It has been described as the "body turning down the hematological thermostat," possibly diverting substrates and energy into channels more critical for survival than hemoglobin.

### INITIAL PATIENT INTERVIEW

The patient interview is an integral part of the screening process. It should be expanded to include not only food preferences but questions about weight change, patterns of eating, changes in appetite, taste, food intolerances, digestive disorders, educational needs, and potential drug–nutrient interactions, in addition to clinical observations indicative of malnutrition or high nutritional risk. Although the time taken for an initial interview does not necessarily need to be extended, to accomplish all these things, observational and interviewing skills need to be maximized if the dietary interview is to serve as an effective instrument of nutritional assessment [9]. Shortcuts such as the use of an abbreviated self-nutrition history may then be compared to a food guide such as the basic four or, if possible, a more comprehensive food guide in order to arrive at a gross estimate of the adequacy of the diet. Limitations of any type of dietary intake are given in table 4. Table 5 is a sample nutrition history. If the preliminary assessment fails to identify a nutritional problem, the data-collection process should stop here with a very brief note in the patient's medical record [9].

### In-Depth Nutritional Assessment

If more information seems to be needed or if a nutritional problem has been identified in preliminary screening, an in-depth nutritional assessment should be performed. A complete assessment includes a comprehensive dietary history as well as more extensive clinical biochemical data. Tables 6 and 7 include parameters of malnutrition useful in the performance of a nutritional assessment.

### CLINICAL DATA

Clinical data include the medical history, physical examination, anthropometric measurements, and dental and radiographic examination. Physical signs indicative of malnutrition include abnormalities of the skin, hair, and mucous membranes. Their manifestation may vary with the age and sex of the person, the season of the year, or geographical location. Clinical signs of malnutrition may be caused by the lack of more than one nutrient or by nonnutritional factors such as poor absorption from the gastrointestinal tract. Interpretation must be made in conjunction with other clinical, dietary, and biochemical data.

The dental examination is an essential part of the physical examination, and the condition of the oral cavity can contribute valuable information about the nutritional status of the person. The radiographic examination can be used to assess skeletal maturity and to assist in the diagnosis of metabolic bone disease and deficiency diseases such as rickets and scurvy.

### Anthropometry and Classification of Weight Loss

The first and most important anthropometric measurements, which should have been performed as part of the initial screening process, are those of the patient's height and weight. These should be compared to ideal weight using a current table [7, 10,11], as opposed to the outdated 1959 insurance statistics frequently cited as a reference. Weight loss should be classified; one method is described in table 8.

### Estimation of Muscle Mass and Fat Stores Using Skinfold Calipers

For in-depth assessment additional anthropometry may be performed on such features as muscle mass and fat stores. Arm muscle circumference is estimated using the following equation:

Arm muscle circumference = arm circumference − (0.314 × triceps skinfold (mm)).

Nomograms for estimating arm muscle circumferences are provided in tables 9 and 10.

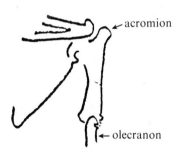

Measurement of arm circumference is taken over belly of muscle (not on lateral or medial side) halfway between acromion and oleocranon on the dominant arm, hanging loosely. Tape measure is held firmly at right angle to the long axis of the arm but does not displace the fat below. The reading is made to the nearest millimeter. Measurement of triceps skinfold is made at the same place as the arm circumference, parallel to axis of arm. The arm is placed at 90° flexion and worked back and forth so that the triceps muscle is not included in skinfold. With arm hanging loosely, use thumb and index finger to pick up skinfold. Calipers are applied approximately 1 cm below where the skinfold is being held so that pressure will be exerted by the calipers. Record after calipers drop once but before they go down again (when they go down the second time fat is being pushed aside); for someone very heavy it may take about 3 sec for the first drop to occur. Record to the nearest millimeter [9]. American standards for anthropometeric measurement have been developed [16].

### Additional Laboratory Measurements

*Visceral protein status*    An approximation of the serum transferrin value can be derived from the total iron-binding capacity (TIBC):

$$serum\ transferrin = (0.8 \times TIBC) - 43.$$

*Immune function—total lymphocyte count*    The total lymphocyte count is equal to the percentage of lymphocytes multiplied by the white blood cell count (WBC):

$$\text{total lymphocyte count} = \frac{\text{percentage of lymphocytes} \times \text{WBC}}{100}$$

*Lean body mass—creatinine height index*    The actual daily urinary creatinine excretion is compared with an ideal value from table 11 to compute the creatinine height index:

$$\text{creatine height index (CHI)} = \frac{\text{actual urinary creatinine}}{\text{ideal urinary creatinine}} \times 100.$$

For example, the ideal urinary creatinine for a man of height 177.8 cm is 1,596 mg/day. If his actual daily urinary creatinine loss is 1,200 mg, then the creatinine height index is equal to $^{1,200}/_{1,596} \times 100$ or 75%. The CHI is an effective measure of muscle mass and allows estimation of lean body mass.

*Nitrogen metabolism*    A measurement of the nitrogen balance is useful in documenting effectiveness of nutritional therapy and is calculated by the formula [6]

$$\text{nitrogen balance} = \frac{\text{protein intake}}{6.25} - (\text{urinary urea nitrogen} + 4).$$

The apparent net protein utilization is generated using the relationship

$$\text{net protein utilization (apparent)} = \frac{\dfrac{\text{protein intake}}{6.25} - \dfrac{\text{urinary urea nitrogen} + 2} - \text{obligatory nitrogen loss.}}{\dfrac{\text{protein intake}}{6.25}}$$

The obligatory nitrogen loss is roughly equal to 0.1 g/kg of body weight. An easy-to-use nomogram has been published for estimating nitrogen balance [7].

*Calorie expenditure*    The calculation of basal energy expenditure (BEE) is performed using the following equations:    [2]

for men:   $\text{BEE} = 66 + (13.7 \times W) + (5 \times H) - (6.8 \times A)$;
for women:   $\text{BEE} = 655 + (9.6 \times W) + (1.7 \times H) - (4.7 \times A)$,

where $W$ = actual weight in kg; $H$ = height in cm; and $A$ = age in years. Using the value for basal energy expenditure, the caloric intakes can be expressed as a multiple of BEE:

$$\text{kilocalorie intake as percentage of BEE} = \frac{\text{caloric intake}}{\text{basal energy expenditure}} \times 100.$$

*Evaluation of caloric intake*    An excellent nomogram has been published that is useful in estimating caloric needs in different clinical conditions [7]. An evaluation of caloric intake can also be obtained using table 12. The effect of fever and infection on nutrient needs should be considered [16–20]. New techniques now being experimented with may make this process more reliable [21–23].

Once the data base is complete and the nutritional assessment performed, the information generated should be used as the basis of the nutritional care plan.

**Table 1.  Maximizing the Time for Patient Nutritional Care Planning**

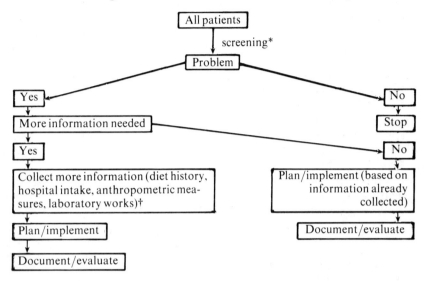

*Source*:   Adapted from Developing an approach to nutritional assessment [9].
* See table 2.
† See table 3.

**Table 2.  Initial Screening of Patients for Nutritional Problems**

Look for the following in medical record or nursing Kardex:

a. Needs for patient education.
b. Those on modified diets causing deficiencies in recommended allowances for more than 3 days (i.e., clear liquid diet) without nutrient supplementation or with inappropriate nutrient supplementation.
c. IV/NPO for more than 3 days without supplementation.
d. Low intakes of formula/tube feedings.
e. Weight 20% above ideal body weight or 10% below (taking into account any edema).
f. Children—inconsistent growth or weight for stature above or below normal limits.
g. Pregnancy—weight gain deviating from normal pattern.
h. Conditions causing increased needs or decreased intake of nutrient—cancer, malabsorption, diarrhea, hyperthyroidism, excessive inflammation, postoperative states, hemorrhage, wounds, burns.
i. Chronic use of any drugs that affect nutritional status.
j. Chewing, swallowing, appetite, taste, smell alterations.
k. Fever consistently above 37°C for more than 2 days.
l. Hct less than 43% (males), 37% (females); Hb less than 14 g/dl (males), 12 g/dl (females), with mean cell volume less than 82 cu or greater than 100 cu (see p. A22 for more details).
m. Absolute decrease in lymphocyte count (below 1,500 cells/mm³).
n. Elevated or decreased cholesterol (above 250 mg/dl or below 130 mg/dl).
o. Serum albumin less than 3 g/dl (in patients without nephrosis, hepatic insufficiency, generalized dermatitis, overhydration).

*Source*:   Reprinted from Developing an approach to nutritional assessment [9].

**Table 3. Laboratory Values in Anemia**

| Description | Iron deficiency | Macrocytic/megaloblastic/pernicious (B₁₂, folate) | Anemia of chronic disease |
|---|---|---|---|
| | Microcytic, hypochromic | Macrocytic (cells have very short life so there are much fewer; cells are larger & laden with Hb) | Usually normocytic, normochromic (sometimes hypochromic; even more rarely, hypochromic & microcytic) |
| Red blood cells (RBC) | May be normal | Decrease | Decrease |
| Hb (grams of Hb/100 ml blood; normal = 13.5–18 g/ml [male], 12–16 g/ml [female]) | Low | Low (esp. in severe disease); although cells are laden with Hb and large, there are fewer of them | Low |
| Hct (volume of packed cells found in 100 ml blood; normal = 40–54% [male], 38–47% [female]) | Low | Low | Low |
| Mean cell volume (describes red cells in terms of individual cell size) (MCV = $\frac{Hct}{RBC}$, normal = 82–100 cu) | $\frac{Hct}{RBC} = \frac{low}{low\ normal}$ = low (less than 80 cu) | $\frac{Hct}{RBC} = \frac{low}{very\ low}$ = high (greater than 94 cu) | $\frac{Hct}{RBC} = \frac{low}{low}$ = normal (80–94 cu) |
| Mean cell Hb (Hb content of each individual red blood cell) (MCH = $\frac{Hb}{RBC}$, normal = 27–32 pg) | $\frac{Hb}{RBC} = \frac{low}{normal}$ = low | $\frac{Hb}{RBC} = \frac{normal\ to\ low}{very\ low}$ = high | $\frac{Hb}{RBC} = \frac{low}{low}$ = normal |
| Mean cell Hb content (concentration of Hb in grams per 100 ml of RBCs) (MCHC = Hb/Hct, normal = 32–36% | $\frac{Hb}{Hct} = \frac{lower}{low}$ = low (less than 30%) | $\frac{Hb}{Hct} = \frac{low\ to\ low\ normal}{low\ to\ low\ normal}$ = normal (sometimes slightly reduced in severe anemia) (more than 30%) normal | $\frac{Hb}{Hct} = \frac{low}{low}$ = normal (greater than 30%) |
| TIBC (sum of plasma Fe & unsaturated iron binding capacity, normal = 250–400 µg/dl | High (low Fe, normal transferrin = less transferrin is bound) | Low (increased destruction of cells; therefore, increased turnover of Fe) | Low (normal Fe, low transferrin = more transferrin is bound) |

*Source:* Adapted from Developing an approach to nutritional assessment [9].

**Table 4. Limitations of Any Type of Dietary Intake**

1. Highly structured questionnaire may gather misinformation due to food omissions or giving the patient the impression he should be eating a particular food; unstructured questioning may be too vague for the sick patient.

2. Patient may be too ill or away from home too long to give accurate information to any type of dietary intake questioning.

3. Patients have a great deal of difficulty quantifying home intakes (those on poor diets may overestimate certain nutrients; those with excess intake may underestimate).

4. When calculating intake, always keep in mind wide variations and error in food composition tables.

5. When estimating dietary intake compare intake not only to normal needs but also to increased needs in disease (i.e., temperature and infection, hyperthyroidism, malabsorption, hemorrhage, trauma (surgery), inflammation).

*Source:* Reprinted from Developing an approach to nutritional assessment [9].

**Table 5.  Sample Nutrition History**

**Nutrition History**

Please fill this questionnaire in to the best of your ability. It will help us assess
your nutritional status and plan for your nutritional care while you are here.

| Name | | Age | Today's date |
|---|---|---|---|
| Occupation | Height | Current weight | Desired weight |

*Have you recently gained or lost weight?*  [    ]  *Yes*  [    ]  *No*      *If yes, how much?* _____  [    ]  *gained*  [    ]  *lost*

*Do you follow any restrictions in your diet?*  [    ]  *Yes*  [    ]  *No*      *If yes, list what they are:* _____  _____

_____

_____

*Do you have any food intolerances or allergies?*  [    ]  *Yes*  [    ]  *No*      *If yes, what are they:* _____

_____

_____

*Do you take any medications?*  [    ]  *Yes*  [    ]  *No*      *If yes, what are they, and how frequently do you take them?* __

_____

_____

*Do you take any vitamins?*  [    ]  *Yes*  [    ]  *No*      *If yes, what kind, and how often?* _____

_____

*Do you have any problems chewing?*  [    ]  *Yes*  [    ]  *No* _____

*Do you have any problems swallowing?*  [    ]  *Yes*  [    ]  *No* _____

*Are your bowels (check one):*  [    ]  *Normal*  [    ]  *Constipated*  [    ]  *Diarrhetic* _____

*Do you eat regularly?*  [    ]  *Yes*  [    ]  *No*      *How many meals a day do you eat?* _____

*Where are most of your meals prepared?* _____

*How often do you eat in restaurants?* _____

*Do you think you diet is nutritionally well-balanced?* _____

*Please go on to the other side.*

Courtesy of Antigone Letsou, R.D., Dept. of Dietetics, New England Medical Center Hospital.

**Table 5** *(Continued)*

Do you include the following in your **daily** diet?
(Answer yes or no, then fill in the **daily** amount.)

| Food | Yes or No | Amount daily |
|---|---|---|
| (1) Milk | [   ] Yes<br>[   ] No | |
| (2) Meat, fish, poultry | [   ] Yes<br>[   ] No | |
| (3) Eggs | [   ] Yes<br>[   ] No | |
| (4) Vegetables | [   ] Yes<br>[   ] No | |
| (5) Fruits | [   ] Yes<br>[   ] No | |
| (6) Bread, potatoes, rice, or other starches | [   ] Yes<br>[   ] No | |
| (7) Butter, margarine, or other fats | [   ] Yes<br>[   ] No | |
| (8) Desserts | [   ] Yes<br>[   ] No | |
| (9) Snacks (What kind and how often?) | [   ] Yes<br>[   ] No | |
| (10) Sanka, tea, or coffee | [   ] Yes<br>[   ] No | |
| (11) Alcohol | [   ] Yes<br>[   ] No | |
| (12) Sugar | [   ] Yes<br>[   ] No | |
| (13) Salt | [   ] Yes<br>[   ] No | |

Do not write below this line:   for dietitian's use only

Nutritional assessment:

| Dietitian | |
|---|---|
| Date | Extension |

**Table 6.   Clinical Signs Used in the Physical Examination for Nutritional Assessment**

|  | *Sign* | *Nutrient considerations* |
|---|---|---|
| Hair | Dry staring<br>Dyspigmented<br>Easily pluckable | Protein-kilocalorie<br>  malnutrition |
| Eyes | Xerophthalmia, keratomalacia<br>Bitot's spots<br>Circumcorneal injection<br>Conjunctival palor | Vitamin A<br>Vitamin A<br>Riboflavin<br>Anemia |
| Lips | Bilateral lesions and scars<br>Cheilosis | Niacin, riboflavin<br>Niacin, riboflavin |
| Gums | Acute peridontal gingivitis<br>  (marginal redness or swelling;<br>  swollen red papillae; bleeding<br>  gums) | Ascorbic acid |
| Tongue | Smooth, pale, atrophic<br>Red, painful, denuded, edema<br>Furrows, serrations, geographic | Anemia<br>Niacin, riboflavin<br>Probably not nutritional |
| Face and neck | Nasolabial seborrhea<br>Bilateral parotid enlargement<br>Goiter | Riboflavin, niacin<br>Protein?<br>Iodine |
| Skin | Petechiae, purpura<br>Symmetrical dermatitis of<br>  exposed skin<br>Thickened pressure points<br>Scrotal dermatitis<br>Follicular hyperkeratosis<br>"Crazy pavement" dermatitis<br>Bilateral dependent edema | Ascorbic acid<br><br>Niacin<br>Niacin<br>Riboflavin<br>Vitamin A<br>Vitamin A, protein<br>Protein, thiamine |
| Skeletal | Costochondral beading<br>Epiphyseal enlargement<br>Cranial bossing, craniotabes<br>Bowed legs | Vitamin C or D<br>Vitamin D<br>Vitamin D<br>Vitamin D |
| Neurologic | Loss of vibratory sense, deep<br>  tendon reflexes, calf tenderness | Thiamine |

Courtesy of Mary B. McCann, M.D. Maine Medical Center.

**Table 7. Table of Current Guidelines for Criteria of Nutritional Status for Laboratory Evaluation**

| Nutrient and units | Age of subject (years) | Criteria of status — Deficient | Criteria of status — Marginal | Criteria of status — Acceptable |
|---|---|---|---|---|
| Hemoglobin (g/100 ml)* | 6–23 mos. | Up to 9.0 | 9.0–9.9 | 10.0+ |
| | 2–5 | Up to 10.0 | 10.0–10.9 | 11.0+ |
| | 6–12 | Up to 10.0 | 10.0–11.4 | 11.5+ |
| | 13–16M | Up to 12.0 | 12.0–12.9 | 13.0+ |
| | 13–16F | Up to 10.0 | 10.0–11.4 | 11.5+ |
| | 16+M | Up to 12.0 | 12.0–13.9 | 14.0+ |
| | 16+F | Up to 10.0 | 10.0–11.9 | 12.0+ |
| | Pregnant (after 6+ mos.) | Up to 9.5 | 9.5–10.9 | 11.0+ |
| Hematocrit (packed cell volume in percent)* | Up to 2 | Up to 28 | 28–30 | 31+ |
| | 2–5 | Up to 30 | 30–33 | 34+ |
| | 6–12 | Up to 30 | 30–35 | 36+ |
| | 13–16M | Up to 37 | 37–39 | 40+ |
| | 13–16F | Up to 31 | 31–35 | 36+ |
| | 16+M | Up to 37 | 37–43 | 44+ |
| | 16+F | Up to 31 | 31–37 | 33+ |
| | Pregnant | Up to 30 | 30–32 | 33+ |
| Serum albumin (g/100 ml)* | Up to 1 | — | Up to 2.5 | 2.5+ |
| | 1–5 | — | Up to 3.0 | 3.0+ |
| | 6–16 | — | Up to 3.5 | 3.5+ |
| | 16+ | Up to 2.8 | 2.8–3.4 | 3.5+ |
| | Pregnant | Up to 3.0 | 3.0–3.4 | 3.5+ |
| Serum protein (g/100 ml)* | Up to 1 | — | Up to 5.0 | 6.0+ |
| | 1–5 | — | Up to 5.5 | 5.5+ |
| | 6–16 | — | Up to 6.0 | 6.0+ |
| | 16+ | Up to 6.0 | 6.0–6.4 | 6.5+ |
| | Pregnant | Up to 5.5 | 5.5–5.9 | 6.0+ |
| Serum ascorbic acid (mg/100 ml)* | All ages | Up to 0.1 | 0.1–0.19 | 0.2+ |
| Plasma vitamin A ($\mu$g/100 ml)* | All ages | Up to 10 | 10–19 | 20+ |
| Plasma carotene ($\mu$g/100 ml)* | All ages | Up to 20 | 20–39 | 40+ |
| | Pregnant | — | 40–79 | 80+ |
| Serum iron ($\mu$g/100 ml)* | Up to 2 | Up to 30 | — | 30+ |
| | 2–5 | Up to 40 | — | 40+ |
| | 8–12 | Up to 50 | — | 50+ |
| | 12+M | Up to 60 | — | 60+ |
| | 12+F | Up to 40 | — | 40+ |
| Transferrin saturation (percent)* | Up to 2 | Up to 15.0 | — | 15.0+ |
| | 2–12 | Up to 20.0 | — | 20.0+ |
| | 12+M | Up to 20.0 | — | 20.0+ |
| | 12+F | Up to 15.0 | — | 15.0+ |
| Serum folacin (ng/ml)† | All ages | Up to 2.0 | 2.1–5.9 | 6.0+ |
| Serum vitamin $B_{12}$ (pg/ml)† | All ages | Up to 100 | — | 100+ |
| Thiamine in urine ($\mu$g/g creatinine)* | 1–3 | Up to 120 | 120–175 | 175+ |
| | 4–5 | Up to 85 | 85–120 | 120+ |
| | 6–9 | Up to 70 | 70–180 | 180+ |
| | 10–15 | Up to 55 | 55–150 | 150+ |
| | 16+ | Up to 27 | 27–65 | 65+ |
| | Pregnant | Up to 21 | 21–49 | 50+ |

**Table 7.  Table of Current Guidelines for Criteria of Nutritional Status for Laboratory Evaluation** *(Continued)*

| *Nutrient and units* | *Age of subject (years)* | *Criteria of status* | | |
|---|---|---|---|---|
| | | *Deficient* | *Marginal* | *Acceptable* |
| Riboflavin in urine (μg/g creatinine)* | 1–3 | Up to 150 | 150–499 | 500+ |
| | 4–5 | Up to 100 | 100–299 | 300+ |
| | 6–9 | Up to 85 | 85–269 | 270+ |
| | 10–16 | Up to 70 | 70–199 | 200+ |
| | 16+ | Up to 27 | 27–79 | 80+ |
| | Pregnant | Up to 30 | 30–89 | 90+ |
| RBC transketolase-TPP-effect (ratio)† | All ages | 25+ | 15–25 | Up to 15 |
| RBC glutathione reductase-FAD-effect (ratio)† | All ages | 1.2+ | — | Up to 1.2 |
| Tryptophan load (mg xanthuronic acid excreted)† | Adults (Dose: 100 mg/kg body weight) | 25+( 6 hr) 75+(24 hr) | — — | Up to 25 Up to 75 |
| Urinary pyridoxine (μg/g creatinine)† | 1–3 | Up to 90 | — | 90+ |
| | 4–6 | Up to 80 | — | 80+ |
| | 7–9 | Up to 60 | — | 60+ |
| | 10–12 | Up to 40 | — | 40+ |
| | 13–15 | Up to 30 | — | 30+ |
| | 16+ | Up to 20 | — | 20+ |
| Urinary N'methyl nicotinamide (mg/g creatinine)* | All ages | Up to 0.2 | 0.2–5.59 | 0.6+ |
| | Pregnant | Up to 0.8 | 0.8–2.49 | 2.5+ |
| Urinary pantothenic acid (μg)* | All ages | Up to 200 | — | 200+ |
| Plasma vitamin E (mg/100 ml)† | All ages | Up to 0.2 | 0.2–0.6 | 0.6+ |
| Transaminase index (ratio)† | | | | |
| EGOT‡ | Adult | 2.0+ | — | Up to 2.0 |
| EGPT§ | Adult | 1.25+ | — | Up to 1.25 |

*Source*:  Reprinted from Nutritional assessment in health programs [6].
* Adapted from the Ten State Nutrition Survey.
† Criteria may vary with different methodology.
‡ Erythrocyte glutamic oxalacetic transaminase.
§ Erythroctye glutamic pyruvic transaminase.

**Table 8.  Evaluation of Weight Change**

| *Time interval* | *Significant weight loss (%)* | *Severe weight loss (%)* |
|---|---|---|
| 1 week | 1.0–2.0 | Greater than 2.0 |
| 1 month | 5.0 | Greater than 5.0 |
| 3 months | 7.5 | Greater than 7.5 |
| 6 months | 10.0 | Greater than 10.0 |

$$\text{Percent weight change} = \frac{(\text{usual weight - actual weight}) \times 100}{\text{usual weight}}$$

*Source*:  Adapted from Nutritional and metabolic assessment of the hopitalized patient [2].

**Table 9. Arm Antrhropometry in Nutritional Assesment: Nomogram for Children**

| Arm circumference (cm) | Arm area (cm²) | Arm muscle circumference (cm) | Arm muscle area (cm²) | Triceps fatfold (mm) |
|---|---|---|---|---|
| 27.0 | 58.0 | 26.0 | | 2 |
| | 56.0 | | 52.0 | |
| 26.0 | 54.0 | | 48.0 | 4 |
| | 52.0 | 24.0 | 44.0 | |
| 25.0 | 50.0 | | | 6 |
| | 48.0 | | 40.0 | |
| 24.0 | 46.0 | 22.0 | 36.0 | 8 |
| | 44.0 | | | |
| 23.0 | 42.0 | 20.0 | 32.0 | 10 |
| | 40.0 | | 28.0 | |
| 22.0 | 38.0 | 18.0 | 24.0 | 12 |
| 21.0 | 36.0 | | | |
| | 34.0 | 16.0 | 20.0 | 14 |
| 20.0 | 32.0 | | | 16 |
| | 30.0 | | 16.0 | |
| 19.0 | 28.0 | 14.0 | | 18 |
| 18.0 | 26.0 | 12.0 | 12.0 | 20 |
| | 24.0 | | | |
| 17.0 | 22.0 | 10.0 | 8.0 | 22 |
| 16.0 | 20.0 | 8.0 | | 24 |
| 15.0 | 18.0 | | 4.0 | 26 |
| 14.0 | 16.0 | 6.0 | | 28 |
| | 14.0 | | 2.0 | |
| 13.0 | 12.0 | 4.0 | | 30 |
| 12.0 | 10.0 | | | 32 |
| 11.0 | | | | |
| 10.0 | 8.0 | | | |
| 9.0 | 6.0 | | | |
| 8.0 | | | | |

To obtain muscle circumference:
1. Lay ruler between values of arm circumference and fatfold.
2. Read off muscle circumference on middle line.

To obtain tissue areas:
1. The arm areas and muscle areas are alongside their respective circumferences.
2. Fat area = arm area − muscle area.

*Source*: Reprinted from Arm anthropometry in nutritional assessment: nomograms for rapid calculation of muscle circumference and cross sectional muscle and fat areas [15].

**Table 10.  Arm Anthropometry in Nutritional Assessment:  Nomogram for Adults**

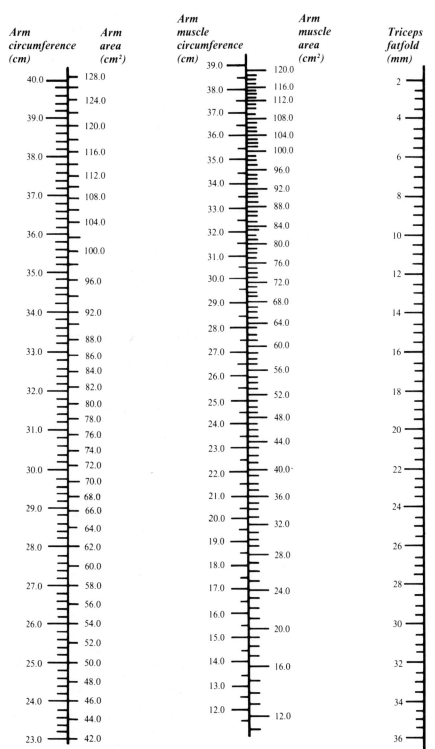

To obtain muscle circumference:
    1. Lay ruler between values of arm circumference and fatfold.
    2. Read off muscle circumference on middle line.
To obtain tissue areas:
    1. The arm areas and muscle areas are alongside their respective circumferences.
    2. Fat area = arm area − muscle area.

*Source*:  Reprinted from Arm anthropometry in nutritional assessment:  nomograms for
          rapid calculation of muscle circumference and cross sectional muscle and fat areas.

### Table 11. Ideal Urinary Creatinine Values

| Men* | | Women† | |
|---|---|---|---|
| Height (cm) | Ideal creatinine (mg) | Height (cm) | Ideal creatinine (mg) |
| 157.5 | 1,288 | 147.3 | 830 |
| 160.0 | 1,325 | 149.9 | 851 |
| 162.6 | 1,359 | 152.4 | 875 |
| 165.1 | 1,386 | 154.9 | 900 |
| 167.6 | 1,426 | 157.5 | 925 |
| 170.2 | 1,467 | 160.0 | 949 |
| 172.7 | 1,513 | 162.6 | 977 |
| 175.3 | 1,555 | 165.1 | 1,006 |
| 177.8 | 1,596 | 167.6 | 1,044 |
| 180.3 | 1,642 | 170.2 | 1,076 |
| 182.9 | 1,691 | 172.7 | 1,109 |
| 185.4 | 1,739 | 175.3 | 1,141 |
| 188.0 | 1,785 | 177.8 | 1,174 |
| 190.5 | 1,831 | 180.3 | 1,206 |
| 193.0 | 1,891 | 182.9 | 1,240 |

*Source*: Reprinted from Nutritional and metabolic assessment of the hospitalized patients [2].
\* Creatinine coefficient (men) = 23 mg/kg of ideal body weight.
† Creatinine coefficient (women) = 18 mg/kg of ideal body weight.

### Table 12. Nutritional Therapy

| A. Energy Requirements | Kilocalories Required (per 24 hr) |
|---|---|
| Type of Therapy | |
| Parenteral anabolic | 1.75 × BEE |
| Oral anabolic | 1.50 × BEE |
| Oral maintenance | 1.20 × BEE |

| B. Prescriptions for Anabolism* | Protein (g/day) | Kilocalories (kcal/day) |
|---|---|---|
| Type of Therapy | | |
| Oral protein-sparing | 1.5 × weight† | |
| Total parenteral nutrition | (1.2–1.5) × weight | 40 × weight |
| Oral hyperalimentation | (1.2–1.5) × weight | 35 × weight |

*Source*: Reprinted from Nutritional and metabolic assessment of the hospitalized patient [2].
\* Levels of protein intake are to be adjusted according to blood urea nitrogen values and nitrogen balance.
† Weight = actual weight in kg.

References

1. Robinson, C. H., and Lawler, M. R.: Normal and Therapeutic Nutrition. 15th ed. New York: Macmillan, 1977.
2. Blackburn, G. L.; Bristrian, B. R; Maini, B. S.; Schlamm, H. T.; and Smith, M. F.: Nutritional and metabolic assessment of the hospitalized patient. J. Paren. Enter. Nutr. 1:11, 1977.
3. Butterworth, C. E., and Blackburn, G. L.: Hospital malnutrition and how to asssess the nutritional status of a patient. Nutr. Today 10:8, Mar./Apr. 1975.
4. Task Force on Nutrition; American College of Obstetricians and Gynecologists: Assessment of maternal nutrition. Available from: American College of Obstetricians and Gynecologists, One East Wacker Drive, Chicago, IL, 60601.
5. Grant, A.: Nutritional assessment: guidelines for dietitians. Available from: Northwest Kidney Center, 1102 Columbia St. Seattle, WA, 98104.
6. Christakis, G.: Nutritional assessment in health programs. Am. J. Pub. Health 63:1, 1973.
7. Wilmore, D. W.: The Metabolic Management of the Critically Ill. New York: Plenum Medical Book Co., 1977.

8. Walters, F. M., and Crumley, S. J.: Patient Care Audit. A Quality Assurance Procedure Manual for Dietitians. Chicago: American Dietetic Association, 1978.

9. Hopkins, C.: Developing an approach to nutritional assessment. Unpublished paper given April 28, 1978, Portland, OR.

10. Davidson, J. K.: Controlling diabetes with diet therapy. Postgrad. Med. 59:114, 1976.

11. Monthly Vital Statistics Report. National Center for Health Statistics HRA-76-1120, Vol. 23(3) (Suppl.), June 22, 1976.

12. Fisher, J. E.: Parenteral and enteral nutrition. Dis. Month. 24(9):3, 1978

13. Walker, W. F.: Nutrition after injury. World Rev. Nutr. Dietet. 19:174, 1974.

14. Zerfas, A. J.; Shorr, I. J.; and Neumann, C. G.: Office assessment of nutritional status. Pediatr. Clin. N. Am. 24:254, 1977.

15. Gurney, J. M., and Jeliffe, D. B.: Arm anthropometry in nutritional assessment: nomograms for rapid calculation of muscle circumference and cross sectional muscle and fat areas. Am. J. Clin. Nutr. 26:912, 1973.

16. Frisancho, A. R.: Triceps skin fold and upper arm muscle size norms for assessment of nutritional status. Am. J. Clin. Nutr. 27:1052, 1974.

17. Bristrian, B. R.: Interaction of nutrition and infection in the hospital setting. Am. J. Clin. Nutr. 30:1228, 1977.

18. Blackburn, G. L.: Nutritional assessment and support during infection. Am. J. Clin. Nutr. 30:1493, 1977.

19. Keusch, G. T.: The consequences of fever. Am. J. Clin. Nutr. 30:1211, 1977.

20. Kinney, J. M.: Energy requirements in injury and sepsis. Acta anaesth. Scand. (suppl.) 55:15, 1974.

21. Nagablushan, V. S. and Rao, N.: Studies on 3-methylhistidine metabolism in children with protein energy malnutrition. Am. J. Clin. Nutr. 31:1322, 1978.

22. Young, V. R.; Haverberg, L. N.; Bilmazes, C.; and Munro, H. N.: Potential use of 3 methylhistidine excretion as an index of progressive catabolism during starvation. Metabolism 22:1429, 1973.

23. Munro, H. N., and Young, V. R.: Urinary excretion of N-methylhistidine (3-methylhistidine): a tool to study metabolic responses in relation to nutrient and normal status in health and disease of man. Am. J. Clin. Nutr. 31:1688, 1978.

# Vegetarian Diets

***Vegan diet or strict vegetarian diet*** One that includes some or all of the following foods: vegetables, fruits, enriched or whole grain breads and cereals, dry peas and beans, lentils, nuts and nutlike seeds, peanuts, and peanut butter. In addition, the diet specifically excludes all foods of animal origin, meat, poultry, fish, eggs, and dairy products such as milk, cheese, and ice cream [1,2,4–6].

***Lactovegetarian diet*** One that includes dairy products plus some or all of the following foods: vegetables, fruits, enriched or whole grain breads and cereals, dry peas, beans, lentils, nuts and nutlike seeds, peanuts, and peanut butter. The diet excludes meat, poultry, fish, and eggs [1].

***Lactoovovegetarian diet*** One that includes eggs and dairy products plus some or all of the following foods: vegetables, fruits, enriched or whole grain breads and cereals, dry peas, beans, lentils, nuts and nutlike seeds, peanuts, and peanut butter. The diet excludes meat, poultry, and fish [1–5].

***Zen macrobiotic diet*** A dietary regimen composed of ten basic diets ranging from the lowest level, diet 3, which includes 10% cereals, 30% vegetables, 10% soup, 30% animal products, 15% salads and fruits, and 5% desserts, to diet 7; the latter is the highest level of the regimen and is 100% cereals [6].

***Characteristics of the diets*** The lactoovovegetarian diet resembles the average Western diet in many ways. The main difference is that it replaces meat with a variety of legumes, meat analogues, cereals, nuts, and generous intakes of milk, milk products, and eggs. In contrast, the pure or strict vegetarian diet is devoid of any animal foods and must be skillfully implemented. Since many plant foods are low in kilocalories, greater quantities of many different varieties of them must be chosen in order to ensure nutritional adequacy. Even given such wise choices, the diet must be supplemented with vitamin $B_{12}$, since plant foods contain no known source of this vitamin [1–4].

***Indications for use*** In addition to the ecological and religious concerns that have prompted an increase in adherence to various forms of vegetarian diets [1–8], the replacement of part of the animal sources of protein with plant sources may have other advantages. For example, vegetarians have lower serum levels of low density lipoprotein (LDL) cholesterol. They also have higher ratios of high density lipoprotein (HDL) cholesterol to low density lipoprotein (LDL) cholesterol than vegetarians who consume greater quantities of foods high in saturated fat [9–12]. In addition, a vegetarian diet is often quite high in dietary fiber [13], whose role in human nutrition is just beginning to be more clearly elucidated.

***Possible adverse reactions*** *Vitamin $B_{12}$ deficiency* Total abstinence from foods of animal origin is known to be associated with low serum vitamin $B_{12}$ levels and the rare occurrence of megaloblastic anemia, subacute degeneration of the spinal cord, or both [14,15]. To a much lesser degree than vegans, some lactovegetarians and lactoovovegetarians may be at risk of developing vitamin $B_{12}$ deficiencies during periods of increased need. Repeated blood loss or blood donations and pregnancy increase the risk. In these instances and for vegetarians with a dietary vitamin $B_{12}$ intake of less than 0.5 $\mu$g per day, supplementation with additional vitamin $B_{12}$ is recommended [16,17].

*Calcium deficiency* Particularly for children, unless milk in some form is included in the diet, it may be difficult to get enough calcium [1–3]. Vegans who do not compensate for the loss of milk in the diet by use of a vitamin and mineral fortified milk substitute and increased use of calcium containing foods run the risk of provoking a calcium deficiency as well as a riboflavin or vitamin $B_{12}$ deficiency.

*Vitamin D deficiency* Children of strict vegetarians who are not exposed to sunlight at regular intervals are prone to develop vitamin D deficiency and rickets unless a source of vitamin D is included in their diets [18–20]. Furthermore, plasma 25-hydroxyvitamin-D levels have been reported to be lower in pregnant vegetarian women than in pregnant nonvegetarian women [21].

**Contraindications** The Zen macrobiotic diet at higher levels is grossly inadequate in many nutrients and has produced disastrous nutritional consequences in some of its younger adherents [22,23]. This version of the vegetarian diet is contraindicated under any and all conditions.

**Suggestions for dietitians** *Guidelines for formulating a lactoovovegetarian diet and lactovegetarian diet [4]*

1. Formulate the diet from a modified version of the basic food groups to fit the needs of the individual:
   a. *Vegetables and fruits* 4 or more servings, including at least 1 citrus fruit and 1 leafy green or yellow vegetable.
   b. *Whole grain breads and cereals* 4 or more servings daily.
   c. *Milk* (at least 2 cups) and *dairy products* such as cheese.
   d. *Protein rich foods* at least 2 servings. Substitute eggs, meat analogues, legumes, nuts, and seeds for meat, poultry, and fish. Although commercial meat analogues are not essential to a well balanced lactoovovegetarian diet, their use facilitates meal planning and adds variety to the diet. Omit eggs on lactovegetarian diet.
2. In modifying the diet of an individual changing from a nonvegetarian to a vegetarian pattern, the intake of low nutrient density foods should be reduced. In their place use high nutrient density foods.
3. If additional kilocalories are needed to meet energy needs, increase the intake of whole grain breads and cereals and milk.
4. Use a wide variety of grains, legumes, nuts, fruits, and vegetables.
5. Use adequate amounts of milk and milk products to meet calcium

needs, at least 2 cups for an adult, 3 cups for an adolescent, and 4 cups for pregnant and lactating women.

6. Provide instruction in making food choices which have complementary amino acid patterns. Specifically, combine a plant protein lacking in one amino acid with another food that contains a large amount of it. Examples of this are the combination of milk which is high in lysine, isoleucine, and methionine with (a) breads and cereals in which lysine is the limiting amino acid, or (b) with nuts and seeds in which lysine and methionine are the limiting amino acids, or (c) vegetables that are deficient in isoleucine and methionine. Combination of nuts and seeds that are low in lysine and isoleucine but adequate in methionine and tryptophan with legumes that are high in lysine and isoleucine but in which methionine and lysine are the limiting amino acids will result in a satisfactory amino acid supply. Using the Equivalent lists for planning vegetarian diets (pp. A36–A37) one may design a variety of combinations of foods that will meet the needs of menu planning for the vegetarian.

7. When indicated, the vegetarian diet can be modified successfully to fit the confines of a number of therapeutic diets. An excellent diet manual has been published which includes many therapeutic vegetarian diets that should prove helpful to the dietitian [24].

*Guidelines for planning a vegan or strict vegetarian diet [4]*

1. Follow suggestions 1, 2, 3, 4, and 6 for planning lacto- and lacotovovegetarian diets with one exception: omit all eggs and dairy products.

2. Stress vigilance in the consumption of sufficient amounts of food to meet caloric needs. Closer nutritional surveillance is needed for adequate implementation of this type of vegetarian diet than for more liberal vegetarian diets. Many plant foods are very low in kilocalories; consequently, the sheer bulk of food required to meet energy needs may constitute a problem for certain individuals.

3. Milk and milk products are excellent sources of protein, riboflavin, calcium, vitamin D, and vitamin $B_{12}$. In the absence of dairy products, it becomes more difficult to obtain adequate amounts of these nutrients. Employ compensatory measures to offset the lack of vitamin $B_{12}$ in the diet and the large nutritional gap left by the omission of dairy products:

   a. Incorporate fortified meat analogues into the diet.
   b. Increase the use of legumes, nuts, and dried fruits.
   c. Increase the use of green leafy vegetables.
   d. Emphasize that regular exposure to sunshine is one way of obtaining vitamin D.
   e. Incorporate a fortified soybean based milk into the diet. This is essential for the young child.
   f. Inactivated yeast may be added to the diet occasionally, although it is not necessary daily.

Daily Food Plan

| FOOD GROUP | AMOUNT |
|---|---|
| Milk | 2 cups or more (use fortified soybean based milk on vegan diets) |
| Protein food equivalents | 5 equivalents (see lists 1 and 2) |
| Nut and seed equivalents | 1 or more equivalent |
| Vegetables and fruits | 4 servings or more, including: 1 citrus fruit, 1 serving legume exchanges, 1 serving dark green or yellow vegetable (use larger portion on vegan diets) |
| Unrefined cereal and breads | 5 or more servings |
| Fats, oils | 1 tbsp or more |

## Protein Food Equivalents: List 1
### (75 kcal, 7 g protein, 5 g fat)

| | *Amount* | *Weight* |
|---|---|---|
| Cottage cheese | ¼ cup | 45 g |
| Cheddar cheese | 1 slice | 30 g |
| Egg | 1 | 50 g |
| Soy cheese (tofu) | ¼ cup | 40 g |
| Peanut butter | 2 tbsp (omit 2 fat) | 30 g |
| *Loma Linda Foods* | | |
| Big Franks | 1 frank | 1½ oz |
| Chili with Beans | ⅓ cup (omit 1 bread, add ½ fat) | 3 oz |
| Dinner Cuts | 1 cut (add 1 fat) | 1½ oz |
| Linketts | 1 linkett | 1¼ oz |
| Little Links | 2 links | 1½ oz |
| Nuteena | 1 slice (⅜″ thick) (omit 1 fat) | 2 oz |
| Proteena | 1 slice (¼″ thick) | 1¼ oz |
| Redi-Burger | 1 slice (¼″ thick) | 1¼ oz |
| Sandwich Spread | 6 tbsp (omit ½ fat and ½ bread) | 2½ oz |
| Stew-Pac | ¼ cup | 1½ oz |
| Soybeans, Boston | ¼ cup (omit ½ bread, add 1 fat) | 2 oz |
| Soybeans, green | ⅓ cup (omit ½ bread, add 1 fat) | 2½ oz |
| Tenderbits | 4 bits | 2½ oz |
| Tender Rounds | 2 rounds | 1½ oz |
| VegeBurger | 3 tbsp (add 1 fat) | 1¼ oz |
| Vegelona | 1 slice (¼″ thick) (add ½ fat) | 1¼ oz |
| VitaBurger (reconstituted) | ¼ cup (add 1 fat) | 2 oz |
| *Worthington Foods* | | |
| Beef Style | 1 slice (add ½ fat) | 1 oz |
| Chicken Style | 1 slice | 1 oz |
| Choplets | ½ chop (add 1 fat) | 1 oz |
| Choplet Burger | 3 tbsp (add 1 fat) | 1½ oz |
| Corned Beef Style | 3 slices (omit ½ fat) | 1½ oz |
| Cutlets | ½ piece (add 1 fat) | 1 oz |
| Fillet | ¾ fillet | 20 g |
| Fried Chicken Style | 1½ pieces (omit ½ fat) | 1½ oz |
| Granburger (rehydrated) | ¼ cup (add 1 fat) | 2 oz |
| Non-meat Balls | 2 balls | 1 oz |
| Prosage | 1 slice (⅜″) | 1 oz |
| Salisbury Steak Style | 1 patty (omit ½ bread) | 2 oz |
| Saucettes | 2 links | 1 oz |
| Smoked Beef Style | 5 slices (add ½ fat) | 1 oz |
| Smoked Turkey Style | 2 slices | 40 g |
| Vegetable Skallops | 1½ pieces (add 1 fat) | 1½ oz |
| Vegetarian Burger | ⅓ cup (add 1 fat) | 70 g |
| Veja-Links | 2 links | 70 g |
| Wham | ¼ cup diced (add 1 fat) | 1 oz |

## Protein Food Equivalents: List 2
(reduced fat; 55 kcal, 7 g protein, 3 g fat)

| | Amount | Weight |
|---|---|---|
| Egg whites | 3 whites | 1½ oz |
| Count Down (Fisher) | 1 slice | 1½ oz |
| Low-fat cottage cheese | ¼ cup | 45 g |
| *Loma Linda Foods* | | |
| Chili with Beans | ⅓ cup (omit 1 bread) | 3 oz |
| Dinner Cuts | 1 cut (add ½ fat) | 1½ oz |
| Soybeans, Boston | ¼ cup (omit ½ bread) | 2 oz |
| Soybeans, green | ⅓ cup (omit ½ bread) | 2½ oz |
| Tender Rounds | 1 round | |
| VegeBurger | 3 tbsp (add ½ fat) | 1¼ oz |
| Vegelona | 1 slice (¼″ thick) | 1½ oz |
| VitaBurger (reconstituted) | ¼ cup (add ½ fat) | 2 oz |
| *Worthington Foods* | | |
| Beef Style | 1 slice | 1 oz |
| Choplets | ½ chop (add ½ fat) | 1 oz |
| Choplet Burger | 3 tbsp (add ½ fat) | 1½ oz |
| Corned Beef Style | 3 slices | 1½ oz |
| Cutlets | ½ piece (add ½ fat) | 1 oz |
| Granburger | ¼ cup (add ½ fat) | 2 oz |
| Vegetable Skallops | 1½ pieces | 1½ oz |
| Vegetarian Burger | ⅓ cup (add ½ fat) | 70 g |
| Wham | ¼ cup diced | 1 oz |

*Source*: Adapted from Diet Manual Utilizing a Vegetarian Diet Plan [24].
*Note*: Other protein foods may be used if the fat is adjusted in the day's menu.


## Nut and Seed Equivalents
(6 g protein, 16 g fat, 6 g carbohydrate)

| FOOD | AMOUNT PER CHOICE |
|---|---|
| *Nuts** | |
| Brazil nuts | 10 nuts |
| Cashew nuts | 12–16 nuts |
| Peanuts | 2 tbsp |
| Peanut butter | 2 tbsp |
| Pistachio nuts | 1 oz or 30 g |
| Walnuts, black | 16–20 nuts |
| *Seeds* | |
| Pumpkin and squash seeds | 2 tbsp |
| Sesame seeds | 3 tbsp or 4 tbsp meal |
| Sunflower seeds | 3 tbsp or 4 tbsp meal |

* Almonds, English walnuts, and pecans may also be added to the diet occasionally. However, they contain more kilocalories and/or fat than the other nuts.


## Legume Equivalents
(approximately 12 g protein, 1 g fat, 30 g carbohydrate)

One equivalent = ¼ to ⅓ cup dry beans (makes ¾ cup to 1 cup cooked)

| | |
|---|---|
| Black beans | Mung beans |
| Broad beans | Pea beans or dried peas |
| Chick peas or garbanzos | Pinto beans |
| Cowpeas including black-eyed peas | Red beans |
| Lentils | Soybeans |
| Lima beans | White beans |

**References**

1. Raper, N. R., and Hill, M. M.: Vegetarian diets. Nutrition Program News. USDA. July–Aug., 1973.
2. Vyhmeister, I. B.; Register, U. D.; and Sonnenberg, L. M.: Safe vegetarian diets for children. Pediatr. Clin. N. Am. 24: 203, 1977.
3. Zmora, E.; Gorodischer, R.; and Bar-Ziv, J.: Multiple nutritional deficiencies in infants from a strict vegetarian community. Am. J. Dis. Child. 133: 141, 1979.
4. Register, U. D., and Sonnenberg, L. M.: The vegetarian diet. J. Am. Diet. Assoc. 62: 253, 1973.
5. Zolber, K.: Producing meals without meat. Hospitals 49:81, June 16, 1975.
6. Council on Foods and Nutrition: Zen macrobiotic diets. JAMA 218: 397, 1971.
7. Erhard, D.: The new vegetarians. Part I. Nutr. Today 8(6): 4, 1973.
8. Erhard, D.: The new vegetarians. Part II. Nutr. Today 9(1): 20, 1974.
9. Hardinge, M. G., and Stare, F. J.: Nutritional studies of vegetarians. 2. Dietary and serum levels of cholesterol. Am. J. Clin. Nutr. 2: 83, 1954.
10. West, R. O., and Hayes, O. B.: Diet and serum cholesterol levels. A comparison between vegetarians and non-vegetarians in a Seventh-Day Adventist group. Am. J. Clin. Nutr. 21: 853, 1968.
11. Sacks, F. M., Castelli, W. P., Donner, A. and Kass, E. H.: Plasma lipids and lipoproteins in vegetarians and controls. N. Engl. J. Med. 292: 1148, 1975.
12. Burslem, J.; Schonfeld, G.; Howald, M. A.; Weidman, S. W.; and Miller, J. P.: Plasma apoprotein and lipoprotein lipid levels in vegetarians. Metabolism 27: 711, 1978.
13. Hardinge, M. G.; Chambers, A. C.; Crooks, H.; and Stare, F. J.: Nutritional studies of vegetarians. III. Dietary levels of fiber. Am. J. Clin. Nutr. 6: 523, 1958.
14. Smith, A. D. M.: Veganism: a clinical survey with observations on vitamin $B_{12}$ metabolism. Br. Med. J. 1: 1655, 1962.
15. Winawer, S. J.; Streiff, R. R.; and Zamcheck, N.: Gastric and hematological abnormalities in a vegan with nutritional vitamin $B_{12}$ deficiency: effect of oral vitamin $B_{12}$. Gastroenterology 53: 130, 1967.
16. Ledbetter, R. B., and Del Pozo, E.: Severe megaloblastic anaemia due to nutritional vitamin $B_{12}$ deficiency. Acta Haematol. 42: 247, 1969.
17. Armstrong, B. K.; Davis, R. E.; Nicol, D. J.; van Merwyk, A. J.; and Larwood, C. J.: Hematological, vitamin $B_{12}$ and folate studies on Seventh-Day Adventist vegetarians. Am. J. Clin. Nutr. 27: 712, 1974.
18. Committee on Nutritional Misinformation, National Academy of Sciences: Can a vegetarian be well nourished? JAMA 233:898, 1975.
19. Finberg, L.: Human choice, vegetable deficiencies and vegetarian rickets. Am. J. Dis. Child. 133: 129, 1979.
20. Dwyer, J. T.; Dietz, W. H.; Hass, G.; and Suskind, R.: Risk of nutritional rickets among vegetarian children. Am. J. Dis. Child. 133: 134, 1979.
21. Dent, C. E., and Gupta, M. M.: Plasma 25-hydroxy-vitamin-D levels during pregnancy in Caucasians and in vegetarian and non-vegetarian Asians. Lancet 2: 1057, 1975.
22. Robson, J. R. K.; Konlande, J. E.; Larkin, F. A.; O'Connor, P. A.; and Liu, H. Y.: Zen macrobiotic dietary problems in infancy. Pediatrics 53: 326, 1974.
23. Erhard, D.: A starved child of the new vegetarians. Nutr. Today 8(6):10, 1973.
24. Beckner, A.; Hayasaka, R.; Jacobsen, R.; Johnson, M.; Oakley, S.; and Vyhmeister, I.: Diet Manual Utilizing a Vegetarian Diet Plan. Loma Linda: Seventh Day Adventist Dietetic Association, 1975.

# Vegetarian Diets

COMMITTEE ON NUTRITIONAL MISINFORMATION,
NATIONAL ACADEMY OF SCIENCES

Can a vegetarian be well nourished?

The current trend in the eating habits of certain young adults, away from the familiar Western food patterns toward vegetarianism, has caused concern about the nutritional implications of such changes. This is a legitimate concern, shared by the parents of teenagers and many other Americans. Most nutritionists agree that vegetarian diets can be adequate, if sufficient care is taken in planning them.

Vegetarian diets may be based only on plant food sources (total vegetarians), plant foods plus dairy products (lactovegetarians), or plant foods plus dairy products and eggs (lactoovovegetarians). As the diet becomes less restrictive as to sources of nutrients, the probability of its meeting nutrient requirements increases. When milk and/or eggs are included the risk of nutritional inadequacies is greatly reduced. The value of diets of varied origin is that they are more likely to provide essential nutrients. Adoption of restrictive diets, such as the Zen macrobiotic diets, without taking into account their nutritional limitations, endangers health.

**Nutritional Issues** Both the quantity and the quality of protein are of central concern in all diets. The quality of proteins in plant foods, notably cereal grains, is generally lower than that of animal proteins. Protein quality is dependent on the amounts and the utilizability of 8 of the 20 constituent amino acids in protein. Protein foods of animal origin contain these 8 amino acids in nearly optimum amounts and in an available form, and thus are said to be high-quality proteins. On the other hand, cereal grain proteins are relatively low in the essential amino acid lysine, and thus provide lower-quality protein. Legumes such as dried beans and peas contain ample lysine, but are relatively low in methionine, so they also provide protein of marginal quality. When cereal and legume proteins are eaten together, the methionine provided by the cereal grain and the lysine provided by the legume improve the "balance" in the amino acid supply and the mixture of proteins is of better quality than that provided by either alone. The worldwide practice of combining cereals and legumes in the food of man and farm animals provides evidence of the supplementary effect of one plant protein food on another. If this mixing of plant protein foods is done judiciously, combinations of lower-quality protein foods can give mixtures of about the same nutritional value as high-quality animal protein foods.

Reprinted from American Journal of Clinical Nutrition 27: 1095, Oct. 1974. A statement of the Food and Nutrition Board, Division of Biological Sciences, Assembly of Life Sciences, National Research Council (prepared by the Committee on Nutritional Misinformation), National Academy of Sciences, May 1974.

Other nutrients likely to be of marginal content in all-plant diets are calcium, iron, riboflavin, vitamin $B_{12}$, and, for children not exposed to sunlight, vitamin D. Milk and eggs provide these nutrients, as well as excellent quality proteins, thus reducing the risk of inadequacy, and should be eaten especially by the preschool child.

Nutritional Status of Vegetarians

Individual pure vegetarians from many populations of the world have maintained seemingly excellent health. This demonstrates that diets of properly selected plant foods can be nutritionally adequate. A study reported by Hardinge and Stare [1] in 1954 involved the nutrient intake and the nutritional status, as indicated by physical examination and laboratory analysis, of 200 subjects in three dietary groups: nonvegetarian, lactoovovegetarian, and total vegetarian. No evidence of deficiency was found and the intake of nutrients by each group equaled or exceeded the Recommended Dietary Allowances of the National Research Council, with the exception of vitamin $B_{12}$, which was low in the total vegetarian diet. It should be pointed out that, had the studies been continued for a much longer period, anemia due to lack of vitamin $B_{12}$ might have become evident.

Planning a Vegetarian Diet

Man's nutrient requirements, with the exception of vitamin $B_{12}$, can be met by all-plant diets [2]. However, more attention should be given to planning when the diet is limited in food products of animal origin. The most important safeguard for average consumers is great variety in the diet. The greatest risk comes from undue reliance on a single plant food source, usually a cereal grain or starchy root crop. Legumes, particularly soybeans, are rich in protein, B vitamins, and iron. Grains are good sources of carbohydrates, proteins, thiamin, iron, and trace minerals. Nuts and other seeds contribute fat, protein, B vitamins, and iron. Dark green, leafy vegetables are sources of calcium, riboflavin, and carotene (a precursor of vitamin A), and should be used liberally by total vegetarians. Plant foods do not contain vitamin $B_{12}$. Milk and eggs are satisfactory sources, but the total vegetarian should consume fortified soybean milk or a vitamin $B_{12}$ supplement. In winter months when exposure to sunlight is limited, infants may receive inadequate vitamin D unless this vitamin is provided.

As with all human diets, vegetarian diets should not contain excessive amounts of "calories only" foods such as those containing chiefly starch, sugars, refined fats and oils, or alcohol. Two daily servings of high-protein meat alternates such as legumes, high-protein nuts, peanut butter, meat analogs, dairy products, or eggs are recommended. If dairy products are not used, calcium and riboflavin can be obtained in adequate amounts by liberal intake of dark green, leafy vegetables or by consumption of fortified soy milk.

Summary

A vegetarian can be well nourished *if* he eats a variety of plant foods and gives attention to the critical nutrients mentioned above. Dairy products and eggs are outstanding sources of the nutrients of greatest concern. Legumes, leafy vegetables, and a source of vitamin $B_{12}$ are important components of the diet containing no foods of animal origin.

References
1. Hardinge, M. G., and Stare, F. J.: Nutritional studies of vegetarians, nutritional, physical and laboratory findings. Am. J. Clin. Nutr. 2: 73, 1954.
2. Register, U. D., and Sonnenburg, L. M.: The vegetarian diet. J. Am. Diet. Assoc. 62: 253, 1973.

# Nutritional Aspects of Vegetarianism, Health Foods, and Fad Diets

COMMITTEE ON NUTRITION, AMERICAN ACADEMY OF PEDIATRICS

The Committee on Nutrition is concerned about the recent increase in nutritional practices that are potentially hazardous to the health of children. The purpose of this statement is to discuss some common dietary patterns which may be harmful and/or which may fail to provide the promised or anticipated benefits. Such diets include those based on religion, life-style, morality, or ecologic concerns (e.g., vegetarianism and Zen macrobiotics), and those in which special virtues of a particular food, foods, or nutrients are exaggerated (e.g., organic, natural, and health foods, or diets supplemented with massive doses of one or more vitamins) [1]. The committee urges that claims for benefit of special diets should be subjected to critical, scientific evaluation before acceptance by the medical community.

Vegetarian Diets    Vegetarianism with may individual modifications is popular, especially among adolescents and young adults. Vegetarian diets may be classified as lactoovovegetarian (plant foods with dairy products and eggs), lactovegetarian (plant foods with dairy products), and pure vegetarian (plant foods only). The term "vegan" refers to a group of individuals who not only eat pure vegetarian diets but also share a philosophy and life-style [2]. The Zen macrobiotic diet does not fit into this classification and will be described separately.

Many individuals and population groups have practiced vegetarianism on a long-term basis and have demonstrated excellent health. Plant-based diets supplemented with milk or with milk and eggs tend to be nutritionally similar to diets containing meat. The National Academy of Sciences' Food and Nutrition Board has emphasized that even pure vegetarians can be well nourished if they select their diets carefully to provide sufficient kilocalories, a good balance of essential amino acids, and adequate sources of calcium, riboflavin, iron, vitamin A, vitamin D, and vitamin $B_{12}$ [3]. Indeed, there are some nutritional benefits of a well-balanced vegetarian diet, such as the rarity of obesity [3] and a tendency toward lower serum cholesterol levels [4]. On the other hand, the more stringent Zen macrobiotic diet is likely to be hazardous and leaves less room for modification [5–10].

### PURE VEGETARIANS AND VEGANS [2,3,6,7,10,11]

A problem with vegetarian diets is the tendency to be so high in bulk that they may not meet caloric needs. Because of diminished kilocalories, protein is used as an energy source; thus, a protein content equivalent to the recommended daily allowance (RDA) becomes marginal. There are several ways to improve protein nutrition. The quantity of protein in the diet is enhanced by using legumes in which the concentration of protein is high. The quality of vegetable proteins is improved by combining in each meal foods that provide the essential amino acids in the optimal ratios. For example, cereal grains (such as wheat and rice) are poor in the essential amino acid lysine and can be effectively combined with legumes, such as varieties of dry beans, soybeans, and peas, which have adequate lysine but little methionine [3,12]. When the two foods are eaten at the same meal, they provide a mixture of protein that is better than either alone.

The risk of other deficiencies is decreased if a large variety of foods is used and undue reliance on a single cereal staple is avoided. An adequate intake of most vitamins, minerals, and other nutrients can be obtained with legumes (including fortified soybean formulas), whole grain products, nuts, seeds, and dark green, leafy vegetables. Legumes provide B vitamins and iron in addition to relatively concentrated protein. Whole grains are a source of thiamine, iron, and trace minerals as well as carbohydrate and protein. Nuts and seeds contain B vitamins and iron, and they provide fat, which tends to be low in vegetarian diets. Dark green, leafy vegetables help to supply adequate calcium and riboflavin, which are lacking when dairy products are excluded. Vitamin $B_{12}$ deficiency occurs in pure vegetarian diets after a variable period because this vitamin is derived exclusively from animal products. The deficiency can be avoided if vitamin $B_{12}$ supplementation is provided in tablet form or in fortified plant foods such as vitamin $B_{12}$-fortified soy or nut "milks" that are usually available in health food stores. Vitamin supplements are acceptable to most vegans.

### ZEN MACROBIOTIC DIET

The Zen macrobiotic diet [5–10] is perhaps the most dangerous of the current diets for growing children. The goals of this rigid nutritional system are largely spiritual. Ten stages of dietary restriction progress from −3 to +7, with gradual elimination of animal products, fruits, and vegetables. The lower-level diets can meet nutritional needs [6,7], but the highest-level diet is composed only of cereals and restricts nutritional balance that is inherent in more diverse diets. In addition, caloric intake is usually low. Strict adherence to the more rigid diets can result in scurvy, anemia, hypoproteinemia, hypocalcemia, emaciation, or even death. Self-treatment of disease is common in this group, and medical consultation is discouraged. In 1971, the Council of Foods and Nutrition of the American Medical Association pointed out the dangers of the Zen macrobiotic diet [5]. Poor growth is the main clinical finding in infancy, as exemplified in a recent report of two infants who had been fed Kokoh (a Zen macrobiotic food mixture for infant feeding) from birth to 7 and 14 months [10]. They were substantially underweight (5 and 6 kg, respectively), and their body lengths were below the third percentile of the Iowa standards, reflecting a caloric intake that was 40% of the RDA. Experience with some parents who use the Zen macrobiotic diet has indicated that they may be more accepting of nutritional advice for their children than for themselves. If parents are told of their infant's poor growth and of the long-term consequences of protein-calorie undernutrition, they may adopt a lower, more nutritionally diverse and adequate step of the diet.

### VITAMIN A

There are unsubstantiated claims that extremely high doses of vitamin A (25,000 to 50,000 IU/day) improve visual acuity in people who work in either bright or dim light. Large doses of vitamin A are also used for the treatment of acne and to prevent infection. Such high doses can produce serious toxic effects in children, including anorexia, desquamation of the skin, increased intracranial pressure, and X-ray changes in the long bones [13,14]. Sufficient vitamin A for infants and children is present in most diets. Caffey has warned [15] that the hazards of vitamin A poisoning from the routine prophylactic feeding of concentrates of vitamins A and D to healthy infants and children who eat good diets are considerably greater than the hazards of vitamin A deficiency in healthy infants and children not fed vitamin concentrates. Ingestion of 20,000 IU/day or more for one or two months is likely to be toxic. A joint statement of this committee and the Committee on Drugs discusses the use and abuse of vitamin A in detail [13].

### VITAMIN C

Pauling recommended a daily dose of vitamin C between 1 and 5 g for the prophylaxis of the common cold [16]. This book has resulted not only in a surge of interest in vitamin C but also in its use in enormous quantities to prevent colds. The Committee on Drugs of the American Academy of Pediatrics stated in 1971 that there was no scientific evidence that vitamin C in the doses recommended by Pauling was either safe or efficacious for the prevention of the common cold [17]. Since that time, a number of carefully controlled, double-blind studies [18–21] suggest that the use of vitamin C has, at best, a small effect on severity and duration of symptoms of the common cold. The report of a recent conference on vitamin C points out discrepancies among these studies and concludes that large doses of vitamin C have not been proven to have widespread usefulness as a cold remedy [22]. Clearly, much more research is needed to confirm whether vitamin C is useful in preventing the common cold and to determine what harmful consequences such large daily doses of the vitamin may have. Large doses of vitamin C can interfere with vitamin $B_{12}$ absorption and metabolism in man, and this problem may not be overcome by extra vitamin $B_{12}$ supplementation [23]. Healthy adults can become conditioned to high doses of ascorbate (0.5 to 1.5 g/day) over a two-week period with the result that they develop lower-than-normal serum and leukocyte ascorbic acid values on returning to a normal intake [24]. A similar phenomenon in the fetus may explain the development of scurvy in normally fed offspring of mothers who have ingested 400 mg of ascorbic acid daily throughout pregnancy [25]. Until more information is available, people should be cautious in substantially exceeding the RDA for vitamin C.

### VITAMIN D

Vitamin D in amounts much greater than the RDA of 400 IU daily has been claimed to build stronger bones, especially when the vitamin is taken in its "natural" form in fish liver oil. We know of no evidence to support such claims. The RDA is adequate for most infants and children and provides an ample margin of safety, even without exposure to sunlight. Overuse of vitamin D in Britain and the European continent, with intakes between 3,000 and 4,000 IU daily, is believed to be related to the idiopathic hypercalcemia of infancy seen relatively frequently during and after World War II [26]. The disease became quite rare after the dietary intake of vitamin D was reduced to less than 1,500 IU daily [26].

### VITAMIN E

Vitamin E has commanded much public attention and controversy. High dietary intakes of vitamin E have been claimed to prolong life, increase sexual potency, and prevent such diseases as mental retardation, heart disease, and cancer. There is little or no basis for these claims. The wide distribution of vitamin E in vegetable oils and cereal grains makes deficiency in humans unlikely [27]. Vitamin E supplementation may be necessary for persons with intestinal malabsorption, such as low-birth-weight infants whose absorption of the vitamin is often decreased for the first 12 months of life [28]. In other situations, an excess of vitamin E may be harmful, although the evidence for this is scant. There is evidence, both in man and in the experimental animal, that excess vitamin E intake can interfere with vitamin K metabolism, result in a prolonged prothrombin time, and predispose to bleeding [29]. Excessive vitamin E intake in the experimental animal decreases the rate of wound healing [30], and in man it has resulted in gastrointestinal symptoms and creatinuria [31].

Health Foods   The terms "organic," "natural," and "health" foods generally carry the following connotations. Organic foods are plant products grown in soil enriched with humus and compost on which no pesticides, herbicides, or inorganic fertilizers have been used, or they are meat and dairy products from animals raised on "natural" feeds and not treated with drugs such as hormones or antibiotics. Natural foods are those made from ingredients of plant or animal origin which are altered as little as possible, and which contain no synthetic or artificial ingredients or additives. Health food is a general term which seems to encompass natural and organic foods. The term includes conventional foods which have been subjected to less processing than usual (such as unhydrogenated nut butters and whole grain flours) and less conventional foods such as brewer's yeast, pumpkin seeds, wheat germ, and herb teas.

### NUTRITIONAL ASPECTS

The nutritional value of foods that reach the consumer depends not only on the composition of the raw materials but also on various changes which occur during processing, storage, and distribution [32]. Nutritional losses occur whether food is processed commercially or at home or is stored in an unprocessed state [33,34]. Variations in the nutrient content of raw foodstuffs will affect the content of vitamins and minerals in the final food product as much as, and sometimes more than, the processing itself. For example, carrots may vary 100-fold in their concentration of carotene (provitamin A), and samples of fresh tomato juice have shown 16-fold differences in vitamin C per serving. Although the data are somewhat sketchy, the raw foods being produced today are not significantly different in terms of vitamin content from those produced two or more decades ago [34]. The food preservation techniques in greatest use today minimize the loss of nutritive value of foods and are safe and well standardized.

There is no test to differentiate organically grown and organically processed food from similar commercial products. Long-term studies have failed to show the nutritional superiority of organically grown crops in comparison with those grown under standard agricultural conditions with chemical fertilizers [35]. If the soil is deficient in nutrients, crop yield rather than the nutritional quality of the plant will be primarily affected.

Other concerns about agricultural practices and food processing procedures may have more validity (e.g., residual hormones and antibiotics in meat, and pesticide residue on dairy, fruit, and vegetable products) [36]. In addition, the variety of food additives in commercial use is large, which makes complete screening of such products for safety difficult for industry and federal agencies [37]. Each of these issues is complicated, unresolved, and beyond the scope of this discussion. It is apparent that concern about these issues is often the basis for use of health foods despite their high cost.

Organically grown foodstuffs cost more than their nonorganic counterparts [38,39]. In a 1976 survey by the U.S. Department of Agriculture in the Washington, D.C., area, a market basket of 33 standard foods bought in a supermarket cost $17.49; 33 counterparts labeled "organic" cost from $23.74 to $28.00 in "natural" food stores [40]. The difference in cost (1⅓ to 1⅔ higher) for foods purchased in "health" stores is of particular concern for low-income families who may have to skimp in quantity or sacrifice other important items in the budget to afford health foods. At this time, there is no compelling evidence that the high cost of these products results in concomitant benefit to the consumer. There are no standard tests to identify organic foods; therefore, the consumer is forced to rely on the integrity of the farmer and distributor for assurance that the products were grown or prepared as claimed.

DIETS FOR ATHLETES

Special diets and dietary supplements for athletes can be briefly considered as a separate category of health foods [41]. There is a widespread misconception that high-protein diets improve athletic performance. This belief is the basis for the ingestion of disproportionately large amounts of rare red meat and milk by many athletes.

In addition, the belief has led to the use of special protein supplements, which is particularly widespread among weight lifters. The major dietary need of athletes is calories, and protein is rarely a limiting factor. With exercise, the need for calories increases roughly in proportion to the increased expenditure of energy. Ordinarily, an athlete will spontaneously increase his food intake to a degree that meets caloric needs, that provides more than adequate protein, and that maintains a relatively constant weight. The requirement for protein does not increase with exercise, except to a slight degree when muscle mass increases. The belief that honey has special merit as a carbohydrate source for athletes has no scientific basis. The intermittent use of stringent diets for a wrestler to meet a lower weight class is nutritionally unsound and seems unduly extreme if competitive athletics are to be viewed as a health-promoting, recreational activity. Other nutritional practices of athletes may be harmful but are not within the scope of this discussion.

Conclusion  Most individuals who adhere to unusual nutritional practices, except for balanced vegetarianism, are aware that their ideas run counter to the mainstream of medical and nutritional opinion. Some adopt such diets as an expression of disillusion with medicine or the "establishment." Physicians and other health professionals should be prepared to encounter strong resistance if they attempt to reverse such practices. Parents are likely to resist the suggestion of major dietary changes, and it is best to focus on those features of the diet that are of greatest potential harm to their children. However, even with the more extreme dietary practices, it is usually possible to prevent serious harm by striving for dietary variety and balance and working within the value system or philosophy of the group or individual.

COMMITTEE ON NUTRITION (1976, 1977)

LEWIS A. BARNESS, M.D., *Chairman*
ALVIN M. MAUER, M.D., *Vice-Chairman*
ARNOLD S. ANDERSON, M.D.
PETER R. DALLMAN, M.D.
GILBERT B. FORBES, M.D.
JAMES C. HAWORTH, M.D.
MARY JANE JESSE, M.D.
BUFORD L. NICHOLS, JR., M.D.
CHARLES R. SCRIVER, M.D.
NATHAN J. SMITH, M.D.
MYRON WINICK, M.D.
*Consultants*
WILLIAM C. HEIRD, M.D.
O. L. KLINE, PH.D.
DONOUGH O'BRIEN, M.D.

References

1. Nutrition misinformation and food faddism. Nutr. Rev. 32 (Suppl. 1), July 1974.
2. McKenzie, J.: Profile on vegans. Plant Foods Hum. Nutr. 2: 79, 1971.
3. Committee on Nutritional Misinformation, Food and Nutrition Board, National Research Council: Vegetarian diets. Am. J. Clin. Nutr. 27: 1095, 1974.
4. West, R. O., and Hayes, O. B.: Diet and serum cholesterol levels: a comparison between vegetarians and non-vegetarians in a Seventh-Day Adventist Group. Am. J. Clin. Nutr. 21: 853, 1968.
5. Council on Foods and Nutrition: Zen macrobiotic diets. JAMA 218: 397, 1971.
6. Register, U. D., and Sonnenberg, L. M.: The vegetarian diet: scientific and practical considerations. J. Am. Diet. Assoc. 62: 253, 1973.
7. Miller, D. S., and Mumford, P.: The nutritive value of Western vegan and vegetarian diets. Plant Foods Hum. Nutr. 2: 201, 1972.
8. Erhard, D.: The new vegetarians: I. Vegetarianism and its medical consequences. Nutr. Today 8: 4, Nov.–Dec. 1973.
9. Erhard, D.: A starved child of the new vegetarians. Nutr. Today 8: 10, Nov.–Dec. 1973.
10. Robson, J. R. K.; Konlande, J. E.; Larkin, F. A.; et al.: Zen macrobiotic dietary problems in infancy. Pediatrics 53: 326, 1974.
11. Brown, P. T., and Bergan, J. G.: The dietary status of "new" vegetarians. J. Am. Diet. Assoc. 67: 455, 1975.
12. Harper, A. E.; Benevenga, N. J.; and Wohlhueter, R. M.: Effect of ingestion of disproportionate amounts of amino acids. Physiol. Rev. 50: 428, 1970.
13. Committee on Drugs and Nutrition: The use and abuse of vitamin A. Pediatrics 48: 655, 1971.
14. Nutrition Committee, Canadian Paediatric Society: The use and abuse of vitamin A. Can. Med. Assoc. J. 104: 521, 1971.
15. Caffey, J.: Chronic poisoning due to excess of vitamin A: description of the clinical and roentgen manifestations in seven infants and young children. Pediatrics 5: 672, 1950.
16. Pauling, L. C.: Vitamin C and the Common Cold. San Francisco: W. H. Freeman, 1970.
17. Committee on Drugs: Vitamin C and the common cold. Am. Acad. Pediatr. Newslett. 22, Nov. 1, 1971.
18. Anderson, T. W.; Reid, D. B. W.; and Beaton, G. H.: Vitamin C and the common cold: a double blind trial. Can. Med. Assoc. J. 107: 503, 1972.
19. Wilson, C. W. M., and Loh, H. S.: Common cold and vitamin C. Lancet 1: 638, 1973.
20. Coulehan, J. L.; Reisinger, K. S.; Rogers, K. D.; and Bradley, D. W.: Vitamin C prophylaxis in a boarding school. N. Engl. J. Med. 290: 6, 1974.
21. Anderson, T. W.; Beaton, G. H.; Corey, P. N.; and Spero, L.: Winter illness and vitamin C: the effect of relatively low doses. Can. Med. Assoc. J. 112: 823, 1975.
22. Second conference on vitamin C: VI. Ascorbic acid and respiratory illness. Ann. NY Acad. Sci. 258: 498, 1975.
23. Herbert, V., and Jacob, E.: Destruction of vitamin $B_{12}$ by ascorbic acid. JAMA 230: 241, 1974.
24. Rhead, W. J., and Schrauzer, G. N.: Risks of long-term ascorbic acid overdosage. Nutr. Rev. 29: 262, 1971.
25. Cochrane, W. A.: Overnutrition in prenatal and neonatal life: a problem? Can. Med. Assoc. J. 93: 893, 1965.
26. Food and Nutrition Board, National Research Council: Hazards of overuse of vitamin D. Am. J. Clin. Nutr. 28: 512, 1975.
27. Food and Nutrition Board, National Research Council: Supplementation of human diets with vitamin E. Nutr. Rev. 32 (Suppl.), July 1974.
28. Melhorn, D. K., and Gross, S.: Vitamin E-dependent anemia in the premature infant: II. Relationships between gestational age and absorption of vitamin E. J. Pediatr. 79: 581, 1971.
29. Hypervitaminosis E and coagulation. Nutr. Rev. 33: 269, 1975.
30. Ehrlich, H. P.; Tarver, H.; and Hunt, T. K.: Inhibitory effects of vitamin E on collagen synthesis and wound repair. Ann. Surg. 175: 235, 1972.
31. Hillman, R. W.: Tocopherol excess in man: creatinuria associated with prolonged ingestion. Am. J. Clin. Nutr. 5: 597, 1957.

32. Expert Panel on Food Safety and Nutrition and the Committee on Public Information, Institute of Food Technologists: The effects of food processing on nutritional values. Nutr. Rev. 33: 123, 1975.

33. Nesheim, R. O.: Nutrient changes in food processing: a current review. Fed. Proc. 33: 2267, 1974.

34. Expert Panel on Food Safety and Nutrition and the Committee on Public Information, Institute of Food Technologists: The effects of food processing on nutritional values. Food Technol. 28: 77, 1974.

35. Alther, L.: Organic farming on trial. Natural History 81: 16, 1972.

36. Hayes, W. J.: Recognized and possible exposure to pesticides. Toxicology of Pesticides. Baltimore: Williams & Wilkins, 1975: 265.

37. Kermode, G. O.: Food additives. Sci. Am. 226 (3): 15, 1972.

38. Jukes, T. H.: The organic food myth. JAMA 230: 276, 1974.

39. Fomon, S. J., and Anderson, T. A., eds.: Practices of Low Income Families in Feeding Infants. Washington, DC: U.S. Government Printing Office, 1972.

40. Cromwell, C.: Organic Foods: An Update. Family Economics Review. Washington, DC: Agricultural Research Service, U.S. Department of Agriculture, 1976: 8–11.

41. Van Itallie, T. B.; Sinisterra, L.; and Stare, F. J.: Nutrition and athletic performance. JAMA 162: 1120, 1956.

# Nutrition

AMERICAN COLLEGE OF OBSTETRICIANS AND GYNECOLOGISTS

A woman's nutritional status during pregnancy is of great importance to her health and to that of her baby. Ideally, nutritional assessment should be made before conception. Failing that, it should be repeated at regular intervals during and after pregnancy.

Growth is a process requiring energy. Maternal energy sources about fifteen percent above average non-pregnant needs are required during pregnancy. This is equivalent to an additional 300 kcal* per day. The actual advisable caloric intake varies within wide limits depending upon maternal age, activity, height, pre-pregnant weight, stage of pregnancy, and amibient temperature. Caloric needs are greater in the last trimesters than the first.

The simplest method of evaluating caloric intake is to observe the pattern of weight gain, which is usually minimal (1 to 2 kg) in the first trimester followed by a relatively linear rate of gain of approximately 0.4 kg per week during the last two trimesters. Therefore, caloric intake should be sufficient to support a total weight gain of at least 10 to 12 kg during the entire pregnancy in all patients regardless of the pre-pregnant weight. Weight reduction diets in pregnancy are not advisable.

Protein requirements in pregnancy should be calculated on a weight basis. This amounts to a total daily protein intake of 1.3 g per kg for the adult woman (approximately 75 g per day), 1.5 g per kg for the adolescent aged 15 to 18 and 1.7 g per kg for younger girls. About two-thirds of the total protein intake should be of high biologic quality such as found in eggs, milk, meat, or soy protein. Adequate total energy intake is essential for optimal protein utilization.

Most women are unable to meet the gestational requirement for iron by diet and iron stores. It is therefore recommended that prophylactic supplements be given in the form of simple ferrous salts in amounts of 30 to 60 mg of elemental iron daily throughout pregnancy and for several months postpartum.

Folic acid is also required in increased amounts during pregnancy. Particularly rich dietary sources of folate include green leafy vegetables, kidney, liver, and peanuts. Since dietary levels of folate may or may not be adequate to meet the demands of pregnancy, some authorities advocate routine supplementation of all patients. If folate supplementation is elected, amounts of 400 to 800 µg per day are appropriate.

Although other vitamins and minerals are generally required in increased amounts during pregnancy, the advisability of routine supplementation is controversial. If vitamin-mineral supplements are

---

* The caloric value of the diet refers to the physiologically available or metabolizable energy yield of foods actually consumed. The unit of measure is the kilocalorie (kcal).

Reprinted from Standards for Ambulatory Obstetric Care (American College of Obstetricians and Gynecologists, 1977).

given, they should not be regarded as substitutes for a balanced diet and continued nutritional counseling.

Sodium is required in pregnancy for the expanded maternal tissue and fluid compartments as well as to provide for fetal needs. The normal patient may use the level of sodium intake she prefers. Routine sodium restriction is not advised.

Unless otherwise indicated by complications of the preceding pregnancy and delivery, a well-balanced diet should be provided during the early puerperium. Fluid should neither be restricted nor markedly increased.

For the woman who chooses to breastfeed her infant, nutrition is particularly important. Lactation requires substantial amounts of energy sources, with at least 500 kcal per day above non-pregnant levels recommended. Calcium and protein are also required in greatly increased amounts during lactation inasmuch as 0.2 to 0.3 g of calcium and 8 to 12 g of protein are contained in each day's production of breast milk. Consumption of one quart of milk daily will provide these needs for the nursing mother. In patients for whom milk is physiologically or psychologically unacceptable, alternative sources of the protein and calcium will be needed.

If weight reduction is indicated because of pre-gestational obesity or excessive weight gain during pregnancy, weight reduction regimens may be instituted after lactation or, for the non-nursing mother, two to four weeks postpartum.

# Salt Intake and Eating Patterns of Infants and Children in Relation to Blood Pressure

COMMITTEE ON NUTRITION, AMERICAN ACADEMY OF PEDIATRICS

Essential hypertension is a major health problem in the adult population in the United States; and its association with heart disease, stroke, and renal failure (particularly among patients in the third and fourth decades) has made efforts for its prevention a matter of high priority [1]. Twenty percent of the adult population has hypertension or hypertensive heart disease [1]. Multiple factors [2–4] contribute to the development of hypertension. The level of dietary salt intake by persons in the United States has been proposed by Dahl and Love [5] as one factor, and they have recommended that dietary salt intake by persons in this country be lowered.

Dahl [6] has suggested that the salt intake of infants and children predisposes to hypertension later in life, and he has focused on the salt content of processed infant foods. This is of concern because dietary intake of salt by infants sometimes exceeds minimum requirements by four to six times [7], and because salt feeding early in life in hypertensive-sensitive rats [8] has induced hypertension more readily than when salt is provided later.

A subcommittee of the Food Protection Committee of the Food and Nutrition Board (NAS-NRC) reviewed the subject [9] and concluded that, whereas average salt intake of infants was indeed several times the minimum requirement, evidence relating salt intake to hypertension later in life was ambiguous. The committee recommended that the salt content of infant foods be reduced. Manufacturers have complied, and subsequent surveys [10] have shown a reduction in salt intake of infants less than 8 months old. However, the salt intake of older infants remains unchanged, and children of all ages appear to have a salt intake well in excess of the estimated minimum requirements. The salt intake of infants and children and its possible relation to hypertension continue to lead to recommendations that dietary salt intake should be decreased [11].

Difficulties arise in attempting to recommend a suitable range for dietary salt because of the tremendous range of biological tolerance in normal human beings, the widely different levels of salt appetite, and the cultural significance which salt has in relation to food [12]. The Committee on Nutrition has reviewed the factors which affect dietary salt intake, including changes in cultural patterns that may alter the quantity of salt ingested. The committee has also reviewed current thinking on the causes of hypertension and the evidence relating salt intake to hypertension. The committee recommends actions that reduce or avoid increasing the present level of salt intake by children in the population at large. Children with a family history

Reprinted from Pediatrics 53: 115, Jan. 1974. Copyright American Academy of Pediatrics 1974.

**Salt Intake and Eating Patterns  /  A53**

of hypertension may benefit from a low salt diet, although the evidence to date is incomplete.

Salt Tolerance and Dietary Patterns

DIETARY SALT INTAKE OF ADULTS

The human adult who is not subjected to unusual salt losses from sweating or losses of gastrointestinal or other body fluids can maintain health and normal activity on little sodium (Na).* Certain societies exist for which virtually no sodium is available [12]. Kempner [13] demonstrated that patients with hypertension could sustain normal activities for months on diets containing as little as 2 meq of Na per day. Hence, the minimum requirement (0.1 meq/100 kcal) for normal adults in a favorable setting is low; it is higher for those experiencing skin losses from sweating and for pregnant and lactating women. The maximum tolerance for adults is high. Japanese and Thai farmers ingest 20 to 25 g of salt, 400 to 500 meq of Na, per day (20 meq/100 kcal), with no signs of salt toxicity, i.e., edema or hypernatremia [3]. A few individuals are reported to ingest 1,000 meq of Na per day habitually without evident harm.

Table 1.  Sodium Intake of Infants at 6 Months of Age

|  | Total meq/day | Dietary salt intake | | Na:K |
|  |  | /kg | /100 kcal |  |
| --- | --- | --- | --- | --- |
| Infant-human milk | 6–8 | 1 | 1 | 0.60 |
| Puyau average [7] | 45±12 | 6 | 6 | 0.70–1.50 |
| Six-month-old infant Purvis [10] |  |  |  |  |
| 1969 survey | 40–45 | 6 | 6 | 1.15 |
| 1972 survey | 25–30 | 3–4 | 3–4 | 0.89 |
| Adult | 150–200 | 2–3 | 6–8 | 1.20–2.00 |

*Source*:  Detailed data from Purvis et al. [10] kindly provided to the committee.

The capacity to adapt to a low intake may derive from man's evolutionary roots as an herbivore [12]; the biological advantages of his tolerance to a high intake are less clear. Access to a high intake provides replacement when salt is lost from the body as sweat or gastrointestinal losses. Historically, salt was a valued preservative, particularly for meat and fish. Other mammals, notably herbivores, seek salt from salt licks but probably do not ingest salt in quantities comparable to modern man. The search for salt derives from an appetite for salt which is stimulated by salt deficiency, notably in herbivores. However, an appetite for salt can be acquired as an individual preference [12].

The ability of humans to adapt to a wide range of sodium intake is due to the renal-endocrine system responsible for regulating body sodium, within narrow limits, by varying urinary excretion of sodium according to sodium intake and nonrenal sodium losses. The hormonal system (renin, angiotensin, and adrenal mineralocorti-

* Salt is used in this paper to refer to sodium chloride; Na refers to the sodium content of the diet. Where Na content is high, the chloride content also is high in nearly every instance.

coids) [14] and the kidney [15] are key factors in the physiological regulation of blood pressure, and there is evidence for considerable genetically determined variability within this control system. Also, regulation of body potassium (K) in response to variation in intake of K is dependent on elements in the sodium control system. Blood pressure is affected by variations in the ratio of Na:K in diet as well as the dietary Na alone.

Food patterns often have changed as a result of the vagaries of history, but they stabilized where food sources became dependable and cultural patterns became set. In the last 100 years, food sources in the United States have undergone vast change, and the process continues. The major element of this change in our society has been linked to the movement of people from a rural setting to cities and suburbs. Coincidentally, established cultural ties often have been disrupted and food sources have changed, with increasing dependence on processed or manufactured foods as the principal food source.

There is some evidence from marketing data that average per capita adult salt consumption has not changed in the last few decades, despite the change in food sources; presently, the average per capita consumption of Na per day is 150 to 200 meq [16]. However, the proportion of Na provided from consumer purchase of salt has declined, and that provided from processed or prepared foods has increased [17]. Salt intake has become increasingly determined by food processors, rather than by individuals.

### SALT INTAKE OF INFANTS

The minimum salt requirement for the infant actually exceeds that of the adult. One to two meq of Na per day is required for growth; skin and gastrointestinal losses for children are estimated to be 2 meq/day. These plus obligatory urinary losses result in a requirement of 6 to 8 meq of Na per day [18,19]. Growth rate, stool composition, and skin losses are more important determinants of the daily salt requirement than body size or caloric need during the first year of life. The traditional source of sodium for the infant has been human milk, which provides 5 to 10 meq of Na per day (1 meq/100 kcal); infants receiving human milk often excrete less than 2 meq of Na per day. The Na:K ratio of human milk (and most mammalian milk) is 0.6 to 0.7 meq. The potassium requirement for growth exceeds the sodium requirement.

Renal mechanisms for conserving and excreting salt are well developed in the infant from 1 month of age. However, extrarenal losses, such as occur in gastroenteritis, are more likely to lead to salt depletion or hyponatremia in infants than in adults. Conversely, the infant with restricted access to water is at greater risk of salt excess and hypernatremia.

Infants, as is true with adults, have a tolerance for a salt intake several times the minimum. Intakes of 100 meq of Na per day (10 meq/100 kcal) without adverse effects are observed [7]. While higher intakes may be possible, the phenomenon of hypernatremia is a greater risk to infants because their access to water may be

**Table 2.  Source of Salt in the U.S. Infant's Diet—1972 Survey of 374 Infants**

*meq of Na per day*

| Age (mo) | 2 | 4 | 6 | 8 | 10 | 12 |
|---|---|---|---|---|---|---|
| *From* | | | | | | |
| Formula | 8.0 | 4.5 | 1.5 | 1.0 | 1.0 | 0 |
| Milk | 2.0 | 7.0 | 12.5 | 13.5 | 12.5 | 12 |
| Baby food | 3.5 | 7.5 | 12.0 | 15.0 | 13.5 | 12 |
| Table food* | 0 | 0 | 3.0 | 9.5 | 24.0 | 39 |
| Total | 13.5 | 19.0 | 29.0 | 38.0 | 51.0 | 63 |
| Estimated sodium of an infant receiving only human milk | 6 | 7 | 8 | 9 | 10 | 12 |

* Sodium content estimated form Handbook No. 8, U.S. Department of Agriculture, December 1963. Does not include table salt.

limited, and higher salt intakes require higher water ingestion for effective renal regulation. Hence, the safe tolerance limits for children appear to be roughly between 8 and 100 meq of Na per day. While this range is considerable, it is less than that of the adult. Except for a few uncommon adrenal disorders, the lower intakes of sodium recommended for infants are compatible with maintenance of normal potassium balances within the range of any normal, dietary intake.

In the past 50 years, the pattern of salt intake among infants has undergone change. Through the first 6 to 9 months of life, infants in the United States used to be fed human milk as the principal source of nutrients; and up until the turn of the century, they received from 5 to 10 meq of Na per day. A trend to adopt modified cows' milk in place of human milk began in the early 1900s and resulted in a two- to threefold increase in sodium intake and a proportional increase in potassium. The introduction of solid food into the young infant's diet also became more popular; as a result, the salt intake increased in varying degrees. Presalted cereals, meats, and vegetables contributed to the sodium intake; fruit did not. The salt was added to the diet in either home or commercial preparations to satisfy the mother's salt appetite. Because infants accept salted and unsalted food in equal amounts [20], the salt content of the food has little effect on its consumption; and it probably reflects the mother's culturally acquired appetite for salt.

Puyau and Hampton [7], who reported the daily Na intake of infants during the first year of life in 1960, found a considerable variation; but the mean intake increased from 30 meq/day at 2 to 3 months to 45 meq at 6 to 8 months and to 60 meq at 11 to 13 months. Table 1 compares salt intake of infants at 6 months of age taken from their diet survey [7] with the results of surveys done in 1969 and 1972 [10], and with the intake of a breast-fed, 6-month-old infant and an average adult. The average intakes exceed those provided from human milk by four- to sixfold; the maximum intake was 100 meq of Na per day. The lower Na intake in the 1972 survey reflects manufacturing changes in 1970, when salt content was reduced. Salt intake of infants compared with adults is higher per kilogram of body weight, but lower in relation to caloric intake. The Na:K ratios are comparable.

Sodium intakes for infants 2 to 12 months of age and the principal food sources from which they are derived are shown in table 2. Dairy milk and table foods increase as principal sources of salt after 8 months of age. Consequently, the impact of any reduction in salt content of infant foods diminishes as the child passes this age.

### SALT INTAKE OF CHILDREN

Beyond infancy, when milk customarily ceases to be the major food, children traditionally eat what their parents do. Hence, salt intake increases with increased intake of family food as the child grows. Family salt intake may be determined by the family's cultural background, and the dietary Na:K ratio of the child reflects his family's. Generally, the Na:K ratio has not exceeded 2.0 [21].

Margaret Mead [22] has pointed out that children no longer learn their modes of behavior from their parents, but rather copy the behavior of their peers or learn from models outside the home, e.g., school, vocation, and chosen adult models. This trend is noticeable in relation to eating patterns. Eating patterns for today's school children and adolescents increasingly are set by fads, by commercial advertising, and by teenage life-styles. The resulting food consumption pattern may consist of school lunches (which in one study [21] contained 15 meq of Na per 100 kcal), quick-service foods, etc. One possible consequence of this development is the tendency for salt intake to be consistently high in all children. Peer group pressures and uniform food sources may make it difficult for a child who desires it to adopt a diet low in salt.

## Salt Intake and the Causes of Hypertension

Because of the prevalence of essential hypertension in adults, there is a major public health concern with its causes; the reviews already cited [2–4] outline a number of predisposing factors. These factors include race, family history, stress, variations in endocrine and kidney function, and body habitus. Salt has also been cited as causing hypertension. There is no question that an increase in salt intake by most hypertensive patients will increase their blood pressure. The converse also is true. The question is whether salt intake induces hypertension and, in particular, whether salt consumption by the general population in this country is a risk.

The evidence that salt intake induces hypertension is based on experimental studies in rats and epidemiological studies in humans.

### EVIDENCE IN RATS RELATING HYPERTENSION TO SALT INTAKE

Hypertension in animals produced by almost any experimental technique was increased when the salt intake was increased [16].

An increase in the salt content of the diet can cause hypertension in rats. Meneely and Ball [23] summarized their observations of blood pressure and other responses to the dietary manipulation of sodium, chloride, and potassium. There were no differences in growth (length and weight), longevity, or blood pressure among animals of 100 g body weight fed between 0.15% and 2.0% salt in their dry rations

(0.5 = 7.0 meq/100 kcal diet). Those fed 2.8% or 5.6% salt (10 or 20 meq of Na per 100 kcal) developed moderate hypertension, grew slightly less, and had a shorter life-span; among those fed 7% or more salt, more severe hypertension and growth retardation resulted, and they had a much shorter life-span. There was cardiac and renal enlargement proportional to the blood pressure elevation; microscopically, arteriolar lesions were seen, particularly in the kidneys of the severely hypertensive rats. Potassium chloride lessened the effects of high NaCl feeding on blood pressure and life-span.

Dahl [24] demonstred that feeding 8% or more (25 to 30 meq/100 kcal) salt to rats in dry rations could result in irreversible hypertension, but with considerable variation in blood pressure response within the general population. He then developed a salt-resistant and a salt-sensitive strain of rats. A salt intake in the salt-sensitive rats of from 0.4% to 11% of the diet correlated with progressive elevation of blood pressure [25]. When rats of this strain were fed 8% salt from weaning to 6 weeks of age, they developed hypertension by 1 year of age and their life-span was shortened [8]. The effect, both in blood pressure and life-span, was less when the extra salt intake was provided between 3 and 6 months of age.

In summary: intakes of 10 to 30 meq of Na per 100 kcal/day (3 to 8 meq/kg/day) induce hypertension in nonselected laboratory rats; lesser amounts induce hypertension in genetically selected rats. Early feeding of salt to sensitive rats predisposes to hypertension later. Adding potassium to the diet to maintain a Na:K ratio < 2.0 protects against the induction of hypertension. Resistant rats tolerate high Na intakes.

### EPIDEMIOLOGICAL STUDIES IN HUMANS

Dahl [16] demonstrated that some cultures show a positive linear relation between average salt intake and the overall prevalence of hypertension. Eskimos, who ingest an average of 30 meq of Na per day, are virtually free of hypertension; some Japanese farmers ingest an average of 500 meq of Na per day, and 40% of them over 40 years old are hypertensive. Average salt consumption in the United States is 150 to 200 meq of Na per day, and there is a 20% prevalence of hypertension among adults over 40 years of age.

Additional studies [26] have confirmed Dahl's findings. When blood pressure and salt intake of two Polynesian groups were compared [27], the prevalence of hypertension was greater with increasing age in the group averaging an intake of 120 to 140 meq of Na per day than in the group averaging 60 meq of Na per day. Disparities have also been observed. For example, the native population in St. Kitt's Island in the West Indies [28] ingests 100 to 150 meq of Na per day and shows a much higher prevalence of hypertension than that occurring in the United States.

Individuals within a culture (population) show only negligible correlation between a single, measured blood pressure and daily salt intake. Dahl [16] first reported higher blood pressures in laboratory workers who regularly added salt to prepared food compared to blood pressures in workers adding little or no salt to prepared food.

Miall [29] assessed salt intake by diet history and urine sodium excretion and found no correlation in males in a Welsh mining community and a negative correlation in females. Prior [27] also noted no correlation between individual blood pressures and salt intake in his "high-salt" Polynesian group. Dawber and his colleagues [30] failed to find correlation in the "Framingham Study" between blood pressure and daily salt intake.

In other studies, no differences in salt excretion were observed between hypertensive and normal patients [31,32].

Dahl [16] expressed the view that salt intake is one of the multiple factors which act in various degrees to cause hypertension. However, if a low salt diet diminishes the risk of developing hypertension and a high salt diet increases the risk, some degree of correlation should be expected between an individual's salt intake and his blood pressure. Little correlation has been found. An important limitation to all the data is the method used to access salt ingestion over the years, i.e., one- or two-day samples of dietary intake by history or sodium excretion in a 24-hour urine sample. A second limitation is the relatively small sample size.

In summary: epidemiological observations suggest a relation between salt ingestion and hypertension but fail to support the hypothesis that salt consumption is a *major* factor in causing hypertension in persons in the United States.

Summary    Approximately 20% of children in this country are at risk of developing hypertension as adults. The factors that will induce hypertension are genetic, which cannot be modified, and environmental, which can be modified. Genetic factors assist in identifying the population at risk, i.e., family history of hypertension, myocardial infarction, stroke, or renal disease. The population with a negative family history is less at risk.

The role of salt intake as an environmental factor in the induction of hypertension has still to be defined. For 80% of the population in this country, present salt intake has not been demonstrated to be harmful; i.e., hypertension has not developed. Salt intake is likely to be only one of the contributing factors for those whose genetic makeup predisposes them to hypertension.

Salt appetite for some is an important expression of personal preference in relation to diet; for others, salt-containing foods have important cultural values. Present evidence does not provide a firm basis for advising a change in the dietary salt intake for the general population. There is a reasonable possibility that a low salt intake begun early in life may protect, to some extent, persons at risk of developing hypertension.

Salt consumption today is being determined to an increasing degree by food manufacturers and processors and quick-service food suppliers. To the extent that salt is added to a food prior to its being served, the individual has an obligatory rather than a selected intake of salt. The consumption of presalted foods may be producing significant changes in salt intake which are not perceived at this time.

**Recommendations**    The committee favors development of guidelines for restraining the use of salt by food processors.

As a public health measure, consumers need more information on the salt content of their diet. The committee believes that information on the amount of salt added to processed foods should be made available to consumers.

The committee recommends the marketing of foods for low salt diets ($< 40$ meq of Na per day, i.e., 1,000-mg Na diet) to make them available at the same cost and convenience as diets which provide more salt.

The committee recommends that nutrition education be directed to increasing public awareness of the potentials for dietary variation that can enhance the cultural and social value of eating and still conform to good nutrition practices. The genetic and cultural heterogeneity of the population in this country justifies a flexible policy with respect to diet recommendations. Salt is but one example of a nutrient that can be enjoyed by many, but must be restricted in some. Dietary modification for persons at risk, rather than for the population at large, is consistent with sound medical and epidemiological practices.

COMMITTEE ON NUTRITION

MALCOLM A. HOLLIDAY, M.D., *Chairman*
ARNOLD S. ANDERSON, M.D.
LEWIS A. BARNESS, M.D.
RICHARD B. GOLDBLOOM, M.D.
JAMES C. HAWORTH, M.D.
ALVIN M. MAUER, M.D.
ROBERT W. MILLER, M.D.
DONOUGH O'BRIEN, M.D.
WILLIAM B. WEIL, JR., M.D.
CHARLES F. WHITTEN, M.D.
*Consultants:*
JOAQUIN CRAVIOTO, M.D.
L. J. FILER, JR., M.D.
O. L. KLINE, PH.D.
ROBERT W. WINTERS, M.D.

**References**    1. Report of Inter-Society Commission for Heart Disease Resources. Circulation 44: A237, 1971.
2. Evans, J. G., and Rose, G.: Hypertension. Br. Med. Bull. 27: 37, 1971.
3. Henry, J. P., and Meehan, J. P.: The Circulation: An Integrative Physiologic Study. Chicago: Year Book Medical Publishers, 1971.
4. Shapiro, A. P.: Essential hypertension—why idiopathic? Am. J. Med. 54: 1, 1973.
5. Dahl, L. K, and Love, R. A.: Etiological role of sodium chloride intake in essential hypertension in humans. JAMA 164: 397, 1957.
6. Dahl, L. K.: Salt in processed baby foods. Am. J. Clin. Nutr. 21: 787, 1968.
7. Puyau, F. A., and Hampton, L. P.: Infant feeding practices, 1966: salt content of the modern diet. Am. J. Dis. Child. 111: 370, 1966.
8. Dahl, L. K.; Knudsen, K. D.; Heine, M. A.; and Leitl, G. J.: Effects of chronic excess salt ingestion. Modification of experimental hypertension in the rat by variations in the diet. Circ. Res. 22: 11, 1968.
9. Filer, L. J., Jr.: Salt in infant foods. Nutr. Rev. 29: 27, 1971.

10. Purvis, G; Wallace, R.; Harper, J. W.; Lovasz, R.; and Stewart, R. A.: The role of supplementary foods in the nutrition of U.S. infants. Ninth International Congress of Nutrition, Abstracts of Short Communications, Mexico, September 1972: 169.

11. Blair-West, J. R.; Coghlan, J. P.; Denton, D. A.; Funder, J. W.; Nelson, J.; Scoggins, B. A.; and Wright, R. D.: Sodium homeostasis, salt appetite and hypertension. Circ. Res. 26–27 (Suppl. 11): 251, 1970.

12. Denton, D.: Instinct, appetites and medicine. Aust. N.Z. J. Med. 2: 203, 1972.

13. Kempner, W.: Treatment of hypertensive vascular disease with rice diet. Am. J. Med. 5: 545, 1948.

14. Laragh, J. H.; Baer, L.; Brunner, H. R.; Buhler, F. R.; Sealey, J. E.; and Vaughan, E. D., Jr.: Renin, angiotensin and aldosterone system in pathogenesis and management of hypertensive vascular disease. Am. J. Med. 52: 633, 1972.

15. Guyton, A. C.; Coleman, T. G.; Cowley, A. W.; Scheel, K. W.; Manning, R. D.; and Norman, R. A.: Arterial pressure regulation: overriding dominance of the kidneys in long term regulation and in hypertension. Am. J. Med. 52: 584, 1972.

16. Dahl, L. K.: Salt and hypertension. Am. J. Clin. Nutr. 25: 231, 1972.

17. Mineral Year Book. Washington, DC: U.S. Bureau of Mines, U.S. Government Printing Office, annually, 1961–71.

18. Gamble, J. L.; Wallace, W. M.; Eliel, L.; Holliday, M. A.; Cushman, M.; Appleton, J.; Shenberg, A.; and Piotti, J.: Effects of large loads of electrolytes. Pediatrics 7: 305, 1951.

19. Fomon, S. J.: Infant Nutrition. Philadelphia: W. B. Saunders, 1967: 141.

20. Fomon, S. J.; Thomas, L. N.; and Filer, L. J., Jr.: Acceptance of unsalted strained foods by normal infants. J. Pediatr. 76: 242, 1970.

21. Droese, W.; Stolley, H.; Schlage, C.; and Wortberg, B.: Significance of salt level in food for infants and children. Nutritio Dieta, No. 18: 215, 1973.

22. Mead, M.: Culture and Commitment: A Study of the Generation Gap. New York: Natural History Press, 1970.

23. Meneely, G. R., and Ball, C. O.· Experimental epidemiology of chronic sodium chloride toxicity and the protective effect of potassium chloride. Am. J. Med. 25: 713, 1958.

24. Dahl, L. K.: Effects of chronic excess salt feeding: induction of self-sustaining hypertension in rats. J. Exp. Med. 114: 231, 1961.

25. Dahl, L. K.; Heine, M.; and Tassinari, L.: Effects of chronic excess salt ingestion. Evidence that genetic factors play an important role in susceptibility to experimental hypertension. J. Exp. Med. 115: 1173, 1962.

26. Isaacson, L. C.; Modlin, M.; and Jackson, W. P. U.: Sodium intake and hypertension. Lancet 1: 946, 1963.

27. Prior, I. A. M.; Evans, J. G.; Harvey, H. P. B.; Davidson, F.; and Lindsey, M.: Sodium intake and blood pressure in two Polynesian populations. New Engl. J. Med. 279: 515, 1968.

28. Schneckloth, R. E.; Corcoran, A. C.; Stuart, K. L.; and Moore, F. E.: Arterial pressure and hypertensive disease in a West Indian Negro population: report of a survey in St. Kitts, West Indies. Am. Heart J. 63: 607, 1962.

29. Miall, W. E.: Follow-up study of arterial pressure in the population of a Welsh mining valley. Br. Med. J. 2: 1204, 1959.

30. Dawber, T. R.; Kannel, W. B.; Kagan, A.; Donabedian, R. K.; McNamara, P. M.; and Pearson, G.: Environmental factors in hypertension. Stamler, J.; Stamler, R.; Pullman, T. N. The Epidemiology of Hypertension. New York: Grune & Stratton, 1967: 225.

31. Ashe, B. I., and Mosenthal, H. O.: Protein, salt and fluid consumption of 1,000 residents of New York. JAMA 108: 1160; 1937.

32. Swaye, P. S.; Gifford, R. W., Jr.; and Berrettoni, J. N.: Dietary salt and essential hypertension. Am. J. Cardiol. 29: 33, 1972.

# Breast-Feeding

NUTRITION COMMITTEE OF THE CANADIAN PAEDIATRIC SOCIETY
AND THE COMMITTEE ON NUTRITION OF THE AMERICAN ACADEMY
OF PEDIATRICS

Despite increasing evidence for the apparent superiority of human milk, formula-feeding has progressively supplanted breast-feeding throughout much of the industrialized world, with the exception of the Soviet Union and Israel [1]. The decline of breast-feeding in industrialized society began about 50 years ago, then spread to developing countries. This change in feeding patterns has had implications for infant morbidity and mortality and for the economy of those nations which can least afford to waste their resources [1].

The need to intensify the promotion of a return to breast-feeding has been stated in several documents [2,3]. A resolution adopted by the World Health Organization in May 1974 urged all member countries to undertake vigorous action [4], and an International Pediatric Association seminar on nutrition in 1975 placed special emphasis on education programs [5].

For much of the population in developing countries, both economic and health considerations speak conclusively for breast-feeding [2,6]. The physiologic role of breast-feeding has received less emphasis in the industrialized world because of the low morbidity and mortality of bottle-fed infants, which has resulted from nutritional and technological advances in the formulation and manufacture of infant formulas [7,8] as well as from the higher standards of housing, sanitation, and public health services in these countries [9]. However, newer information suggests that significant advantages still exist for the breast-fed infant [10,11], including one study in which a lower morbidity was reported during the first year of life [12]. Therefore, it seemed timely to examine and evaluate present-day information, to provide up-to-date guidance for physicians in counseling mothers with regard to feeding their infants, to discuss factors related to the decline of breast-feeding in the United States and Canada, and to propose ways and means to encourage breast-feeding if the advantages of breast-feeding prove compelling.

## Nutritional and Physiological Properties of Human Milk

On teleological grounds, it is reasonable to suppose that the milk of each species is well adapted to the particular needs of that species. On this basis, the various properties of human milk will be compared with those of infant formulas.

### NUTRITION

Differences in the composition of human milk and unmodified cow's milk have been known for many years [13,14]. Early attempts to substitute unmodified cow's milk for human milk were unsatisfactory for feeding infants. Heat treatment, homogenization, and the addition of carbohydrate to cow's milk improved to some extent its usefulness and tolerance by infants, but protein and ash levels were still unphysiologically high, and the fat was absorbed poorly.

Newer knowledge of nutritional and physiological needs of infants and advances in technology have led to the development of newer infant formulas which provide many of the nutritional and physiological characteristics of breast milk [7,8]. However, there are still differences between infant formulas and breast milk [11], and we believe human milk is nutritionally superior to formulas for the following reasons.

### Fat and Cholesterol

Lipids of human milk are better absorbed by infants than those of cow's milk [15], mainly because of the fatty acid composition and the position of the fatty acids on the glycerol molecule. Human milk has a high oleic acid content [16], and the palmitate residue is mainly in the 2-position of the glycerol molecule [17]. This improves its digestibility. The presence of significant lipolytic activity in human milk may also help fat absorption [18]. Human milk lipids are better absorbed than those of earlier marketed infant formulas [15,19,20]. Vegetable oils, which replace butterfat in newer infant formulas [7,8], have significantly improved fat absorption [16]—even in the first month of life—to practically the level achieved with breast milk [15].

In preterm newborn infants fed formulas, fat malabsorption may still be as high as 25% to 30% [21]. Medium-chain triglycerides (MCT) permit fat absorption similar to that from breast milk [22,23]. Poor fat absorption makes it difficult for preterm infants to meet energy requirements, and nitrogen retention may also be decreased. Breast milk or MCT-containing infant formulas help overcome this problem.

When the butterfat of milk is replaced by vegetable oils in infant formulas to provide better fat absorption, most of the cholesterol is removed. Thus, these formulas are practically devoid of cholesterol, but human milk contains cholesterol. Cholesterol may play a significant role in early feeding of the infant. Even though humans synthesize cholesterol efficiently, some authors have suggested that exogenous cholesterol for formation of nerve tissue or for synthesis of bile salts may be useful to the infant. It would be difficult to determine this experimentally. Another question is prompted by animal studies suggesting that the ingestion of cholesterol during infancy may induce enzymes that can subsequently better metabolize cholesterol and thereby result in lower serum cholesterol levels early in life [24,25]. This has not been confirmed in other animal studies or retrospective and cross-sectional studies carried out in infants. High cholesterol feeding did not protect the subjects against high serum cholesterol levels later in life [26,27]. An ongoing, prospective, longitudinal study in the Boston area [28] seems to show that 30-year-old adults who were exclusively breast-fed for at least two months had significantly lower serum cholesterol levels than those who had been breast-fed for less than two months. This finding is now being tested in a larger group of subjects from four other longitudinal studies. Because subjects in the Boston study had received evaporated cow's milk (which does contain cholesterol), it is difficult to attribute the findings to cholesterol per se. Active research is needed to determine the effects of dietary cholesterol or breast-feeding on serum cholesterol level and the incidence of arterial disease in later life.

A recent concern about the fat composition of infant formulas is the relatively high polyunsaturated fatty acid content of most of them. Vegetable oils, which are well absorbed by the infant, are usually higher in polyunsaturated fatty acid content than the fat in "average" breast milk. Linoleic acid or polyunsaturated fatty acid levels in human milk vary from 8% to 20% of the fat [14,29], depending on the type of fat consumed by the mother, but the average level for human milk in recent years is considered to be about 14% [30]. The physiologic consequences of feeding the full-term infant a formula which has a linoleic acid content two or three times the average in human milk are not known. However, in preterm infants, formulas with high levels of polyunsaturated fatty acids may cause a relative or absolute deficiency of vitamin E [31] (characterized by hemolytic anemia) as a result of increased lipid peroxidation, particularly when iron supplements are also given. This is reviewed in a recent statement on feeding low-birth-weight infants [32].

### Protein

The neonatal and suckling periods are characterized by a level of anabolic activity almost never equaled later in life. This is especially true in low-birth-weight infants. Clearly then, it is vital to provide an optimum source and level of nitrogen intake [33,34]. Most formulas used for full-term and preterm infants are based on cow's milk protein [7]. Recent studies [35,36] suggest that current estimates of protein requirements of preterm infants may be too high because they are based on cow's milk protein rather than on human milk protein. The total level of protein in formulas is higher than in human milk to provide a margin of safety for the infant.

The proteins in human milk differ qualitatively from those in cow's milk. In the latter, the casein/albumin-globulin whey ratio is approximately 76:24; in human milk it is approximately 40:60. The major fraction of albumin-type protein in cow's milk whey is composed of $\beta$-lactoglobulin, which is not present in human milk [37]. The major albumin of human milk whey is $\alpha$-lactoglobulin. Some milk-based formulas have been made from demineralized whey and milk to provide a casein/whey ratio similar to that in human milk. The sulfur amino acids in cow's milk are provided mainly by methionine, with a small amount of cystine; relatively more cystine is present in human milk. Because of this lower protein content, human milk also contains less aromatic amino acids than cow's milk. Thus, the amino acid composition of human milk is particularly suited to the metabolic peculiarities of the newborn infant, especially those of the preterm infant, whose liver is inefficient in converting methionine to cystine and in metabolizing tyrosine [35]. There are notable differences between the plasma amino acid patterns of preterm infants fed human milk and those fed cow's milk-based infant formulas [36], but the importance of this remains unclear.

Breast milk also contains a variety of nucleotides [38]. They provide a source of nonprotein nitrogen which has been postulated to play a role in anabolism and growth. In this context, it is interesting to note that recent analyses of human milk from well-nourished mothers who had been lactating for two to three months showed that the average protein concentration was only 0.88 g/dl, representing about 75% of the total nitrogen; the remaining 25% was supplied as nonprotein nitrogen [39]. Previous estimates of breast milk protein were based on determination of total nitrogen by Kjeldahl N-analysis, which did not distinguish protein nitrogen from nonprotein nitrogen. In cow's milk, only 6% of the total nitrogen is supplied as nonprotein nitrogen [40]; the remainder is supplied as intact protein. Whether some of the factors in the nonprotein nitrogen in human milk are of nutritional significance to the infant remains to be studied.

*Iron*

The iron content of milk from all mammalian species is low. In a recent study [41], an average of 0.2 to 0.3 $\mu$g/ml was found in term human milk. Teleologically, the low iron concentration in human milk may be extremely useful because there are two bacteriostatic proteins in human milk [42]—lactoferrin and transferrin—which lose their bacteriostatic properties when saturated with iron. A review of the relation of the iron content of milk to the incidence of infection was recently published [43]. Lactoferrin is present in human milk in much higher quantities than in cow's milk [44]. The small amount in milk used to make infant formulas is denatured, and its bacteriostatic properties have been lost in processing the formula.

Data suggest that about 50% of the iron in human milk is absorbed; iron in pasteurized cow's milk is less well absorbed [45–47]. McMillan et al. [46] recently reported that the iron in human milk is sufficient to meet the iron requirements of the exclusively breast-fed, full-term infant until he triples his birth weight. It has been postulated that the better availability of iron in human milk, as compared to cow's milk, may be the result of the lower content of protein and phosphorus and the higher levels of lactose and vitamin C [46]. Present-day infant formulas include most of these advantages (i.e., lower protein and phosphorus and a greater lactose and vitamin C content). Heat treatment in making the formula has also significantly improved iron absorption [48]. In 1970, Gross found that about 50% of the iron in infant formula containing 1.4 $\mu$g/ml was retained by infants [49]. The infant fed pasteurized cow's milk too early in life is prone to iron deficiency partly because the milk is a poor source of iron and partly because cow's milk which has not been properly heat-treated causes significant gastrointestinal blood loss in some infants [50]. This is not found with heat-treated formulas.

### OVERFEEDING AND THE OBESITY QUESTION

The relationship between infant feeding and obesity in later life is still poorly understood, but it has been the subject of many conferences and papers [51]. Obesity is extremely prevalent in Canada [52]; 10% of the men and 30% of the women are obese. Obesity is also prevalent in the United States, where current estimates indicate that 25% to 33% of the population is overweight or obese [53]. The effects of obesity probably include decreased life expectancy, but evidence for increased mortality from hypertension and cardiovascular disease is still conflicting [54].

Some studies have shown a higher prevalence of obesity in formula-fed infants than in breast-fed infants [2]; other studies show no difference between formula-fed and breast-fed infants [55]. Studies have suggested that obese infants may be at increased risk of becoming obese children [56] and adults [57,58], but the evidence is fragmentary and at times conflicting. Although animal studies suggest that early overfeeding increases the cellularity of the adipose tissue, there is also evidence that fat-cell multiplication in humans continues throughout childhood [59]. In any event, because the first few years of life may be a critical time for adipose tissue development, excessive weight gain should be avoided during this time and throughout childhood. Overfeeding in infants may affect food habits and regulation of energy intake later in childhood and adult life [40,60]. Although current infant feeding practices are associated with a high prevalence of obesity in infants, the extent to which this predisposes to obesity in childhood and adult life is still uncertain.

There are several reasons why breast-feeding may better control caloric intake than formula-feeding. Milk intake by the breast-fed infant is determined primarily by the amount needed to satisfy the infant; the mother of the formula-fed infant may see some formula left in the bottle and induce the infant to consume more [40]. In addition, recent studies have shown that milk samples from nursing mothers at the end of feeding contain much higher levels of lipid and protein than at the beginning of the feeding; this change in composition may satiate the infant or in some way signal a cessation of feeding [61].

However, a more significant fact may be that the early introduction of solid foods, which adds greatly to the caloric intake of the infant, has paralleled the use of infant formulas. In a study in England, twice as many bottle-fed infants as breast-fed infants were receiving solid foods at age 2 months [62].

### IMMUNOLOGIC CONSIDERATIONS

At birth the newborn infant is suddenly transferred from a regulated environment to one in which prompt adaptation is required for survival. He must receive adequate nourishment and quickly develop immunologic mechanisms to enable him to exist in a hostile environment. There is increasing evidence that newborn infants can acquire certain important elements of host resistance from breast milk while maturation of his own immune system is taking place [63]. The human breast secretes antibodies to some intestinal micro-organisms, and this may help protect breast-fed infants from enteric infections [64–66]. An important recent observation has established the presence of an enteromammary system by which enteric antigen-stimulated mucosal plasma cells in the mother migrate to breast tissue, where they secrete antibodies, or are secreted directly into breast milk, where antibodies are produced [67]. Most of the factors contributing to immunologic protection *cannot* be supplied by heat-treated formula.

The critical role of breast-feeding in the prevention of gastroenteritis in infants in developing countries has been demonstrated. Although gastroenteritis is less common in infants in industrialized countries, breast-fed infants have been shown to be less susceptible [68]. A recent study [69] further suggests that breast-feeding is protective against intestinal infections, but only when it is an ongoing process. Respiratory infections, meningitis, and Gram-negative sepsis are also reported to be less frequent among breast-fed infants [12,70,71]. However, a small study in an affluent community has shown no difference in resistance to infection between breast- and formula-fed infants [72]. A study in a Canadian Eskimo population concluded that children who had been breast-fed for at least one year had an incidence of chronic otitis media that was one-eighth that of children who had been bottle-fed as infants [73].

The newborn infant does not receive a full complement of antibodies transplacentally. Immunoglobulin G (IgG) is provided in this manner; IgA and IgM are not. The serum levels of these three immunoglobulins are significantly higher in colostrum-fed infants. Some intestinal absorption of these macromolecules may take place [74], although, unlike other animal species, human colostral antibodies are not absorbed from the intestine in significant quantities during the neonatal period. In colostrum and breast milk, secretory IgA is the dominant immunoglobulin [75]. It is resistant to proteolysis and confers passive mucosal protection of the gastrointestinal tract against the penetration of intestinal organisms and antigens [76].

Breast milk is also a source of the iron-binding whey protein, lactoferrin. It is normally about one third saturated with iron and has an inhibitory effect on *Escherichia coli* in the intestine. Its bacteriostatic effect is diminished as it becomes saturated with iron [47,77]. Heating also results in loss of its iron-binding capacity, as well as of its inhibitory effect on *E. coli*. Arguments against the fortification of infant formula with iron, on the basis of saturating lactoferrin, have no validity because heat-treated infant formula has no inhibitory effect on the growth of *E. coli* when compared to fresh, unprocessed human or cow's milk. The addition of iron (12 mg/litre) does not change the rate of growth of *E. coli* in formula [78]. There is no evidence of an increased incidence of infection in infants fed iron-fortified formulas compared with those fed unfortified formulas.

Lysozymes are bacteriolytic enzymes which are more abundant in human milk than in cow's milk [79]. Bacterial lysis by IgA antibodies does not occur unless lysozymes are present [80]. The biologic importance of low concentrations of specific complement fractions C3 and C4 in human milk is unknown at present.

Living leukocytes are normally present in human colostrum [79, 81]. Macrophages comprise about 90% of the cells and are found in a concentration of about 2,100/mm³. These cells have the ability to synthesize complement, lysozyme, and lactoferrin. Lymphocytes comprise 10% of the cells; some are T cells which may have the ability to transfer delayed hypersensitivity from the mother to her infant; others are B cells which synthesize IgA. Although the biologic importance of the colostral cells to the infant has yet to be determined, pregnant women orally immunized with a nonpathogenic strain of *E. coli* during the last month of gestation produce colostrum with IgA-producing plasma cells that can synthesize antibodies to *E. coli* liposaccharide [82].

Another component of the possible "nutritional immunity" conferred by breast milk is the maintenance of a microflora in which *Lactobacillus bifidus* is predominant [83]. The alimentary canal is sterile at birth; within a few hours bacterial colonization occurs. After three or four days, more than 99% of the flora consists of the anaerobic *L. bifidus*, with a paucity of putrefactive bacteria such as the Gram-negative anaerobes (*Bacteroides, Proteus, Clostridium,* and *E. coli*). The mechanisms by which a wholly breast-fed infant is able to maintain an acid stool with *L. bifidus* as the predominant organism are poorly understood, but they probably involve several complex, interdependent factors, including the low buffering capacity of breast milk [84], the high lactose content of milk [84], specific *L. bifidus* growth-promoting factors [38], and the destruction of ingested *E. coli* by lactoferrin in the alkaline pH of the small intestine [79]. Even though most infant formulas provide a lactose content similar to that of human milk and a buffering capacity almost as low as that of human milk, the predominantly *L. bifidus* flora is not maintained. With the introduction of supplementary milk feedings or solid foods in breast-fed infants, the microflora changes to the usual adult type.

Breast milk also spares the gastrointestinal tract from exposure to foreign food antigens at a time when macromolecules may be readily absorbed [85] and may cause a local reaction. Evidence suggests that allergic manifestations later in childhood (such as eczema, rhinitis, and asthma) are more prevalent in bottle-fed infants than in breast-fed infants, presumably because of the early exposure to cow's milk and other food antigens [86–88]. The incidence of cow's milk allergy is low, but, when it does occur, it may cause a wide spectrum of clinical symptoms and affect the jejunal mucosal histology and growth [89,90]. In a Boston study [28], a slightly reduced occurrence of allergic manifestations during childhood and adult life was found in persons who were wholly breast-fed up to 2 months of age. This reduction was more evident when breast-feeding was coupled with a negative history of allergy. A recent study has noted a reduction in allergic disease in breast-fed infants with a strong family history of allergy, strict environmental control, and delayed immunization [91].

Immunologic immaturity of the gut is considered to be a factor of possible importance in the pathogenesis of necrotizing enterocolitis [92]. This frequently fatal condition is rare in low-birth-weight, breast-fed neonates. Its frequency is apparently increased in preterm infants fed hypertonic formulas [93]. A similar disorder can be produced experimentally in goats by feeding dialyzed milk of higher osmolality [94]. Fresh rat breast milk is protective in the newborn rat subjected daily to hypoxia [92]. However, the degree of protection offered by breast milk against necrotizing enterocolitis in the human infant is not yet known. At a recent workshop on human milk in premature infant feeding, the need for active research to determine if it is protective and to identify the properties most important for such protection was emphasized [95].

Much remains to be learned about the role of the secretory immunoglobulin system and its relationship to viral, bacterial, and food antigens in the early months of life.

The sudden infant death syndrome (SIDS) is the most frequent cause of death in infants between 1 and 12 months of age [96]. It has been reported by some [97,98] to occur significantly less often in breast-fed infants, although others [99,100] have found no association with the type of feeding. SIDS is probably a multifactorial condition of presently unknown etiology and pathogenesis.

MISCELLANEOUS

The low renal solute load in breast milk provides a margin of safety for the young infant with physiologically immature renal function [2]. This was extemely important some years ago when high-protein, high-solute formulas were fed. It is of less consequence today because infant formulas now provide renal solute loads which are not greatly in excess of those of breast milk. In low-birth-weight infants weighing less than 1,500 g, the low sodium [101] and calcium [102] content of formulas, and perhaps of pooled term human milk [103], may lead to hyponatremia and impaired growth and provide insufficient calcium for skeletal mineralization. Based on these considerations, some increases in mineral levels might be made in formulas intended for use by premature infants to achieve a mineral retention equivalent to that in utero [32].

At a global level, breast-feeding may play a role as a means of contraception [104], but it is not reliable for the individual mother. There may be a significant delay in ovulation in many mothers when infants are fully breast-fed. Ovulation and menstruation are delayed for at least ten weeks in some women, and up to six months in others [1,104,105]. In some cultures, the contraceptive effect is attributed in part to the taboo of sexual intercourse while the mother is breast-feeding the infant [1,106]. Although earlier oral contraceptives—which contained large doses of both estrogen and progestins—tended to suppress lactation, the newer preparations—which contain progestins alone—do not interfere with milk secretion and may even increase it [104].

Many drugs ingested by a lactating mother will be present in her milk and excreted in amounts depending on various factors, such as blood levels, dissociation constants, and fat solubility. This subject has been well reviewed [107]. Drugs such as antithyroid compounds, antimetabolites, anticoagulants, and most cathartics may be hazardous to the nursing infant, and a nursing mother should be advised not to take these drugs [108]. Recent findings of organochlorine insecticides such as DDT, polychlorinated biphenyls (PCBs), and other environmental pollutants in breast milk have raised questions which have not as yet been resolved in regard to the safety of breast-feeding by all mothers [109]. The restriction of the use of DDT resulted in a decrease in the concentrations found [110,111]. No such change has been seen for PCBs, but banning of the compound is more recent [111].

Early and prolonged contact between a mother and her newborn infant can be an important factor in mother-infant "bonding" and in the development of a mother's subsequent behavior to her infant [112,113]. It has been reported that mothers who have had prolonged physical ("skin-to-skin") contact with their newborn infants exhibit greater soothing behavior, engage in more eye-to-eye contact with the infant later in infancy, and are more reluctant to leave their infants with someone else than mothers who have had the lesser amount of contact which prevails in most maternity wards [113]. Breast-feeding may promote maternal-infant bonding, particularly when this contact is desired by the mother [10].

Epidemiology of Breast-Feeding

A steady decline in breast-feeding was documented in both developed and developing countries until recently. Before 1950, in the industrialized world, breast-feeding was more common among the lower social classes. However, in the past 10 to 15 years the decline in breast-feeding as a concomitant of socioeconomic development has changed. Data from the United States show that breast-feeding is even less commonly practiced among lower income groups than among higher income groups [114]. In the 1940s, approximately 65% of the infants in the United States were breast-fed while in the hospital [115]. By 1972, only 28% and 15% were nursed by their mothers by the time they reached the age of 1 week and 2 months, respectively [116]. Statistics from the United Kingdom also reveal a significant decline, with figures of 60% in 1948 and a little more than 40% in 1968 [117]. In a marketing survey completed in 1973 by Ross Laboratories in Canada, 35% of the infants were breast-fed during the first week of life; by 3 and 6 months, only 17% and 6%, respectively, were still breast-fed. *Consumer Reports* states that, in 1975 in the United States, 38% of the women leaving the hospital after childbirth reported they were breast-feeding. In 1976, surveys by Mead Johnson Company and Ross Laboratories found that 53% of infants in the United States and 48% of those in Canada were breast-fed at the time of discharge from the hospital.

Factors Responsible for the Decline of Breast-Feeding

Historically, bottle-feeding was intended to replace the wet nurse when breast-feeding by the mother was not possible, because many wet nurses were irresponsible and only the wealthy could afford a healthy wet nurse [118]. Pasteurization of milk helped initiate sanitation practices which permitted some substitution of cow's milk for breast-feeding. Late in the nineteenth century, heat treatment of evaporated milk reduced curd tension; the addition of carbohydrate early in the twentieth century decreased excessive protein and electrolyte levels, which further improved bottle-feeding. The technologic progress and nutritional discoveries of more recent decades made bottle-feeding a viable alternative. Bottle-feeding gradually replaced breast-feeding and resulted in the development of infant formulas which provide the best alternative for meeting nutritional needs during the first year when breast-feeding is unsuccessful, inappropriate, or stopped early [10].

With the profound social transformations which have taken place in the Western world, breast-feeding is frequently considered incompatible with modern life-styles or with work outside the home. Furthermore, the advantages of breast-feeding in terms of nutrition, immunity, and psychophysiologic interaction between the mother and her offspring are frequently considered to be outweighed by possible inconvenience, by fear or failure of lactation, and by anxieties concerning infection and/or cosmetic effects on the breasts. In addition, the act of breast-feeding is frequently regarded as a source of embarrassment or shame, and it is usually carried out privately. It is a curious commentary on our society that we tolerate all degrees of explicitness in our literature and mass media as regards sex and violence, but the normal act of breast-feeding is taboo.

When breast-feeding was universal, as it still is in some societies, the "art" was handed down through the generations. This familiar personal heritage was comforting and reassuring to the young mother. In Western societies, the new mother frequently receives little encouragement to breast-feed from her husband, relatives, friends, and even physicians. Furthermore, because formula-feeding is safe, acceptable, and promoted as "nearly identical" in nutritional composition to breast milk, the new mother may have little inclination to breast-feed.

Nowadays, mothers in many maternity wards are expected to formula-feed their infants for the convenience of the hospital staff. If the new mother is to be enabled to breast-feed, she needs free access to her infant, knowledgeable help, encouragement, and instruction. Recent studies have shown a dramatic increase in breast-feeding with in-hospital instruction from staff and mothers [119–121]. Sedgwick [122] has found that 96% of the mothers were able to breast-feed successfully when circumstances were favorable.

Successful lactation is the result of reflex interactions between mother and her offspring [123]. Stimulation of the breast, the areola, and the nipple leads to the secretion of prolactin in the mother's circulation and to milk secretion in the alveoli [124]. The suckling stimulus brings about the release of oxytocin, which contracts myoepithelial cells around the alveoli, thereby ejecting milk into lacteals [125]. Emotional tension and stress readily inhibit this reflex; therefore, the anxieties of the young mother during a short stay on an obstetric ward—where she often receives inadequate instruction and little emotional support—may explain why success is elusive, even when the mother wishes to breast-feed. The main cause of lactation failure is thought to be inhibition of the "milk ejection reflex."

Drugs such as chlorpromazine and oxytocin nasal spray [105] can be used for a short period to assist a mother who is having difficulty with "let down" in establishing successful lactation. The reasons for stopping breast-feeding after the mother goes home include cracked nipples and infection [126] or erroneous advice to adhere to a rigid three- to four-hour feeding schedule [105,112]. Many infants cry to be fed every two to three hours during the first two weeks of life. This can lead some mothers to feel that they have an inadequate supply of milk. If mothers resort to supplemental feeding, lactation may cease within a week or so because the development of full milk production is dependent on emptying the breasts [105,127]. This is also the problem with the advice to feed "ten minutes on each breast," which may deprive the infant of the nutritional benefits of milk of a somewhat different composition at the end of a feed [61]. Good breast-feeding techniques are described in detail by Applebaum [105]; when they are practiced, breast-feeding can be a convenient and pleasant way for the majority of women to feed their infants [112,128].

Ways to Increase Breast-Feeding Breast-feeding is strongly recommended for full-term infants, except in the few instances where specific contraindications exist. Ideally, breast milk should be practically the only source of nutrients for the first four to six months for most infants. When the nursing mother is healthy and well fed, fluoride and possibly vitamin D may be the only supplements which need to be provided to the infant. Iron may also be given after about four months [47].

Because the decision to breast-feed or not is the result of many factors—including education, cultural background, and personality—information about breast-feeding should be included in nutrition and sex education in schools [129,130]. This information and education should also be provided for boys because the husband's attitudes are important in successful lactation [5,129].

There is also a need for all physicians to become much more knowledgeable about infant nutrition and the physiology, value, and technique of breast-feeding. Education about breast-feeding should be directed to the undergraduate curriculum of physicians and nurses and to the residency training program of obstetricians and pediatricians.

The routine in many hospitals makes breast-feeding difficult; therefore, efforts should be made to change obstetrical ward and neonatal unit practices to increase the opportunity for successful lactation. Changes may include the following:

1. Decrease the amount of sedation and/or anesthesia given to the mother during labor and delivery because large amounts can impair suckling in the infant [105].
2. Avoid separation of the mother from her infant during the first 24 hours.
3. Breast-feed infants on an "on demand" schedule rather than on a rigid three- to four-hour schedule, and discourage routine sup-

plementary formula feedings.

4. Reappraise physical facilities to provide easy access of the mother to her infant. Rooming-in of mother and infant is important to successful lactation.

Many women require encouragement to foster the "milk ejection reflex" [126]; therefore, the personnel involved in the care of pregnant women and new mothers should be psychologically oriented toward breast-feeding and should be well informed about the preparation of the breast, lactation, and the management of breast-feeding. Nursing personnel with personal experience in breast-feeding can be extremely helpful [131]. In addition, mothers should be taught the details of breast-feeding during prenatal classes as well as during the postpartum period. Consultation between maternity services and members of La Leche League International (9616 Minneapolis Avenue, Franklin Park, IL 60131) or the Human Lactation Center Ltd. (666 Sturgis Highway, Westport, CT 06880) may be helpful in encouraging breast-feeding.

The availability of infant formulas and other infant foods has influenced infant feeding practices throughout the world. Apathy and lack of knowledge about infant nutrition by health professionals and the medical profession have been important problems. Effective and, at times, unfair publicity of formula-feeding, lack of financial support from governments in developing countries, and the need for many women to work outside the home have also been contributory factors. These factors have resulted in a decrease in breast-feeding in sections of society where formula use may not be suitable [1,3,132, 133]. Breast-feeding and provision of inexpensive "multi-mix" weaning foods have been suggested as two immediate priorities in developing countries. Also, supplies of infant formulas similar in nutritional quality to breast milk must be available for infants who cannot breast-feed; particular care must be paid to ensure safe water and sanitary conditions for mothers using these formulas.

Many women in both industrialized and developing countries now work outside the home, for either economic or personal reasons. Increasing numbers of married women have a full-time career that they are either reluctant or unable to give up. Therefore, it is recommended that countries adopt legislation to enable new mothers to obtain three to four months of leave after delivery to care for their infants. In addition, studies need to be carried out to determine whether it is feasible or practical for mothers to continue to breast-feed their infants—possibly in day nurseries adjacent to places of work—after returning to work.

Summary
1. Full-term newborn infants should be breast-fed, except if there are specific contraindications or when breast-feeding is unsuccessful.
2. Education about breast-feeding should be provided in schools for all children, and better education about breast-feeding and infant nutrition should be provided in the curriculum of physicians and nurses. Information about breast-feeding should also be presented in public communications media.
3. Prenatal instruction should include both theoretical and practical

information about breast-feeding.

4. Attitudes and practices in prenatal clinics and in maternity wards should encourage a climate which favors breast-feeding. The staff should include nurses and other personnel who are not only favorably disposed toward breast-feeding but also knowledgeable and skilled in the art.

5. Consultation between maternity services and agencies committed to breast-feeding should be strengthened.

6. Studies should be conducted on the feasibility of breast-feeding infants at day nurseries adjacent to places of work subsequent to an appropriate leave of absence following the birth of an infant.

COMMITTEE ON NUTRITION

LEWIS A. BARNESS, M.D., *Chairman*
ALVIN M. MAUER, M.D.
ARNOLD S. ANDERSON, M.D.
PETER R. DALLMAN, M.D.
GILBERT B. FORBES, M.D.
BUFORD L. NICHOLS, JR., M.D.
CLAUDE ROY, M.D.
NATHAN J. SMITH, M.D.
W. ALLAN WALKER, M.D.
MYRON WINICK, M.D.

Initiated by the Nutrition Committee of the Canadian Paediatric Society, this statement was prepared by both the Committee on Nutrition of the American Academy of Pediatrics and the Nutrition Committee of the Canadian Paediatric Society.

References

1. Berg, A.: The Nutrition Factor: Its Role in National Development. Washington, DC: Brookings Institute, 1973: 89–106
2. Committee on Medical Aspects of Food Policy: Present-Day Practice in Infant Feeding: Report on Health and Social Subjects No. 9. Report of a Working Party of the Panel on Child Nutrition, Great Britain Department of Health and Social Security. London: Her Majesty's Stationery Office, 1974.
3. Jelliffe, D. B., and Jelliffe, E. F. P.: Human milk, nutrition, and the world resource crisis. Science 188: 557, 1975.
4. Twenty Seventh World Health Assembly, Part I: Infant Nutrition and Breast Feeding. Official Records of the World Health Organization, No. 217: 20, 1974.
5. Recommendations for action programmes to encourage breast feeding. Acta Paediatr. Scand. 65: 275, 1976.
6. Wade, N.: Bottle-feeding: adverse effects of a western technology. Science 184: 45, 1974.
7. Lindquist, B.: Standards and indications for industrially produced infant formulas. Acta Paediatr. Scand. 64: 677, 1975.
8. Sarett, H. P.: Nutritional value of commercially produced foods for infants. Bibl. Nutr. Dieta 18: 246, 1973.
9. Latham, M. C.: Nutrition and infection in national development. Science 188: 561, 1975.
10. Committee on Nutrition: Commentary on breast feeding and infant formulas, including proposed standards for formulas. Pediatrics 57: 278, 1976.
11. Vahlquist, B.: New knowledge concerning the biological properties of human milk. Bull. Int. Pediatr. Assoc. 6: 22, Apr. 1976.
12. Cunningham, A. S.: Morbidity in breast-fed and artificially fed infants. J. Pediatr. 90: 726, 1977.
13. Hess, J. H.: Infant Feeding: A Handbook for a Practitioner. Chicago: American Medical Association, 1923.

14. Macy, I. G.; Kelly, H. G.; and Sloan, R. E.: The Composition of Milks. Publ. 254. Washington, DC: National Academy of Science—National Research Council, 1953.
15. Fomon, S. J.; Ziegler, E. E.; Thomas, L. N.; et al.: Excretion of fat by normal full-term infants fed various milks and formulas. Am. J. Clin. Nutr. 23: 1299, 1970.
16. Williams, M. L.; Rose, C. S.; Morrow, G. III; et al.: Calcium and fat absorption in neonatal period. Am. J. Clin. Nutr. 23: 1322, 1970.
17. Filer, L. J.; Mattson, F. H.; and Fomon, S. J.: Triglyceride configuration and fat absorption by the human infant. J. Nutr. 99: 293, 1970.
18. Hernell, O.: Human milk lipases: III. Physiological implications of the bile-salt stimulated lipase. Eur. J. Clin. Invest. 5: 267, 1975.
19. Widdowson, E. M.: Absorption and excretion of fat, nitrogen and minerals from "filled" milks by babies one week old. Lancet 2: 1099, 1965.
20. Hanna, F. M.; Navarrete, D. A.; and Hsu, F. A.: Calcium-fatty acid absorption in term infants fed human milk and prepared formulas simulating human milk. Pediatrics 45: 216, 1970.
21. Zoula, J.; Melichar, V.; Novak, M.; et al.: Nitrogen and fat retention in premature infants fed breast milk, "humanized" cow's milk or half skimmed cow's milk. Acta Paediatr. Scand. 55: 26, 1966.
22. Tantibhedhyangkul, P., and Hashim, S. A.: Clinical and physiologic aspects of medium-chain triglycerides: alleviation of steatorrhea in premature infants. Bull. NY Acad. Med. 47: 17, 1971.
23. Roy, C. C.; Ste-Marie, M.; Chartrand, L.; et al.: Correction of the malabsorption of the preterm infant with a medium-chain triglyceride formula. J. Pediatr. 86: 446, 1975.
24. Reiser, R., and Sidelman, Z.: Control of serum cholesterol homeostasis by cholesterol in the milk of the suckling rat. J. Nutr. 102: 1009, 1972.
25. Hahn, P., and Kirby, L.: Immediate and late effects of premature weaning and of feeding a high fat or high carbohydrate diet to weanling rats. J. Nutr. 103: 690, 1973.
26. Friedman, G., and Goldberg, S. J.: Concurrent and subsequent serum cholesterols of breast- and formula-fed infants. Am J. Clin. Nutr. 28: 42, 1975.
27. Glueck, C. J.; Tsang, R.; Balistreri, W.; and Fallat, R.: Plasma and dietary cholesterol in infancy: effects of early low or moderate dietary cholesterol intake on subsequent response to increased dietary cholesterol. Metabolism 21: 1181, 1972.
28. Vladian, I., and Reed, R. B.: Adult health related to child growth and development: a follow-up of the longitudinal studies of child health and development. Harvard School of Public Health. Unpublished data.
29. Potter, J. M., and Nestel, P. J.: The effects of dietary fatty acids and cholesterol on the milk lipids of lactating women and the plasma cholesterol of breast-fed infants. Am. J. Clin. Nutr. 29: 54, 1976.
30. Guthrie, H. A.; Picciano, M. F.; and Sheehe, D.: Fatty acid patterns of human milk. J. Pediatr. 90: 39, 1977.
31. Williams, M. L.; Shott, R. J.; O'Neal, P. L.; and Oski, F. A.: Role of dietary iron and fat on vitamin E deficiency anemia of infancy. N. Engl. J. Med. 292: 887, 1975.
32. Committee on Nutrition: Nutritional needs of low birth weight infants. Pediatrics 60: 519, 1977.
33. Ghadimi, H.; Arulanantham, K.; and Rathi, M.: Evaluation of nutritional management of the low birth weight newborn. Am. J. Clin. Nutr. 26: 473, 1973.
34. Winick, M., and Noble, A.: Cellular response in rats during malnutrition at various ages. J. Nutr. 89: 300, 1969.
35. Raiha, N. C. R.: Biochemical basis for nutritional management of preterm infants. Pediatrics 53: 147, 1974.
36. Raiha, N. C. R.; Heinonen, K.; Rassin, D. K.; and Gaull, G. E.: Milk protein quantity and quality in low-birth weight infants: I. Metabolic responses and effects on growth. Pediatrics 57: 659, 1976.
37. Bell, K., and McKenzie, H. A.: $\beta$-lactoglobulins. Nature 204: 1275, 1964.
38. Gyorgy, P.: The uniqueness of human milk: Biochemical aspects. Am. J. Clin. Nutr. 24: 970, 1971.
39. Lonnerdal, B.; Forsum, E.; and Hambraeus, L.: The protein content of human milk: I. A transversal study of Swedish normal material. Nutr. Rep. Int. 13: 125, 1976.

40. Fomon, S. J.: Infant Nutrition. 2d ed. Philadelphia: W. B. Saunders, 1974: 20–23.
41. Picciano, M. F., and Guthrie, H. A.: Copper, iron and zinc contents of mature human milk. Am. J. Clin. Nutr. 29: 242, 1976.
42. Bullen, J. J.; Rogers, H. J.; and Griffiths, E.: Iron binding proteins and infection. Br. J. Haematol. 23: 389, 1972.
43. Committee on Nutrition: Relationship between iron status and incidence of infection in infancy. Pediatrics 62: 246, 1978.
44. Masson, P. L., and Heremans, J. F.: Lactoferrin in milk from different species. Comp. Biochem. Physiol. 39B: 119, 1971.
45. Mackay, H. M. M.: Nutritional Anemia in Infancy With Special Reference to Iron Deficiency. Publ. 157. Medical Research Council Special Report Series. London: Her Majesty's Stationery Office, 1931.
46. McMillan, J. A.; Landaw, S. A.; and Oski, F. A.: Iron sufficiency in breast-fed infants and the availability of iron from human milk. Pediatrics 58: 686, 1976.
47. Saarinen, U. M.; Siimes, M. A.; and Dallman, P. R.: Iron absorption in infants: high bioavailability of breast milk iron as indicated by the extrinsic tag method of iron absorption and by the concentration of serum ferritin. J. Pediatr. 91: 36, 1977.
48. Theuer, R. C.; Martin, W. H.; Wallander, J. F.; and Sarett, H. P.: Effects of processing on availability of iron salts in liquid infant formula products: experimental milk-based formulas. J. Agric. Food Chem. 21: 482, 1973.
49. Report of the Sixth-second Ross Conference on Pediatric Research: Iron Nutrition in Infancy. Columbus, OH: Ross Laboratories, 1970.
50. Wilson, J. F.; Lahey, M. E.; and Heiner, D. C.: Studies on iron metabolism: V. Further observations on cow's milk-induced gastrointestinal bleeding in infants with iron-deficiency anemia. J. Pediatr. 84: 335, 1974.
51. Weil, W. B., Jr.: Current controversies in childhood obesity. J. Pediatr. 91: 175, 1977.
52. Nutrition Committee: Nutrition Canada, National Survey: A National Priority: Report to the Department of National Health and Welfare. Ottawa: Information Canada, 1973.
53. Report of the President's Biomedical Research Panel: I. Appendix A: The Place of Biomedical Science in Medicine and the State of Science. Publ. (OS) 76–50. Washington, DC: U.S. Department of Health, Education and Welfare, April 30, 1976.
54. Mann, G. V.: The influence of obesity on health, parts I and II. N. Engl. J. Med. 291: 178, 226, 1974.
55. deSwiet, M.; Fayers, P.; and Cooper, L.: Effect of feeding habit on weight in infancy. Lancet 1: 892, 1977.
56. Eid, E. E.: Follow-up study of physical growth of children who had excessive weight gain in first six months of life. Br. Med. J. 2: 74, 1970.
57. Lloyd, J. K.; Wolff, O. H.; and Whelen, W. S.: Childhood obesity: a long-term study of height and weight. Br. Med. J. 2: 145, 1961.
58. Charney, E.; Goodman, H. C.; McBride, M.; et al.: Childhood antecedents of adult obesity: Do chubby infants become obese adults? N. Engl. J. Med. 295: 6, 1976.
59. Brook, C. G. D., and Dobbing, J.: Fat cells in childhood obesity. Lancet 1: 224, 1975.
60. Myres, A. W.: Obesity: is it preventable in infancy and childhood? Can. Family Physician 21: 73, April 1975.
61. Hall, B.: Changing composition of human milk and early development of an appetite control. Lancet 1: 779, 1975.
62. Sleigh, G., and Ounsted, M.: Present-day practice in infant feeding. Lancet 1: 753, 1975.
63. Garrard, J. W.: Breast-feeding: Second thoughts. Pediatrics 54: 757, 1974.
64. Ste-Marie, M. T.; Lee, E. M.; and Brown, W. R.: Radioimmunologic measurements of naturally occurring antibodies: III. Antibodies reactive with *Escherichia coli* or *Bacteroides fragilis* in breast fluids and sera of mothers and newborn infants. Pediatr. Res. 8: 815, 1974.
65. Mata, L. J., and Wyatt, R. G.: Host resistance to infection. Am. J. Clin. Nutr. 24: 976, 1971.
66. Stoliar, O. A.; Kaniecki-Green, E.; Pelley, R. P.; et al.: Secretory IgA against enterotoxins in breast-milk. Lancet 1: 1258, 1976.
67. Goldblum, R. M.; Ahlstedt, S.; Carlsson, B.; and Hanson, L. A.: Antibody production by human colostrum cells, abstracted. Pediatr. Res. 9: 330, 1975.

68. Ironside, A. G.; Tuxford, A. F.; and Heyworth, B.: A survey of infantile gastroenteritis. Br. Med. J. 3: 20, 1970.
69. Larsen, S. A., Jr., and Homer, D. R.: Relation of breast versus bottle feeding to hospitalization for gastroenteritis in a middle-class U.S. population. J. Pediatr. 92: 417, 1978.
70. Mellander, O.; Vahlquist, B.; and Mellbin, T.: Breast feeding and artificial feeding: a clinical serological and biochemical study in 402 infants, with a survey of the literature: the Norrbotten study. Acta Paediatr. Scand. 48 (Suppl. 116): 1, 1959.
71. Winberg, J., and Wessner, G.: Does breast milk protect against septicaemia in the newborn? Lancet 1: 1091, 1971.
72. Adebonojo, F. O.: Artificial vs. breast feeding: relation to infant health in a middle class American community. Clin. Pediatr. 11: 25, 1972.
73. Schaefer, O.: Otitis media and bottle feeding: an epidemiological study of infant feeding habits and incidence of recurrent and chronic middle ear disease in Canadian Eskimos. Can. J. Public Health 62: 478, 1971.
74. Iyengar, L., and Selvaraj, R. J.: Intestinal absorption of immunoglobulins by newborn infants. Arch. Dis. Child. 47: 411, 1972.
75. Hanson, L. A., and Winberg, J.: Breast milk and defense against infection in the newborn. Arch. Dis. Child. 47: 845, 1972.
76. Walker, W. A., and Isselbacher, K. J.: Physiology in medicine: intestinal antibodies. N. Engl. J. Med. 297: 767, 1977.
77. Iron and resistance to infection. Lancet 2: 325, 1974.
78. Baltimore, R. S.; Vecchitto, J. S.; and Pearson, H. A.: Growth of *Escherichia coli* and concentration of iron in an infant feeding formula. Pediatrics. In press.
79. Goldman, A. S., and Smith, C. W.: Host resistance factors in human milk. J. Pediatr. 82: 1082, 1973.
80. Glynn, A. A.: Lysozyme: antigen, enzyme and antibacterial agent. Scientific Basis of Medicine, annual review, 1968: 31.
81. Gotoff, S. P.: Neonatal immunity. J. Pediatr. 85: 149, 1974.
82. Walker, W. A.: Host defense mechanisms in the gastrointestinal tract. Pediatrics 57: 901, 1976.
83. Mata, L. J.; Mejicanos, M. L.; and Jimenez, F.: Studies on the indigenous gastrointestinal flora of Guatemalan children. Am. J. Clin. Nutr. 25: 1380, 1972.
84. Bullen, C. L., and Willis, A. T.: Resistance of the breast-fed infant to gastroenteritis. Br. Med. J. 3: 338, 1971.
85. Gray, G. M., and Cooper, H. L.: Protein digestion and absorption. Gastroenterology 61: 535, 1971.
86. Gerrard, J. W.; MacKenzie, J. W. A.; Goluboff, N.; et al.: Cow's milk allergy: prevalence and manifestations in an unselected series of newborns. Acta Paediatr. Scand., Suppl. 234, 1973.
87. Taylor, B.; Norman, A. P.; Orgel, H. A.; et al.: Transient IgA: deficiency and pathogenesis of infantile atopy. Lancet 2: 111, 1973.
88. Matthew, D. J.; Taylor, B.; Norman, A. P.; et al.: Prevention of eczema. Lancet 1: 321, 1977.
89. Freier, S.; Kletter, B.; Gery, I.; et al.: Intolerance to milk protein. J. Pediatr. 75: 623, 1969.
90. Eastham, E. J., and Walker, W. A.: Effect of cow's milk on the gastrointestinal tract: A persistent dilemma for the pediatrician. Pediatrics 60: 477, 1977.
91. Hamburger, R. N., and Orgel, H. A.: The prophylaxis of allergy in infants debate, abstracted. Pediatr. Res. 10: 387, 1976.
92. Barlow, B.; Santulli, T. V.; Heird, W. C.; et al.: An experimental study of acute neonatal enterocolitis: the importance of breast milk. J. Pediatr. Surg. 9: 587, 1974.
93. Herbst, J. J.: Diet and necrotizing enterocolitis. Moore, T. D., ed.: Necrotizing Enterocolitis in the Newborn Infant: Report of the 68th Ross Conference on Pediatric Research. Columbus, OH: Ross Laboratories, 1975: 71.
94. De Lemos, R. A.; Rogers, J. H., Jr.; and McLaughlin, G. W.: Experimental production of necrotizing enterocolitis in newborn goats, abstracted. Pediatr. Res. 8: 380, 1974.
95. Fomon, S. J.: Human milk in premature infant feeding: Report of a second workshop. Am. J. Public Health 67: 361, 1977.
96. Committee on Infant and Preschool Child: The sudden-infant-death syndrome. Pediatrics 50: 964, 1972.

97. Enquiry Into Sudden Death in Infancy, Reports on Public, Health and Medical Subjects No. 113. London: Her Majesty's Stationery Office, 1965.

98. Tonkin, S.: Epidemiology of SIDS in Auckland, New Zealand, in Robinson R., ed.: *SIDS, 1974:* Proceedings of the Francis E. Camps International Symposium on Sudden and Unexpected Death in Infancy. Toronto: Canadian Foundation for the Study of Infant Deaths, 1974: 169.

99. Froggatt, P.; Lynas, M. A.; and MacKenzie, G.: Epidemiology of sudden unexpected death in infants ("cot death") in Northern Ireland. Br. J. Prev. Soc. Med. 25: 119, 1971.

100. Naeye, R. L.; Ladis, B.; and Drage, J. S.: Sudden infant death syndrome: A prospective study. Am. J. Dis. Child 130: 1207, 1976.

101. Chance, G. W.; Radde, I. C.; Willis, D. M.; et al.: Postnatal growth of infants of < 3 kg birth weight: Effects of metabolic acidosis, of caloric intake and of calcium, sodium, and phosphate supplementation. J Pediatr. 91: 787, 1977.

102. Day, G. M.; Chance, G. W.; Radde, I. C.; et al.: Growth and mineral metabolism in very low birth weight infants: II. Effects of calcium supplementation on growth and divalent cations. Pediatr. Res. 9: 568, 1975.

103. Atkinson, S. A.; Bryand, M. H.; Radde, I. C.; et al.: Effect of premature birth on total nitrogen and mineral concentration in human milk. Read before the Western Hemisphere Nutrition Congress V, Quebec City, Aug. 1977.

104. Jelliffe, D. B., and Jelliffe, E. F. P.: Lactation, conception, and the nutrition of the nursing mother and child. J. Pediatr. 81: 829, 1972.

105. Applebaum, R. M.: The obstetrician's approach to the breasts and breastfeeding. J. Reprod. Med. 14: 98, 1975.

106. Morley, C.: Paediatric priorities in the developing world, in Apley J., ed.: Postgraduate Paediatric Series. London: Butterworth, 1973: 103.

107. Arena, J. M.: Contamination of the ideal food. Nutr. Today 5: 2, 1970.

108. Catz, C. S., and Giacoia, G. P.: Drugs and metabolites in human milk, in Galli, C.; Jacini, G.; and Pecile, A., eds.: Dietary Lipids and Postnatal Development. New York, Raven Press, 1973: 247.

109. Polychlorinated Biphenyls, Department of National Health and Welfare— Committee Report, Information Letter DD-24. Ottawa: Department of National Health and Welfare, Mar. 31, 1978.

110. Jonsson, V.; Liu, G. J. K.; Armbruster, J.; et al.: Chlorohydrocarbon pesticide residues in human milk in greater St. Louis, Missouri, 1977. Am. J. Clin. Nutr. 30: 1106, 1977.

111. Holdrinet, M. V.; Braun, H. E.; Frank, R.; et al.: Organochlorine residues in human adipose tissue and milk from Ontario residents, 1969–1974. Can. J. Public Health 68: 74, 1977.

112. Newton, N.: Psychologic differences between breast and bottle feeding. Am. J. Clin. Nutr. 24: 993, 1971.

113. Klaus, M. H.; Jerauld, R.; Kreger, N. C.; et al.: Maternal attachment: Importance of the first post-partum days. N. Engl. J. Med. 286: 460, 1972.

114. Fomon, S. J., and Anderson, T. A.: Practices of Low-Income Families in Feeding Infants and Small Children With Particular Attention to Cultural Subgroups, Publication 725605. US Dept of Health, Education and Welfare, Maternal and Child Health Service, 1972.

115. Bain, K.: The incidence of breast-feeding in hospitals in the United States. Pediatrics 2: 313, 1948.

116. Martinez, G. A., cited by Fomon, S. J.: Infant Nutrition, ed. 2. Philadelphia: W. B. Saunders, 1974: 8.

117. Vahlquist, B.: Amningssituationem i i-och u-land: Tid for onwardering: Semper Nutrition symposium. Naringsforskning 17 (Suppl. 8): 17, 1973.

118. Levin, S. S.: A Philosophy of Infant Feeding. Springfield, IL: Charles C. Thomas, 1963.

119. Nunnally, D. M.: A new approach to helping mothers breastfeed. JOGN Nurs. 3: 34, July/Aug. 1974.

120. Bird, I. S.: Breast-feeding classes on the post-partum unit. Am. J. Nurs. 75: 456, 1975.

121. Sloper, K.; McKean, L.; and Baum, J. D.: Factors influencing breast-feeding. Arch. Dis. Child 50: 165, 1975.

122. Sedgwick, J. P.: A preliminary report of the study of breast-feeding in Minneapolis. Am. J. Dis. Child 21: 455, 1921.

123. Jelliffe, D. B., and Jelliffe, E. F. P.: Doulas, confidence and the science of lactation. J. Pediatr. 84: 462, 1974.

124. Kolodny, R. D.; Jacobs, L. S.; and Daughaday, W. H.: Mammary stimulation causes prolactin secretion in non-lactating women. Nature 238: 284, 1972.
125. Wolstenholme, G., and Knight, J., eds.: Lactogenic Hormones: Ciba Foundation Symposium, 1972. Edinburgh, Scotland: Churchill Livingstone, 1972.
126. Ladas, A. K.: How to help mothers breast feed: Deductions from a survey. Clin. Pediatr. 9: 702, 1970.
127. Davies, D. P., and Thomas, C.: Why do women stop breast-feeding? Lancet 1: 420, 1976.
128. Tompson, M.: The convenience of breast feeding. Am. J. Clin. Nutr. 24: 991, 1971.
129. Eastham, E.; Smith, D.; Poole, D.; and Neligan, G.: Further decline of breast-feeding. Br. Med. J. 1: 305, 1976.
130. Bacon, C. J., and Wylie, J. M.: Mothers' attitudes to infant feeding at Newcastle General Hospital in summer 1975. Br. Med. J. 1: 308, 1976.
131. Weichert, C.: Breast feeding: First thoughts. Pediatrics 56: 987, 1975.
132. Jelliffe, D. B.: Commerciogenic malnutrition. Nutr. Rev. 30: 199, 1972.
133. The infant-food industry. Lancet 2: 503, 1976.

# The Use and Abuse of Vitamin A

COMMITTEES ON DRUGS AND ON NUTRITION,
AMERICAN ACADEMY OF PEDIATRICS

Vitamin A is an essential nutrient necessary for maintenance of normal epithelial tissue and for optimal growth [1,2]. Impaired dark-adaptation and night blindness are well-known manifestations of vitamin A deficiency. Although vitamin A is present in many foods, it cannot be assumed that all individuals receive adequate amounts. Preliminary reports from the recent 10-state nutrition survey* show that a significant proportion of the population has a low intake of vitamin A and low plasma vitamin A levels. Thus it would appear important to improve the diet of a considerable segment of the population or provide a vitamin A supplement for them.

Vitamin A is found in food in carotenoids, which are converted to vitamin A in the intestine; or it may be preformed, as in foods from animal sources (or in diet supplements). There is no danger of excessive intake of vitamin A when carotenoids are ingested.

The recommended daily allowances of vitamin A are: for infants and children up to age 12 years, from 1,500 to 4,500 IU; for adults, 5,000 IU; and for pregnant women 6,000 IU [3,4]. Although diets of many individuals provide higher levels of vitamin A, there are no known advantages in exceeding these allowances in normal individuals.

Thus, for prophylactic use or as a safeguard against inadequate intake, there are properly formulated supplements available on the market, i.e., those that contain 1,500 to 4,000 IU for infants and children, 5,000 IU for adults, and 6,000 IU for pregnant women.

However, excessive intake of preformed vitamin A may result in serious and potentially toxic effects. The easy availability of vitamin A in large doses without prescription exposes individuals to the danger of severe clinical toxicity. Physicians should be aware of the circumstances in which vitamin A toxicity may occur and its clinical manifestation.

Doses of 25,000 IU or more of vitamin A, which are present in some vitamin preparations, should not be used, unless severe deficiency of vitamin A, documented by an abnormally low blood level, exists. These doses taken daily for an extended period of time pose a risk, particularly to the pregnant woman and fetus. Studies in pregnant animals have shown that large doses of vitamin A produce central nervous system anomalies with hydrocephalus, encephalocoele, and other teratological effects in the offspring [5,6]. Infants may develop a bulging fontanel or hydrocephalus when given about 10 times the recommended daily allowance of vitamin A for several weeks [7–9]. The older child or adult with hypervitaminosis A manifests pseudotumor cerebri, a syndrome that may simulate the

* Proceedings of Workshop on Vitamin A. Food and Nutrition Board, Jan. 28, 29, 1971.

presence of an intracranial neoplasm, with signs and symptoms of unlocalized increased intracranial pressure [10–18], such as headache, nausea, vomiting, lethargy, tinnitus, and diplopia. Physical findings are usually limited to the eyes, with sixth nerve paresis, papilledema, and, in long-standing cases, optic atrophy and even blindness. Ingestion of as little as 25,000 to 50,000 IU of vitamin A per day for as short a period as 30 days can induce signs of increased intracranial pressure. Nonspecific findings encountered at all ages include dry skin and mucous membranes, sparse hair, brittle nails, myalgia, bone pain, arthralgia, abdominal pain, splenomegaly, and hypoplastic anemia with leukopenia.

Despite awareness of the potential dangers of vitamin A toxicity, the incidence of hypervitaminosis A appears to be increasing. Hypervitaminosis A may result through easy availability of high potency vitamin preparations without prescription and through the overzealous parent who frequently administers vitamins under the popular premise, that, if one is good, two are better. The problem may be compounded by the use of bizarre, highly fortified health foods.

Serious problems of hypervitaminosis A have arisen in the use of large doses of vitamin A in treatment of acne vulgaris in adolescents. The clinical impression that high doses of vitamin A (50,000 IU to 150,000 IU per day) over a prolonged period are beneficial treatment for acne vulgaris has not been validated by well-controlled clinical trials, nor is the rationale for this method of treatment clear [19].

Vitamin supplements with proper levels of vitamin A for infants, children, adults, and pregnant women are available on the market. These should be prescribed when indicated. Vitamin supplements containing more than the daily doses recommended (6,000 IU) should not be used.

Conclusion    The grave risks resulting from the unrestricted sale of high concentrations of vitamin A make it imperative that an active curb, by appropriate legislation if necessary, be placed on the over-the-counter marketing of *high potency* vitamin A preparations. Physicians should be aware of the vitamin A content in the preparations they prescribe for their patients. They also should caution parents regarding the dangers of overdosage of this vitamin.

COMMITTEE ON DRUGS

SUMNER J. YAFFE, M.D., *Chairman*

COMMITTEE ON NUTRITION

L. J. FILER, JR., M.D., *Chairman*

References    1. Roels, O. A.: Vitamin A physiology. JAMA 214: 1097, 1970.
2. Meharen, D.: The vitamins. Bondy P., ed. Duncan's Metabolism, 6th ed. Philadelphia: W. B. Saunders, 1969: 1280.
3. Food and Nutrition Board, National Research Council: Recommended Dietary Allowances, rev. 7th ed. Publ. 1064. Washington, DC: National Academy of Sciences, 1968.
4. Committee on Nutrition: Proposed changes in food and drug administration regulations concerning formula products and vitamin-mineral dietary supplements for infants. Pediatrics 40: 916, 1967.

5. Cohlan, S. Q.: Excessive intake of vitamin A as a cause of congenital anomalies in the rat. Science 117: 535, 1953.

6. Cohlan, S. Q.: Congenital anomalies in the rat produced by excessive intake of vitamin A during pregnancy. Pediatrics 13: 556, 1954.

7. Arena, J. M.; Sarazen, P., Jr.; and Baylin, G. J.: Hypervitaminosis A, report of an unusual case with marked craniotabes. Pediatrics 8: 788, 1951.

8. Marie, J., and See, G.: Acute hypervitaminosis A of the infant: its clinical manifestation with benign acute hydrocephalus and pronounced bulge of the fontanelle; a clinical and biologic study. Am. J. Dis. Child. 87: 731, 1954.

9. Persson, B.; Tunell, R.; and Ekengren, K.: Chronic vitamin A intoxication during the first half year of life. Description of 5 cases. Acta Paediatr. Scand. 54: 49, 1965.

10. Gribitz, D.; Silverman, S. H.; and Sobel, A. E.: Vitamin A poisoning. Pediatrics 7: 372, 1951.

11. Sulzberger, M. D., and Lagar, M. P.: Hypervitaminosis A: report of a case in an adult. JAMA 146: 788, 1951.

12. Gerber, A.; Raab, A. P.; and Sobel, A. E.: Vitamin A poisoning in adults. Am. J. Med. 16: 729, 1954.

13. Oliver, T. K., Jr., and Havener, W. H.: Eye manifestations of chronic vitamin A intoxication. Arch. Ophthal. 60: 19, 1958.

14. Oliver, T. K., Jr.: Chronic vitamin A intoxication. Am. J. Dis. Child. 95: 57, 1958.

15. Morrice, G., Jr.; Havener, W. H.; and Kapetansky, F.: Vitamin A intoxication as a cause of pseudotumor cerebri. JAMA 173: 1802, 1960.

16. Feldman, M. H., and Schlezinger, N. S.: Benign intracranial hypertension associated with hypervitaminosis A. Arch. Neurol. 22: 1, 1970.

17. Fedotin, M. S.: Hypervitaminosis A causing pseudotumor cerebri. JAMA 212: 628, 1970.

18. Lascari, A. D., and Bell, W. E.: Pseudotumor cerebri due to hypervitaminosis A: toxic consequences of self-medication for acne in an adolescent girl. Clin. Pediatr. 9: 627, 1970.

19. Anderson, J.; Anderson, D.; and Stokoc, J. H., recorders: Vitamin A in acne vulgaris (Report of the Southeast Scotland Faculty of the College of General Practitioners). Br. Med. J., Issue 5352: 294, 1963.

# Hazards of Overuse of Vitamin D

COMMITTEE ON NUTRITIONAL MISINFORMATION,
NATIONAL ACADEMY OF SCIENCES

An excess intake of vitamin D can result in serious toxicity. Vitamin D is stored in the fatty tissues of the body and is present in the circulating plasma. Because vitamin D promotes absorption of calcium from the intestine, a large excess of stored vitamin D can cause excessive quantities of calcium in the blood (hypercalcemia) persisting for months after intake of vitamin D has been discontinued. Chronic hypercalcemia causes calcification of soft tissues with particularly serious injury to the kidney; associated general symptoms are weakness, lethargy, anorexia, and constipation. The sensitivity of individuals to an excess of vitamin D is quite variable so that it is not possible to state the minimal toxic dose. Overuse of vitamin D in England and the European continent during the 1940s and 1950s is thought to be the cause of a serious disorder of infancy called "idiopathic hypercalcemia" that was seen with unusual frequency in that period. Following reduction of vitamin D intake to levels approximating those considered adequate in this country, "idiopathic hypercalcemia" has become quite rare.

Vitamin D is an unusual nutrient in that its major natural source is not food, but rather the 7-dehydrocholesterol in the skin, which is converted to vitamin D by the shortwave ultraviolet component of sunshine. The usual foods of infants, including breast milk, contain little vitamin D. Without exposure to sunshine or fortification of the diet with vitamin D, vitamin D deficiency results in infants. In some industrial cities of the temperate zones infants may not get sufficient exposure to ultraviolet light because of the combination of climatic conditions and atmospheric smog. Smog absorbs most of the sun's shortwave ultraviolet light radiation even on sunny days. For this reason rickets, the disease resulting from defective mineralization of bone due to lack of vitamin D, was once extremely common in infants and children in northern Europe and the United States. Because of the widespread use of vitamin D-fortified milk and infant feeding preparations, rickets has become an exceedingly rare disease in this country.

The vitamin D requirement of infants during the rapidly growing period of the first 6 months of life, can be, and has been, accurately determined. In this age period a daily intake of 400 IU of vitamin D is adequate with an ample margin of safety for normal biological variation. For most infants 100 IU/day in milk would probably suffice. Vitamin D is also required by older children and adults but determination of the true requirement beyond infancy is extremely difficult, and the assumption has been made that a daily intake of 400

Reprinted from American Journal of Clinical Nutrition 28: 512, May 1975. A statement of the Food and Nutrition Board, Division of Biological Sciences, Assembly of Life Sciences, National Research Council. Prepared by the Committee on Nutritional Misinformation, National Academy of Sciences, Nov. 1974.

units meets the needs beyond infancy as well. This seems justified by our present experience. In the adult, the poor mineralization of bone resulting from vitamin D deficiency is termed osteomalacia. Nutritional osteomalacia due to lack of vitamin D has been described particularly in elderly patients on highly restricted diets estimated to provide less than 100 IU of vitamin D/day. The normal child, the adult, and the pregnant or lactating woman do not require more than 400 IU of vitamin D/day. These normal requirements are met by exposure to sunshine and consumption of such foods as vitamin D-fortified milk, egg yolk, and fish, such as salmon, sardines, herring, and tuna. The use of vitamin D concentrates is necessary for breast fed infants and infants on nonfortified milk but is rarely required for the proper vitamin D nutrition of other infants, children, or adults.

Use of highly concentrated preparations of vitamin D may be required by patients with specific diseases requiring unusual amounts of vitamin D. This treatment must be closely supervised by a physician. Vitamin D must be metabolized in the liver and kidney before it becomes the active compound that regulates the calcium and phosphate metabolism of the body and ensures normal bone mineralization. The vitamin D requirements of patients with liver disease and kidney disease must be separately determined, and such patients may require much greater amounts of this vitamin than is normally given. Because of poor absorption of vitamin D by patients with intestinal malabsorption, increased amounts of dietary vitamin D are needed in their treatment.

In summary, excessive amounts of vitamin D are hazardous and only individuals with diseases affecting vitamin D absorption or metabolism require more than 400 IU/day. Such needs should be established by clinical evaluation, and treatment should be specifically recommended and supervised by physicians.

References

1. American Academy of Pediatrics Committee on Nutrition: The relation between infantile hypercalcemia and vitamin D—public health implications in North America. Pediatrics 40: 1050, 1967.
2. Gough, K. R.; Lloyd, O. C.; and Willis, M. R.: Nutritional osteomalacia. Lancet 2: 1261, 1964.
3. Harrison, H. E.: Calcium Metabolism in Pediatrics. 15th ed. Edited by H. L. Barnett. New York: Appleton-Century-Crofts, 1972.

# Supplementation of Human Diets with Vitamin E

COMMITTEE ON NUTRITIONAL MISINFORMATION,
NATIONAL ACADEMY OF SCIENCES

Among all the vitamins probably none has commanded more public attention or been the subject of more clinical controversy than vitamin E. The list of ailments claimed to be relieved by this vitamin includes most noninfectious diseases, e.g., heart disease, sterility, muscular weakness, cancer, ulcers, skin disorders, burns, and shortness of breath. As for apparently healthy subjects, vitamin E has been claimed to promote physical endurance, enhance sexual potency, prevent heart attacks, protect against the health-related effects of air pollution, and slow the aging process and alleviate its accompanying ailments.

How did these claims come about? To some extent they arose from a misinterpretation of the results of research on experimental animals. Vitamin E was shown to be among the factors required to prevent sterility in male rats and to permit normal pregnancy in female rats. This discovery naturally led to examination of the possible beneficial effect of the vitamin in connection with various problems of reproduction in men and women. The relevant tests on human subjects are difficult to evaluate because they cannot be conducted in a laboratory setting in which the effects of other factors can be eliminated. Some instances of beneficial effects were reported but, on the basis of results obtained over the past 35 years, leading scientific and medical opinion does not support the view that supplemental vitamin E has any value in preventing male impotency or sterility or in altering the outcome of pregnancy. Advocates of vitamin E supplementation in human beings overlook the fact that an effect on reproduction in animals can be demonstrated only when the animals have been fed for long periods on diets free of vitamin E. The widespread presence of the vitamin in human diets has prevented a deficiency, such as seen in animals under experimental conditions, from developing in man.

In most animal species that have been studied, severe vitamin E deficiency causes muscle wasting or dystrophy. Understandably, vitamin E has therefore been tested as a treatment for various muscle diseases of man, including hereditary muscular dystrophy. Again, results have been negative. The muscles of persons with dystrophy contain normal amounts of vitamin E, and there is no evidence that the condition in man is associated with a dietary deficiency of this vitamin.

Abnormalities in the heart muscle of vitamin E-deficient animals are less common and less severe than those seen in the skeletal muscle. In cattle and sheep, however, heart-muscle abnormalities can be severe, whereas severely deficient monkeys with skeletal dystrophy

Reprinted from Nutrition Reviews (Suppl.): 37, July 1974. A statement of the Food and Nutrition Board, Division of Biology and Agriculture, National Research Council. Prepared by the Committee on Nutritional Misinformation, National Academy of Sciences.

and bone-marrow failure have shown no cardiac involvement. Similarly, there is no evidence that cardiac disease is a consequence of vitamin E deficiency in man and, to date, extensive tests have failed to demonstrate therapeutic benefit from supplemental vitamin E.

Why has supplemental vitamin E been so ineffective in treatment of disease? Clearly, it is because the reproductive failure, heart disease, and muscular dystrophy observed in man are not attributable to dietary deficiency of this vitamin. Likewise, there is no satisfactory scientific or clinical evidence that supplemental dietary vitamin E is beneficial in the treatment of such other conditions as burns, skin disorders, poor physical performance, and cancer.

Surveys of the United States population indicate that adequate amounts of vitamin E are supplied by the usual diet. The recommended daily dietary allowances of this vitamin range from 5 to 30 international units, depending upon age, sex, and physiologic state, and are deemed to exceed the actual needs of most individuals. Dietary vitamin E is supplied in substantial amounts by most vegetable oils as well as by margarine and shortening made from these oils, and significant inputs are made by many vegetables and by whole grain cereals. Meats, fish, poultry, milk, eggs, legumes, fruits, and nuts also contribute to the dietary supply. Thus, supplementation of the diet with vitamin E is unlikely to be useful in alleviating any of the ailments mentioned above.

Are there any special cases in which supplementary vitamin E is beneficial? Some physicians prescribe vitamin E for premature infants, who frequently have low blood levels of the vitamin because of limited transfer from the mother's blood before birth. Patients afflicted with conditions that interfere with normal digestion or absorption of fats and fat-soluble vitamins require supplements of these vitamins, one of which is vitamin E. Such individuals should be under the care of a physician; for others vitamin E supplements are unnecessary. Self medication with vitamin E in the hope that a more or less serious condition will be alleviated may indeed be hazardous, especially when appropriate diagnosis and treatment may thereby be delayed or avoided.

Summary Misleading claims that vitamin E supplementation of the ordinary diet will cure or prevent such human ailments as sterility, lack of virility, abnormal termination of pregnancy, heart disease, muscular weakness, cancer, ulcers, skin disorders, and burns, are not backed by sound experimentation or clinical observations. Some of these claims are based upon deficiency symptoms observed in other species. Careful studies over a period of many years attempting to relate these symptoms to vitamin E deficiency in human beings have been unproductive. The wide distribution of vitamin E in vegetable oils, cereal grains, and animal fats makes a deficiency in humans very unlikely. Premature infants or individuals with impaired absorption of fats may require supplemental vitamin E, but they should, in any event, be under the care of a physician.

References    Binder, H. J., and Spiro, H. M.:   Am. J. Clin. Nutrition 20: 594, 1967.
Mason, K. E., and Horwitt, M. K.:   Sebrell, W. H., and Harris, R. S., eds.   The Vitamins Vol. 5. New York:   Academic Press, 1972:   293–309.

# Megavitamin Therapy for Childhood Psychoses and Learning Disabilities

COMMITTEE ON NUTRITION, AMERICAN ACADEMY OF PEDIATRICS

Vitamins have long been recognized for their unique role in human nutrition. Most of these low-molecular weight, organic substances are precursors of coenzymes, and adequate amounts to meet the known nutritional needs of healthy persons of all ages have been defined by the Food and Nutrition Board of the National Academy of Sciences as the "Recommended Dietary Allowances" (RDA). The consistent opinion of the Committee on Nutrition of the American Academy of Pediatrics has been that normal children receiving a normal diet do not need vitamin supplementation [1] over and above RDA levels.

However, there are a variety of clinical entities in which the daily intake of vitamins needs to be significantly increased. This is true, for example, with the fat-soluble vitamins A, D, E, and K in the steatorrhoeas [2] and in the autosomally recessive selective malabsorption of vitamin $B_{12}$ [3]. Rarely, children treated with isoniazid require increased pyridoxine; and, when treated with diphenylhydantoin sodium (Dilantin), they need increased folic acid and vitamin D [4]. Finally, there are a number of rare inborn errors of metabolism affecting the apoenzyme at the cofactor binding site or involving the metabolism of the vitamin itself to its biologically active derivative [5]. In these so-called dependency syndromes, the metabolic defect may completely or partially be overcome by greatly increasing vitamin or cofactor availability.

Set against a background of wide public belief in the benefits of vitamins, the accounts of dramatic amelioration of deficiency states, the easy and relatively inexpensive availability of these substances, and the occasional remarkable benefit of large doses (both in the dependency syndromes and in certain other clinical situations), it is not surprising that a cult developed in the use of large doses of water-soluble vitamins to treat a wide spectrum of disease states. In particular, "megavitamin" therapy came to be applied to the use of large amounts of nicotinic acid or nicotinamide in the treatment of schizophrenia. Pauling, in 1968 [6], coined the term "orthomolecular medicine," meaning the treatment or prevention of diseases by altering body concentrations of certain normally occurring substances. Pauling's term now encompasses the additional use of nicotinamide adeinine dinucleotide (NAD), riboflavin, ascorbic acid, pyridoxine, calcium panthotenate, vitamin $B_{12}$, folic acid, and trace minerals in doses considerably in excess of the RDA for a wide range of problems including arthritis, neuroses, geriatric problems, hyperlipidemia, and depression.

Reprinted from Pediatrics 58: 910, December 1976. Copyright American Academy of Pediatrics 1976.

This "orthomolecular" approach has been used in children primarily in the treatment of nonspecific mental retardation, psychoses, autism, hyperactivity, dyslexia, and other learning disorders reminiscent of an earlier advocacy of large doses of glutamic acid for Down's syndrome [7–10]. The substantially anecdotal evidence of therapeutic benefit in these and other conditions should be viewed with skepticism until vigorous evidence of benefit has been obtained and published in peer reviewed journals.

As an example of this approach, Cott [11] reports giving niacin (1 to 2 g/24 hr), ascorbic acid (1 to 2 g/24 hr), pyridoxine (200 to 400 mg/24 hr), and calcium pantothenate (400 to 600 mg/24 hr) to more than 500 children with psychoses and learning disabilities. The author claims that the treatment shows promise and is sometimes dramatic; however, no precise data are given on which any objective assessment of results can be made.

Although no comparable evaluation has been carried out on children for autism and learning disabilities, the claims of orthomolecular psychiatrists in the treatment of adult schizophrenia have recently been carefully examined in a report to the American Psychiatric Association by a Task Force on Vitamin Therapy in Psychiatry [12,13]. Their conclusions were emphatic that orthodox, properly controlled, and well-standardized trials found nicotinic acid therapy to be without value. Moreover, there is some evidence that long-term administration of high doses of nicotinic acid in man may lead to persistent skin erythema, pruritis, tachycardia, liver damage, hyperglycemia, and hyperuricemia [14].

There are a number of situations in pediatric practice where a specific vitamin deficiency can be demonstrated by biochemical tests and increased amounts of vitamins can be shown to resolve these conditions. Vitamin therapy under these conditions is justified, and it is reasonable to expect that other conditions of this type will be identified. In contrast, megavitamin therapy as a treatment for learning disabilities and psychoses in children, including autism, is not justified on the basis of documented clinical results.

COMMITTEE ON NUTRITION

LEWIS A. BARNESS, M.D., *Chairman*
ALVIN M. MAUER, M.D., *Vice-Chairman*
ARNOLD S. ANDERSON, M.D.
PETER R. DALLMAN, M.D.
GILBERT B. FORBES, M.D.
JAMES C. HAWORTH, M.D.
MARY JANE JESSE, M.D.
CHARLES R. SCRIVER, M.D.
MYRON WINICK, M.D.
*Consultants*
WILLIAM C. HEIRD, M.D.
O. L. KLINE, PH.D.
DONOUGH O'BRIEN, M.D.
*Technical Advisory Group*
RUDOLPH M. TOMARELLI, PH.D., *Chairman*

DUANE A. BENTON, PH.D.
IVY M. CELENDER, D.SC.
GEORGE A. PURVIS, PH.D.
SIDNEY SAPERSTEIN, PH.D.
ROBERT E. SMITH, PH.D.
*Liaison Representatives*
BETTY E. ANDERSON
MYRTLE L. BROWN, PH.D.
MARGARET CHENEY, PH.D.
JOGINDER CHOPRA, M.D.
WILLIAM J. DARBY, M.D., PH.D.
MARY C. EGAN
J. MICHAEL LANE, M.D.
HAROLD T. MCLEAN
MERRILL S. READ, PH.D.
HERBERT P. SARETT, PH.D.
L. J. TEPLY, PH.D.
PHILIP L. WHITE, SC.D.

References

1. Committee on Nutrition: Proposed changes in Food and Drug Administration regulations concerning formula products and vitamin-mineral dietary supplements for infants. Pediatrics 40: 916, 1967.
2. Silverman, A.; Roy, C. C.; and Cozzetto, F. J.: Pediatric Clinical Gastroenterology. St. Louis: C. V. Mosby, 1975: 514.
3. Bell, M.; Harries, J. T.; Wolff, O. H.; et al.: Familial selective malabsorption of vitamin $B_{12}$. Arch. Dis. Child. 48: 896, 1973.
4. Christiansen, C.; Rodbro, P.; and Nielsen, C. T.: Iatrogenic osteomalacia in epileptic children: a controlled therapeutic trial. Acta Pediatr. Scand. 64: 219, 1975.
5. Scriver, C. R.: Vitamin-responsive inborn errors of metabolism. Metabolism 22: 1319, 1973.
6. Pauling, L.: Orthomolecular psychiatry. Science 160: 265, 1968.
7. Green, G.: Subclinical pellagra, its diagnosis and treatment. Schizophrenia 2: 70, 1970.
8. Hoffer, A.: Treatment of hyperkinetic children with nicotinamide and pyridoxine. Can. Med. Assoc. J. 107: 111, 1972.
9. Hoffer, A.: Vitamin B-3 dependent child. Schizophrenia 3: 107, 1971.
10. Rimland, B.: Megavitamin treatment in children. Hawkins, D., and Pauling, L., eds.: Orthomolecular Psychiatry. San Francisco: W. H. Freeman, 1973.
11. Cott, A.: Megavitamins: the orthomolecular approach to behavioral disorders and learning disabilities. Acad. Ther. 7: 245, 1972.
12. Megavitamin and Orthomolecular Therapy in Psychiatry: Task Force Report No. 7. Washington, DC: American Psychiatry Association, 1973.
13. Megavitamin and orthomolecular therapy in psychiatry: excerpts from the Report of the Task Force on Vitamin Therapy in Psychiatry. Nutr. Rev. 32: 44, 1974.
14. Winter, S. L., and Boyer, J. L.: Hepatic toxicity from large doses of vitamin $B_3$ (nicotinamide). N. Engl. J. Med. 289: 1180, 1973.

# PART B    Modifications in
## Consistency and Texture

# Clear Liquid Diet

*Definition*     A diet that includes only those foods which are clear and are liquid or liquefy at room temperature, such as fat free broth, bouillon, coffee, tea, decaffeinated coffee, strained fruit juices, flavored gelatin, carbonated beverages [1], and popsicles.

*Characteristics of the diet*     The diet is highly restrictive and is of little nutritive value; it provides some electrolytes, mainly sodium chloride and potassium, and a small amount of kilocalories, mainly in the form of carbohydrate. The amount of fluid in a given feeding is usually restricted to 30–60 ml/hr at first, with gradually increasing amounts being given as the patient's tolerance improves.

*Purpose of the diet*     To provide an oral source of fluids and small amounts of kilocalories and electrolytes as a means of preventing dehydration and reducing colonic residue to a minimum. Fluid replacement and the maintenance of the body's water balance become matters of prime concern whenever an acute illness produces a marked intolerance for food. Fluid and electrolyte losses may occur in diarrheal diseases or in adults with prolonged gastric drainage or poor intake [2].

*Indications for use*     A clear liquid diet may be used as a progression between intravenous feeding and a full liquid or solid diet following certain types of surgery [3]. Its use may also be indicated as the first step in oral feedings for fluid and electrolyte replacement in diarrheal diseases; to reduce the amount of residue in the colon as a preparation for bowel surgery or for a barium enema [4,5]; following colonic surgery; or as the first step in oral alimentation of the severely debilitated patient.

*Possible adverse reactions*     The diet is inadequate in kilocalories and most nutrients. Its continued use leads to weight loss, tissue wasting, and multiple nutritional deficiences, particularly if instituted in individuals with increased caloric needs or those whose nutritional status is marginal.

*Contraindications*     The diet is contraindicated in any condition when used on a long-term basis as the sole means of nutritional support. In such cases the use of semisynthetic liquid diets may be indicated.

*Suggestions for dietitians*     Although commercial gelatin products and commercial sweetened beverage mixtures are good sources of water and provide some kilocalories, their electrolyte content is insufficient to permit them to be of practical value as vehicles for the replacements of electrolytes lost in vomitus and diarrheal fluid [6,7]. On the other hand, one bouillon cube provides 424 mg sodium, and three servings of bouillon make a significant contribution to the replacement of sodium losses when indicated. If well tolerated, strained fruit juices, particularly orange juice, provide excellent sources of potassium and vitamin C.

If a restricted sodium clear liquid diet is required, salt free broth should be substituted for bouillon. Following gastric surgery or myocardial infarction, it may be desirable to eliminate caffeine containing beverages such as coffee and tea and colas; caffeine stimulates hydrochloric acid secretion, as well as increasing heart rate [8].

## Clear Liquid Diet

**Sample menu**

**A.M.**

4 oz apple juice
1 cup cherry flavored gelatin
8 oz ginger ale
Coffee or tea with sugar

**BETWEEN MEALS**

½ cup lemon flavored gelatin

**NOON**

1 cup bouillon
4 oz strained orange juice
½ cup grape flavored gelatin
Coffee or tea with sugar

**BETWEEN MEALS**

8 oz ginger ale

**P.M.**

1 cup bouillon
4 oz sweetened cranberry juice
½ cup lime flavored gelatin
Coffee or tea with sugar

**BEDTIME**

½ cup pineapple flavored gelatin

## References

1. Turner, D.: Handbook of Diet Therapy, 5th ed. Chicago: University of Chicago Press, 1970.
2. Mason, E. E.: Fluid, Electrolytes and Nutrient Therapy in Surgery. Philadelphia: Lea & Febiger, 1974.
3. Larsen, R. B.: Dietary needs of patients following general surgery. Hospitals 39: 133, July 16, 1965.
4. Goldberg, H. I., and Moss, A. A.: Roentographic methods of colonic examination. Sleisinger, M. H., and Fordtran, J. S., eds. Gastrointestinal Disease. Philadelphia: W. B. Saunders, 1973.
5. Randall, H. T.: Enteric feeding. Ballinger, W. F.; Collins, J. A.; Drucker, W. R.; and Zappa, R., eds. Manual of Surgical Nutrition. Philadelphia: W. B. Saunders, 1975.
6. Brusilow, S. W., and Cooke, R. E.: Fluid therapy of diarrhea and vomiting. Pediatr. Clin. N. Am. 11: 889, 1964.
7. Scanlon, J. W.: Electrolyte content of commercial gelatin products and sweetened liquid mixtures in treatment of diarrhea. Clin. Pediatr. 9: 508, 1970.
8. Ritchie, J. M.: Central nervous system stimulants II. The xanthines. Goodman, L. S., and Gilman, A., eds. The Pharmacological Basis of Therapeutics. 5th ed. New York: Macmillan, 1975.

# Full Liquid Diet

*Definition*      A diet consisting of foods that are liquid or liquefy at room temperature [1].

*Characteristics of the diet*      A variety of foods may be used, including milk, plain frozen desserts, pasteurized eggs, fruit juices, vegetable juices, cereal gruels, broth, and milk and egg substitutes. The diet provides 1,800–2,000 kcal and 80 g protein per day. Nourishments are served between meals to increase the caloric intake.

*Purpose of the diet*      To provide an oral nourishment that is well tolerated by patients who are acutely ill or who are unable to swallow or chew solid foods.

*Indications for use*      Nourishment in the form of full liquids may be necessary following oral surgery or plastic surgery of the face and neck, in other postoperative states as a transition between a clear liquid and a fiber restricted or regular diet [2], in patients with esophageal strictures, and following mandibular fractures.

*Possible adverse reactions*      Particularly if meat soups and brewer's yeast are not used, the diet is inadequate in folic acid, iron, and vitamin $B_6$.

*Contraindications*      Patients who, after surgery, demonstrate nausea, vomiting, distension, or diarrhea when given a full liquid diet may temporarily be lactose intolerant [3]. Because of the 6 cups of milk included, the diet is high in lactose and would be contraindicated in cases of severe lactose intolerance. The lactose content may be lowered by substituting lactose hydrolyzed milk [4] or lactose free products. In addition, the diet is high in cholesterol and should not be used on a long-term basis in patients with hypercholesterolemia unless it is modified.

*Suggestions for dietitians*      Individuals on a full liquid diet for more than 2 or 3 days should receive high kilocalorie, high protein supplements. For additional kilocalories butter or fortified margarine may be added to hot liquids, and powdered glucose or glucose polymers may be dissolved in fruit juices [5]. The use of a sugar such as glucose, which is not as sweet as sucrose, will permit larger amounts to be added. For additional protein nonfat dry milk may be incorporated into certain foods, such as milk and puddings. Lactose free supplements are available for those who are lactose intolerant. Most individuals are able to tolerate 1 or 2 oz of finely homogenized strained meat added to bouillon or tomato juice.

If a low sodium diet is indicated, low sodium soups, eggnogs, and custard should be used. If the diet is to be used following tonsillectomy or adenoidectomy, the use of straws is usually prohibited.

In order to prevent the danger of salmonella infection, raw eggs should not be used. In addition, there is a possibility that raw egg white, containing a heat labile protein called avidin, interferes with the body's absorption of biotin [6].

For long-term use in a patient with hypercholesterolemia, substitute skim milk for whole milk, and use polyunsaturated fats and oils.

| Foods allowed | Foods excluded |
|---|---|

*Beverages*

Milk, milk drinks, milk substitutes, carbonated beverages, cocoa, coffee, tea, decaffeinated coffee, eggnogs, milkshakes, instant breakfast, cereal beverages, sweetened liquid beverages, liquid dietary supplements, complete liquid diets, infant formula

*Beverages*

Any containing raw eggs or egg white, fruits, or other prohibited foods

*Breads*

None

*Breads*

All

*Cereals*

Refined cooked cereals, strained whole grain cereals in gruels

*Cereals*

All others

*Desserts*

Cornstarch puddings, custard, gelatin, plain ice cream, sherbet, fruit ices, popsicles, Bavarian cream

*Desserts*

Any dessert containing solid foods such as nuts, fruits, seeds, etc.

*Eggs*

Eggs cooked in custards, egg substitutes, puddings, ice cream, etc., or pasteurized eggs used in eggnogs or cooking, salmonella free frozen eggs

*Eggs*

Raw eggs and egg whites or unpasteurized eggs

*Soups*

Bouillon, consommé, broth; strained vegetable, meat, or cream soups containing finely homogenized meat

*Soups*

All others

*Vegetables*

Vegetable juices and vegetable purees that are strained and diluted in cream soups, mashed white potato diluted in cream soups

*Vegetables*

All others

*Miscellaneous*

Honey, sugar, syrup, glucose, lactose, sucrose, salt, flavorings, chocolate syrup, cinnamon, nutmeg, brewer's yeast

*Miscellaneous*

All others

## Full Liquid Diet

**Daily food plan**

6 cups fluid milk
3 eggs in custards or puddings or pasteurized in eggnog
1 cup strained cooked cereal
½ cup citrus juice
¼ cup finely strained vegetable puree diluted in cream soup
2 servings broth, bouillon, or cream soup
1 tbsp butter or fortified margarine
3 tsp sugar
Tea, coffee, carbonated beverages as desired

**Sample menu**

A.M.

½ cup orange juice
1 cup farina with 2 tsp fortified margarine, 1 tsp sugar, and milk
Coffee or tea with sugar
1 cup pasteurized eggnog

BETWEEN MEALS

1 cup pasteurized eggnog

NOON

½ cup apricot nectar
1 cup cream of potato soup with fortified margarine or butter
1 cup milk
½ cup Bavarian cream
Coffee or tea with sugar

BETWEEN MEALS

Blenderized milkshake with 4 oz milk, 2 tsp chocolate syrup, 2 oz ice cream (plain), and 2 tsp sugar

P.M.

½ cup pineapple juice
1 cup strained cream of vegetable soup with 1 tsp fortified margarine or butter
1 cup milk or pasteurized eggnog
½ cup caramel custard
Coffee or tea with sugar

BEDTIME

½ cup lemon gelatin
1 cup pasteurized eggnog

References
1. Turner, D.: Handbook of Diet Therapy. 5th ed. Chicago: University of Chicago Press, 1970.
2. Larsen, R. B.: Dietary needs of patients following general surgery. Hospitals 39: 133, July 16; 1965.
3. Randall, H. T.: Enteric feeding. Ballinger, W. F., Collins, J. A.; Drucker, W. R.; and Zeppa, R., eds. Manual of Surgical Nutrition. Philadelphia: W. B. Saunders, 1975.
4. Turner, S. J.; Daly, T.; Hoyrigan, J. A.; Rand, A. G.; and Thayer, W. R.: Utilization of a low lactose milk. Am. J. Clin. Nutr. 29: 739, 1976.
5. University of Iowa Hospitals and Clinics. Recent Advances in Therapeutic Diets. Ames: Iowa State University Press, 1973.
6. Goodhart, R. S.: Biotin. Goodhart, R. S., and Shils, R. E., eds. Modern Nutrition in Health and Disease. 5th ed. Philadelphia: Lea & Febiger, 1973.

# Modified Fiber Diets: Terms Related to Fiber

*Crude fiber*    That portion of a feeding material which remains after treatment with boiling sulfuric acid, alkali, water, alcohol, and ether. Although it may include some not readily soluble hemicelluloselike materials, it is mainly a measure of the cellulose content of food [1–3]. The crude fiber intake of nonvegetarians has been estimated to be between 8 and 12 g/day, and the estimated daily adult requirement is 6 g [4].

*Dietary fiber*    Also referred to as purified dietary fiber and purified plant fiber [5]—that portion of plant materials taken in our diet which is resistant to digestion by the secretions of the human gastrointestinal tract [6,7]. In addition to cellulose and lignin, it includes certain homopolysaccharides formerly classified as hemicelluloses [1] and pectins [5].

*Nonpurified plant fiber*    Also referred to as nonpurified dietary fiber [5]—any fibrous material in its natural state with all cell wall ingredients present: polysaccharides, lignin, cutins, minerals, unavailable lipids, etc. It has been suggested that this term be used when referring to the nonpurified fibrous fraction of alfalfa, wheat, and other grains; fruits and vegetables; and the like [5].

*Synthetic nonnutritive fiber*    That portion of plant materials not usually consumed by man as part of his diet, including materials such as cellophane, highly refined cellulose from wood pulp, and other highly refined materials [5] [8,9].

*Residue*    The total solid of feces made up of undigested and unabsorbed food and metabolic and bacterial products [10].

*Residue vs. fiber*    Kramer has proposed the abandonment of the term *residue* in reference to diets because of its dual meaning. It is used to refer to two phenomena interchangeably: (1) the indigestible content of food such as found in dietary fiber, and (2) increases in fecal output regardless of whether any portion of the food being referred to remains in the colon after digestion. For example, in spite of the fact that prune juice yields no residue upon chemical digestion, it is still classified as a high residue food: although it does not contribute directly to colonic residue, it contains a laxative that indirectly increases the volume of the stool [11].

References
1. Cummings, J. H.:   Progress report:   dietary fiber.   Gut 14: 69, 1973.
2. Southgate, J. A.:   The definition and analysis of dietary fiber.   Nutr. Rev. 35: 31, 1977.
3. Theander, O.:   The chemistry of dietary fibers.   Nutr. Rev. 35: 23, 1977.
4. Hardinge, M. G.; Chambers, A. C.; Crooks, H.; and Stare, F.:   Nutritional studies of vegetarians. III. Dietary levels of fiber.   Am. J. Clin. Nutr. 6: 523, 1958.
5. Spiller, G. A., and Amen, R. J.:   Plant fibers in nutrition:   need for better nomenclature.   Am. J. Clin. Nutr. 28: 675, 1975.
6. Trowell, H.:   Crude fiber, dietary fiber and atherosclerosis.   Atherosclerosis. 16: 138, 1972.
7. Trowell, H.:   Definitions of fiber.   Lancet 1: 503, 1974.

8. Kritchevsky, D., and Story, J. A.:   Binding of bile salts in vitro by nonnutritive fiber.   J. Nutr. 104: 458, 1974.
9. Kritchevsky, D,; Tepper, S. A.; and Story, J. A.:   Nonnutritive fiber and lipid metabolism.   J. Food Sci. 40: 12, 1975.
10. Turner, D.:   Handbook of Diet Therapy. 5th ed. Chicago:   University of Chicago Press, 1970.
11. Kramer, P.:   The meaning of high and low residue diets.   Gastroenterology. 47: 649, 1964.

# Dietary Fiber Content of Foods

| | Total dietary fiber (g/100) | Noncellulose poly-saccharides (g/100) | Cellulose (g/100) | Lignin (g/100) | Portion sizes | Weight (g) | Total dietary fiber/serving |
|---|---|---|---|---|---|---|---|
| **FRUITS** | | | | | | | |
| Apples (flesh only) | 1.42 | 0.94 | 0.48 | 0.01 | 1 med. | 141 | 2.00 |
| (peel only) | 3.71 | 2.21 | 1.01 | 0.49 | 1 med. | 11 | 0.41 |
| Bananas | 1.75 | 1.12 | 0.37 | 0.26 | one 6 in. | 100 | 1.75 |
| Cherries (flesh and skin) | 1.24 | 0.92 | 0.25 | 0.07 | 25 sm./med. 15 lg. | 100 | 1.24 |
| Grapefruit (canned) | 0.44 | 0.34 | 0.04 | 0.55 | ½ cup | 120 | 0.53 |
| Guavas (canned)* | 3.64 | 1.67 | 1.17 | 0.80 | 1 med. | 10 | 3.64 |
| Mandarin oranges (canned)* | 0.29 | 0.22 | 0.04 | 0.03 | ½ cup | 100 | 0.29 |
| Mangoes (canned)* | 1.00 | 0.65 | 0.32 | 0.03 | ½ cup | 83 | 0.83 |
| Peaches (flesh and skin) | 2.28 | 1.46 | 0.20 | 0.62 | 1 med. | 100 | 2.28 |
| Pears (flesh only) | 2.44 | 1.32 | 0.67 | 0.45 | ½ med. | 87 | 1.12 |
| (peel only) | 8.59 | 3.72 | 2.18 | 2.67 | ½ med. | 11 | 0.95 |
| Plums (flesh and skin) | 1.52 | 0.99 | 0.23 | 0.30 | 2 med. | 100 | 1.52 |
| Rhubarb (raw) | 1.78 | 0.93 | 0.70 | 0.15 | ½ cup | 60 | 1.07 |
| Strawberries (raw) | 2.12 | 0.98 | 0.33 | 0.81 | 10 lg. | 100 | 2.12 |
| (canned)* | 1.00 | 0.48 | 0.20 | 0.33 | ⅜ cup | 100 | 1.00 |
| Sultanas | 4.40 | 2.40 | 0.83 | 1.17 | | | |
| **NUTS** | | | | | | | |
| Brazils | 7.73 | 3.60 | 2.17 | 1.96 | ¼ cup | 35 | 2.71 |
| Peanuts | 9.30 | 6.40 | 1.69 | 1.21 | 1 tbsp | 9 | 0.84 |
| **PRESERVES** | | | | | | | |
| Jam, plum | 0.96 | 0.80 | 0.14 | 0.03 | 1 tbsp | 20 | 0.19 |
| strawberry | 1.12 | 0.85 | 0.11 | 0.15 | 1 tbsp | 20 | 0.22 |
| Lemon curd | 0.20 | 0.18 | 0.02 | tr. | | | |
| Marmalade | 0.71 | 0.64 | 0.05 | 0.01 | 1 tbsp | 20 | 0.14 |
| Mincemeat | 3.19 | 2.09 | 0.60 | 0.50 | | | |
| Peanut butter | 7.55 | 5.64 | 1.91 | tr. | 1 tbsp | 15 | 1.13 |
| Pickles | 1.53 | 0.91 | 0.50 | 0.12 | | | |
| **DRIED SOUPS** | | | | | | | |
| Minestrone | 6.61 | 4.60 | 1.91 | 0.10 | | | |
| Oxtail | 3.84 | 2.89 | 0.94 | 0.01 | | | |
| Tomato | 3.32 | 1.95 | 1.33 | 0.04 | 1 serv. | 16 | 0.53 |
| **BEVERAGES** | | | | | | | |
| Cocoa | 43.27 | 11.25 | 4.13 | 27.90 | 1 oz | 28 | 12.12 |
| Chocolate drink | 8.20 | 2.61 | 1.16 | 4.43 | 1 oz | 28 | 2.30 |
| Coffee and chicory essence | 0.79 | 0.73 | 0.02 | 0.04 | | | |
| Instant coffee | 16.41 | 15.55 | 0.53 | 0.33 | 1 serv. | 2 | 0.33 |
| **EXTRACTS** | | | | | | | |
| Bovril | 0.91 | 0.85 | 0.03 | 0.03 | | | |
| Marmite | 2.69 | 2.60 | 0.03 | 0.06 | | | |
| **LEAFY VEGETABLE** | | | | | | | |
| Broccoli tops (boiled) | 4.10 | 2.92 | 0.85 | 0.03 | ½ cup | 73 | 2.99 |
| Brussels sprouts | 2.86 | 1.99 | 0.80 | 0.07 | ½ cup | 70 | 2.00 |
| Cabbage | 2.83 | 1.76 | 0.69 | 0.38 | ½ cup | 73 | 2.07 |
| Cauliflower | 1.80 | 0.67 | 1.13 | tr. | ½ cup | 63 | 1.13 |
| Lettuce (raw) | 1.53 | 0.47 | 1.06 | tr. | ½ cup | 55 | 0.84 |
| Onions (raw) | 2.10 | 1.55 | 0.55 | tr. | one 2 ¼ in. | 100 | 2.10 |
| **LEGUMES** | | | | | | | |
| Beans (baked) canned | 7.27 | 5.67 | 1.41 | 0.19 | ⅓ cup | 85 | 6.18 |
| Beans (runner) boiled | 3.35 | 1.85 | 1.29 | 0.21 | ½ cup | 50 | 1.67 |
| Peas, frozen (raw) | 7.75 | 5.48 | 2.09 | 0.18 | ½ cup | 73 | 5.66 |
| garden (canned)† | 6.28 | 3.80 | 2.47 | 0.01 | | | |
| processed (canned)† | 7.85 | 5.20 | 2.30 | 0.35 | ½ cup | 67 | 5.26 |
| **ROOT VEGETABLES** | | | | | | | |
| Carrots, young (boiled) | 3.70 | 2.22 | 1.48 | tr. | ½ cup | 75 | 2.78 |
| Parsnips (raw) | 4.90 | 3.77 | 1.13 | tr. | ½ lg. | 100 | 4.90 |
| Swedes (raw) | 2.40 | 1.61 | 0.79 | tr. | | | |
| Turnips (raw) | 2.20 | 1.50 | 0.70 | tr. | ⅔ cup | 86 | 1.89 |

* Fruit and syrup.
† Drained.

| | Total dietary fiber (g/100) | Noncellulose polysaccharides (g/100) | Cellulose (g/100) | Lignin (g/100) | Portion sizes | Weight (g) | Total dietary fiber/serving |
|---|---|---|---|---|---|---|---|
| POTATO | | | | | | | |
| Main crop (raw) | 3.51 | 2.49 | 1.02 | tr. | one 2 ¼ in. | 100 | 3.51 |
| Chips, fried | 3.20 | 2.05' | 1.12 | 0.03 | 10 pcs. | 20 | 0.64 |
| Crisps | 11.90 | 10.60 | 1.07 | 0.32 | 3 ½ oz | 10 | 11.90 |
| Canned (solid and liquid) | 2.51 | 2.23 | 0.28 | tr. | ⅖ cup | 10 | 2.51 |
| PEPPERS (cooked) | 0.93 | 0.59 | 0.24 | tr. | ½ cup | 68 | 0.63 |
| TOMATOES (fresh) | 1.40 | 0.65 | 0.45 | 0.30 | 1 small | 10 | 1.40 |
| TOMATOES (canned)† | 0.85 | 0.45 | 0.37 | 0.03 | ½ cup | 12 | 1.02 |
| SWEET CORN cooked | 4.74 | 4.31 | 0.31 | 0.12 | ½ ear | 50 | 2.37 |
| canned† | 5.69 | 4.97 | 0.64 | 0.08 | ½ cup | 83 | 4.72 |
| FLOURS | | | | | | | |
| White, breadmaking | 3.15 | 2.52 | 0.60 | 0.03 | ½ cup | 60 | 1.89 |
| Brown | 7.87 | 5.70 | 1.42 | 0.75 | | | |
| Whole meal | 9.51 | 6.25 | 2.46 | 0.80 | ½ cup | 67 | 6.28 |
| Bran | 44.0 | 32.70 | 8.05 | 3.23 | ½ cup | 30 | 13.20 |
| BREADS | | | | | | | |
| White | 2.72 | 2.01 | 0.71 | tr. | 1 slice | 23 | 0.63 |
| Brown, Boston | 5.11 | 3.63 | 1.33 | 0.15 | 1 slice | 35 | 1.79 |
| Hovis | 4.54 | 2.99 | 1.01 | 0.04 | | | |
| Whole meal | 8.50 | 5.95 | 1.31 | 1.24 | 1 slice | 23 | 1.96 |
| BREAKFAST CEREALS | | | | | | | |
| All Bran | 26.70 | 17.82 | 6.01 | 2.88 | ¾ cup | 42 | 11.20 |
| Cornflakes | 11.00 | 7.26 | 2.42 | 1.32 | ¾ cup | 19 | 2.09 |
| Grapenuts | 7.00 | 5.14 | 1.28 | 0.58 | ¾ cup | 84 | 5.88 |
| Readibrek | 7.60 | 5.39 | 0.99 | 1.22 | | | |
| Rice Krispies | 4.47 | 3.47 | 0.78 | 0.22 | ¾ cup | 21 | 0.94 |
| Puffed wheat | 15.41 | 10.35 | 2.59 | 2.47 | ¾ cup | 9 | 1.39 |
| Sugar Puffs | 6.08 | 4.00 | 0.99 | 1.09 | | | |
| Shredded wheat | 12.26 | 8.79 | 2.63 | 0.84 | 1 bisc. | 22 | 2.70 |
| Special K | 5.45 | 3.68 | 0.72 | 1.05 | ¾ cup | 12 | 0.65 |
| Swiss Breakfast | 7.41 | 5.31 | 1.36 | 0.74 | | | |
| Weetabix | 12.72 | 9.18 | 2.35 | 1.19 | ¾ cup | 42 | 5.34 |
| MISCELLANEOUS | | | | | | | |
| Choc. digestine ½ coated | 3.50 | 2.13 | 0.59 | 0.78 | | | |
| Choc. fully coated | 3.09 | 1.36 | 0.42 | 1.31 | 1 cook. | 11 | 0.34 |
| Chrispbread, rye | 11.73 | 8.33 | 1.66 | 1.74 | 2 crax | 13 | 1.48 |
| Crispbread, wheat | 4.83 | 3.34 | 0.94 | 0.55 | | | |
| Ginger biscuits | 1.99 | 1.45 | 0.30 | 0.24 | 1 snap | 4 | 0.08 |
| Matzo | 3.85 | 2.72 | 0.70 | 0.43 | 1 pc. | 20 | 0.77 |
| Oatcakes | 4.00 | 3.16 | 0.40 | 0.44 | | | |
| Semisweet | 2.31 | 1.76 | 0.33 | 0.22 | | | |
| Short-sweet | 1.66 | 1.42 | 0.11 | 0.13 | 1 cook. | 7 | 0.12 |
| Wafers (filled vanilla) | 1.62 | 1.08 | 0.47 | 0.07 | 1 wafer | 3 | 0.05 |

*Source:* Adapted from Southgate, D. A. T.; Bailey, B.; Collinson, E.; and Walker, A. F.: A guide to calculating intakes of dietary fiber. J. Hum. Nutr. 30: 303, 1976.

\* Fruit and syrup.
† Drained.

# Fiber Restricted Diet

***Definition***    A diet that contains a minimum of fiber and connective tissue. Until more complete and accurate tables of composition are published regarding the dietary fiber content of foods, diets must provisionally be described in qualitative terms [1].

***Characteristics of the diet***    The low fiber diet presented here is based on available tables of composition which report mainly the crude fiber content of foods [2,3] and give only very limited data on dietary fiber content [4]. Indigestible carbohydrate is reduced by using young immature vegetables, ripe canned or well cooked fruits, and certain raw fruits and vegetables low in dietary fiber content. Tender meat or meat made tender in the cooking process is used to decrease the amount of connective tissue.

***Purpose of the diet***    To prevent the formation of an obstructing bolus by high fiber foods in patients with narrowed intestinal or esophageal lumens [5,6].

***Effects of the diet***    In general, low fiber diets decrease the weight and bulk of the stool and lead to delayed intestinal transit [7]. However, a low fiber diet is not necessarily synonymous with a low residue diet. Colonic residue is also increased by such low fiber foods as milk and prune juice, which increase stool weight by other mechanisms [8,9].

***Indications for use***    There is a limited place for the use of low fiber diets during acute phases of diverticulosis, ulcerative colitis, or infectious enterocolitis, when the bowel is markedly inflamed. In these instances any distension caused by bulky food and bowel movements may cause pain [10]. The diet is indicated whenever inflammatory changes have progressed to stenosis of the intestinal or esophageal lumen or in some instances of esophageal varices. Barring such complications, there is little evidence to support continued long-term use of a low fiber diet in the treatment of regional enteritis, ulcerative colitis, or pyloric stenosis [5,11–13].

The diet may be used as a soft diet in the transition between a completely liquid diet and a normal diet in patients convalescing from surgery, trauma, or other illnesses. It should be individualized to suit specific patient tolerances, depending on the type of surgery or illness.

Use of a "low residue diet" has been suggested in managing certain complications of radiotherapy that result in stenosis of the intestinal lumen [14].

***Possible adverse reactions***    Fiber deficient diets are associated with prolonged intestinal transit and small infrequent stools. Painter has suggested that continued use of a low fiber diet containing large amounts of highly refined carbohydrates may be associated with diverticular disease of the colon. According to this theory, the reduced bulk of the diet eventually results in the narrowing of the colonic lumen. The small compact stool produced by low fiber diets causes the colon to contract more tightly around it, thus decreasing the size of the lumen and increasing intraluminal pressures. These pressure increases may lead to herniation of the colonic muscle and the characteristic diverticula of the disorder [15].

Upon the basis of epidemiological data, fiber deficient diets have been linked to a variety of other diseases afflicting Western civilization, such as cancer of the colon [16]. At this time, however, proof of any cause and effect relationship has not been forthcoming [17].

*Contraindications*    A low fiber diet may actually aggravate the symptoms and is contraindicated in the irritable colon syndrome or in diverticulosis unless the lumen of the colon is narrowed or stenosed [15].

*Suggestions for dietitians*    *Adjusting the diet to permit greater reductions in colonic residue*    The amount of colonic residue produced can be further decreased by including only the following fruits and vegetables in the diet: strained fruit and vegetable juices, such as tomato juice, and white potatoes without skin. All other fruits and vegetables in any form, including prune juice, should be eliminated. There is limited evidence that milk, which contains no crude fiber, may indirectly contribute to fecal residue. Thus, in certain patients, it may be wise to restrict milk intake to 2 cups a day. The excluded or restricted foods either contribute directly to the residue in the colon or increase it by other mechanisms, such as a laxative action, e.g., diphenyllisatin in prune juice.

## Fiber Restricted Diet

| Foods allowed | Foods excluded |
|---|---|
| *Beverages* | *Beverages* |
| Milk, carbonated beverages, Postum, cider, coffee, tea | Drinks made from vegetables and fruits not allowed or other foods not allowed |
| *Bread and cereal products* | *Bread and cereal products* |
| White bread and toast; melba toast; crackers; bagels; cereals; waffles; French toast; refined cereals such as Cream of Wheat, Cream of Rice, cornflakes, puffed rice | Coarse whole grain breads and cereals; any not on allowed lists, especially bran flakes, cracked wheat, Post Grape-Nuts, Post Grape-Nuts Flakes |
| *Desserts* | *Desserts* |
| Plain cakes and cookies; gelatin; plain puddings; custard; any plain desserts made from allowed foods without nuts or coconut, e.g., ice cream, ices, popsicles, etc. | Coconut or nuts, or any desserts made with other foods not allowed |
| *Fats* | *Fats* |
| Butter, margarine, salad oils, mayonnaise, cream, crisp bacon, plain gravies, plain salad dressings with allowed foods | Nuts, olives |
| *Fruits* | *Fruits* |
| Strained fruit juices, except prune, and canned fruit, except those not allowed | Any not allowed, especially dates, figs, prunes, boysenberries, blackberries, blueberries, kumquats, pineapple, rhubarb, avocados, grapes, apples, peaches, pears, guavas, fresh grapefruit and orange sections |

**Foods allowed**

*Meat and meat substitutes*

Ground or well cooked tender beef, ham, veal, lamb, pork, poultry, tender steak and chops, fish, oysters, shrimp, lobster, clams, liver, crab, organ meats, eggs, cheese

**Food excluded**

*Meat and meat substitutes*

Tough fibrous meats with gristle; peanut butter, smooth or chunky

*Soups and miscellaneous*

Any soups made from allowed foods or strained soups; arrowroot; candy, such as butterscotch, jelly beans, marshmallows, plain hard candy; cornstarch; gelatin; honey; molasses; sugar; tomato catsup; vinegar; prepared mustard; plus the following spices, which contain less than 0.015 g fiber/⅛ tsp: [18]:

| | |
|---|---|
| Allspice | Oregano |
| Basil | Paprika |
| Bay leaves | Parsley flakes |
| Celery salt, powder, or leaves | Pepper, black, ground |
| Cinnamon | Rosemary |
| Cumin powder | Sage |
| Ginger | Savory |
| Mace | Tarragon |
| Marjoram | Thyme |
| Onion powder | Tumeric |

*Soups and miscellaneous*

Chocolate nut bars or peanut brittle, pickles, sesame seed, any soup made from vegetables not on allowed lists; and any other foods not on allowed lists

*Vegetables*

Strained vegetable juice; lettuce; cooked asparagus, beets, green beans, tomato; eggplant; acorn squash without seeds; lima beans, spinach

*Vegetables*

Any not allowed, especially peas, parsnips, rutabagas, broccoli, brussels sprouts, cabbage, onions, carrots, turnips, cauliflower, baked beans, fresh tomatoes, zucchini, corn

## Fiber Restricted Diet  Sample Menu

### A.M.

½ cup orange juice
1 soft cooked egg
1 slice white toast with 1 tsp butter or fortified margarine
1 cup cornflakes
1 cup milk
Coffee or tea

### Noon

7 oz chicken vegetable soup
1 hamburger on bun
1 tsp catsup
½ cup asparagus
1 small banana
½ cup milk
Coffee of tea

### P.M.

3–4 oz tender broiled steak
1 baked potato without skin
1 cup cooked spinach
½ cup canned grapefruit sections

2 slices rye bread
1 tsp butter or fortified margarine
½ cup milk
Coffee or tea

References

1. Trowell, H.:  Definitions of fiber.  Lancet 1: 503, 1974.
2. Composition of Foods—Raw, Processed, Prepared.  Agricultural Handbook No. 8. Washington, DC:  Agriculture Research Service, U.S. Department of Agriculture, 1963.
3. Hardinge, M. G.; Swarner, J. B.; and Crooks, H.:  Carbohydrates in foods.  J. Am. Diet. Assoc. 46: 197, 1965.
4. Southgate, D. A. T.; Bailey, B.; Collinson, E.; and Walker, A. F.:  A guide to calculating intakes of dietary fiber.  J. Hum. Nutr. 30: 303, 1976.
5. Williams, C. N.:  Diet and disease of the gastrointestinal tract. N. S.  Med. Bull. 52: 211, 1973.
6. Donaldson, R. M.:  The muddle of diets for gastrointestinal disorders. JAMA 225: 1243, 1973.
7. Parks, T. G.:  The role of dietary fiber in the prevention and treatment of diseases of the colon.  Proc. R. Soc. Med. 66: 681, 1973.
8. Kramer, P.:  The meaning of high and low residue diets.  Gastroenterology 47: 649, 1964.
9. Hosoi, K.; Alvarez, W. C.; and Mann, F. C.:  Intestinal absorption. A search for a low residue diet.  Arch. Intern. Med. 41: 112, 1928.
10. Goldstein, F.:  Diet and colonic disease.  J. Am. Diet. Assoc. 60: 499, 1972.
11. Manier, J. W.:  Diet in gastrointestinal diseases.  Med. Clin. N. Am. 54: 1357, 1970.
12. Meyer, J. H.:  Ulcerative colitis. Sleisinger, M. H., and Fordtran, J. S., eds.  Gastrointestinal Disease. Philadelphia:  W. B. Saunders, 1973.
13. Donaldson, R. M.:  Regional enteritis. Sleisinger, M. H., and Fordtran, J. S., eds.  Gastrointestinal Disease. Philadelphia:  W. B. Saunders, 1973.
14. Olson, M. H.:  Managing the complications of radiotherapy.  Am. Fam. Phys. 9: 136, Apr. 1974.
15. Painter, N. S., and Burkitt, D. P.:  Diverticular disease of the colon:  a deficiency disease of Western civilization.  Br. Med. J. 2: 450, 1971.
16. Burkitt, D. P.; Walker, A. R. P.; and Painter, N. S.:  Dietary fiber and disease.  JAMA 229: 1068, 1974.
17. Eastwood, M. A.; Fisher, N,; Greenwood, C. T.; and Hutchinson, J. B.:  Perspectives of the bran hypothesis.  Lancet 1: 1029, 1974.
18. American Spice Trade Association:  Nutritional Composition of Spices. American Spice Trade Association, 1973.

# High Fiber Diet

***Definition*** A diet that contains increased amounts of cellulose, hemicellulose, lignin, and pectin and provides approximately 13 or more g crude fiber daily.

***Characteristics of the diet*** Emphasis is placed on modifying the normal diet by increasing the intake of whole grain breads and cereals and fresh fruits and vegetables that are high in fiber content. The intake of highly refined carbohydrates is reduced to the extent that they are replaced by unrefined foods. The caloric content of the diet is not substantially different from that of a normal diet.

***Purpose of the diet*** High fiber diet therapy is directed toward one or more of the following aims:

1. Increasing the volume and weight of the residue that reaches the distal colon [1];
2. Increasing gastrointestinal motility in those in whom it has been decreased [2];
3. Decreasing intraluminal colonic pressures in patients with increased pressures [3,4]. Specifically, a high fiber diet has been shown to provide relief from the symptoms of diverticulosis and to result in decreased intraluminal colonic pressures in these patients [2,5]. Increased fiber intake may help maintain the normal size of the colonic lumen and thus prevent further segmentation of diverticular disease [2,6].

Furthermore, high fiber diet therapy has been demonstrated to prevent the gradual return of excessively high preoperative intraluminal pressures in patients who have undergone myotomies [7] (a myotomy is an operative procedure that divides the thickened circular muscle layer in diverticular disease and at least temporarily lowers intraluminal colonic pressures).

***Effects of increased fiber intake on the intestine*** *Increased motility* The bulk of the food itself mechanically stimulates intestinal motility. However, there is controversy as to whether this effect occurs to a significant degree only in patients with decreased motility. Two studies performed in individuals with normal intestinal transit times indicate that a high fiber diet may not significantly affect gastrointestinal motility [8] or transit [9]. A more recent study, however, indicates that wheat bran increases motility in normal subjects [10].

*Production of volatile fatty acids* Foods high in fiber content, particularly hemicellulose and to a lesser extent cellulose, are broken down by intestinal bacteria to volatile fatty acids that act as potent cathartics [11]. This could be an important factor in increasing stool weight [12], shortening transit time, and increasing flatulence.

*Water absorption* Crude fiber imbibes water or acts as a hygroscopic agent [4,13]. It appears to modify the stool by acting as a vehicle for molecular or gel water in normal people and for interstitial water in people with diverticular disease [4].

*Decreased intraluminal colonic pressures*    As previously mentioned, a high fiber diet has been shown to decrease the high intraluminal colonic pressures found in people with diverticular disease.

*Action as a weak cation exchange resin*    The fact that fiber has the ability to act like a weak cation exchange resin may have physiological significance. This property suggests that the electrolyte content of the stool could be influenced by the diet [13]. It is an area that warrants further investigation for a possible link between cancer of the colon and fiber deficient diets.

*Changes in bile salt metabolism*    Pectin has been reported to lower serum cholesterol levels [14]. There are other indications that bile salt metabolism may be altered by dietary fiber [15–17], although there is lack of general agreement on this point [12,14,18–20]. One theory proposes that the binding of bile salts in the intestine may inhibit cholesterol absorption and decrease serum cholesterol levels. *In vitro* studies indicate that fiber derived from bran is much less effective as a binder of bile salts than that derived from such vegetables as carrots and peas [21–24].

*Insulin and carbohydrate response*    Insulin response to a high fiber–high carbohydrate diet is half that of a low fiber–high carbohydrate diet; carbohydrate induced hyperlipemia may not occur on a high fiber–high carbohydrate diet [25].

**Indications for use**    Increasing fiber intake may be beneficial in atonic constipation, uncomplicated diverticulosis, and the irritable bowel syndrome or whenever it may be desirable to increase the volume of the stool [3,26–32].

*Bran vs. cereals, fruits and vegetables*
The inclusion of a high fiber diet in this section is by no means intended to promulgate its use as either the most effective or the only method of increasing dietary fiber intake. Daily consumption of bran supplements is easy, inexpensive, and the most widely recommended form of high fiber diet therapy. For patients who are already eating a well balanced diet, who cannot afford extra servings of fruits and vegetables, and who tolerate such supplements well, bran may be the treatment of choice.

Because of its higher fiber content and greater indigestibility than many fruits and vegetables, bran has a more pronounced laxative effect [33]. The degree of effect of fruits and vegetables varies with source and age and maturity of cell walls; older, more mature fruits and vegetables produce a greater effect. Despite the observed variation, however, the laxative effect of fruit and vegetable fiber in humans is quantitatively important and should not be discounted [34,35]. Furthermore, dietary fiber is made up of several components each of which may have a *different* effect upon the gastrointestinal tract.

Vegetable fiber that is high in pectin has been reported to lower serum lipids, whereas wheat fiber such as bran has no effect on lipids [21–24]. One study on the effects of bran as compared to another type of fiber called bagasse (residue found in grapes, beet pulp, or sugar cane) reported that although both types of fiber increased the weight and volume of stools, they had dissimilar metabolic effects [36]. More attention needs to be paid to the testing of the specific effects of the different components of dietary fiber from a variety of sources prior to any recommendation to increase intake of one form of dietary fiber, such as bran, at the expense of another.

***Possible adverse reactions*** *Osmotic diarrhea* Volatile fatty acids produced by the action of bacteria on large amounts of fiber in the intestine may result in an irritating osmotic diarrhea and increased flatus production [12].

*Decreased serum levels of iron, calcium, etc.* Exclusive reliance on large quantities of foods high in phytate content to increase dietary fiber intake, as opposed to a mixed high fiber diet, may have undesirable nutritional consequences [37]. Bran or breads made from unprocessed flour have been reported to lower serum levels of calcium [38,39], zinc [39], iron [40,41] and serum folate [31]. The observed effect is the result of the formation of insoluble phytates in the intestine and is also related to the uronic acid content of the food [42].

***Contraindications*** The diet is contraindicated when changes due to inflammation have caused stenosis or narrowing of the intestinal lumen [6,8,43].

***Suggestions for dietitians*** No attempt should be made to institute a high fiber diet in a patient with diverticulosis prior to his instruction in the nutritional goals and effects of the diet. Particularly in the patient who has been maintained on a low fiber diet for years, high fiber diet therapy will require threatening changes in eating behavior that are often difficult to accept. Frequent reassurance from the dietitian about the value of the diet may be needed to allay the patient's fears, particularly if minor side effects, such as increased flatus production, occur. Achievement of patient involvement and cooperation are essential if the learning process is to culminate in the desired behavioral changes and the realization of the goals of the diet.

Suggested High Fiber Diet    **Sample menu**

A.M.

4 stewed prunes
½ cup or more Nabisco 100% Bran
1 soft cooked egg
1 tsp fortified margarine or butter
1 slice whole wheat bread, toasted
1 cup milk
Coffee or tea

Noon

Ham and cheese sandwich with 2 slices whole wheat bread and 1 tsp fortified margarine
1 sliced tomato salad
1 piece blueberry pie (1/6 of 9 in. pie)
½ cup milk
Coffee or tea

P.M.

3–4 oz roast beef and gravy
1 large stalk broccoli
1 ear corn on the cob, 4 in. long
1 slice pineapple
1 whole wheat roll with 1 tsp fortified margarine or butter
½ cup milk
Coffee or tea

Between meals

1 fresh pear 3 × 2½ in.

References

1. Leeb, P. M., and Sleisinger, M. H.: Diverticular disease of the colon. Sleisinger, M. H., and Fordtran, J. S., eds. Gastrointestinal Disease. Philadelphia: W. B. Saunders, 1973.
2. Parks, T. G.: The role of dietary fiber in the prevention and treatment of diseases of the colon. Proc. R. Soc. Med. 66: 681, 1973.
3. Painter, N. S., and Burkitt, D. P.: Diverticular disease of the colon: a deficiency disease of Western civilization. Br. Med. J. 2: 450, 1971.
4. Findlay, J. M.; Mitchell, W. D.; Smith, A. N.; Anderson, A. J.; and Eastwood, M. A.: Effects of unprocessed bran on colon function in normal subjects and in diverticular disease. Lancet 1: 146, 1974.
5. Painter, N. S.; Almeida, A. Z.; and Colebourne, K. W.: Unprocessed bran in the treatment of diverticular disease of the colon. Br. Med. J. 2: 137, 1972.
6. Donaldson, R. M.: Regional enteritis. Sleisinger, M. H., and Fordtran, J. S., eds. Gastrointestinal Disease. Philadelphia: W. B. Saunders, 1973.
7. Smith, A. N.; Kirwan, W. O.; and Shariff, S.: Motility effects of operations performed for diverticular disease. Proc. R. Soc. Med. 67: 1041, 1974.
8. Eastwood, M. A.; Kirkpatrick, J. R.; Mitchell, W. D.; Bone, A.; and Hamilton, T.: Effects of dietary supplements of wheat bran and cellulose on faeces and bowel function. Br. Med. J. 4: 392, 1973.
9. Payler, D. K.; Pomare, E. W.; Heaton, K. W.; and Harvey, R. F.: The effect of wheat bran on intestinal transit. Gut 16: 209, 1975.
10. Weinreich, J.; Pederson, D.; and Dinesen, K.: Role of bran in normals. Acta Med. Scand. 202: 125, 1977.
11. Manier, J. W.: Diet in gastrointestinal diseases. Med. Clin. N. Am. 54: 1357, 1970.
12. Cummings, J. H.: Progress report: dietary fiber. Gut 14: 69, 1973.
13. McConnell, A. A.; Eastwood, M. A.; and Mitchell, W. D.: Physical characteristics of vegetable foodstuffs that could influence bowel function. J. Sci. Food Agric. 25: 1457, 1974.
14. Durrington, P. N.; Manning, A. P.; Bolton, C. H.; and Hartog, M.: Effect of pectin on serum lipids and lipoproteins, whole gut transit time and stool weight. Lancet 2: 394, 1976.
15. Kay, R. M. and Truswell, A. S.: Effect of citric pectin on blood lipids and fecal steroid excretion in man. Am. J. Clin. Nutr. 30: 171, 1977.

16. Hepner, G. W.: Altered bile acid metabolism in vegetarians. Am. J. Dig. Dis. 20: 935, 1975.
17. Pomare, E. W., and Heaton, K. W.: Alteration of bile salt metabolism by dietary fiber (bran). Br. Med. J. 4: 262, 1973.
18. Reilly, R. W., and Kirsner, J. B.: Fiber deficiency and colonic disorders. Am. J. Dig. Dis. 20: 49, 1975.
19. Tarpila, S.; Miettinen, T. A.; and Metsaranta, L.: Effects of bran on serum cholesterol, faecal mass, fat bile acids and neutral steroids and biliary lipids in patients with diverticular disease of the colon. Gut. 19: 137, 1978.
20. Connell, A. M.; Smith, C. L.; and Somsel, M. L.: Absence of effect of bran on blood lipids. Lancet 1: 496, 1975.
21. Story, J. A., and Kritchevsky, D.: Comparison of the binding of various bile acids and bile salts in vitro by several types of fiber. J. Nutr. 106: 1292, 1976.
22. Eastwood, M. A.; Anderson, R.; Mitchell, W. D.; Robertson, J.; and Pocock, S.: A method of measure for the absorption of bile salts to vegetable fiber of different water holding capacity. J. Nutr. 106: 1429, 1976.
23. Eastwood, M. A.: Fiber and enterohepatic circulation. Nutr. Rev. 35: 42, Mar. 1977.
24. Truswell, A. S.: Food fiber and blood lipids. Nutr. Rev. 35: 51, Mar. 1977.
25. Albrink, M. J.; Newman, T.; and Davidson, P. C.: Effect of high and low fiber diets on plasma lipids and insulin. Am. J. Clin. Nutr. 32: 1486, 1979.
26. Smits, B. J.: Irritable bowel syndrome. Practitioner 213: 37, 1974.
27. Shapiro, J. L.: Diverticular disease of the colon. South. Med. J. 67: 710, 1974.
28. Painter, N. S.: The high fiber diet in the treatment of diverticular disease of the colon. Postgrad. Med. J. 50: 629, 1974.
29. Brodribb, A. J. M., and Humphreys, D. M.: Diverticular disease: three studies. Part I. Relation to other disorders and fiber intake. Br. Med. J. 1: 424, 1976.
30. Brodribb, A. J. M., and Humphreys, D. M.: Diverticular disease: three studies. Part II. Treatment with bran. Br. Med. J. 1: 425, 1976.
31. Brodribb, A. J. M., and Humphreys, D. M.: Diverticular disease: three studies. Part III. Metabolic effect of bran in patients with diverticular disease. Br. Med. J. 1: 428, 1976.
32. Mendeloff, A. I.: Dietary fiber. Nutr. Rev. 33: 321, 1975.
33. Hoppert, C. A., and Clark, A. J.: Digestibility and effect on laxation of crude fiber and cellulose in certain common foods. J. Am. Diet. Assoc. 21: 157, 1945.
34. Van Soest, P. J., and McQueen, R. W.: The chemistry and estimation of fibre. Proc. Nutr. Soc. 32: 123, 1973.
35. Kelsay, J. L. Behall, K. M. and Prather, E. S.: Effect of fiber from fruits and vegetables on metabolic responses of human subjects. I. Bowel transit time, number of defecations, fecal weight, urinary excretions of energy and nitrogen and apparent digestibilities of energy, nitrogen and fat. Am. J. Clin. Nutr. 31: 1149, 1978.
36. Walters, R. L.; McLean Baird, I.; Davies, P. S.; Hill, M. J.; Drasar, B. S.; Southgate, D. A. T.; Green, J.; and Morgan, B.: Effects of two types of dietary fibre on faecal steroid and lipid excretion. Br. Med. J. 2: 536, 1975.
37. Reinhold, J. G.; Faradj, B.; Abadi, P.; and Ismail-Beigi, F.: Decreased absorption of calcium, magnesium, zinc and phosphorous by humans due to increased fiber and phosphorous consumption as wheat bread. J. Nutr. 106: 493, 1976.
38. Heaton, K. W., and Pomare, E. W.: Effect of bran on blood lipids and calcium. Lancet 1: 49, 1974.
39. Reinhold, J. G.; Nasr, K.; Lahimgarzadeh, A.; and Hedayati, H. L.: Effect of purified phytate and phytate rich bread upon metabolism of zinc, calcium, phosphorous and nitrogen in man. Lancet 1: 283, 1973.
40. Jenkins, D. J. A.; Hill, M. S.; and Cummings, J. H.: Effect of wheat fiber on blood lipids, fecal steroid excretion and serum iron. Am. J. Clin. Nutr. 28: 1408, 1975.
41. Bjorn-Rasmussen, E.: Iron absorption from wheat bread. Influence of various amounts of bran. Nutr. Metab. 16: 101, 1974.
42. Branch, W. J.; Southgate, D. A. T.; and James, W. P. T.: Binding of calcium by dietary fibre: its relationship to unsubstituted uronic acids. Proc. Nutr. Soc. 34: 120a, 1975.
43. Donaldson, R. M.: The muddle of diets for gastrointestinal disorders. JAMA 225: 1243, 1973.

# American Dietetic Association Position Paper on Bland Diet in the Treatment of Chronic Duodenal Ulcer Disease

The bland diet and its modifications have been used for many years as part of the treatment for duodenal ulcer and other gastrointestinal disorders. It has most often been defined as one which is chemically and mechanically nonirritating [1, 2]; however, there is considerable lack of agreement as to which foods are actually nonirritating. Review of diet manuals from many states reveals regional differences as to foods allowed [3]. A review of the literature reveals that much of the rationale for the bland diet is based on tradition and even folklore [3–8].

The American Dietetic Association, in its commitment to interpret and apply the science of nutrition in the promotion of individual, group, and community health:

1. Recognizes that the rationale (chemically and mechanically nonirritating) for the bland diet is not sufficiently supported by scientific evidence.

   a. Spices, condiments, and highly seasoned foods are usually omitted on the basis that they irritate the gastric mucosa. However, experiments have indicated that no significant irritation occurs, even when most condiments are applied directly on the gastric mucosa [1–3]. Exceptions are those items which do cause gastric irritation, including black pepper, chili powder, caffeine, coffee, tea, cocoa, alcohol, and drugs [2,3,6,9].

   b. Milk has been the basis of diets for duodenal ulcer for many years. One of the primary aims in dietary management of duodenal ulcer disease is to reduce acid secretion and neutralize the acid present [8]. While milk does relieve duodenal ulcer pain, the acid neutralizing effect is slight [1,7,10]. Its buffering action could be outweighed by its ability to stimulate acid production [10]. Most foods stimulate acid secretion to some extent; protein provides the greatest buffering action and is also the most powerful stimulus to acid secretion [3,5,7,11–13]. The use of milk therapy has been greatly reduced over the past decade, owing to a better knowledge of its side effects and allergic reactions [1,7,10,14]. The controversy regarding the use of milk still continues. There are those who still advocate the regular use of milk [2,5], primarily during the active stage of acute duodenal ulcer; however, strict insistence on its use during remission is unwarranted [7,10,14,15].

   c. Roughage, or coarse food, has been excluded from the diet on the basis that it aggravates the inflamed mucosal area. There is no evidence that such foods as fruit skins, lettuce, nuts, and celery, when they are well masticated and mixed with saliva,

Approved by the Executive Board, May 21, 1971, as Position Paper Number 000011.

will scrape or irritate the duodenal ulcer [12,14]. Grinding or pureeing of foods is necessary only when the teeth are in poor condition or missing.

d. The effect of a bland diet on the healing of duodenal ulcer has been studied extensively. Investigations have compared various bland diets with regular or free-choice diets [1,3–8,16,17]. The results indicate that a bland diet made no significant difference in healing the ulcer. One such study [8] demonstrated that the acidity of the gastric contents was frequently lower when a free-choice diet was taken. Many foods have been incriminated as the cause of gastric discomfort and are subsequently eliminated from the patient's diet. Studies done on patients with and without documented gastrointestinal disease indicate that those with gastrointestinal disease cannot be distinguished by food intolerance [14]. Symptoms of intolerance were more related to individual response than to intake of specific food or the presence of disease.

2. Believes that scientific investigation supports the validity of frequent, small feedings in the management of patients with duodenal ulcer disease [8]. These have been found to offer the most comfort to the patient [6]; additionally, acidity of the gastric contents is lower with small-volume, frequent feedings. It must also be recognized that rest, preferably in bed, rapidly reduces duodenal ulcer symptoms [5,7,15]. This is a specially important factor in the healing of the ulcer.

3. Believes the following points should be of major consideration in developing a dietary plan for duodenal ulcer patients:

a. Individualization of the dietary plan, since patients differ as to specific food intolerances, living patterns, life-styles, work hours, and education.

b. Utilization of small-volume, frequent feedings.

c. Provision of educational materials relative to dietary support.

4. Advocates the continued pursuit of current research and recommends that valid information be utilized in updating dietary regimens.

5. Suggests that dietetic practitioners be cognizant of the possible harmful effects of a milk rich bland diet in patients who have a tendency towards hypercalcemia and/or atherosclerosis.

References

1. Kramer, P., and Caso, E. K.:  Is the rationale for gastrointestinal diet therapy sound?  J. Am. Diet. Assoc. 42: 505, 1963.
2. Shull, H. J.:  Diet in the management of peptic ulcer.  JAMA 170: 1068, 1959.
3. Weinstein, L.; Olson, R.; Van Itallie, T.; Caso, E.; Johnson, D.; and Ingelfinger, F.:  Diet as related to gastrointestinal function.  JAMA 176: 935, 1961.
4. Buchman, E.; Kaung, D.; and Knapp, R.:  Dietary treatment in duodenal ulcer.  Am. J. Clin. Nutr. 22: 1536, 1969.
5. Diet and duodenal ulcer.  Br. Med. J. 3: 727, 1969.
6. Diets for peptic ulcer.  Br. Med. J. 4: 834, 1965.
7. Gillespie, I.:  Disease of the digestive system. Duodenal ulcer.  Br. Med. J. 4: 281, 1967.
8. Lennard-Jones, J. E., and Barbouris, N.:  Effect of different foods on the acidity of the gastric contents in patients with duodenal ulcer. Part I. A comparison between two "therapeutic" diets and freely-chosen meals.  Gut 6: 113, 1965.

9. Spiro, H. M.: Clinical Gastroenterology. New York: Macmillan, 1970.
10. Piper, D. W.: Milk in the treatment of gastric disease. Am. J. Clin. Nutr. 22: 191, 1969.
11. Code, C. F.: Stimulating effects of various foods on gastric-acid secretion. Am. J. Dig. Dis. 6: 50, 1953.
12. Kotrba, C., and Code, C. F.: Gastric acid secretory response to some purified foods and to addition of sucrose or olive oil. Am. J. Dig. Dis. 14: 1, 1969.
13. Williams, C. B.; Forrest, A. P.; and Campbell, H.: Buffering capacity of food in relation to stimulation of gastric secretion. Gastroenterology 55: 567, 1968.
14. Kock, J. P., and Donaldson, R. M.: A survey of food intolerances in hospitalized patients. N. Engl. J. Med. 271: 657, 1964.
15. Tanner, N. C.: The care of peptic ulcer patients. Bristol Medicochir. J. 84: 179, 1969.
16. Buchman, E.; Kaung, D.; and Knapp, R. N.: Unrestricted diet in the treatment of duodenal ulcer. Gastroenterology 56: 1016, 1969.
17. Ingelfinger, F. J. ed.: Controversy in Internal Medicine. Philadelphia: W. B. Saunders, 1966: 159–180.

Additional References    Dotevall, G., and Walan, A.: Antacids in the treatment of peptic ulcer. Acta Med. Scand. 182: 529, 1967.

George, J. D.: Gastric acidity and motility. Am. J. Dig. Dis. 13: 376, 1968.

Kramer, P.; Kearney, M.; and Ingelfinger, F. S.: The effect of specific foods and water loading on the ileal excreta of ileostomized human subjects. Gastroenterology 42: 535, 1962.

Rae, J. W., and Allison, R. S.: The effect of diet and regular living conditions on the natural history of peptic ulcer. Q. J. Med. 22: 439, 1953.

Wintrobe, M. M.; Thorn, G. W.; Adams, R. D.; Bennet, I. L.; Braunwald, E.; Isselbacher, K. J.; and Pettersdorf, R. G., eds.: Harrison's Principles of Internal Medicine. 6th ed. New York: McGraw-Hill, 1970: 1444–55.

# Bland Diet:   Supplementary Information

Various stages of aversive and restrictive bland diets continue to be in widespread use despite the absence of any scientific basis for them [1]. Because of its protein and calcium content, milk results in increased gastric acid secretion, which often coincides with the onset of postprandial pain in persons with ulcers [2-4]. Homogenization, mincing, or pureeing of foods may actually *increase* rather than *decrease* gastric acid secretion [5]. Individuals with hiatal hernia and/or reflux esophagitis should avoid the following foods since they have been documented to cause decreased lower esophageal sphincter pressure and/or have an irritating effect on the esophageal mucosa: tomatoes, tomato juice, citrus juices, chocolate, peppermint, and excessively fatty foods [6]. Decaffeinated coffee [7], red pepper [8], and cola beverages [9] should be added to the list of foods that stimulate gastric secretion; beyond this restriction, little new information has been forthcoming to incriminate any food as a gastric irritant. Fortunately for the patients, however, effective drug therapy to reduce gastric acid secretion looms on the therapeutic horizon as an alternative to less rational forms of diet therapy [10–16].

References

1. Ingelfinger, F. J.; Ebert, R. V.; Finland, M.; and Relman, A. S.:   Controversy in Internal Medicine II. Philadelphia:   W. B. Saunders, 1974.
2. Ippoliti, A. F.; Maxwell, V.; and Isenberg, Jon I.:   The effect of various forms of milk on gastric acid secretion, studies in patients with duodenal ulcer and normal subjects.   Ann. Intern. Med. 84: 286, 1976.
3. Behar, J.; Hitchings, M.; and Smyth, R. D.:   Calcium stimulation of gastrin and gastric acid secretion; effect of small doses of calcium carbonate.   Gut 18: 442, 1977.
4. Brodie, M. J.; Ganguli, P. C.; Fine, A.; and Thomson, T. J.:   Effects of oral calcium gluconate on gastric acid secretion and serum gastrin concentration in man.   Gut 18: 111, 1977.
5. Hunt, D. R., and Forrest, A. P. M.:   The role of the antrum in determining the acid secretory response to meals of different consistency.   Gut 16: 774, 1975.
6. Castell, D. O.:   Medical measures that influence the gastroesophageal junction.   South. Med. J. 71: 26, 1978.
7. Cohen, S., and Booth, G. H.:   Gastric acid secretion and lower esophageal sphincter pressure in response to coffee and caffeine.   N. Engl. J. Med. 293: 897, 1975.
8. Solanke, T. F.:   The effect of red pepper (capsicum frutescens) on gastric acid secretion.   J. Surg. Res. 15: 385, 1973.
9. Groisser, D. S.:   A study of caffeine in tea. I. A new spectophotometric micro method. II. Concentration of caffeine in various strengths, brands, blends and types of teas.   Am. J. Clin. Nutr. 31: 1727, 1978.
10. Barbezat G. O., and Bank, S.:   Effect of prolonged cimetidine therapy on gastric acid secretion in man.   Gut 19: 151, 1978.
11. Winship, D. H.:   Cimetidine in the treatment of duodenal ulcer.   Gastroenterology 74: 402, 1978.
12. Isenberg, Jon I:   Peptic ulcer disease.   Postgrad. Med. 57: 163, Jan. 1975.
13. Celestin, L. R.; Harvey, V.; Saunders, J. H. B.; Wormsley, K. G.; Forrest, J. A. H.; Logan, R. F. A.; Sherman, J. C.; Haggie, S. J.; Wyllie, J. H.; Albinus, M.; Thompson, M. H.; Venables, C. W.; Burland, W. L.; Duncan, W. A. M.; Hawkins, B. W.; and Sharpe, P. C.:   Treatment of duodenal ulcer by metiamide.   Lancet 2: 779, 1975.

14. Ziegler, R.; Minne, H.; Hotz, J.; and Goebel, H.: Inhibition of gastric secretion in man by oral administration of calcitonin. Digestion 11: 157, 1974.
15. Wilson, D. E.; Winnan, G.; Quertermus, J.; and Tao, P.: Effects of an orally administered prostaglandin analogue (16,16-dimethyl prostaglandin $E_2$) on human gastric secretion. Gastroenterology 69: 607, 1975.
16. Isenberg, J. I.: Therapy of peptic ulcer. JAMA 233: 540, 1975.

# Tube Feedings

*Definition*    Liquid or blenderized diets designed to provide essential nutrients in a form that will easily pass through a tube.

*Characteristics of the diet*    Tube feedings can be conveyed either by the nasogastric route, via a pharyngostomy, or through a gastrostomy or jejunostomy. They may vary from a homogenized or blenderized mixture of foods selected from a normal diet to food combinations carefully formulated to meet specific therapeutic needs [1]. In addition, three basic types of commercially prepared and presterilized feedings are available: (1) milk or casein based formulas, (2) blenderized diet feedings, and (3) synthetic fiber free liquid diets. The dilution most often recommended is 1 kcal/ml; more concentrated solutions may not easily pass through the tube or may be poorly tolerated [2].

The ideal tube feeding should possess the following characteristics [2]:
1) Low cost
2) Bacteriologic safety
3) Relatively low osmolality
4) Caloric density equivalent to 1 kilocalorie per ml
5) Suitable protein–kilocalorie ratio
6) Adequate but not excessive nutrient intake with nutrients present in non toxic ratios and amounts
7) Balanced nutrient composition, including electrolyte composition, proper balance of amino acids, and well utilized supplementary sources of nutrients
8) Nutritional adequacy for short term use and when indicated for long term feeding
9) Convenience and ease of administration
10) Suitable viscosity and homogenization

*Purpose of the diet*    To provide a source of complete nutrition in a form that will easily pass through a tube in patients in whom oral feeding methods are contraindicated or not tolerated. Such a diet should adequately maintain nutritional status and physical well-being over a period of time, if necessary [3].

*Indications for use*
1. As a means of enteral alimentation when the normal swallowing mechanism has been inhibited or interfered with, as in:
   a. Head and neck surgery involving resection of muscles used in swallowing, in particular, surgical treatment of carcinoma of the maxillo-facial, pharyngeal, or cervical areas [4]
   b. Mandibular fractures
   c. In certain instances following head and neck irradiation or palliative chemotherapy [4]
   d. In severe comatose or unconscious states when the patient cannot eat [5]
   e. Following strokes, paralysis, or trauma to the oral pharyngeal cavity [5]

2. To meet the increased requirements of severly burned patients who will not or cannot consume enough food to meet their needs [6]
3. To control hypoglycemia by continuous intragastric feeding in type I glycogen storage disease [7]
4. For early feeding of low birth weight infants in an attempt to counter hypoglycemia, acidemia, and hyperbilirubinemia and to support brain growth [8]. However, this clinical application is a controversial one because of potential hazards involved [9].

The choice of a tube feeding to meet the specific needs of the patient should be made only with an understanding of the patient's physical condition, including any abnormalities in his metabolic profile, and should be preceded by a detailed study of the previous diet and his tolerance to it. Results of fat tolerance and lactose tolerance tests are of particular value, as are, among, others, determinations of blood urea nitrogen, hemoglobin, hematocrit, glucose levels, serum cholesterol, albumin, sodium, potassium, iron, zinc, magnesium, vitamin $B_{12}$ and osmolality, urinary calcium, forminoglutamic acid and osmolality [10].

***Possible adverse reactions*** *Diarrhea* Diarrhea complicating a tube feeding can be either bacterial or osmotic in origin. Nausea and vomiting may also occur. Pain and diarrhea can also occur if a nasogastric tube is passed into the duodenum. The use of too concentrated a solution or one that is very hypertonic, particularly when given rapidly, will cause an influx of water into the intestine and produce a watery diarrhea. Excessive sugars, free amino acids, and excess electrolytes all contribute to increased osmolality, causing diarrhea and dehydration [2]. The large amounts of lactose present in certain milk based tube feedings may also precipitate an osmotic diarrhea [11].

In addition, improper handling or unsanitary practices may cause bacterial contamination of the feeding. Tube feedings provide an excellent medium for bacterial growth, and for this reason presterilized, canned tube feedings may be more desirable than other types [12].

*Hypertonicity* Hypertonicity due to solute loading may occur as a result of inadequate water intake in patients receiving feeding mixtures that are too high in protein and electrolytes in relation to their water content [13]. Unless the kidney can excrete urine of very high specific gravity and eliminate the excess urea and electrolytes in a volume of water smaller than that administered, both hypernatremia and azotemia will result [14]. In severely affected patients the serum sodium level may reach 170 meq/litre as compared to the normal 138–45 meq/litre [13]. Thus, high protein tube feedings with high osmolar loads may actually hinder nutrition; if the patient cannot adequately excrete the increased nitrogen load, he will develop a water deficit and hypernatremia. Patients with a decrease in body fluid have decreased skin turgor and dry mucous membranes. Dry, sticky membranes may reflect sodium excess [15]. All tube fed patients should be given additional water, as an inadequate water intake produces serious consequences. Serious losses of water and electrolytes may result with tube feeding in patients with serious malabsorption secondary to bowel fistulas or damaged or resected small intestines [16].

*Fluid overload or overhydration* The use of large amounts of water to clear tubing after each feeding or to dilute a mixture may result in fluid overload or overhydration. Decreases in levels of serum osmolality, serum sodium, blood urea nitrogen, and hematocrit occur in tube fed patients who are over-hydrated [15,17]. On the other hand, increases in these levels above the normal range suggest dehydration. Flat neck veins are associated with an increase of extracellular fluid [15].

*Intestinal perforation* Intestinal perforation is a hazard of nasojejunal feeding of young infants, particularly if polyvinyl feeding tubes are used. It has been suggested that these tubes become hard and less pliable after a time in the intestine [18].

*Changes in duodenal microflora and enterocolitis* Qualitative changes in the duodenal microflora of young infants may occur after long-term intubation; bacterial con-tamination of the upper small intestine may result [19]. Neonatal staphylococcal enterocolitis has been reported in infants in whom a nasogastric or gastric catheter was inserted through a site colonized by staphylococcus aureus [20].

*Aspiration pneumonia* There is a risk of aspiration pneumonia as a result of regurgitation of stomach contents in tube fed patients who are comatose [21]. The potential hazard is increased in debilitated patients having depressed cough reflexes, particularly when there is a preexisting pulmonary problem [16]. In elderly or unconscious patients, elevation of the head of the bed of an angle of 30° may prevent the occurrence of this complica-tion. It may also be wise to discontinue feeding at night in elderly or very weak patients who may aspirate if supine [21].

*Nausea* Nausea in a tube fed patient can be the result of improper location of the tube tip, exces-sive rate of feeding, feeding too large a volume, feeding too soon after intubation, or anxiety.

*Esophagitis and esophageal stricture* Because of prolonged use of large caliber feeding tubes via nasopha-ryngeal tube or esophagostomy tube [16].

*Hyperosmolar nonketatic coma* Can occur in individuals with diabetes fed excessively high car-bohydrate containing formulas when adequate precautions are not taken [16].

*Metabolic derangements in patients with renal or hepatic disorders* [16].

*Inadequate dietary selenium intake* A recent analysis of twenty formulas designed for adult use con-cluded that only 3 of them provided an amount of selenium similar to that consumed in a typical U. S. diet. [22].

**Contraindications** Tube feedings are contraindicated in pa-tients who develop intestinal obstructions [16] or paralytic ileus, such as certain severely burned patients [6] or postoperative patients who have no evidence of restored peristaltic function. Any form of enteral alimentation is contraindicated until peristalsis is reestablished, and bowel sounds are heard with the aid of a stethoscope.

*Suggestions for dietitians*      *Hints for planning and implementation of tube feedings*      In general the diet should be planned so that nor more than 20% of the total kilocalories are derived from protein; a higher protein intake will result in excessively high solute loads requiring excretion by the kidney [2,23]. Patients receiving synthetic diets with the protein in the form of free amino acids will often be able to tolerate even less protein. Care should be taken in planning or choosing a tube feeding for a person with diabetes so that the carbohydrate content is not disproportionately high. One suggested guide is that the feeding have a caloric distribution of approximately 40% fat [5]. Special attention should be given to proper sanitary practices in the preparation, storage, handling, and administration of tube feeding mixtures. Raw eggs should never be used as part of the diet because of the danger of a salmonella infection. The unused portion of any feeding that is in an opened can or has been made or mixed in the institution should be discarded within 24 hours. Enteral hyperalimentation or large amounts of nutrients in excess of varied requirements is facilitated by a special pump or by a simple apparatus specially designed for this purpose [24]. Detailed explanations of the proper administration of tube feedings have been published elsewhere [4,25,26].

Continuous pump infusion of liquid diets through a small caliber feeding tube into the distal duodenum or proximal jejunum is superior to previous methods of bolus tube feedings through a large tube into the stomach [27]. The lower the osmolality of the formula, the more rapidly the infusion may be given [28]. Jejunostostomy feedings should be isotonic and administered more slowly then nasogastric feedings because diarrhea and gastric regurgitation are common with their use [26].

Tube feedings should not be warmed before use. A cold formula can be fed without problems if administered slowly. Warming the mixture may result in destruction of water soluble vitamins, coagulation of proteins, clogging of nasogastric tubes, coagulation of the formula, or more rapid growth of bacteria.

*Monitoring the effects of the tube feeding*      Total water intake in all tube fed patients should be monitored carefully on a daily basis. Particularly when synthetic diets with a high osmolality are used as tube feedings, care should be taken to assure that an adequate fluid intake is provided. A daily record of the intake of all nutrients, including water, should be kept. Reduced or missing nutrients or an intake rendered inadequate by excessive dilution or poor tolerance should be brought to the physician's attention and recorded in the medical record [2,29,30].

# Composition of Some Commonly Used Commercial Tube Feedings

## MILK OR CASEIN BASED FEEDINGS

| Product | Manufacturer | Caloric distribution (%) | Composition | Remarks |
|---|---|---|---|---|
| **Sustagen** (powder)<br><br>1 lb cans<br>2½ lb cans<br>5 lb cans | Mead Johnson and Co., Evansville, IN 47721 | 24 protein<br>8 fat<br>68 carbohydrate | Corn syrup solids, concentrated skim milk, powdered whole milk, calcium caseinate, dextrose, vanilla flavor, lecithin, vitamins and minerals; chocolate flavor also contains sucrose and cocoa | Used as oral or tube feeding<br>Recommended dilution for oral use: 1:1 with water<br>A high protein, high carbohydrate, low fat feeding<br>When used as tube feeding, use with caution |
| **Meritene** (powder)<br><br>1.14 oz envelopes<br>1 lb cans<br>4½ lb cans | Doyle Pharmaceutical Co., Minneapolis, MN 55416 | When mixed with skim milk:<br>36 protein<br>2 fat<br>62 carbohydrate<br>When mixed with whole milk:<br>26 protein<br>29 fat<br>45 carbohydrate | Specially processed nonfat dry milk, corn syrup solids, natural and artificial flavors, lecithin, vitamins and minerals | Recommended dilution 4 level tbsp powder to 8 oz skim or 8 oz whole milk or 1 envelope to 8 oz milk powder<br>When used as tube feeding, use with caution |
| **Meritene** (liquid)<br><br>10 oz (300 ml) cans | Doyle Pharmaceutical Co. | 24 protein<br>30 fat<br>46 carbohydrate | Concentrated sweet milk, corn syrup solids, vegetable oil, sodium caseinate, sucrose, natural and artificial flavoring, salt, stabilizers, vitamins and minerals | Used as oral or tube feeding<br>Ready to serve<br>Presterilized<br>A high protein feeding |
| **Sustacal** (liquid)<br><br>12 oz cans (360 ml) cans<br>12 cans per case | Mead Johnson and Co. | 24 protein<br>21 fat<br>55 carbohydrate | Sugar, concentrated sweet skim milk, corn syrup solids, partially hydrogenated soy oil, sodium caseinate, calcium caseinate, soy protein isolate, artificial flavor, vegetable stabilizers, vitamins and minerals | Used as oral or tube feeding<br>Should be diluted when used by tube to ½ strength on the first day and ¾ strength on the second day in order to permit the body to adjust to the protein load<br>Ready to serve<br>Presterilized<br>6 g lactose per 12 oz of a high protein feeding |
| **Sustacal** (powder)<br><br>1.9 oz packets<br><br>In units of 4, 12 units per case | Mead Johnson and Co. | When mixed with 8 oz whole milk:<br>24 protein<br>21 fat<br>55 carbohydrate | Nonfat dry milk, sugar, corn syrup solids, artificial flavor, vitamins and minerals | Recommended dilution: 1.9 oz packet per 8 oz whole milk<br>30.9 g lactose when mixed with 8 oz whole milk |
| **Isocal**<br><br>8 fl oz cans<br>12 fl oz cans<br>12 cans per case<br><br>Also in tube feeding sets | Mead Johnson and Co. | 13 protein<br>37 fat<br>50 carbohydrate<br>7 kilocalories as MCT<br>30 kilocalories as soy oil | Corn syrup solids, soy oil, calcium caseinate, sodium caseinate, soy protein isolate, lecithin, vitamins and minerals plus MCT oil | Ready to serve<br>Presterilized<br>Lactose free<br>Contains MCT |

## MILK OR CASEIN BASED FEEDINGS

| Product | Manufacturer | Caloric distribution (%) | Composition | Remarks |
|---|---|---|---|---|
| **Nutri-1000**<br><br>32 oz (960 ml)<br>cans<br>6 cans per<br>case | Cutter Laboratories,<br>Berkeley, CA 94710 | 17 protein<br>39 fat<br>44 carbohydrate | Skim milk, sucrose, soy oil, hydrogenated coconut oil, dextrinmaltose, mono- and diglycerides, soy lecithin, vanilla extract, salts, vitamins and minerals | Used as oral or tube feeding<br>Ready to serve<br>Presterilized<br>5.3 g lactose per 100 ml<br>Renal solute load:<br>230 mOsm/litre |
| **Nutri-1000<br>LF** | Cutter Laboratories | Vanilla flavor:<br>17 protein<br>39 fat<br>44 carbohydrate | Water, corn syrup solids, corn oil, sugar, calcium caseinate, soybean oil (partially saturated), mono- and triglycerides, potassium citrate, soy lecithin, calcium citrate calcium carrageenan, artificial flavor | Lactose free<br>Ready to serve |
| **Ensure**<br><br>8 oz cans<br>32 oz cans<br>8 oz tube-<br>feeding sets | Ross Laboratories,<br>Columbus, OH 43216 | 14 protein<br>31 fat<br>55 carbohydrate | Water, corn syrup solids, sucrose, corn oil, sodium caseinate, calcium caseinate, soy protein isolate, potassium citrate, magnesium chloride, soy lecithin, carrageenan, artificial flavoring, vitamins and minerals | Used as oral or tube feeding<br>Ready to serve<br>Presterilized<br>Lactose free<br>Low in iodine |
| **Ensure Plus**<br><br>8 oz cans<br>32 oz cans | Ross Laboratories | 15 protein<br>32 fat<br>53 carbohydrate | Water, corn syrup solids, sodium and calcium caseinates, corn oil, sucrose, soy protein isolate, potassium citrate, magnesium chloride, calcium carbonate, soy lecithin, vitamins and minerals, carrageenan, artificial flavoring | Ready to serve<br>Used as oral or tube feeding<br>Vanilla flavor<br>1.5 kcal/ml |
| **Ensure Plus<br>Osmolyte** | Ross Laboratories | 14 protein<br>32 fat (15 MCT)<br>54 carbohydrate | Water, corn syrup solids, sodium and calcium caseinates, medium chain triglycerides, corn oil, soy protein isolate, soy oil, potassium citrate, soy lecithin, vitamins and minerals, carrageenan | Lactose free<br>Low residue<br>Contains glucose polymers—less sweet than similar products<br>Useful in certain types of fat malabsorption |
| **Support-M<br>#325**<br><br>12 fl oz bottles | Hospital Diet Products<br>Corp., Buena Park, CA<br>90621 | 12 protein<br>36 fat<br>52 carbohydrate | Water, sucrose, corn syrup solids, soy oil, nonfat dry milk, modified whey powder, soy protein isolate, artificial flavor, mono- and diglycerides, vitamins and minerals | Used as oral or tube feeding<br>A blend of various foods to meet U.S. RDA for protein and all essential vitamins in 1,800 kcal (5 bottles) |
| **Low Sodium<br>Provida<br>#128**<br><br>12 fl oz bottles | Hospital Diet Products<br>Corp. | 24 protein<br>27 fat<br>49 carbohydrate | Water, sucrose, low sodium nonfat dry milk, calcium caseinate, corn syrup solids, soy oil, coconut oil, artificial flavor, mono- and diglycerides, vitamins and minerals | Ready to serve |

**Composition of Some Commonly Used Commercial Tube Feedings** *(Continued)*

BLENDERIZED DIET FEEDINGS

| Product | Manufacturer | Caloric distribution (%) | Composition | Remarks |
|---|---|---|---|---|
| **Formula 2**<br><br>6.75 fl oz or<br>200 ml jars | Cutter Laboratories | 15 protein<br>36 fat<br>49 carbohydrate | Water, nonfat dry milk, beef, sucrose, carrots, corn oil, orange juice concentrate, egg yolks, green beans, farina, cellulose gum, magnesium sulfate, artificial flavor, sodium ascorbate, vitamins and minerals | 3.74% lactose or 7.48 g/200 ml<br>Ready to serve<br>Presterilized |
| **Vitaneed**<br><br>12 fl oz bottles | Hospital Diet Products Corp. | 14 protein<br>35 fat<br>51 carbohydrate | Water, corn syrup solids, puree beef, soy oil, puree green beans, puree peaches, sucrose, soy protein isolate, puree carrots, mono- and diglycerides, propylene glycol alginate, vitamins and minerals | Used as oral or tube feeding<br>Low cholesterol<br>Lactose free |
| **Compleat B**<br><br>13.6 oz<br>(400 ml) cans | Doyle Pharmaceutical Co. | 16 protein<br>36 fat<br>48 carbohydrate | Deionized water, beef puree, maltodextrin, green bean puree, pea puree, nonfat dry milk, corn oil, sucrose, peach puree, orange juice, sodium tripolyphosphate, lecithin, carrageenan, vitamins and minerals | Ready to serve<br>Presterilized |
| **Carnacal #145**<br><br>12 fl oz bottles | Hospital Diet Products Corp. | 16 protein<br>36 fat<br>48 carbohydrate | Water, corn syrup solids, puree beef, sucrose, soy oil, puree green beans, puree peaches, nonfat dry milk, modified whey powder, soy protein isolate, mono- and diglycerides, vitamins and minerals | Ready to use |

SOY-WHEY-MEAT BASED FEEDINGS

| Product | Manufacturer | Caloric distribution (%) | Composition | Remarks |
|---|---|---|---|---|
| **Vital** | Ross Laboratories | 17 protein<br>9 fat<br>74 carbohydrate | Glucose oligo- and polysaccharides, enzymatically hydrolyzed proteins (soy, whey, and meat), sucrose, cornstarch, sunflower oil, dipotassium phosphate, calcium glycerophosphate, natural and artificial banana and vanilla flavor, 1-amino acids, vitamins and minerals, ferrous gluconate | Used as oral or tube feeding 91% nitrogen derived from partially hydrolyzed whey, soy, and beef protein (⅓ from each) with remaining 9% as essential amino acids |

SOY BASED FEEDINGS

| Product | Manufacturer | Caloric distribution (%) | Composition | Remarks |
|---|---|---|---|---|
| **Renu** | Hospital Diet Products Corp. | 13 protein<br>36 fat<br>51 carbohydrate | Water, corn syrup solids, soy oil, soy protein isolate, sucrose, oat powder, artificial flavor, mono- and diglycerides. 1-methionine, vitamins and minerals | Osmolality of 345 mOsm/kg water<br>Lactose free<br>Ready to use |

Composition of Commercially Available Tube Feedings per 100 ml

| | Sustacal* | Isocal* | Liquid Meritene† | Nutri-1000‡ | Compleat B† | Formula 2‡ | Ensure§ | Renu⊥ | Nutri-1000 LF‡ |
|---|---|---|---|---|---|---|---|---|---|
| Osmolality (mOsm per litre) | Vanilla 650 Choc. 650 | 300 | Vanilla 560 Choc. 610 | 500 | 390 | 435–510 | 450 | 345 | 380 |
| Kilocalories per ml | 1.00 | 1.06 | 1.00 | 1.06 | 1.00 | 1.00 | 1.06 | 1.00 | 1.06 |
| Protein (g) | 6.03 | 3.42 | 6.00 | 4.00 | 4.00 | 3.75 | 3.67 | 3.33 | 3.94 |
| Fat (g) | 2.30 | 4.46 | 3.30 | 5.50 | 4.00 | 4.00 | 3.67 | 3.89 | 12.35 |
| Carbohydrate (g) | 13.80 | 13.00 | 11.50 | 10.10 | 12.00 | 12.20 | 14.29 | 13.06 | 9.98 |
| Vitamin A (IU) | 463.90 | 264.00 | 416.67 | 260.00 | 312.00 | 250.00 | 260.42 | 323.89 | 260.42 |
| Vitamin D (IU) | 36.90 | 21.00 | 33.30 | 21.00 | 25.00 | 24.00 | 20.83 | 27.78 | 20.83 |
| Vitamin E (IU) | 2.80 | 4.00 | 2.50 | 1.57 | 1.90 | 2.10 | 3.13 | 1.83 | 1.56 |
| Ascorbic acid (mg) | 5.60 | 15.80 | 7.50 | 4.67 | 5.60 | 3.90 | 15.62 | 5.83 | 4.69 |
| Folic acid (mg) | 0.04 | 0.02 | 0.03 | 0.02 | 0.02 | 0.02 | 0.02 | 0.04 | 0.02 |
| Thiamine (mg) | 0.14 | 0.20 | 0.19 | 0.11 | 0.14 | 0.08 | 0.16 | 0.14 | 0.10 |
| Riboflavin (mg) | 0.17 | 0.23 | 0.22 | 0.11 | 0.16 | 0.08 | 0.18 | 0.16 | 0.10 |
| Niacin (mg) | 1.94 | 2.60 | 1.67 | 1.03 | 1.25 | 1.00 | 2.08 | 1.47 | 1.04 |
| Vitamin $B_6$ (mg) | 0.19 | 0.26 | 0.25 | 0.11 | 0.19 | 0.14 | 0.20 | 0.17 | 0.10 |
| Vitamin $B_{12}$ ($\mu$g) | 0.60 | 0.80 | 0.50 | 0.32 | 0.38 | 0.30 | 0.63 | 0.44 | 0.31 |
| Biotin (mg) | 0.03 | 0.02 | 0.02 | 0.02 | 0.02 | — | 0.02 | 0.03 | 0.02 |
| Pantothenic acid (mg) | 0.97 | 1.32 | 0.83 | 0.53 | 0.62 | 0.48 | 0.52 | 0.72 | 0.52 |
| Calcium (mg) | 100.00 | 63.60 | 125.00 | 119.60 | 62.50 | 110.00 | 52.08 | 36.94 | 52.08 |
| Phosphorus (mg) | 91.70 | 53.00 | 125.00 | 93.60 | 168.80 | 95.00 | 52.08 | 41.67 | 52.08 |
| Iodine ($\mu$g) | 13.90 | 8.10 | 12.50 | 7.80 | 9.38 | 7.50 | 7.81 | 13.89 | 7.81 |
| Iron (mg) | 1.67 | 0.95 | 1.50 | 0.93 | 1.10 | 1.26 | 0.94 | 1.19 | 0.94 |
| Magnesium (mg) | 37.50 | 21.20 | 33.30 | 20.83 | 25.00 | 20.00 | 20.83 | 27.78 | 20.83 |
| Copper (mg) | 0.19 | 0.11 | 0.17 | 0.11 | 0.12 | 0.10 | 0.10 | 0.17 | 0.10 |
| Zinc (mg) | 1.39 | 1.05 | 1.25 | 0.77 | 0.94 | 0.75 | 1.56 | 0.92 | 0.78 |
| Manganese (mg) | 0.28 | 0.25 | 0.33 | 0.13 | 0.25 | 0.02 | 0.21 | — | 0.13 |
| Potassium (mg) | 205.60 | 132.50 | 166.70 | 133.33 | 130.00 | 191.00 | 125.00 | 46.11 | 145.83 |
| Sodium (mg) | 92.50 | 53.00 | 91.70 | 52.08 | 156.20 | 63.00 | 72.91 | 64.72 | 70.83 |
| Vitamin $K_1$ ($\mu$g) | — | 13.25 | — | 9.00 | — | — | 98.95 | — | 15.63 |
| Choline (mg) | — | 26.50 | 8.30 | 19.79 | 18.80 | — | 52.08 | — | 19.79 |
| Chloride (mg) | — | 106.00 | 166.70 | 120.00 | 80.00 | 190.00 | 104.16 | — | — |

* Mead Johnson and Co., Evansville, IN 47721.
† Doyle Pharmaceutical Co., Minneapolis, MN 55416.
‡ Cutter Laboratories, Berkeley, CA 94710.
§ Ross Laboratories, Columbus, OH 43216.
⊥ Hospital Diet Products Corp., Buena Park, CA 90621.

**Composition of Commercially Available Tube Feedings per 100 ml** *(Continued)*

| | Ensure Plus§ | Ensure Plus Osmolyte§ | Vital§ | Low Sodium Provida #128⊥ | Support-M #325⊥ | Carnacal #145⊥ | Vitaneed⊥ |
|---|---|---|---|---|---|---|---|
| Osmolality (mOsm per litre) | 600 | 300 | 450 | 628 | 475 | 625 | 435 |
| Kilocalories per ml | 1.50 | 1.06 | 1.00 | 1.00 | 1.00 | 1.00 | 1.02 |
| Protein (g) | 5.42 | 3.67 | 4.20 | 6.00 | 3.00 | 4.00 | 3.50 |
| Fat (g) | 5.25 | 3.79 | 1.00 | 3.00 | 4.00 | 4.00 | 4.00 |
| Carbohydrate (g) | 19.71 | 14.30 | 18.50 | 12.00 | 13.00 | 12.20 | 13.00 |
| Vitamin A (IU) | 260.42 | 260.42 | 333.30 | 500.00 | 350.00 | 400.00 | 350.00 |
| Vitamin D (IU) | 20.83 | 20.83 | 26.70 | 40.00 | 30.00 | 30.00 | 25.00 |
| Vitamin E (IU) | 4.69 | 3.12 | 2.00 | 3.00 | 2.50 | 2.00 | 3.00 |
| Ascorbic acid (mg) | 15.63 | 16.66 | 6.00 | 7.50 | 6.50 | 7.50 | 7.50 |
| Folic acid (mg) | 0.02 | 0.02 | 0.03 | 0.04 | 0.04 | 0.04 | 0.04 |
| Thiamine (mg) | 0.26 | 0.16 | 0.10 | 0.15 | 0.15 | 0.15 | 0.13 |
| Riboflavin (mg) | 0.27 | 0.18 | 0.11 | 0.18 | 0.17 | 0.17 | 0.15 |
| Niacin (mg) | 3.13 | 2.08 | 1.33 | 2.00 | 2.00 | 1.80 | 1.80 |
| Vitamin $B_6$ (mg) | 0.31 | 0.21 | 0.13 | 0.20 | 0.20 | 0.20 | 0.20 |
| Vitamin $B_{12}$ ($\mu$g) | 0.94 | 0.63 | 0.40 | 0.50 | 0.50 | 0.50 | 0.50 |
| Biotin (mg) | 0.03 | 0.02 | 0.02 | 0.04 | 0.03 | 0.03 | 0.02 |
| Pantothenic acid (mg) | 0.83 | 0.52 | 0.67 | 1.00 | 0.80 | 1.00 | 0.80 |
| Calcium (mg) | 62.50 | 54.16 | 70.00 | 145.00 | 46.00 | 72.00 | 57.50 |
| Phosphorus (mg) | 62.50 | 54.16 | 70.00 | 85.00 | 44.00 | 71.00 | 52.50 |
| Iodine ($\mu$g) | 10.42 | 7.92 | 10.00 | 15.00 | 15.00 | 15.00 | 15.00 |
| Iron (mg) | 1.41 | 0.92 | 1.20 | 1.80 | 1.30 | 1.50 | 1.20 |
| Magnesium (mg) | 31.25 | 20.83 | 26.70 | 40.00 | 35.00 | 30.00 | 30.00 |
| Copper (mg) | 0.16 | 0.10 | 0.13 | 0.25 | 0.20 | 0.20 | 0.15 |
| Zinc (mg) | 2.35 | 1.54 | 1.00 | 1.50 | 1.00 | 1.00 | 1.00 |
| Manganese (mg) | 0.21 | 0.21 | 0.13 | — | — | — | — |
| Potassium (mg) | 187.50 | 87.50 | 120.00 | 155.00 | 67.00 | 115.00 | 65.00 |
| Sodium (mg) | 104.16 | 54.16 | 40.00 | 32.50 | 62.50 | 110.00 | 55.00 |
| Vitamin $K_1$ ($\mu$g) | 158.33 | 100.00 | 0.13 | — | — | — | — |
| Choline (mg) | 52.08 | 54.16 | 13.30 | — | — | — | — |
| Chloride (mg) | 158.33 | 79.16 | 70.00 | — | — | — | — |

§ Ross Laboratories, Columbus, OH 43216.
⊥ Hospital Diet Products Corp., Buena Park, CA 90621.

**Sodium-Restricted Blenderized Tube Feeding**

***Description***    Foods low in sodium content are blenderized to a consistency which will pass through a nasogastric tube or pour into a gastrostomy tube. To prevent solute loading, the average patient requires ½ ml water/ml tube feeding, given at the same time as the tube feeding. For optimal protein utilization, the tube feeding provides approximately 25 non-protein kilocalories per gram of protein.

This formula is not suitable for jejunostomy feeding. Diarrhea may result from insufficient water and/or lactose intolerance.

***Order as***    Sodium Restricted Blenderized Tube Feeding ml per day. A minimum of 2,000 ml/day (2,000 kcal, 20 meq Na) is recommended.

***Approximate composition***

|  | 1 litre | 2 litres | 3 litres |
|---|---|---|---|
| Kilocalories | 1,000 | 2,000 | 3,000 |
| Carbohydrate | 124 g | 248 g | 372 g |
| Protein | 32 g | 65 g | 97 g |
| Fat | 48 g | 96 g | 144 g |
| Calcium | 492 mg | 984 mg | 1,475 mg |
| Iron | 15 mg | 29 mg | 44 mg |
| Sodium | 10 meq (231 mg) | 20 meq (463 mg) | 30 meq (695 mg) |
| Potassium | 25 meq (964 mg) | 49 meq (1,928 mg) | 74 meq (2,893 mg) |
| Magnesium* | 6 meq | 12 meq | 18 meq |
| Vitamin A | 5,750 IU | 11,500 IU | 17,250 IU |
| Vitamin C | 62 mg | 124 mg | 186 mg |
| Vitamin D | 100 IU | 200 IU | 300 IU |
| Thiamine | 459 $\mu$g | 917 $\mu$g | 1,376 $\mu$g |
| Riboflavin | 760 $\mu$g | 1,520 $\mu$g | 2,280 $\mu$g |
| Niacin | 7 mg | 14 mg | 21 mg |
| Cholesterol | 75 mg | 150 mg | 225 mg |
| Fiber | 0.5 g | 1 g | 1.5 g |
| Lactose | 12 g | 24 g | 36 g |
| Osmolality* | 410 mOsm | 410 mOsm | 410 mOsm |
| Osmolality (plus 500 ml water/litre)* | 300 mOsm | 300 mOsm | 300 mOsm |
| Sucrose | Insignificant amounts | | |

\* Values determined by Rhode Island Hospital Laboratory, 1969.
*Source*:  Reprinted from Manual of Surgical Nutrition [31].
*Notes*:   The 1980 RDA include recommendations for vitamin E, phosphorus, magnesium, and zinc. These diets have not been analyzed for these substances. Blenderized tube feedings may be calculated with restrictions in protein and potassium.

**Formula for Tube Feeding**

|  | 1 litre | 2 litres | 3 litres |
|---|---|---|---|
| SF instant Cream of Wheat, cooked | 115 g | 230 g | 345 g |
| SF strained beef | 100 g | 200 g | 300 g |
| Unsweetened frozen orange juice | 120 ml | 240 ml | 360 ml |
| SF strained carrots | 50 g | 100 g | 150 g |
| Fortified instant nonfat milk powder | 23 g | 46 g | 69 g |
| SF bread | 50 g | 100 g | 150 g |
| Corn syrup | 70 g | 140 g | 210 g |
| Corn oil | 40 g | 80 g | 120 g |
| Water is added to reach the desired volume. | | | |

*Notes*:  Values determined by Rhode Island Hospital Laboratory, 1969.
SF = salt free.

*CAUTION: The 1980 Recommended Daily Dietary Allowances of the National Research Council are not met by this diet for:*

### 1 litre

| | |
|---|---|
| Kilocalories | Children, males, females, and pregnant and lactating women |
| Protein | Children 7 to 10 years of age |
| | Males, females, and pregnant and lactating women |
| Niacin | Children 1 to 10 years of age |
| | Males, females, and pregnant and lactating women |
| Riboflavin | Children 4 to 10 years of age |
| | Males, females, and pregnant and lactating women |
| Thiamine | Children, males, females, and pregnant and lactating women |
| Calcium | Children, males, females, and pregnant and lactating women |
| Iron | Males 11 to 18 years of age |
| | Females 11 to 22 years of age |
| | Pregnant and lactating women |

### 2 litres

| | |
|---|---|
| Kilocalories | Children 7 to 10 years of age |
| | Males |
| | Females 11 to 22 years of age |
| | Pregnant and lactating women |
| Thiamine | Children 7 to 10 years of age |
| | Males, females, and pregnant and lactating women |
| Calcium | Males 11 to 18 years of age |
| | Females 11 to 18 years of age |
| | Pregnant and lactating women |

## Protein Restricted Formula

DESCRIPTION: This tube feeding contains approximately 15 g protein per litre.

ADEQUACY: This feeding fails to meet the Recommended Dietary Allowances for all nutrients except kilocalories and fat.

APPROXIMATE NUTRITIVE VALUE OF 1 LITRE OF FORMULA:

| | | | |
|---|---|---|---|
| Kilocalories | 1,000.0 | Thiamine (mg) | 0.4 |
| Protein (g) | 15.0 | Riboflavin (mg) | 0.7 |
| Fat (g) | 45.0 | Niacin equiv. (mg) | 1.5 |
| Carbohydrate (g) | 140.0 | Ascorbic acid (mg) | 50.0 |
| Calcium (mg) | 300.0 | Vitamin D (IU) | 55.0 |
| Iron (mg) | 5.0 | Sodium (mg) | 300.0 |
| Vitamin A (IU) | 1,400.0 | Potassium (mg) | 1,000.0 |

INGREDIENTS IN 1 LITRE OF FORMULA (g):

| | |
|---|---|
| Milk | 244 |
| Cooked enriched farina | 200 |
| Grape juice | 100 |
| Dextrose | 40 |
| Pureed vegetable | 100 |
| Pureed fruit | 200 |
| Orange juice | 100 |
| Vegetable oil | 35 |

Ingredients are blended at high speed until mixture is of a thick pouring consistency.

*Source*: Adapted from Recent Advances in Therapeutic Diets [32].

## Approximate Kilocalorie: Nitrogen Ratios of Some Common Tube Feedings

| | Total kcal:nitrogen ratio | Nonprotein kcal:nitrogen ratio |
|---|---|---|
| Vitaneed | 180 | 160 |
| Carnacal ( #145) | 160 | 135 |
| Support-M ( #325) | 210 | 185 |
| Low Sodium Provida ( #128) | 105 | 80 |
| Ensure | 180 | 155 |
| Ensure Plus | 170 | 145 |
| Nutri-1000 | 165 | 140 |
| Nutri-1000 LF | 265 | 240 |
| Isocal | 190 | 165 |
| Meritene | 105 | 80 |
| Compleat B | 155 | 130 |
| Sustacal | 105 | 80 |
| Formula 2 | 165 | 140 |
| Renu | 190 | 165 |
| Ensure Plus Osmolyte | 180 | 155 |
| Vital | 150 | 125 |

## References

1. Turner, D.: Handbook of Diet Therapy. 5th ed. Chicago: University of Chicago Press, 1970.
2. Gormican, A., and Liddy, E.: Nasogastric tube feedings: practical considerations in prescription and evaluation. Postgrad. Med. 53: 71, 1973.
3. Gormican, A.; Liddy, E.; and Thrush, L. B.: Nutritional status of patients after extended tube feeding. J. Am. Diet. Assoc. 63: 247, 1973.
4. Noone, R. B., and Graham, W. P. III: Nutritional care after head and neck surgery. Postgrad. Med. 53: 80, 1973.
5. Kaiser, C. M.: Nutritional care of patients receiving tube feedings. Chicago: American Dietetic Association, 1969.
6. Love, R. T.: Nutrition in the burned patient. J. Miss. State Med. Assoc. 13: 391, 1972.
7. Burr, I. M.; O'Neil, J. A.; Karzon, D. T.; Howard, L. J.; and Greene, H. L.: Comparison of the effects of total parenteral nutrition, continuous intragastric feeding, and portacaval shunt on a patient with type I glycogen storage disease. J. Pediatr. 85: 792, 1974.
8. Landwirth, J.: Continuous nasogastric infusion feedings of infants of low birth weight. Clin. Pediatr. 13: 603, 1974.
9. Chen, J. W., and Wong, P. W. K.: Intestinal complications of nasojejunal feeding in low birth weight infants. J. Pediatr. 85: 109, 1974.
10. Gormican, A.: Tube feeding. Dietetic Currents 2(2), April, May, June, 1975.
11. Walike, J. W., and Walike, B. C.: Lactose content of tube feeding diets as a cause of diarrhea. Laryngoscope 83: 1109, 1973.
12. Gormican, A.: Prepackaged tube feedings. Hospitals 44: 58, September 1, 1970.
13. Randall, H. T.: Nutrition in the care of the surgical patient. Goodhart, R. S., and Shils, M. E., eds. Modern Nutrition in Health and Disease. Philadelphia: Lea & Febiger, 1973.
14. McCarter, D.: Nourishing the solute sensitive patient. Am. J. Nurs. 73: 1935, 1973.
15. Grant, M. M., and Kubo, W. M.: Assessing a patient's hydration status. Am. J. Nurs. 75: 1306, 1975.
16. Shils, M. E.: Enteral nutrition by tube. Cancer Res. 57: 2432, 1977.
17. Kubo, W.; Grant, M.; Walike, B.; Bergstrom, N.; Wong, H.; Hanson, R.; and Padilla, G.: Fluid and electrolyte problems of tube-fed patients. Am. J. Nurs. 76: 912, 1976.
18. Boros, S. J., and Reynolds, J. W.: Duodenal perforation: a complication of neonatal nasojejunal feeding. J. Pediatr. 85: 107, 1974.
19. Challacombe, D.: Bacterial microflora in infants receiving nasojejunal tube feeding. J. Pediatr. 85: 113, 1974.
20. Gutman, L. T.; Idriss, Z. H.; Gehlbach, S.; and Blackmon, L.: Neonatal staphylococcal enterocolitis: association with indwelling feeding catheters and S. aureus colonization. J. Pediatr. 88: 836, 1976.
21. Dhar, P.; Zamcheck, N.; and Broitman, S. A.: Nutrition in diseases of the pancreas. Goodhart, R. S., and Shils, M. E., eds. Modern Nutrition in Health and Disease. Philadelphia: Lea & Febiger, 1973.

22. Zabel, N. L.; Harland, J.; Gormican, A. T.; and Ganther, H. E.: Selenium content of commercial formula diets. Am. J. Clin. Nutr. 31: 850, 1978.
23. Mason, E. E.: Fluid Electrolyte and Nutrient Therapy in Surgery. Philadelphia: Lea & Febiger, 1974.
24. Gougeon, F. W.: Enteral hyperalimentation: a new apparatus for administration. Surgery 79: 697, 1976.
25. Kaminski, M. W.: Tube Feeding: Tips and Techniques. Norwich: Eaton Laboratories, 1973.
26. Fischer, J. E.: Parental and enteral nutrition. Dis. Month. 24 (9): 3, 1978.
27. Dobbie, R., and Butterick, D. D.: Continuous pump/tube enteric hyperalimentation. Use in esophageal disease. JPEN 1: 100, 1977.
28. Shils, M. E.; Bloch, A. S.; and Chernoff, R.: Liquid formulas for oral and tube feeding. JPEN 1: 89, 1977.
29. Padilla, G. V.; Grant, M.; Wong, H.; Hansen, B. W.; Hanson, R. L.; Bergstron, N.; and Kubo, W. R.: Subjective distresses of nasogastric tube feeding. Gastroenterology 3: 53, 1979.
30. Heymsfield, S. B.; Bethel, R. A.; Ansley, J. D.; Nixon, D. W.; and Rudman, D.: Enteral Hyperalimentation: An alternative to central venous hyperalimentation. Ann. Inter. Med. 90: 63, 1979.
31. Ballinger, W. F.; Collins, J. A.; Drucker, W. R.; Dudrick, S. J.; and Zeppa, R.: Manual of Surgical Nutrition. Philadelphia: W. B. Saunders, 1975.
32. University of Iowa Hospitals and Clinics: Recent Advances in Therapeutic Diets. 2nd ed. Ames: Iowa State University Press, 1973.

# Semisynthetic Fiber Free Liquid Diets

*Definition*    Liquid dietary formulations that contain no source of fiber and that provide most of their essential nutrients in a predigested, more easily absorbable form than ordinary diets. Many of these preparations are virtually completely absorbed in the proximal intestine (jejunum and duodenum), leaving a minimum amount of residue to reach the large bowel [1,2].

*Characteristics of the diet*    The nitrogen source is provided either as synthetic L-amino acids or as egg albumen or as a protein hydrolysate such as casein (supplemented with tryptophan, tyrosine, and methionine). By combining individual amino acids with nonessential amino acids, nitrogen can be provided in a very simple form. Carbohydrate is provided in the form of glucose and glucose oligosaccharides (two to ten glucose units linked together) [3] or as a mixture of glucose and partially hydrolyzed starch. Electrolytes are added, as well as fat soluble and water soluble vitamins. Most of these diets contain less than 1% fat. The concentration generally used for adults is 25% wt/vol, which provides approximately 1 kcal/ml [4].

*Purpose of the diet*    To provide a form of liquid nutrition that is easily digested, absorbed, and assimilated, and that permits a positive nitrogen balance while reducing the frequency and volume of stools in patients in whom normal diets are poorly tolerated, not well assimilated, or contraindicated.

*Effects of the diet*    *Decrease in frequency and volume of stools* Because of the absence of fiber, colonic residue is reduced to an endogenous minimum by these diets [5–8]. This effect makes them potentially useful in pre- and postoperative conditions in which it is desirable to rest the lower bowel while maintaining or replenishing nutritional reserves.

*Reduction in fecal flora*    There is a lack of general agreement about the specific alterations in fecal flora produced by synthetic diets [5–11]. In one small group of patients fed a synthetic diet, the concentrations of lactobacteria spore forming bacilli and yeasts decreased rapidly and did not increase again until normal food was supplied [9]. Winitz et al. have reported that synthetic diets with a glucose base substantially reduce fecal flora, while those with a sucrose base appear to be less effective [10]. However, other studies have failed to confirm these results [12]. A report of a trial of an MCT and sucrose based diet indicated no change in total anaerobes, aerobes, and coliforms per stool but a significant decrease in the number of enterococci [5].

The mechanism for the reduction in numbers of bacteria observed by some investigators may be starvation of the bacteria, since all nutrients are absorbed in the small intestine [2]; the reduced amount of fecal material may result in fewer resident sites for bacterial colonization. Yet another study has noted an alteration in the degree of degradation of fecal steroids and bile acid excretion, which may be related to a change in anaerobia flora [13].

*Changes in gastric acid secretion*    Two recent studies in animals [14] and in tube fed patients [15] have reported significant reductions in gastric acid secretion in response to semisynthetic fiber free liquid diets. Another author has reported that the osmolar load results in increased rather than decreased gastric secretions (in an attempt to maintain normal osmolality), since the stomach is the primary defense against hyperosmolar concentrations [16].

*Decreased gastrointestinal motility*    The administration of hyperosmolar solutions will result in decreased gastric motility. The introduodenal or intragastric administration of hyperosmolar synthetic diets results in the release of vasoactive intestinal peptide, a hormone of the glucagon family with inhibitory effects on gastric secretion and presumably gastric emptying time as well [16–18].

*Decreased pancreatic secretions*    Pancreatic secretions produced on semisynthetic fiber free liquid diets have been reported to be "enzyme poor" [19,20]. One study performed in dogs noted a 60% reduction in total pancreatic flora with a resulting total reduction in pancreatic enzyme content [21]. Normally, pancreatic enzyme secretions are evoked by the release of secretin and pancreozymin from the small intestine [14]. The release of these hormones is in turn brought about by the presence of whole proteins, peptones, and acid chyme in the duodenum and probably amino acids as well [22]. Synthetic diets that are associated with decreased gastric acid secretion might also be expected to produce fewer pancreatic secretions than ordinary diets [14].

There are several as yet unresolved controversies as to the efficacy of these diets and their effect upon pancreatic enzyme output [23–25]. For example, the intrajejunal administration at neutral pH of an amino acid based synthetic diet diminished pancreatic stimulation in one particular patient [26]. This effect was not corroborated, however, by a subsequent investigation in which the product was administered in a normal manner permitting its passage through the duodenum [23]. Synthetic diets fed via the intrajejunal route have been reported to provoke fewer pancreatic secretions than those fed by other means and may account for some of the noted differences [17]. However, a recent study disputes this claim [24]. Blackburn and his co-workers have reported clinical improvement in an uncontrolled study of patients with severe acute pancreatitis fed an egg albumen based synthetic diet [27].

The optimal form of protein in these diets has yet to be clearly established. A study of one patient with only 120 cm functioning small bowel concluded that in conditions of simple loss of intestinal absorption surface and in normal pancreatic and biliary function, a synthetic diet containing fat and protein hydrolysate may result in better intestinal absorption of fluids and nutrients than fat free diets based on amino acids and simple carbohydrates [28]. Badly needed are well controlled comparative studies of the effects of different types of synthetic diets to be undertaken not in normal healthy persons but in *groups* of people in whom the diets are clearly indicated for use.

*Decreased fluid output from certain gastrointestinal fistula* The efficacy of these diets in the feeding of patients with external pancreatic [23] and ileal [29] fistulas appears to be less controversial; beneficial changes have been noted. The ileal fistula output of trypsin, bile acids, fluids, and electrolytes appears to be diminished, and the corrosive nature of the discharge is reduced. However, fiber free semisynthetic diets appear to be more effective in patients with ileal fistulas than in those with jejunal or mid-bowel fistulas [30].

*Changes in the composition of serum and urine* The following have been noted in patients receiving semisynthetic fiber free liquid diets:

1. Decreased urinary nitrogen excretion. This effect has permitted positive nitrogen balance even in catabolic states in some instances [1].
2. Serum urea nitrogen and urinary acid and urea are decreased [31,32].
3. Serum cholesterol is initially diminished [31], although in one study this reduction was followed by a gradual rise in serum cholesterol to hypercholesterolemic levels [32].

*Decreased fecal bile acid excretion* An amino acid based synthetic diet has been noted to reduce fecal bile acid excretion significantly in a group of patients with bile acid induced diarrhea [33]. A marked improvement in the diarrhea occurred [33].

**Indications for use** Semisynthetic fiber free liquid diets may be indicated for interim periods between the use of parenteral feedings and more normal diets in certain patients who have sufficient function of the gastrointestinal tract to permit their utilization. Their use has been reported in a variety of protein depleted, hypermetabolic, and catabolic states in patients who might not otherwise be able to meet their nutritional needs, including the following: severe burns [34], bile acid induced diarrhea [33], gastrointestinal fistulas [35–38], pancreatitis after ileus is cleared [4,19,27], inflammatory bowel disease [4,35,38–41], and radiation enteritis [1,4,42]. When these diets were utilized as a dietary preparation for hemorrhoidectomy, postoperative bowel movements were delayed and diminished with less incidence of pain and complications [43]. Another possible clinical application for these diets is as an alternative to complete starvation in the treatment of obesity [32]. When used as tube feedings, they can be given via smaller nasogastric tubes than ordinary tube feedings [38,44]. There is lack of general agreement as to the value of these diets as preoperative bowel preparations [2,45] and in the nutritional management of the short bowel syndrome [46–48], particularly in patients with less than 100 cm of small bowel remaining [47].

**Possible adverse reactions** *Fluid imbalances such as hyperos-*

*molar dehydration, hypertonic nonketotic coma, and fluid retention* In normal dilutions of 25% wt/vol these diets are hypertonic solutions that may produce severe symptoms of osmotic dehydration in certain volume sensitive individuals, such as infants [34].

*Aspiration* Aspiration pneumonitis has been reported to be an infrequent possible complication produced by these diets [34,35].

*Hypoprothrombinemia* This condition may occur in patients receiving synthetic diets that are not supplemented with vitamin K [34,49,50].

*Hyperglycemia* Diabetics fed these diets should have blood glucose monitored carefully; urinary glucose levels and serum electrolytes should be checked frequently in all patients receiving these diets [4].

*Gastrointestinal disturbances* Diarrhea, nausea, and delayed gastric emptying may occur in certain individuals, particularly if the diet is given too rapidly. The rate of administration should be slow for the first few days in order to prevent this complication [51].

*Hair changes* In one long-term study using a very low fat synthetic diet, hair changes were noted in some of the patients. The head hair became thin and sparse with a faint red tinge and tended to fall out more rapidly [32]. These changes were attributed to insufficient intakes of fatty acids.

**Contraindications** Semisynthetic fiber free liquid diets may be contraindicated in instances of severe metabolic stress or ileus [18] and in any condition in which a high osmolar load may be dangerous, such as uncompensated hepatic or renal disease or in patients with the dumping syndrome. Concentrations above 12% wt/vol are contraindicated in children under 10 months of age [4]. Infants under 3 months of age do not tolerate any hypertonic feeding and should not be fed these diets whether diluted or not [18]. In addition, patients with jejunal fistulas are difficult to feed either above or below the fistula and may have insufficient absorptive surface. Such fistulas are often aggravated by improper attempts to use these diets [18].

**Suggestions for dietitians** *Selecting the semisynthetic fiber free liquid diet best suited to the specific clinical condition* Although there are many similarities among different synthetic diets, there are also differences that may affect their selection for a specific patient. Sources of protein, fat, and carbohydrate vary. The advantages to be derived from the use of the more expensive, less palatable, amino acid based preparations over hydrolysates or egg albumen should be questioned. Complete answers have yet to be provided in specific clinical conditions.

Responses to two synthetic diets differing in protein source, e.g., egg albumen vs. an amino acid based diet, were not statistically different in a group of normal healthy volunteers [52]. Other studies in healthy persons indicate that whole protein preparations containing casein or egg albumen may be as well absorbed as amino acid mixtures [53–56]. In normal patients, the human ileum may play a role in the absorption of peptides [57]. However, the optimal protein source of these diets has yet to be established in patients with clinical conditions who would most benefit from their use.

These diets are all lactose and gluten free, and several, but not all, are also soy free. Preparations containing medium chain triglycerides are indicated in certain conditions in which long chain triglycerides are poorly tolerated. A more concentrated formula with improved palatability may have certain psychological advantages when the patient has difficulty consuming adequate amounts of liquids. In patients sensitive to high osmotic loads, osmolality of the product may be the critical component governing its selection for use. Certain diets may not be as well suited as others to long-term use without supplementation of vitamins and minerals [50]. A comparative analysis of the advantages and disadvantages of these diets as well as of their composition and nutritional effects should precede their utilization in any patient [58].

*Palatability and osmolality* The unflavored semisynthetic diets are preferable for use in tube feedings because of their lower osmolality, but their lack of palatability is a disadvantage in oral use. They are particularly distasteful when served warm or at room temperature. Semisynthetic diets are now available in different flavors, and additional flavorings can also be added to improve their taste. However, improvements in palatability are sometimes achieved at the expense of increased osmolality. Conversely, lowered osmolality may be achieved at the expense of the use of more complex constituents, which produce fewer osmotically active particles but which may also not be as readily absorbable, thus defeating the purpose of the diet.

*Proper administration of semisynthetic fiber free liquid diets*

1. *In adults* Most patients should be started on these diets gradually to permit them to adjust to the composition without side effects. A common mistake is to administer the diet too aggressively and then withdraw it completely when gastrointestinal symptoms occur. A half strength solution (10 to 12.5% wt/vol) should be used initially and, if administered by tube, infused at the rate of 40–60 ml/hr [59]. The feeding should be drawn from a small reservoir (500–1,000 ml) and kept at ice temperature to avoid the growth of microorganisms [59]. If this strength is tolerated without nausea, vomiting, distension, or diarrhea, the concentration can be slowly increased to three-quarter strength (18% wt/vol) after 24 hours and then gradually to a full strength solution. For comatose and grossly debilitated patients, the head of the bed is elevated 30° and the infusion may be stopped during the night [18]. When they are fed orally, semisynthetic diets should be served well chilled or over ice and sipped slowly in gradually increasing amounts of less than 100 ml [4] to a maximum of 300 ml [59]. They may also be served frozen as a slush for variety in consistency. Never should semisynthetic diets be served at room temperature. In general, large increases of both concentration and volume should not be made on the same day. Initial jejunostomy feedings should be

isotonic and administered very slowly—40 ml/hr [18].

2. *In infants*     In infants and small children it is necessary to start with even more dilute feedings, and the concentration should be increased with great care [59]. Infants should be started slowly at a roughly isotonic concentration of 7 to 7.5% wt/ vol or a one-fourth strength solution. The concentration should be slowly increased over 4 to 5 days to the level of tolerance, which is usually about 10% and not more than 12% [4]. Newborn infants generally poorly tolerate concentrations above 10% wt/vol, and the risk of diarrhea is increased with higher concentrations [59]. Concentrations of about 12% wt/vol are contraindicated in children under 10 months of age [4]. Young children may accept a synthetic diet from a nursing bottle [59]. In children older than 10 months, concentrations up to 25% are well tolerated if the diet is started slowly in small amounts that are gradually increased [4].

3. *Nutritional monitoring*     Whether synthetic diets are fed orally or by tube, careful attention must be given to adequate fluid intake and to nutritional monitoring of the patient. A record of nutrients and water actually consumed is most useful when used in conjunction with biochemical findings.

   All patients should have their hemoglobin, BUN, blood glucose, and probably serum proteins and serum electrolytes determined prior to the onset of semisynthetic fiber free liquid diet therapy and periodically thereafter. In patients with significant malabsorption, magnesium, calcium, phosphorus, hepatic enzymes, and prothrombin time values should be obtained as well. Fractional urines should be obtained initially for determinations of glucose, acetone, and pH, and 24-hr urinary electrolyte and nitrogen excretion should be periodically measured. Diabetic patients should be monitored more closely, as changes in blood glucose levels induced by the diet may require adjustment of insulin dosage [59].

   Patients should be weighed daily at first and then biweekly thereafter. Fluid retention should be suspected in patients who are gaining weight on low kilocalorie intake or who have otherwise unexplained decreases in serum sodium levels. Fluid and electrolyte loss through fistulas should be estimated and recorded and supplementation given to replace losses when necessary. Extra water may be indicated in patients whose water requirements have been increased by fever, metabolic disturbances, or vomiting or whose serum osmolality determinations are higher than 300 mOsm.

4. *Proper storage*     Once reconstituted, the feedings are perishable and should be refrigerated. The unused portions should be discarded after 24 hr [4], as they make good culture media. When kept below 60° F, they can be stored up to 12 months in the dry state [60]. External tubing and container should be changed every 24 hr [59].

**Semisynthetic Fiber-Free Liquid Diets**

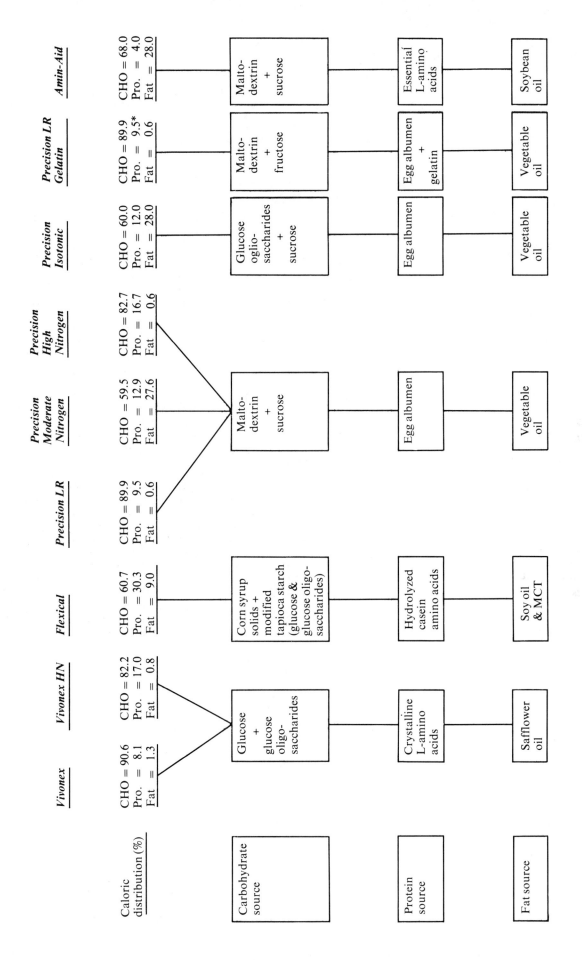

| | Vivonex | Vivonex HN | Flexical | Precision LR | Precision Moderate Nitrogen | Precision High Nitrogen | Precision Isotonic | Precision LR Gelatin | Amin-Aid |
|---|---|---|---|---|---|---|---|---|---|
| Caloric distribution (%) | CHO = 90.6<br>Pro. = 8.1<br>Fat = 1.3 | CHO = 82.2<br>Pro. = 17.0<br>Fat = 0.8 | CHO = 60.7<br>Pro. = 30.3<br>Fat = 9.0 | CHO = 89.9<br>Pro. = 9.5<br>Fat = 0.6 | CHO = 59.5<br>Pro. = 12.9<br>Fat = 27.6 | CHO = 82.7<br>Pro. = 16.7<br>Fat = 0.6 | CHO = 60.0<br>Pro. = 12.0<br>Fat = 28.0 | CHO = 89.9<br>Pro. = 9.5*<br>Fat = 0.6 | CHO = 68.0<br>Pro. = 4.0<br>Fat = 28.0 |
| Carbohydrate source | Glucose + glucose oligosaccharides | | Corn syrup solids + modified tapioca starch (glucose & glucose oligosaccharides) | Maltodextrin + sucrose | | | Glucose oliosaccharides + sucrose | Maltodextrin + fructose | Maltodextrin + sucrose |
| Protein source | Crystalline L-amino acids | | Hydrolyzed casein amino acids | Egg albumen | | | Egg albumen | Egg albumen + gelatin | Essential L-amino acids |
| Fat source | Safflower oil | | Soy oil & MCT | Vegetable oil | | | Vegetable oil | Vegetable oil | Soybean oil |

\* Not including gelatin protein.

**Semisynthetic Fiber Free Liquid Diets**

| | Vivonex | | Vivonex HN | | Flexical | | Precision LR | |
|---|---|---|---|---|---|---|---|---|
| Osmolality (mOsm per litre) | Unflavored 550 | | Unflavored 810 | | Banana 550 | | Cherry 525 | |
| | With flavor packets: | | With flavor packets: | | Fruit punch 550 | | Lemon 525 | |
| | Beef broth 678 | | Beef broth 920 | | Orange 550 | | Lime 525 | |
| | Orange 610 | | Orange 850 | | Vanilla 550 | | Orange 525 | |
| | Grape 610 | | Grape 850 | | | | | |
| | Strawberry 610 | | Strawberry 850 | | | | | |
| | Vanilla 610 | | Tomato 910 | | | | | |
| | Tomato 580 | | | | | | | |
| Kilocalories per ml | 1.0 | | 1.0 | | 1.0 | | 1.1 | |
| **Quantity** | 100 ml | 1,800 ml | 100 ml | 3,000 ml | 100 ml | 2,000 ml | 100 ml | 1,727 ml |
| Carbohydrate (g) | 23.00 | 414.00 | 21.10 | 633.00 | 15.24 | 304.80 | 24.70 | 427.00 |
| Protein (g) | 2.04 | 36.75 | 4.38 | 129.90 | 2.25 | 45.00 | 2.60 | 45.00 |
| Nitrogen (g) | 0.33 | 5.88 | 0.67 | 20.10 | 0.40 | 8.00 | 0.40 | 7.20 |
| Fat (g) | 0.15 | 2.61 | 0.09 | 2.60 | 3.40 | 67.90 | 0.08 | 1.40 |
| Vitamin A (IU) | 277.78 | 5,000.04 | 167.00 | 5,000.00 | 250.00 | 5,000.00 | 290.00 | 5,000.00 |
| Vitamin D (IU) | 22.20 | 399.60 | 13.30 | 400.00 | 20.00 | 400.00 | 23.20 | 400.00 |
| Vitamin E (IU) | 1.67 | 30.06 | 1.00 | 30.00 | 2.20 | 45.00 | 1.70 | 30.00 |
| Vitamin K ($\mu$g) | 3.72 | 66.96 | 2.23 | 66.90 | 12.50 | 250.00 | — | — |
| Ascorbic acid (mg) | 3.33 | 59.94 | 2.00 | 60.00 | 15.00 | 300.00 | 5.20 | 90.00 |
| Thiamine (mg) | 0.08 | 1.44 | 0.05 | 1.50 | 0.19 | 3.80 | 0.13 | 2.25 |
| Riboflavin (mg) | 0.09 | 1.62 | 0.06 | 1.80 | 0.22 | 4.30 | 0.15 | 2.25 |
| Niacin (mg) | 1.11 | 19.98 | 0.67 | 20.10 | 2.50 | 50.00 | 1.16 | 20.00 |
| Pyridoxine (mg) | 0.11 | 2.00 | 0.07 | 2.10 | 0.25 | 5.00 | 0.17 | 3.00 |
| Vitamin B$_{12}$ ($\mu$g) | 0.33 | 5.94 | 0.17 | 6.00 | 0.75 | 15.00 | 0.35 | 6.00 |
| Folic acid (mg) | 0.02 | 0.36 | 0.01 | 0.30 | 0.02 | 0.40 | 0.02 | 0.40 |
| Biotin (mg) | 0.02 | 0.36 | 0.01 | 0.30 | 0.02 | 0.30 | 0.02 | 0.30 |
| Pantothenate (mg) | 0.56 | 10.00 | 0.33 | 9.90 | 1.24 | 25.00 | 0.58 | 10.00 |
| Inositol (mg) | 6.50 | 116.50 | 3.90 | 116.50 | — | — | — | — |
| Choline (mg) | 4.09 | 73.62 | 2.46 | 73.80 | 25.00 | 500.00 | 5.80 | 100.00 |
| Potassium (mg) | 117.00 | 2,105.00 | 70.00 | 2,100.00 | 125.00 | 2,500.00 | 86.80 | 1,500.00 |
| Sodium (mg) | 86.00 | 1,548.00 | 77.02 | 2,310.06 | 35.00 | 700.00 | 69.50 | 1,200.00 |
| Calcium (mg) | 56.00 | 1,008.00 | 33.00 | 990.00 | 60.00 | 1,200.00 | 57.90 | 1,000.00 |
| Magnesium (mg) | 22.20 | 399.60 | 13.30 | 399.00 | 20.00 | 400.00 | 23.20 | 400.00 |
| Manganese (mg) | 0.16 | 2.81 | 0.09 | 2.81 | 0.25 | 5.00 | 0.23 | 4.00 |
| Iron (mg) | 1.00 | 18.00 | 0.60 | 18.00 | 0.90 | 18.00 | 1.00 | 18.00 |
| Copper (mg) | 0.11 | 1.94 | 0.07 | 2.10 | 0.10 | 2.00 | 0.12 | 2.00 |
| Zinc (mg) | 0.83 | 14.94 | 0.50 | 15.00 | 1.00 | 20.00 | 0.87 | 15.00 |
| Iodine (mg) | 0.01 | 0.14 | tr. | 0.14 | 0.01 | 0.15 | 0.01 | 0.15 |
| Phosphorus (mg) | 56.00 | 1,008.00 | 33.02 | 990.00 | 50.00 | 1,000.00 | 57.90 | 1,000.00 |
| Chloride (mg) | 183.68 | 3,306.25 | 185.80 | 5,573.00 | 100.00 | 2,000.00 | 110.00 | 1,900.00 |
| Sulfur (mg) | 0.64 | 11.50 | 0.38 | 11.50 | — | — | — | — |

| | Precision Moderate Nitrogen | | Precision HN | | Precision Isotonic | | Precision LR Gelatin | | Amin-Aid* | |
|---|---|---|---|---|---|---|---|---|---|---|
| Osmolality (mOsm per litre) | Vanilla 395<br>Citrus 395 | | Citrus fruit 557 | | 300 | | Orange 700 | | 1,050 mOsm/kg | |
| Kilocalories per ml | 1.2 | | 1.05 | | 1.0 | | 1.12† | | 2.06 | |
| **Quantity** | 100 ml | 1,680 ml | 100 ml | 2,850 ml | 100 ml | 1,500 ml | 1(5 oz) serv. | 12 (5 oz) serv. | 100 ml | 680 ml |
| Carbohydrate (g) | 17.90 | 300.00 | 21.80 | 620.00 | 15.00 | 225.00 | 35.60 | 427.00 | 34.70 | 236.00 |
| Protein (g) | 3.90 | 65.00 | 4.40 | 125.00 | 3.00 | 45.00 | 3.75‡ | 45.00‡ | 1.90 | 12.90 |
| Nitrogen (g) | 0.62 | 10.40 | 0.70 | 20.00 | 0.50 | 7.50 | 0.60 | 7.20 | 0.24 | 1.60 |
| Fat (g) | 3.70 | 62.00 | 0.05 | 1.40 | 3.10 | 47.00 | 0.10 | 1.40 | 6.50 | 44.20 |
| Vitamin A (IU) | 298.00 | 5,000.00 | 175.00 | 5,000.00 | 333.00 | 5,000.00 | 417.00 | 5,000.00 | — | — |
| Vitamin D (IU) | 23.80 | 400.00 | 14.00 | 400.00 | 26.70 | 400.00 | 33.30 | 400.00 | — | — |
| Vitamin E (IU) | 1.80 | 30.00 | 1.00 | 30.00 | 2.00 | 30.00 | 2.50 | 30.00 | — | — |
| Vitamin K ($\mu$g) | 6.00 | 100.00 | — | — | 6.70 | 100.00 | 8.30 | 100.00 | — | — |
| Ascorbic acid (mg) | 5.40 | 90.00 | 3.20 | 90.00 | 6.00 | 90.00 | 7.50 | 90.00 | — | — |
| Thiamine (mg) | 0.13 | 2.25 | 0.08 | 2.25 | 0.15 | 2.25 | 0.19 | 2.25 | — | — |
| Riboflavin (mg) | 0.15 | 2.60 | 0.09 | 2.60 | 0.17 | 2.60 | 0.22 | 2.60 | — | — |
| Niacin (mg) | 1.19 | 20.00 | 0.70 | 20.00 | 1.33 | 20.00 | 1.67 | 20.00 | — | — |
| Pyridoxine (mg) | 0.18 | 3.00 | 0.10 | 3.00 | 0.20 | 3.00 | 0.25 | 3.00 | — | — |
| Vitamin B$_{12}$ ($\mu$g) | 0.36 | 6.00 | 0.21 | 6.00 | 0.40 | 6.00 | 0.50 | 6.00 | — | — |
| Folic acid (mg) | 0.02 | 0.40 | 0.01 | 0.40 | 0.03 | 0.40 | 0.03 | 0.40 | — | — |
| Biotin (mg) | 0.02 | 0.30 | 0.01 | 0.30 | 0.02 | 0.30 | 0.02 | 0.03 | — | — |
| Pantothenate (mg) | 0.59 | 10.00 | 0.35 | 10.00 | 6.67 | 10.00 | 0.83 | 10.00 | — | — |
| Inositol (mg) | — | — | — | — | — | — | — | — | — | — |
| Choline (mg) | 6.00 | 100.00 | 3.50 | 100.00 | 6.70 | 100.00 | 8.30 | 100.00 | — | — |
| Potassium (mg) | 89.30 | 1,500.00 | 91.20 | 2,600.00 | 100.00 | 1,500.00 | 125.00 | 1,500.00 | 23.00 | 156.40 |
| Sodium (mg) | 101.20 | 1,700.00 | 98.20 | 2,800.00 | 80.00 | 1,200.00 | 100.00 | 1,200.00 | 12.00 | 81.60 |
| Calcium (mg) | 59.50 | 1,000.00 | 35.10 | 1,000.00 | 67.00 | 1,000.00 | 83.30 | 1,000.00 | — | — |
| Magnesium (mg) | 23.80 | 400.00 | 14.00 | 400.00 | 26.70 | 400.00 | 33.30 | 400.00 | — | — |
| Manganese (mg) | 0.24 | 4.00 | 0.14 | 4.00 | 0.27 | 4.00 | 0.33 | 4.00 | — | — |
| Iron (mg) | 1.07 | 18.00 | 0.63 | 18.00 | 1.20 | 18.00 | 1.50 | 18.00 | — | — |
| Copper (mg) | 0.12 | 2.00 | 0.07 | 2.00 | 0.13 | 2.00 | 0.17 | 2.00 | — | — |
| Zinc (mg) | 0.89 | 15.00 | 0.53 | 15.00 | 1.00 | 15.00 | 1.25 | 15.00 | — | — |
| Iodine (mg) | 0.01 | 0.15 | tr. | 0.15 | 0.01 | 0.15 | 0.01 | 0.15 | — | — |
| Phosphorus (mg) | 59.50 | 1,000.00 | 35.10 | 1,000.00 | 67.00 | 1,000.00 | 83.30 | 1,000.00 | — | — |
| Chloride (mg) | 107.10 | 1,800.00 | 119.30 | 3,400.00 | 107.00 | 1,600.00 | 158.30 | 1,900.00 | — | — |
| Sulfur (mg) | — | — | — | — | — | — | — | — | — | — |

‡ In addition to the protein listed here, provided as egg protein, PLR gelatin has 1.8 g gelatin protein per serving (21.4 g per 12 servings).
* Specifically designed for use in patients with liver and renal disease. Unsuited for long-term use unless supplemented with vitamins and minerals.
† The extra gelatin protein present will add an extra 0.05 kcal/ml or 7.2 kcal per serving of gelatin.

**Approximate Kilocalorie and Nitrogen Ratios of Some Common Semisynthetic Fiber Free Liquid Diets**

| | *Total kcal:nitrogen ratio* | *Nonprotein kcal:nitrogen ratio* |
|---|---|---|
| Vivonex | 310 | 285 |
| Vivonex HN | 155 | 125 |
| Flexical | 280 | 255 |
| Precision LR | 265 | 240 |
| Precision MN | 195 | 170 |
| Precision HN | 150 | 125 |
| Precision Isotonic | 200 | 175 |
| Precision LR Gelatin* | 265 | 240 |
| Amin-Aid | 855 | 820 |
| Precision LR Gelatin† | 275 | 240 |

\* Without gelatin protein included.
† With gelatin protein included.

**References**

1. Nealon, T. F.; Grossi, C. E.; and Steier, M.: Use of elemental diets to correct catabolic states prior to surgery. Ann. Surg. 180: 9, 1974.
2. Johnson, W. C.: Oral elemental diet. Arch. Surg. 108: 32, 1974.
3. Lehninger, A. L.: Biochemistry. New York: Worth, 1970.
4. Randall, H. T.: Diet and nutrition in the care of the surgical patient. Goodhart, R. S., and Shils, M. E. eds. Modern Nutrition in Health and Disease. 5th ed. Philadelphia: Lea & Febiger, 1973.
5. Bounous, G., and Devroede, G. J.: Effects of an elemental diet on human fecal flora. Gastroenterology 66: 210, 1974.
6. Winitz, M.: Factors affecting studies with chemically defined diets. Am. J. Clin. Nutr. 26: 785, 1973.
7. Spiller, G. A.; Saperstein, S.; Beigler, M. A.; and Amen, R. J.: Effect on fecal output of various dietary nitrogen sources in pig-tailed monkeys (Macaca nemestrina) fed fiber-free semisynthetic diets. Am. J. Clin. Nutr. 28: 502, 1975.
8. Bornside, G. H., and Cohn, I.: Stability of normal human fecal flora during a chemically defined, low residue liquid diet. Ann. Surg. 181: 58, 1975.
9. Zollner, N.; Ruckdeschel, G.; and Wolfram, G.: Verhalten der darmflora des menschen bei formeldiäten mit wechselndem kohlenhydratgehalt. Nutr. Metab. 18: 127, 1975.
10. Winitz, M.; Adams, R. F.; Seedman, D.A.; Davis, P. N.; Jayko, L. G.; and Hamilton, J. A.: Studies in metabolic nutrition employing chemically defined diets. II. Effects on gut microflora populations. Am. J. Clin. Nutr. 23: 546, 1970.
11. Attebery, H. R.; Sutter, V. L.; and Finegold, S. M.: Effect of a partially chemically defined diet on normal human fecal flora. Am. J. Clin. Nutr. 25: 1391, 1972.
12. Gurry, J. F., and Ellis-Pegler, R. B.: An elemental diet as preoperative preparation of the colon. Br. J. Surg. 63: 969, 1976.
13. Crowther, J. S.; Drasar, B. S.; Goddard, P.; Hill, M. J.; and Johnson, K.: The effect of a chemically defined diet on the faecal flora and faecal steroid concentration. Gut 14: 790, 1973.
14. Rivilis, J.; McArdle, A. H.; Wlodek, G. K.; and Gurd, F. N.: Effect of an elemental diet on gastric secretion. Ann. Surg. 179: 226, 1974.
15. Bury, K. D., and Jambunathan, G.: Effects of elemental diets on gastric emptying and gastric secretion in man. Am. J. Surg. 127: 59, 1974.
16. Fischer, J. F.: Parenteral and enteral nutrition. Dis. Month. 24 (9): 3, 1978.
17. Shils, M. E.: Enteral nutrition by tube. Cancer Res. 37: 2432, 1977.
18. Bury, K. D.: Elemental diets. Fischer, J. F., ed. Total Parenteral Nutrition. Boston: Little, Brown, 1976.
19. Voitk, A.; Brown, R. A.; Echave, V.; McArdle, A. J.; Gurd, F. N.; and Thompson, A. G.: Use of an elemental diet in the treatment of complicated pancreatitis. Am. J. Surg. 125: 223, 1973.
20. Cassim, M. M., and Allardyce, D. B.: Pancreatic secretion in response to jejunal feeding of elemental diet. Am. J. Surg. 180: 228, 1974.
21. McArdle, A. H.; Echave, W.; Brown, R. A.; and Thompson, A. G.: Effect of elemental diet on pancreatic secretion. Am. J. Surg. 128: 690, 1974.

22. Go, V. L. W.; Hofmann, A. F.; and Summerskill, W. H. J.: Pancreozymin bioassay in man based on pancreatic enzyme secretion: potency of specific amino acids and other digestive products. J. Clin. Invest. 49: 1558, 1970.

23. Wolfe, B. M.; Keltner, R. M.; and Kaminski, D. L.: The effect of an intraduodenal elemental diet on pancreatic secretion. Surg. Gynecol. Obstet. 140: 241, 1975.

24. Vidon, N.; Hecketsweiler, P.; Butel, J.; and Bernier, J. J.: Effect of continuous jejunal perfusion of elemental and complex nutritional solutions on pancreatic enzyme secretion in human subjects. Gut 19: 194, 1978.

25. Perrault, J., and Hoffman, H. N.: Apparent controversies related to chemically defined diets. Gastroenterology 70: 634, 1976.

26. Ragins, H.; Levenson, S. M.; Signer, R.; Stamford, W.; and Seifter, E.: Intrajejunal administration of an elemental diet at neutral pH avoids pancreatic stimulation. Am. J. Surg. 126: 606, 1973.

27. Blackburn, G. L.; Williams, L. F.; Bistrian, B. R.; Stone, M. S.; Phillips, E.; Hirsch, E.; Clowes, G. H. A.; and Gregg, J.: New approaches to the management of severe acute pancreatitis. Am. J. Surg. 131: 114, 1976.

28. Simko, V., and Linschfer, W. G.: Absorption of different elemental diets in a short bowel syndrome lasting 15 years. Am. J. Dig. Dis. 21: 419, 1976.

29. Hill, G. L.; Mair, W. S. J.; Edwards, J. P.; and Goligher, J. C.: Decreased trypsin and bile acids in ileal fistula drainage during the administration of a chemically defined liquid elemental diet. Br. J. Surg. 63: 133, 1976.

30. Wolfe, B. M.; Keltner, R. M.; and Kaminski, D. I.: Surgical metabolism, nutrition and endocrinology. Modification of intestinal fistula output by elemental and intravenous alimentation. Surg. Forum 24: 53, 1973.

31. Young, D. S.; Epley, J. A.; and Goldman, P.: Influence of a chemically defined diet on the composition of serum and urine. Clin. Chem. 17: 765, 1971.

32. Baird, I. M.; Parsons, R. I.; and Howard, A. N.: Clinical and metabolic studies of chemically defined diets in the management of obesity. Metabolism 23: 645, 1974.

33. Nelson, L. M.; Carmichael, H. A.; Russell, R. I.; and Atheston, S. T.: Use of an elemental diet (Vivonex) in the management of bile acid induced diarrhea. Gut. 18: 792, 1977.

34. Bury, K. D.; Stephens, R. V.; and Randall, H. T.: Use of a chemically defined, liquid, elemental diet for nutritional management of fistulas of the alimentary tract. Am. J. Surg. 121: 174, 1971.

35. Voitk, A. J.; Brown, R. A.; McArdle, A. H.; Hinchey, E. J.; and Gurd, F. N.: Clinical uses of an elemental diet—preliminary studies. Can. Med. Assoc. J. 107: 123, 1972.

36. Voitk, A. J.; Echave, V.; Brown, R. A.; McArdle, A. H.; and Gurd, F. N.: Elemental diet in the treatment of fistulas of the alimentary tract. Surg. Gynecol. Obstet. 137: 68, 1973.

37. Rocchio, M. A.; Cha, C. J. M.; Haas, K. F.; and Randall, H. T.: Use of chemically defined diets in the management of patients with high output gastrointestinal cutaneous fistulas. Am. J. Surg. 127: 148, 1974.

38. Voitk, A. J.; Echave, V.; Feller, J. H.; Brown, R. A.; and Gurd, F. N.: Experience with elemental diet in the treatment of inflammatory bowel disease. Arch. Surg. 107: 329, 1973.

39. Rocchio, M. A.; Cha, C. J. M.; Haas, K. F.; and Randall, H. T.: Use of chemically defined diets in the management of patients with acute inflammatory bowel disease. Am. J. Surg. 127: 469, 1974.

40. Giorgini, G. L.; Stephens, R. V.; and Thayer, W. R.: The use of "Medical By-pass" in the therapy of Crohn's disease: report of a case. Am. J. Dig. Dis. 18: 153, 1973.

41. Bounous, G.; Devroede, G.; Haddad, H.; Beaudry, R.; Perey, B.; and Lejeune, L. P.: Use of an elemental diet for intestinal disorders and for the critically ill. Dis. Colon Rectum 17: 157, 1974.

42. Haddad, H.; Bounous, G.; Tahan, W. T.; Devroede, G.; Beaudry, R.; and Lafond, R.: Long-term nutrition with an elemental diet following intensive abdominal irradiation. Dis. Colon Rectum 17: 373, 1974.

43. Rosser, R. G.: Dietary preparation for hemorrhoidectomy. Advantages of a nutritionally complete, chemically defined low residue diet. Am. J. Surg. 130: 78, 1975.

44. Voitk, A. J.: The place of elemental diet in clinical nutrition. Br. J. Clin. Pract. 29: 55, 1975.

45. Cooney, D. T.; Wassner, J. D.; Grosfeld, J. L.; and Jesseph, J. E.: Are elemental diets useful in bowel preparation? Arch. Surg. 109: 206, 1974.
46. Voitk, A. J.; Echave, V.; Brown, R. A.; and Gurd, F. N.: Use of elemental diet during the adaptive stage of short gut syndrome. Gastroenterology 65: 419, 1973.
47. Wright, H. K., and Tilson, M. D.: Postoperative disorders of the gastrointestinal tract. New York: Grune & Stratton, 1973.
48. Weser, E.: The management of patients after small bowel resection. Gastroenterology 71: 146, 1976.
49. Kark, R. M.: Liquid formula and chemically defined diets. J. Am. Diet. Assoc. 64: 476, 1974.
50. Young, E. A.; Heuler, N.; Russell, P.; and Weser, E.: Comparative nutritional analysis of chemically defined diets. Gastroenterology 69: 1338, 1975.
51. Stephens, R. V., and Randall, H. T.: Use of a concentrated, balanced, liquid elemental diet for nutritional management of catabolic states. Ann. Surg. 170: 642, 1969.
52. Clark, H. E.; Stuff, J. T.; Moon, W. H.; and Bailey, L. B.: Nitrogen retention and plasma amino acids of men who consumed isonitrogenous diets containing egg albumen or mixtures of amino acids. Am. J. Clin. Nutr. 28: 316, 1975.
53. Silk, D. B. A.; Marrs, T. C.; Addison, J. M.; Burston, D.; Clark, M. L.; and Matthews, D. M.: Absorption of amino acids from an amino acid mixture simulating casein and a tryptic hydrolysate of casein in man. Clin. Sci. Mol. Med. 45: 715, 1973.
54. Kim, Y. S.; Nicholson, J. A.; and Curtis, K. J. Intestinal peptide hydrolases: peptide and amino acid absorption. Med. Clin. N. Am. 58: 1397, 1974.
55. Fairclough, P. D.; Silk, D. B. A.; Clark, M. L.; and Dawson, A. M.: New evidence for intact di- and tripeptide absorption. Gut 16: 843, 1975.
56. Silk, D. B. A.: Progress report. Peptide absorption in man. Gut 15: 494, 1974.
57. Silk, D. B. A.; Webb, J. P.; Lane, A. E.; Clark, M. L.; and Dawson, A. M.: Functional differentiation of human jejunum and ileum: a comparison of the handling of glucose, peptides, and amino acids. Gut 15: 444, 1974.
58. Alexander, F. W.; Clayton, B. E.; and Delves, H. T.: Mineral and trace-metal balances in children receiving normal and synthetic diets. Q. J. Med. 43: 89, 1974.
59. Randall, H. T.: Enteric Feeding. Committee on Pre and Postoperative Care, American College of Surgeons. Manual of Surgical Nutrition. Philadelphia: W. B. Saunders, 1975.
60. Russell, R. I.: Progress report. Elemental diets. Gut 16: 68, 1975.

# Total Parenteral Nutrition

***Parenteral feeding*** A means of providing nutrients by subcutaneous, intramuscular, or intravenous routes or other than through the gastrointestinal tract [1].

***Total parenteral nutrition (TPN)*** The administration, usually through a central venous catheter, of protein hydrolysates or amino acids plus glucose and other essential nutrients in amounts sufficient to meet normal caloric and nitrogen needs [2].

***Enteral hyperalimentation*** The oral or tube feeding of essential nutrients in a caloric concentration appreciably in excess of normal requirements.

***Intravenous hyperalimentation*** The administration by central venous catheter of simple essential nutrients, such as protein hydrolysates or amino acids plus glucose, vitamins, and minerals, in a caloric concentration in excess of normal requirements [2,3]. Many, but not all, persons receiving central venous feedings have increased nutritive requirements because of preexisting malnutrition or hypermetabolic states.

***Characteristics of total parenteral nutrition and intravenous hyperalimentation*** *Composition of TPN solutions* Exact details of the composition and preparation of TPN solutions have been published elsewhere [2–4]. In general, most solutions are based upon the mixing of a 50% solution of glucose with a 5–10% solution of protein hydrolysate or amino acids, which yields a solution of 25% glucose and 3–4% protein [5], providing 1,000 kcal and approximately 6 g nitrogen/litre.

Administered amounts of nutrient solutions are determined on the basis of surface area, specific nutrient needs, and water requirements. Most patients can tolerate an initial volume of 2 litres without complications [6]. Since most adults tolerate 35–50 ml water/kg of body weight daily without overhydration [7], total intake is often increased to 3 litres or more daily [8]. Factors such as extensive water loss, high fever, renal failure, and cardiac decompensation modify water requirements [8].

Solutions utilized in total parenteral nutrition should be formulated to meet the nutritional needs of the individual. In general, 30 kcal/kg of body weight/day are necessary to maintain the ideal weight of the adult with restricted activity. Kilocalories should be increased appropriately to permit weight gain in individuals who are significantly underweight or to meet other needs. Infants require 100–130 kcal/kg of body weight per day [2,3], while patients with burns may need to be hyperalimented with 5,000 or more kilocalories per day [7].

*Carbohydrate, hypertonicity, and the use of central venous catheters* Glucose is the most effective and frequently used carbohydrate source in TPN solutions. Because of high glucose content, most TPN solutions are hypertonic, except for those which

Prepared with the collaboration of John Seashore, M. D., Yale School of Medicine.

incorporate fat as a substitute for some of the glucose kilocalories [2,9,10]. Hypertonic TPN solutions must be delivered through a central venous catheter in order to minimize the risk of phlebitis and thrombosis [3]. Use of the catheter permits prolonged administration of the solutions into a region of high blood flow where they are rapidly diluted.

*Protein sources*     A synthetic crystalline L-amino acid solution is the usual nitrogen source for TPN. Enzymatic hydrolysates of casein and fibrin are also available [11]. Although they are cheaper than amino acids, protein hydrolysates contain 30–40% peptides, which are lost in the urine in large quantities and are less well utilized than amino acids [8].

Recommended Dietary Allowances are approximately 0.8 g protein per kilogram of body weight for a healthy adult, but in practice TPN should provide 1 to 1.5 g/kg/day of protein to most adults to assure that positive nitrogen balance will be achieved [2]. Preexisting malnutrition, ongoing protein loss, major trauma, sepsis, severe burns, neoplasms, and other hypermetabolic conditions may increase protein requirements to even higher levels (up to 4 g/kg/day in extensive burns). Adequate caloric intake is also necessary to achieve positive nitrogen balance and anabolism.

The Recommended Dietary Allowance for protein in infants is 2.0 to 2.5 g/kg/day [12]. Historically, TPN solutions for infants have provided much larger amounts. However, as complications of excessive protein intake, including metabolic acidosis, hyperammoniemia, plasma amino acid imbalances, and cholestatic jaundice have been recognized more frequently [13], there has been a trend toward providing less protein in TPN solutions [14]. One recent study suggests that there is no advantage to intakes greater than 2.5 g/kg/day for the newborn infant [14]. Protein requirements for older children fall somewhere between those for infants and adults, except for teenagers, who need larger amounts to sustain the normal adolescent growth spurt.

*Kilocalorie:nitrogen ratio*     The optimum kilocalorie:nitrogen ratio has not been determined. A ratio of 150:1 has been suggested to be a safe guide [15], but patients with burns, sepsis, and major trauma may need lower ratios, while patients who need only normal nutritional maintenance may do well with ratios of 200–225:1. In general, sicker patients need lower ratios, since protein losses increase more rapidly than the metabolic rate.

*Fat*     Fat is a highly desirable energy source, since it has a high caloric density (9 kcal/g) and provides essential fatty acids. Intravenous fat emulsions used 20–30 years ago were shown to be highly toxic and were withdrawn from the market. More recently, a 10% soybean oil emulsion stabilized with egg yolk phospholipid (Intralipid*) has proven to be safe and effective [9,10,16–18]. The solution is made isotonic by the addition of glycerol and contains 1.1 kcal/ml. Intralipid can be given by peripheral vein in amounts up to 2 g fat per kilogram per day. If a 5% glucose, 4% protein solution is administered simultaneously, adequate *maintenance*

* Cutter Laboratories, Berkeley, CA 94710.

nutrition (2,100 kcal and 60 g protein) can be provided entirely by peripheral vein, thus avoiding the risks of an indwelling central venous catheter. Peripheral TPN with fat is a major advance, but this system is not suitable for patients whose nutrient requirements are significantly greater than maintenance.

*Vitamins, minerals, trace elements* Precise knowledge of principles of correct vitamin, mineral, and trace element supplementation for patients on TPN is meager [8], and needs vary with the specific clinical state of the individual. The clinical manifestations of trace mineral deficiencies are poorly defined, and serum concentrations are not necessarily a reliable guide to adequate replacement. Copper and zinc deficiencies have been well documented [19] in patients receiving TPN. Current recommendations for trace mineral supplementation are based on a few carefully done balance studies [20].

**Purpose of total parenteral nutrition** The provision, in a readily utilized form, of adequate supplies of water, electrolytes, kilocalories, protein, nitrogen, vitamins, and trace minerals in persons in whom conventional methods of enteral alimentation or intravenous feeding are either inadequate or contraindicated [2,10,21]. The primary nutritional goals of total parenteral nutrition are to conserve lean body mass and maintain nutritional equilibrium. The more far-reaching aims of intravenous hyperalimentation are (1) to meet caloric or nutrient needs in excess of normal requirements [22], (2) to compensate for ongoing losses of nutrients [23], and (3) to provide nutritional rehabilitation of the wasted patient [2,24]. Reversal of growth arrest in children is possible if intake is sufficient to establish a sustained positive kilocalorie and nitrogen balance [25].

**Indications for use** TPN is indicated when adequate enteral nutrition is not possible for a "significant" period of time, which is dependent upon the individual's age, nutritional status, and metabolic status. Even 1 or 2 days of starvation may be significant for a wasted, hypermetabolic patient, whereas a healthy, well-nourished, nonstressed adult may tolerate several weeks of semistarvation without important consequence. Most hospitalized patients have at least some stress and should not be allowed to have inadequate nutrition for more than 10 days. Infants and children are normally hypermetabolic relative to adults and should not have more than 5–7 days of inadequate nutrition.

Specific nutritional assessment techniques may help determine the need for TPN (or enteral hyperalimentation). Serum albumin 3.0 g/dl or less, serum transferrin 180 mg/dl or less, nonreactivity to a battery of common skin test antigens (anergy), and deficits of somatic protein determined by anthropometric measurements all correlate with protein-caloric malnutrition and increased morbidity and mortality [26]. Details of these techniques and tables of normal values have been published elsewhere [27].

Specific conditions for which total parenteral nutrition may be indicated include: (1) enterocutaneous fistulas [21,28–30], (2) gastrointestinal and abdominal wall malformations in neonates, (3) intractable diarrhea in infants, (4) necrotizing enterocolitis, (5) sepsis,

(6) peritonitis, (7) burns, (8) other catabolic or hypermetabolic states, (9) short gut syndrome [24], (10) severe inflammatory bowel disease [25,31–34], (11) chylous ascites [35], (12) major trauma, and (13) prolonged positive pressure ventilation. Solutions of essential amino acids mixed with glucose have been used successfully in patients with disorders of nitrogen metabolism [36–38] such as renal or hepatic failure, for whom the usual types of solutions are contraindicated. These solutions provide adequate kilocalories and essential amino acids, and the patient's own urea (in renal disease) or ammonia (in hepatic failure) is the source of nitrogen for synthesis of nonessential amino acids [37].

***Possible adverse reactions*** *Sepsis* An indwelling central venous catheter is always a potential source of sepsis. Infection may enter around the catheter insertion site or through the catheter because of improper handling of the catheter, the intravenous tubing, or their junction. Bacteremia from other sources may seed the catheter tip, which then becomes a nidus for continued septicemia. Persistent unexplained fever, clinical sepsis, or a positive blood culture mandate removal of the catheter and culture of its tip. Meticulous technique in the placement and care of the catheter should keep the incidence of catheter sepsis below 5%.

*Venous thrombosis* The hypertonic fluid may chemically irritate the endothelium of the vein and produce thrombosis or thrombophlebitis [39].

*Complications related to catheter insertion* (1) Pneumothorax, (2) hydrothorax, (3) arterial injury, (4) hematoma, (5) thoracic duct laceration, (6) air embolism, (7) embolization of severed catheter tips, (8) cardiac arrhythmias, and (9) cardiac perforation and pericardial tamponade [8,40].

*Metabolic complications [41–53]* Hyperglycemia, osmotic diuresis, and hyperosmolar coma may result from glucose intolerance (diabetes, prematurity) or from a too rapid increase in the rate of infusion of hypertonic glucose. Fluid and electrolyte imbalance are fairly common in patients who have severe stress, ongoing fluid loss, renal disease, or cardiac disease, and in premature infants. Hypophosphatemia may occur abruptly when hypertonic glucose infusions are started and may impair oxygen transport. Acidosis, alkalosis, hypocalcemia, hypomagnesemia, and anemia may occur.

Close biochemical and clinical monitoring can prevent serious complications [54–56]. Early detection of abnormalities allows correction by minor adjustments in the nutrient solution without the need for resort to radical measures. Accurate intake and output records and thrice-daily urine glucose determinations are essential. Serum glucose, urea nitrogen, and electrolytes are measured daily during the initial adjustment to hypertonic glucose infusions and the anabolic state. Fluid and electrolyte abnormalities are uncommon after the first week if the patient is otherwise stable, and so monitoring can be less frequent.

Clinical fatty acid deficiency (scaly rash, hair falling out) may occur after 2–3 months of fat free TPN. Biochemical evidence of essential fatty acid deficiency occurs within 2–3 weeks in adults [48,57,58] and 1 week in children [59] and may have unknown consequences. Deficiency can be prevented by twice-weekly administration of Intralipid or by daily cutaneous application of sunflower oil or safflower seed oil in liberal amounts [60].

Excessive doses of Intralipid or inadequate plasma clearance of fat emulsion causes a significant rise in serum cholesterol, triglycerides, phospholipids, and prebeta lipoproteins [53]. Decreased pulmonary diffusing capacity, impairment of immune mechanisms, and thrombocytopeimia may result [20].

Abnormalities of hepatic function have been associated with TPN. Hyperammoneimia is common in children and is occasionally seen in adults, probably because of a relative arginine deficiency [61]. Cholestatic jaundice has been described in children, especially premature infants [62]. Liver dysfunction is less common in adults, and the histologic appearance is usually fatty infiltration [52].

*Contraindications*    (1) if the risks inherent in the procedure exceed the nutritional benefits to be derived, (2) if the alimentary tract can be utilized as a route of nutritional supply [24], (3) if feeding by the intravenous route is needed only for short periods of time in patients whose nutritional status has been good [2], (4) in patients with less than 8 cm of small bowel whose condition will not improve despite prolonged periods of parenteral nutrition [24] and who are not probable candidates for long-term hyperalimentation at home [63], (5) during periods of cardiovascular instability or severe metabolic derangement requiring control or correction [24], (6) for long-term use in patients with pathological hyperlipemia, bleeding, coagulation disturbances, or severe liver damage [8].

*Suggestions for dietitians*    Institutions utilizing total parenteral nutrition should organize a total parenteral nutrition team that includes the physician and nurses involved in the care of these patients, pharmacists who usually prepare the solutions, an epidemiologist to help in development of infection control procedures, and the dietitian. The dietitian should provide information about nutrient needs, composition data, and nutrition histories of specific patients that may help to illuminate present nutritional states, as well as general nutrition education for other team members. One of the first charges of such a team should be the development of a very specific protocol for the use of TPN solutions. The team should evaluate procedures and policies continually and serve as an advisory group in the supervision of parenteral feeding and possibly the use of fiber free semisynthetic liquid diets as well [64]. As the practice of total parenteral nutrition at home becomes more widespread [52,63, 65], dietitians can assist in the education of these patients as well.

**Nutritional Composition of Typical Parenteral Feedings: Working Draft of Suggested Composition for Intravenous Multiviamin Preparation for Daily Maintenance of Adequate Vitamin Status**

| | | Formulations | |
|---|---|---|---|
| *Vitamin* | *Units* | *Pediatric (from infancy to 10 years)* | *Adult (11 years and older)* |
| A | IU | 2,500.0 | 4,000.0 |
| D | IU | 400.0 | 400.0 |
| E | IU | 7.0 | 15.0 |
| Thiamin | mg | 1.2 | 3.0 |
| Riboflavin | mg | 1.4 | 3.6 |
| Niacin | mg | 17.0 | 40.0 |
| $B_6$ | mg | 1.0 | 4.0 |
| Pantothenic acid | mg | 6.0 | 15.0 |
| Folacin | μg | 140.0 | 800.0 |
| Ascorbic acid | mg | 100.0 | 90.0 |
| $B_{12}$ | μg | 0.7 | 6.0 |
| Biotin | μg | 20.0 | 60.0 |

*Source*: Reprinted from FDA regulatory practices and philosophy [66].

**Trace Elements (suggested approximate daily intravenous requirements)**

| | *Adults (mg/day)* | *Infants and children (μg/kg/day)* |
|---|---|---|
| Zinc | 2.50–4.00 | 150–300 |
| Copper | 0.50–1.50 | 20 |
| Manganese | 0.15–0.80 | 2–10 |
| Chromium | 0.01–0.02 | 0.14–0.20 |
| Fluoride | 0.02–0.40 | 10–40 |
| Iodine | 0.05–0.10 | 5 |
| Iron | 0.80–1.50 | 75–100 |

*Source*: Dr. Maurice Shils, personal communication.

**Standard Adult Solution with Crystalline Amino Acids (approximate composition/litre)**

| | |
|---|---|
| Protein equivalent | 42 g |
| Dextrose | 250 g |
| Sodium | 40 meq |
| Potassium | 35 meq |
| Chloride | 77 meq |
| Calcium | 4.8 meq |
| Magnesium | 8 meq |
| Phosphate | 21 meq |
| Acetate | 26 meq |
| Kilocalories | 1,156 |

*Note*: This solution is prepared by mixing 500 ml of 8.5% Travasol (Travenol Laboratories, Deerfield, IL) with 500 ml of 50% dextrose in water and adding appropriate electrolytes. Five millilitres of multivitamin concentrate (MVI, USV Pharmaceutical Corp., Tuckahoe, NY), 1 mg folic acid, and 5 mg vitamin K are added to *one* litre each day.

## Composition of Protein Hydrolysates and Amino Acid Solutions per Litre

| | Crystalline amino acid solutions | | | Protein hydrolysate | |
|---|---|---|---|---|---|
| | FreAmine II* 8.5% | AminoSyn† 7% | Travasol‡ 8.5% | Amigen§ 5% (casein) | Aminosol⊥ 5% (fibrin) |
| Protein equivalent (g/litre) | 78 | 70.0 | 85 | 40.6 | 41.1 |
| Sodium (meq) | 10 | 0.0 | 0 | 35.0 | 10.0 |
| Potassium (meq) | 0 | 5.4 | 0 | 19.0 | 17.0 |
| Chloride (meq) | 0 | 0.0 | 34 | 20.0 | 0.0 |
| Calcium (meq) | 0 | 0.0 | 0 | 5.0 | 0.0 |
| Magnesium (meq) | 0 | 0.0 | 0 | 2.0 | 0.0 |
| Phosphate (meq) | 20 | 0.0 | 0 | 30.0 | 0.0 |

* McGaw Laboratories, Irvine, CA 92705.
† Abbot Laboratories, North Chicago, IL 60064.
‡ Travenol Laboratories, Deerfield, IL 60015.
§ Baxter Laboratories, Morton Grove, IL 60053.
⊥ Cutter Laboratories, Berkeley, CA 94710.

**Standard Adult Solution with Protein Hydrolysate (approximate composition/litre)**

| | |
|---|---|
| Protein equivalent | 40 g |
| Dextrose | 250 g |
| Sodium | 50 meq |
| Potassium | 34 meq |
| Chloride | 60 meq |
| Magnesium | 8 meq |
| Phosphate | 32 meq |
| Kilocalories | 1,162 |

*Note*: This solution is prepared by mixing 500 ml of 10% Amigen (Travenol Laboratories, Deerfield, IL) with 500 ml of 50% dextrose in water and adding appropriate electrolytes. Five millilitres of multivitamin concentrate (MVI, USV Pharmaceutical Corp., Tuckahoe, NY), 1 mg folic acid, and 5 mg vitamin K are added to *one* litre each day. Amigen and other protein hydrolysates already contain some of the electrolytes.

### Standard Infant Solution with Crystalline Amino Acids

|  | Approx. composition per litre | | Amount/kg/day at rate of 135 ml/kg/day | |
|---|---|---|---|---|
| Protein equivalent | 19.6 | g | 2.6 | g |
| Dextrose | 200 | g | 27 | g |
| Sodium | 25 | meq | 3.4 | meq |
| Potassium | 24 | meq | 3.2 | meq |
| Chloride | 35 | meq | 4.7 | meq |
| Calcium | 11.3 | meq | 1.5 | meq |
| Magnesium | 4.8 | meq | 0.7 | meq |
| Phosphorus | 8.5 | mM | 1.1 | mM |
| Lactate | 10 | meq | 1.4 | meq |
| Acetate | 12 | meq | 1.6 | meq |
| Zinc | 2.2 | mg | 0.3 | mg |
| Copper | 150 | $\mu$g | 20.3 | $\mu$g |
| Manganese | 110 | $\mu$g | 14.9 | $\mu$g |
| Chromium | 1.5 | $\mu$g | 0.02 | $\mu$g |
| Iodine | 37 | $\mu$g | 5 | $\mu$g |
| Vitamins A | 5000 | IU | 675 | IU |
| D | 500 | IU | 67.5 | IU |
| E | 2.5 | IU | 0.34 | IU |
| K | 0.2 | mg | — | |
| Folate | 0.25 | mg | — | |
| Kilocalories | 880 | | 118 | |

*Note:* This solution is prepared by mixing 230 ml of 8.5% Travasol (Travenol Laboratories, Deerfield, IL) with 400 ml of 50% dextrose in water and adding appropriate electrolytes, vitamins, trace metals, and sterile water (quantum sufficit to 1 litre). Vitamins A, D, and E plus water soluble vitamins added 2.5 ml (MVI, USV Pharmaceutical Corp., Tuckahoe, NY).

References

1. Lagua, R. T.; Claudion, V. S.; and Thiele, V. F.: Nutrition and Diet Therapy Reference Dictionary. 2d ed. St. Louis: C. V. Mosby, 1974.
2. Shils, M. E.: Total parenteral nutrition. Goodhart, R. S., and Shils, M. E., eds. Modern Nutrition in Health and Disease. Philadelphia: Lea & Febiger, 1973.
3. Shils, M. E.: Guidelines for total parenteral nutrition. JAMA 220: 1721, 1972.
4. Munro, H. N.: Protein hydrolysates and amino acids. White, P. L., and Nagy, M. E., eds. Total Parenteral Nutrition. Acton: Publishing Sciences Group, 1974.
5. Wright, H. K., and Tilson, M.D.: Postoperative Disorders of the Gastrointestinal Tract. New York: Grune & Stratton, 1973.
6. Van Wey, C. W. III; Meng, H. C.; and Sandstead, H. H.: Nitrogen balance in postoperative patients receiving parenteral nutrition. Arch. Surg. 110: 272, 1975.
7. Thiele, V. F.: Clinical Nutrition. St. Louis: C. V. Mosby, 1976.
8. Meng, H. C.: Parenteral nutrition: principles, nutrient requirements, and techniques. Geriatrics 30: 97, 1975.
9. Deitel, M., and Kaminsky, V.: Total nutrition by peripheral vein—the lipid system. Can. Med. Assoc. J. 111: 152, 1974.
10. Coran, A. G.: Total intravenous feeding of infants and children without the use of a central venous catheter. Ann. Surg. 179: 445, 1974.
11. Frey, G.: Hyperalimentation—a review. Ariz. Med. 30: 613, 1973.
12. Fomon, S. J.: Infant Nutrition. Philadelphia: W. B. Saunders, 1974.
13. Dale, G.; Panter-Brick, M.; Wagget, J.; and Young, G.: Plasma amino acid changes in the postsurgical newborn during intravenous nutrition with a synthetic amino acid solution. J. Pediatr. Surg. 11: 17, 1976.
14. Seashore, J. H., and Seashore, M. R.: Protein requirements of infants receiving total parenteral nutrition. J. Pediatr. Surg. 11: 645, 1976.
15. Kinney, J. M.: Calories: nitrogen: disease and injury relationships. White, P. L., and Nagy, M. E., eds. Total Parenteral Nutrition. Acton: Publishing Sciences Group, 1974.

16. Wilmore, D. W.; Moylan, J. A.; Helmkamp, G. M.; and Pruitt, B. A.: Clinical evaluation of a 10% intravenous fat emulsion for parenteral nutrition in thermally injured patients. Ann. Surg. 178: 503, 1973.

17. Puri, P.; Guiney, E. J.; and O'Donnell, B.: Total parenteral feeding in infants using peripheral veins. Arch. Dis. Child. 50: 133, 1975.

18. Gazzaniga, A. B.; Bartlett, R. H.; and Shobe, J. B.: Nitrogen balance in patients receiving either fat or carbohydrate for total intravenous nutrition. Ann. Surg. 182: 163, 1975.

19. Solomons, N. W.; Layden, T. J.; Rosenberg, I. H.; Vo-Khactu, K.; and Sandstead, H. H.: Plasma trace metals during total parenteral alimentation. Gastroenterology 70: 1022, 1976.

20. Dr. Maurice Shils, personal communication.

21. Peaston, M. J. T.: Intravenous feeding. Practitioner 212: 552, 1974.

22. Popp, M. B.; Law, E. J.; and Macmillan, B. G.: Parenteral nutrition in the burned child. Ann. Surg. 179: 219, 1974.

23. Rudman, D.; Millikan, W. J.; Richardson, T. J.; Bisler, T. J. II; Stackhouse, W. J.; and McGarrity, W. C.: Elemental balances during intravenous hyperalimentation of underweight adult subjects. J. Clin. Invest. 55: 94, 1975.

24. Dudrick, S. J.; Ruberg, R. L.; Long, J. M.; Allen, T. R.; and Steiger, E.: Uses, Non-uses and Abuses of Intravenous Hyperalimentation. Philadelphia: Lea & Febiger, 1972.

25. Layden, T.; Rosenberg, J.; Nemchausky, B.; Elson, C.; and Rosenberg, I.: Reversal of growth arrest in adolescents with Crohn's disease after parenteral alimentation. Gastroenterology 70: 1017, 1976.

26. Pietsch, J. B.; Meakins, J. L.; and MacLean, L. D.: The delayed hypersensitivity response: application in clinical surgery. Surgery 82: 349, 1977.

27. Blackburn, G. L.; Bristrian, B. R.; Maini, B. S.; Schlamm, H. T.; and Smith, M. F.: Nutritional and metabolic assessment of the hospitalized patient. JPEN 1: 11, 1977.

28. Bryan, H.; Shennan, A.; Griffin, E.; and Angel, A.: Intralipid—its rational use in parenteral nutrition of the newborn. Pediatrics 58: 787, 1976.

29. Aguirre, A.; Fischer, J. E.; and Welch, C. E.: The role of surgery and hyperalimentation in therapy of gastrointestinal cutaneous fistulae. Ann. Surg. 180: 393, 1974.

30. Weisz, G. M.; Hampel, N.; Gersh, I.; Schramek, A.; and Barzilai, A.: Total intravenous hyperalimentation in the management of cecal fistulas. Dis. Colon Rectum 17: 476, 1974.

31. Fischer, J. E.; Foster, G. S.; Abel, R. M.; Abbott, W. M.; and Ryan, J. A.: Hyperalimentation as primary therapy for inflammatory bowel disease. Am. J. Surg. 125: 165, 1973.

32. Myers, R. N., and Goldstein, F.: Parenteral hyperalimentation—five years' clinical experience. Am. J. Gastroenterol. 62: 313, 1974.

33. Eisenberg, H. W.; Turnbull, R. B.; and Weakley, F. L.: Hyperalimentation as preparation for surgery in transmural colitis (Crohn's disease). Dis. Colon Rectum 17: 469, 1974.

34. Vogel, C. M.; Corwin, T. R.; and Baue, A. E.: Intravenous hyperalimentation in the treatment of inflammatory diseases of the bowel. Arch. Surg. 108: 460, 1974.

35. Viswanathan, U., and Putnam, T. C.: Therapeutic intravenous alimentation for traumatic chylous ascites in a child. J. Pediatr. Surg. 9: 405, 1974.

36. Abel, R. M.; Abbott, W. M.; Beck, C. H.; Ryan, J. A.; and Fischer, J. E.: Essential L-amino acids for hyperalimentation in patients with disordered nitrogen metabolism. Am. J. Surg. 128: 317, 1974.

37. Deitel, M.; Sanderson, I.; and Petsoulas, T.: A system of intravenous hyperalimentation. Int. Surg. 58: 670, 1973.

38. Rudman, D.; Galambos, J. T.; Smith, R. B. III; Salam, A. A.; and Warren, W. D.: Comparison of the effect of various amino acids upon the blood ammonia concentration of patients with liver disease. Am. J. Clin. Nutr. 26: 916, 1973.

39. Wilkinson, A. W.: Complications of parenteral feeding. Wilkinson, A. W. Parenteral Nutrition. Baltimore: Williams & Wilkins, 1972.

40. Ryan, J. A.; Abel, R. M.; Abbott, W. M.; Hopkins, C. C.; McCheeney, T.; Colley, R.; Phillips, K.; and Fischer, J. E.: Catheter complications in total parenteral nutrition. N. Engl. J. Med. 290: 757, 1974.

41. Heird, W. C.; Winters, R. W.; and Dudrick, S. J.: Metabolic complications of total parenteral nutrition. Bode, H. H., and Warshaw, J. B. Parenteral nutrition in infancy and childhood. Adv. Exp. Med. Biol. 46: 256, 1974.

42. Sanderson, I., and Deitel, M.: Insulin response in patients receiving concentrated infusions of glucose and casein hydrolysate for complete parenteral nutrition. Ann. Surg. 179: 387, 1974.
43. Craddock, P. R.; Yawata, Y.; Vansanten, L.; Gilberstadt, S.; Silvis, S.; and Jacob, H. S.: Acquired phagocyte dysfunction—a complication of the hypophosphatemia of parenteral hyperalimentation. N. Engl. J. Med. 290: 1403, 1974.
44. Lichtman, M. A.: Hypoalimentation during hyperalimentation. N. Engl. J. Med. 290: 1432, 1974.
45. Altschule, M. D.: Adverse effects of prolonged intravenous alimentation. Med. Counterpoint 34: 21, 1973.
46. Sheldon, G. F.: Defective hemoglobin function: a complication of hyperalimentation. J. Trauma 13: 971, 1973.
47. Vilter, R. W.; Bozian, R. C.; Hess, E. V.; Zellner, D. C.; and Petering, H. C.: Manifestations of copper deficiency in a patient with systemic schlerosis or intravenous hyperalimentation. N. Engl. J. Med. 291: 188, 1974.
48. Richardson, T. J., and Sgoutas, D.: Essential fatty acid deficiency in four adult patients during total parenteral nutrition. Am. J. Clin. Nutr. 28: 258, 1975.
49. Schulze, V. E.: Supraventricular arrhythmias caused by parenteral hyperalimentation. JAMA 228: 341, 1974.
50. Ricour, C.; Millot, M.; and Balsan, S.: Phosphorus depletion in children on long-term total parenteral nutrition. Acta Paediatr. Scand. 64: 385, 1975.
51. Thompson, S. W.: The Pathology of Parenteral Nutrition with Lipids. Springfield: Charles C. Thomas, 1974.
52. Jejeebhoy, K. N.; Zohrab, W. J.; Langer, B.; Phillips, M. J.; Kuksis, A.; and Anderson, C. M.: Total parenteral nutrition at home for 23 months, without complication and with good rehabilitation. Gastroenterology 65: 811, 1973.
53. Forget, P. P.; Fernandes, J.; and Haverkamp Begemann, P.: Utilization of fat emulsion during total parenteral nutrition in children. Acta Paediatr. Scand. 64: 377, 1975.
54. Ruberg, R. L.: Hospital practice of total parenteral nutrition. White, P. L., and Nagy, M. E., eds. Total Parenteral Nutrition. Acton: Publishing Sciences Group, 1974.
55. Parsa, M. H.; Ferrer, J. M.; and Habif, D. V.: Safe Central Venous Nutrition. Guidelines for Prevention and Management of Complications. Springfield: Charles C. Thomas, 1974.
56. Shils, M. E.: Minerals. White, P. L., and Nagy, M. E., eds. Total Parenteral Nutrition. Acton: Publishing Sciences Group, 1974.
57. Riella, M. C.; Broviac, J. W.; Wells, M.; and Scribner, B. H.: Essential fatty acid deficiency in human adults during total parenteral nutrition. Ann. Intern. Med. 83: 786, 1975.
58. Wene, J. D.; Connor, W. E.; and DenBesten, L.: The development of essential fatty acid deficiency in healthy men fed fat-free diets intravenously and orally. J. Clin. Invest. 56: 127, 1975.
59. Friedman, Z.; Danon, A.; Stahlman, M. T.; and Oates, J. A.: Rapid onset of essential fatty acid deficiency in the newborn. Pediatrics 58: 640, 1976.
60. Friedman, Z.; Schochat, S. J.; Maisels, J.; Marks, K. H.; and Lamberth, E. L.: Correction of essential fatty acid deficiency in newborn infant by cutaneous application of sunflower-seed oil. Pediatrics 58: 650, 1976.
61. Heird, W. C.; Nicholson, J. F.; Driscoll, J. M.; Schullinger, J. M; and Winters, R. W.: Hyperammonemia resulting from intravenous alimentation using a mixture of synthetic L-amino acids. J. Pediatr. 81: 162, 1972.
62. Touloukian, R. J., and Seashore, J. H.: Hepatic secretory obstruction with total parenteral nutrition in the infant. J. Pediatr. Surg. 10: 353, 1975.
63. Shils, M. E.: A program for total parenteral nutrition at home. Am. J. Clin. Nutr. 28: 1479, 1975.
64. Johnson, F. Q.: The therapeutic dietitian's role in the alimentation group. J. Am. Diet. Assoc. 62: 648, 1973.
65. Broviac, J. W., and Scribner, B. H.: Prolonged parenteral nutrition in the home. Surg. Gynecol. Obstet. 139: 24, 1974.
66. DeMerre, L. J.: FDA regulatory practices and philosophy. White, P. L., and Nagy, M. E., eds. Total Parenteral Nutrition. Acton: Publishing Sciences Group, 1974.

PART C      Modifications in Protein Content

# High Protein, High Kilocalorie Diet

*Definition*    A diet that provides a level of total kilocalories and protein substantially above that which is normally required. A typical high protein, high kilocalorie diet for an adult may include 1,000 or more supplemental kilocalories daily. It should provide a minimum of 1.5 g protein per kilogram of body weight. For the adult the usual range is between 100 and 120 g protein daily. The Recommended Dietary Allowance for protein for adults is 0.8 g/kg of body weight [1].

*Characteristics of the diet*    The diet is essentially a normal one supplemented with high protein foods. Additional servings of milk, meat, and eggs are included, and special high protein, high kilocalorie proprietary liquid supplements may also be utilized. When kilocalories must be increased to inordinately high levels, as in the severely burned patient, it is inevitable that the diet will be high in carbohydrate and fat as well as protein.

*Purpose of the diet*    (1) to provide for the nutritional rehabilitation of the protein and kilocalorie malnourished patient or (2) to prevent weight loss and tissue wasting in conditions under which normal protein and kilocalorie requirements are greatly increased.

*Effects of the diet*    If continued for a sufficient period of time, a high protein, high kilocalorie diet will reverse the effects of weight loss and tissue wasting associated with protein–kilocalorie malnutrition. It also has a partially restorative effect on immune responses altered by severe malnutrition. If protein and kilocalorie deficits are severe and prolonged, weight loss and protein wasting will progress to atrophy of the thymus gland, delayed hypersensitivity reactions, and altered cell mediated immune responses [2,3]. In one study involving very young infants, high protein, high kilocalorie diet therapy partially but not completely normalized immune responses that had been depressed by severe malnutrition [4]. However, the specific effects of protein depletion on immune responses in man remains obscure and controversial.

*Indications for use*    *Protein–kilocalorie undernutrition*    Replenishment of nutritional reserves via a high kilocalorie, high protein diet adjusted to the needs and tolerances of the individual is indicated in many forms of primary or secondary protein-kilocalorie malnutrition [5–7]. In constructing these diets attention should be paid to the relationship between nonprotein kilocalories and protein nitrogen. A high kilocalorie, low protein diet will distort body composition, while a high protein diet without extra kilocalories from nonprotein sources will permit much of the nitrogen to be wasted. The optimal kilocalorie:nitrogen ratio is approximately 100–200 kcal/g of nitrogen intake [7]. A commonly used kilocalorie: nitrogen ratio is 150 nonprotein kilocalories per every gram of nitrogen [8].

Tissue proteins are depleted before changes in serum albumin are detectable. Therefore, the need for a high kilocalorie, high protein diet should be anticipated before blood changes have occurred [9]. The diet may be especially indicated in preparing a nutritionally wasted patient for surgery. Surgical procedures often result in a catabolic loss of body nitrogen [10], and the protein status of many surgical patients is poor [11]. Although not conclusive, animal studies have suggested that nutrition may play an important role in the adaptation of the small intestine after massive resection [12], that the protein and caloric content of the diet may influence response to the hemorrhagic shock of surgery [13], and that malnutrition severely impairs colonic healing [13]. According to one author, a serum albumin below 3 g/100 ml is indicative of a state of malnutrition so severe that it should be corrected by diet before elective surgery is attempted [8].

*In hypermetabolic or catabolic states* Additional protein and kilocalories should be provided in conditions such as fevers or thyrotoxicosis [7]. High protein, high kilocalorie diet therapy is also indicated in the severely burned patient in order to compensate for greatly increased nutritional requirements and losses of protein salts and fluids from the burn site [15–17]. A combination of several forms of nutritional support may be necessary to achieve the required intakes of protein and kilocalories. The optimum diet for a severely burned patient should contain 2,000–2,200 kcal/m$^2$ of body surface area daily, or approximately 4,000 kcal and 15 g nitrogen/m$^2$ daily, or approximately 30 g nitrogen daily, or 187.5 g protein, as well as supplemental vitamins [15].

*In anorexia nervosa* Restoration of proper nutrition is associated with a reversal of leukopenia, elevated blood urea nitrogen, and some of the other abnormalities associated with anorexia nervosa [18].

**Possible adverse reactions** *Elevated lipid levels in susceptible individuals* The diet is high in lactose, cholesterol, and saturated fat and may produce elevated levels of serum lipids in susceptible individuals if continued over a long period of time. However, adjustments can be made to lower cholesterol, saturated fat intake, and lactose.

*Negative calcium balances* Very high protein diets adversely affect calcium balance, resulting in increased urinary calcium excretion and in some instances negative calcium balances [19,20]. The mechanism of the calciuretic effect of dietary protein is unknown but may be related to alterations of calcium absorption in the gastrointestinal tract [20].

*Vitamin A deficiency* Under certain conditions protein supplements given to patients with kwashiorkor may provoke symptoms of vitamin A deficiency. A high protein diet results in a greater demand by the body for vitamin A. Those patients with kwashiorkor whose liver stores of vitamin A are low should not be treated solely with nonfat milk supplements low in vitamin A. The increased dietary protein will increase the requirement for vitamin A and may mobilize the last reserves of vitamin A from the liver, thus precipitating vitamin A deficiency [21,22]. The vitamin A content of the high protein, high kilocalorie diet presented here is adequate. However, any adjustments made by dietitians in the diet should be made in such a manner as to ensure a sufficient intake of vitamin A.

*Hepatic coma in susceptible individuals* In a few susceptible individuals with severe hepatitis, usually those with massive necrosis, a high protein diet may induce the syndrome of hepatic coma [23].

*Contraindications* The diet is contraindicated in hepatic coma or hyperammoniemia [24] (a blood ammonia level above 150 $\mu$g/100 ml), in uremia, or in any condition in which the renal glomerular rate has been seriously impaired [25]. Despite weight loss and delayed maturation and growth associated with certain inborn errors of protein metabolism, such as methylmalonic acidura, arginosuccinic acidura, proprionicacidemia, hyperammoniemia, maple syrup urine disease, etc., a high protein diet is contraindicated [26–30]. Treatment of choice is either selective amino acid or protein restricted diets [26–30].

*Suggestions for dietitians* Select at least one-half of the day's protein allowance from complete protein foods. Include some complete protein food at each meal. For those persons following a vegetarian high protein diet, an excellent one has been published [31].

With severely burned patients or those whose intakes must be extremely high, it may be necessary to use commercial proprietary supplemental formulas, such as Citrotein,* Sustacal,† or Meritene,* etc. Extra powdered milk may be added to creamed potatoes, cream soups, gravies, and cottage cheese, provided that the vitamin A content of the diet is kept at a high level in patients with low vitamin A stores.

Glucose and glucose polymers may be used as a sweetening agent instead of sucrose. Particularly in a polymerized form, glucose is less sweet than sucrose and more of it may be incorporated in foods without causing them to be overly sweet.

Distribution of meals should be planned for maximum food consumption by the specific patient. In some instances, an increased number of feedings may be indicated. In others, fewer feedings may result in a better appetite.

* Doyle Pharmaceutical Co., Minneapolis, MN 55416.
† Mead Johnson and Co., Evansville, IN 47721.

**Daily food plan (include at least the following foods or their nutritive equivalents)**
**Approximate composition: protein, 125 g; fat, 115 g; carbohydrate, 245 g; kcal, 2,500**

1 qt whole milk
8 oz medium fat meat, fish, poultry, cheese, or substitute (cooked weight)
2 eggs
4 servings vegetables, including:
     1 serving green or yellow vegetable
     1–2 servings potato or substitute
     1–2 servings other vegetable
3 servings fruit, including 1 citrus fruit
1 serving whole grain or enriched cereal
6 servings whole grain or enriched bread
5 tsp butter or fortified margarine
2 tbsp sugar, jam, jelly, or honey

*Note:* See exchange lists, pp. F20–F25, except for last item.

**Sample menu**

A.M.

½ cup orange juice
½ cup farina with milk and sugar
2 eggs scrambled in 2 tsp fortified margarine or butter
1 slice enriched bread with fortified margarine or butter and 1 tbsp jam
1 cup milk
Coffee or tea with 1 tsp sugar

Noon

4 oz roast turkey on 2 slices whole wheat bread
Tomato salad with French dressing
½ cup fruit cocktail
1 cup milk
Coffee or tea with 1 tsp sugar

P.M.

4 oz round steak
1 baked potato
½ cup spinach
2 slices enriched bread
2 tsp fortified margarine or butter
1 banana
1 cup milk
Coffee or tea with 1 tsp sugar

Between meals

1 cup milk
1 slice enriched bread with 1 tsp fortified margarine or butter

References

1. Food and Nutrition Board, National Research Council:   Recommended Dietary Allowances. 9th ed. Washington, D. C.: National Academy of Sciences, 1980.
2. Worthington, B. S.:   Effect of nutritional status on immune phenomena.   J. Am. Diet. Assoc. 65: 123, 1974.
3. Schlesinger, L., and Stekel, A.:   Impaired cellular immunity in marasmic infants.   Am. J. Clin. Nutr. 27: 614, 1974.
4. Ferguson, A. C.; Lawlor, G. J.; Neumann, C. G.; Oh, W.; and Stiehm, R.:   Decreased rosette-forming lymphocytes in malnutrition and intrauterine growth retardation.   J. Pediatr. 85: 717, 1974.
5. Viteri, F. E., and Arroyave, G.:   Protein-calorie malnutrition. Goodhart, R. S., and Shils, M. E., eds. Modern Nutrition in Health and Disease. 5th ed. Philadelphia:   Lea & Febiger, 1973.
6. Robinson, C. H., and Lawler, M. L.:   Normal and Therapeutic Nutrition. 15th ed. New York:   Macmillan, 1977.
7. Moore, F. D., and Brennan, M. F.:   Surgical injury:   body composition and neuroendocrinology. Ballinger, W. F.; Collins, J. A.; Drucker, W. R.; Dudrick, S. J.; and Zeppa, R. eds. Manual of Surgical Nutrition. Philadelphia:   W. B. Saunders, 1975.
8. Kinney, J. M.:   Calories, nitrogen, disease and injury relationships. White, P. L., and Nagy, M. E., eds. Total Parenteral Nutrition. Acton:   Publishing Sciences Group, 1974.
9. Mason, E. E.:   Fluid, Electrolyte and Nutrient Therapy in Surgery. Philadelphia:   Lea & Febiger, 1974.
10. O'Keefe, S. J.; Sender, P. M.; and James, W. P. T.:   Catabolic loss of body nitrogen in response to surgery.   Lancet 2: 1035, 1974.
11. Bistrian, B. R.; Blackburn, G. L.; Hallowell, E.; and Heddle, R.:   Protein status of general surgical patients.   JAMA 230: 858, 1974.
12. Wilmore, D. W.; Dudrick, S. J.; Daly, J. M.; and Vars, H. M.:   The role of nutrition in the adaptation of the small intestine after massive resection.   Surg. Gynecol. Obstet. 132: 673, 1971.
13. Drucker, W. R.; Howar, P. L.; and McCoy, S.:   The influence of diet on response to hemorrhagic shock.   Ann. Surg. 181: 698, 1975.

14. Irwin, T. T., and Hunt, T. K.: Effect of malnutrition on colonic healing. Ann. Surg. 180: 765, 1974.
15. Wilmore, D. W.: Nutrition and metabolism following thermal injury. Clin. Plast. Surg. 1: 603, 1974.
16. Curreri, P. W.; Richmond, D.; Marvin, J.; and Baxter, C. R.: Dietary requirements of patients with major burns. J. Am. Diet. Assoc. 65: 415, 1974.
17. Love, R. T.: Nutrition in the burned patient. J. Miss. State Med. Assoc. 13: 391, 1972.
18. Silverman, J. A.: Anorexia nervosa: clinical observations in a successful treatment plan. J. Pediatr. 84: 68, 1974.
19. Rekha Anand, C., and Linkswiler, H. M.: Effect of protein intake on calcium balance of young men given 500 mg. calcium daily. J. Nutr. 104: 695, 1974.
20. Margen, S.; Chu, J. Y.; Kaufmann, N. A.; and Calloway, D. H.: Studies in calcium metabolism. I. The calciuretic effect of dietary protein. Am. J. Clin. Nutr. 27: 584, 1974.
21. Arroyave, G.: Interrelations between protein and vitamin A and metabolism. Am. J. Clin. Nutr. 22: 1119, 1969.
22. Roels, W. A., and Lui, N. S. T.: The vitamins. Vitamin A and carotene. Goodhart, R. S., and Shils, M. E., eds. Modern Nutrition in Health and Disease. 5th ed. Philadelphia: Lea & Febiger, 1973.
23. Davidson, C. S.: Diseases of the liver. Goodhart, R. S., and Shils, M. E., eds. Modern Nutrition in Health and Disease. 5th ed. Philadelphia: Lea & Febiger, 1973.
24. Scharachmidt, B. F.: Approaches to the management of fulminant hepatic failure. Med. Clin. N. Am. 59: 927, 1975.
25. Burton, B. T.: Current concepts of nutrition and diet in diseases of the kidney. J. Am. Diet. Assoc. 65: 623, 1974.
26. Scriver, C. R., and Rosenberg, L. E.: Amino Acid Metabolism and Its Disorders. Philadelphia: W. B. Saunders, 1973.
27. Lancaster, G.; Mamer, O. A.; and Scriver, C. R.: Branched-chain alpha-keto acids isolated as oxime derivatives: relationship to the corresponding hydroxy acids and amino acids in maple syrup urine disease. Metabolism 23: 257, 1974.
28. Nyhan, W. L.; Fawcett, N.; Ando, T.; Rennert, O. W.; and Julius, R. L.: Response to dietary therapy in $B_{12}$ unresponsive methymalonic acidemia. Pediatrics 51: 539, 1973.
29. Brandt, I. K.; Hsia, E. Y.; Clement, D. H.; and Provence, S. A.: Proprionicacidemia (ketotic hyperglycinemia): dietary treatment resulting in normal growth and development. Pediatrics 53: 391, 1974.
30. Hartlage, P. L.; Coryell, M. E.; Knowlton Hall, W.; and Hahan, D.: Argininosuccinic aciduria: perinatal diagnosis and early dietary management. J. Pediatr. 85: 86, 1974.
31. Beckner, A.; Hayasaka, R.; Jacobsen, R.; Johnson, M.; Oakley, S.; and Vyhmeister, J.: Diet Manual Utilizing a Vegetarian Diet Plan. Loma Linda: Seventh Day Adventist Dietetic Association, 1975.

# Controlled Protein, Potassium, and Sodium Diet

***Definition*** A diet in which the dietary intake of sodium, potassium, and protein are carefully regulated from day to day.

***Characteristics of the diet*** The diet is based on a specialized list of foods that details the amounts of protein, sodium, and potassium each particular food item contains; it permits the substitution of other food items within the list as long as the total protein, sodium, potassium, and fluids do not exceed the limits of the diet prescription [1]. The level of each restriction ordered is not static but is dependent upon the patient's clinical and biochemical status at any particular time [2].

Particularly at lower levels of protein intake, protein containing foods of high biological value, such as milk and eggs, are preferentially used over other sources of protein; they should supply about three-fourths of the daily protein allowance [3]. As milk, meats, and fruits and vegetables are all good sources of potassium, they must be restricted. When a fluid restriction is also necessary, all foods should be served well drained, including canned fruits. Low protein foods are provided in liberal amounts in order to provide adequate kilocalories. On lower levels of protein intake, wheat starch products are used in baking; a low protein pasta, Aproten,* and carbohydrate supplements, such as Cal-Power,* Hy Cal,† Controlyte,‡ and Polycose,§ all provide extra kilocalories. The inclusion of supplements of essential amino acids, such as Amin-Aid⊥ or other essential amino acid solutions tailored to the specific needs of these patients, is most beneficial at levels of protein intake of less than 30 g/day [4–7].

***Purpose of the diet*** (1) To achieve and maintain adequate nutritional status; (2) to lighten the work of a diseased kidney by reducing the urea, uric acid, creatinine, and electrolytes (especially potassium, sodium, and phosphate) that must be excreted; (3) to replace substances, e.g., protein and sodium, that are lost to the body in abnormal amounts because of the impaired renal function [2]; or (4) to replace protein lost in dialysis. Achievement of these goals requires regulation of protein intake, regulation of fluid intake to balance output, regulation of potassium and phosphate intake, insistence upon an adequate caloric intake, and supplementation with appropriate vitamins [2].

Nutritional priorities in the treatment of acute renal failure include preservation of body cell mass, especially visceral protein status, and provision of sufficient energy to permit maintenance of vital functions and of sufficient protein to replace amino acids lost from catabolism [4] and dialysis.

***Kilocalories*** The diet will not be effective unless a full complement of kilocalories is provided [3,5–8]. Nitrogen balance is

* Dietary Specialties, Henkel Corporation, Minneapolis, MN 55435.
† Beecham-Massengill Pharmaceuticals, Melrose, MA 02176.
‡ Doyle Pharmaceutical Co., Minneapolis, MN 55416.
§ Ross Laboratories, Columbus, OH 43216.
⊥ McGaw Laboratories, Irvine, CA 92705.

influenced by both energy and protein intakes [7]. It has been shown that the optimum improvement in nitrogen balance is achieved with a caloric intake of 55 kcal/kg of body weight per day [8]. A minimum of 35–45 kcal/day is required for adults [9]. Children need 1,500 kcal/m² of body surface area [10]. Restoration of body weight in the malnourished child requires 1½ to 2 times normal energy requirements [11].

*Protein in acute renal failure* Protein needs in acute renal failure are often greatly increased by hypercatabolic states such as sepsis, hemorrhage, or open, draining wounds [12]. Until recently, however, severe or total restriction of dietary protein was common. Present practice involves early, frequent dialysis to prevent uremia. In addition, a high protein, high kilocalorie, high water soluble vitamin intake may decrease muscle wasting and improve clinical status [13].

When adequate nourishment cannot be provided orally, the use of parenteral nutrition may be considered. One guide recommends early and vigorous use of hypertonic glucose with 25–40 g/day of high biological value mixtures of crystalline amino acids and a kilocalorie: nitrogen ratio of 300:to 450. It is not certain whether exclusion of nonessential amino acids is beneficial [12].

*Protein in chronic renal failure* Protein intake should be adjusted to avoid induction of uremic toxicity on the one hand and malnutrition on the other [13]. There is no consensus as to whether diets providing less than 0.6 g protein per kilogram of body weight are nutritionally adequate and capable of preventing the wasting syndrome [14]. Agreement about the point in renal disease at which protein restriction should begin is also lacking [9,13].

Since many uremia symptoms appear only when the serum urea nitrogen (SUN) is greater than 90 mg/100 ml, one author recommends protein restriction to maintain a SUN level below 90 mg/100 ml or preferably below 60 mg/100 ml. There is a direct relationship between the ratio of SUN level to creatinine concentration and protein intake in individuals not undergoing dialysis. The optimal protein intake may be estimated using an equation that represents this relationship as $y = 0.13x + 0.77$, where $y = $ SUN level divided by serum creatinine concentration and $x$ represents estimated protein needs [13]. (Example: if SUN = 60 and serum creatinine concentration = 6, then $y = 60/10$, or 6; and $0.13x + 0.77 = y$, or 6; and $0.13x = 6 - 0.77$; and $x$, or estimated protein needs = $5.23/0.13$). Therefore, as in the example, when SUN equals 60 and serum creatinine concentration equals 10, estimated protein needs equal 40 g/day.

The degree of protein restriction needed may also be determined from the glomerular filtration rate (GFR). Restriction is rarely necessary until the glomerular filtration rate falls below 25 ml/min. When GFR is 20–25 ml/min, a protein intake of up to 90 g may be indicated; at a level of 10–15 ml/min, protein intake should be no more than 50 g; for a GFR of 4–10 ml/min, the intake should be 40 g protein [13]. In children, protein should never be restricted below 1.0 to 2.0 g/kg of body weight of high biological value protein [15]. A diet with a large proportion of its protein of high biological value is used more efficiently than one with lower quality proteins high in nonessential amino acids. A low protein diet high in essential amino acids and low in nonessential amino acids promotes recycling of urea nitrogen for protein synthesis. However, the total amount of urea nitrogen recycled has been determined to be much less than previous estimates and of little practical nutritional significance [16].

The abnormalities of amino acid and protein metabolism that occur in chronic renal failure should be considered in the planning of diets for renal disease; essential amino acid supplements or hyperalimentation solutions may be needed [17,18]. Serum concentrations of albumin; transferrin; and plasma concentrations of valine, leucine, isoleucine, lysine, and tryptophan are reduced in chronic renal failure. The conversion of phenylalanine to tyrosine is impaired [19]. Therefore, tyrosine intake should be increased, while phenylalanine excess should be avoided. Histidine can not be transaminated and acts as an essential amino acid [20,21]. Excess histidine should also be avoided as it will increase serum phenylalanine levels [18]. Any excess of methionine or of the other sulfur containing amino acids should be avoided because they slow down the repletion processes [18].

One recommendation for a supplemental formula diet suggests the following ratios of amino acids: for each milligram of threonine, 1.3 mg isoleucine, 1.8 mg leucine, 1.5 mg valine, 7 mg phenylalanine, 1.2 mg tyrosine, 0.4 mg methionine, 0.4 mg cystine, 0.24 mg tryptophan, 1.1 mg lysine, and 0.5 mg histidine. Total amounts to be provided would depend upon patient needs [18].

Although dietary protein prescriptions in the range of 30–50 g are not universal, the problems imposed should be emphasized. It becomes increasingly important to provide adequate kilocalories and protein of high biological value. Weight loss, precipitated by an inadequate caloric intake, initiates a detrimental catabolic process involving breakdown of tissue protein and mobilization of intracellular potassium; thus, the dietary restrictions become ineffective and counterproductive [22].

*Protein in maintenance hemodialysis*    Protein wasting and impaired anabolic response are common findings in patients undergoing hemodialysis [13]. Although the cause is multifaceted, nutritional factors play an important role. Patients undergoing hemodialysis thrice weekly should receive at least 1.0 g protein/kg of body weight per day. An additional 0.2 g/kg/day either as protein or as essential amino acids may also be recommended [13].

*Protein in maintenance peritoneal dialysis*    Protein losses into the dialysate during peritoneal dialysis are much greater than those associated with hemodialysis [23]. A daily protein intake of 1.0 to 1.5 g [23] or 1.2 to 1.5 g [13] may be required, with at least half of this amount from high biological value proteins [23].

*Carbohydrate and fat intake*    Of individuals with chronic renal disease, including those undergoing dialysis, 40–60% develop type IV hyperlipidemia with elevated levels of serum triglycerides and very low density lipoproteins (VLDL) [13,24,25], and increased concentrations of triglycerides in both low density lipoproteins (LDL), and very low density lipoproteins (VLDL). In nondialyzed individuals with chronic renal failure [26] and in those on hemodialysis [27] fasting plasma triglyceride levels decreased in response to dietary intervention that provided a reduction in the proportion of carbohydrate from 50 to 35% of total daily kilocalories. Conflicting results have been reported by other investigators, however [28], and before widespread recommendations are made, long-term studies with larger groups of subjects should be undertaken to define clearly the role of both dietary carbohydrate and fat in the hyperlipidemia of renal disease.

*Sodium and potassium intakes*   Optimal sodium and potassium intakes in patients with renal disease are dependent upon individual circumstances and can be determined only by repeated measurements of these electrolytes in the serum and urine [2]. Frequent determinations of weight, blood pressures taken in the supine and standing positions, serum creatinine, and 24-hour urinary excretion of sodium are necessary for deciding optimal sodium intakes [29]. Sodium excretion should be measured after the patient has been on a 40 meq or 920-mg sodium diet for 4 days. The loss of this electrolyte in the urine accompanied by weight loss and decrease in renal function indicates that additional sodium is needed in the diet. On the other hand, weight gain on a maintenance diet with constant caloric intake is indicative of sodium and water retention [30].

*Sodium and potassium in acute renal failure*   Potassium requirements vary in acute renal failure depending upon the degree of hypermetabolism caused by stress, infection, fever, and pain and upon the hemodynamic status, which is the key to perfusion of cells in tissue anabolism [4]. Serum potassium levels should be maintained at 3.5 to 4.0 meq/litre. When renal failure fluid therapy is combined with dialysis [4], sodium and chloride may be required. Acidosis is best treated by the administration of sodium and potassium acetate salts, while alkalosis responds best to sodium and potassium chloride salts [4].

*Sodium and potassium in chronic renal failure*   In the presence of edema and hypertension (diastolic blood pressure greater than 110 mm mercury), sodium intake may be restricted to levels as low as 40 meq or 920 mg/day [29]. In patients with low body sodium levels (especially after diuretic therapy, vomiting, or diarrhea), as well as normotension or orthostatic hypotension, sodium intakes should be increased to 90 meq or 2,070 mg or more daily [29].

Hypertension is more likely to occur in patients with glomerulonephritis, while patients with polycystic kidney disease, pyelonephritis, or disease affecting the renal tubules where sodium is reabsorbed are more likely to have salt wasting syndromes [29]. In children with hypertension and edema due to chronic glomerulonephritis, daily sodium intake in the range of 45–130 meq or 1,035–3,000 mg/day has been recommended [15]. Dietary restriction of sodium usually becomes necessary when the glomerular filtration rate falls below 4–10 ml/min, or even earlier in the presence of coexisting conditions such as congestive heart failure, liver disease, and the nephrotic syndrome [13].

When urinary volume is adequate, a normal blood level of potassium is maintained. However, in renal insufficiency potassium loads are not excreted in a normal manner. In end stage renal disease, hyperkalemia can occur because of cell catabolism that releases potassium into the blood [30]. Hyperkalemia is exaggerated in the presence of metabolic acidosis. Potassium is generally restricted to 40–60 meq or 1,560–2,340 mg/day [30].

*Sodium and potassium in maintenance hemodialysis*     Daily sodium intake should be limited to 65–87 meq or 1,500–2,000 mg daily to control body fluid retention and hypertension, which may precipitate pulmonary edema and congestive heart failure [9]. Individuals with severe oliguria need more rigid restrictions.

The degree of potassium restriction must be individualized and depends upon the patient's urine volume, serum potassium prior to dialysis, the presence or degree of acidosis, and the amount of potassium in the dialysate bath. One guide suggests that a daily intake of approximately 52 meq or 2,030 mg potassium is typical if the dialysate bath contains 2.6 meq or 100 mg, while another recommends a daily limit of 70 meq or 2,730 mg potassium a day [13]. Patients with diabetes who are dialyzed are more sensitive to potassium excess than others.

*Sodium and potassium in maintenance peritoneal dialysis*     Mild to moderate restrictions of sodium and potassium are indicated for persons on home peritoneal dialysis. An 87–130 meq or 2–3 g sodium intake is reasonable, allows some flexibility in menu planning, and generally prevents excessive thirst. Reductions in sodium content of the dialysate are also helpful in controlling postdialysis thirst [23]. Dietary potassium intake is limited to 75–90 meq or 2,925–3,500 mg daily. It is difficult to reduce potassium intake further, as a high protein and a very low potassium diet are mutually exclusive. Most protein rich foods of high biological value are also high in potassium [23].

*Water balance and fluid restriction in acute renal failure*     Fluid tolerance must be ascertained prior to the start of renal failure fluid therapy [4], particularly in instances of oliguria. Insensible water losses will allow for a total fluid intake of 700–800 ml/day. Once urine output is satisfactory, the optimal intake of 1,500–2,000 ml/day may be achieved [4]. Nasogastric fistula and stool losses will also increase fluid tolerance.

*Water balance and fluid restriction in chronic renal failure and dialysis*     Fluid intake should balance output in the person with renal failure who is not being dialyzed. Daily fluid intake is limited to 400–600 ml, which compensates for water lost from the lungs and the skin [24]. To this should be added fluid equivalent to the amount (if any) lost in the urine or gastrointestinal tract [9]. Fluid intake for the patient on dialysis is usually less than 1 litre/day [3].

*Calcium and phosphorous intakes*     In order to prevent hypocalcemia and renal osteodystrophy secondary to elevations in serum phosphate concentration, calcium supplements may be given in chronic renal failure. In children, oral calcium supplementation with 1–2 g or 50–100 meq elemental calcium per day as calcium carbonate should be started when the glomerular filtration rate reaches 20–25 ml/min [31].

Dietary phosphorus can be effectively controlled by the use of aluminum hydroxide or aluminum carbonate gels, which bind phosphorus in the gastrointestinal tract, decreasing its absorption [9,32, 33]. When the glomerular filtration rate is below 25 ml/min, dietary phosphorus should be restricted to 700–800 mg or 45–52 meq/day, and phosphate binding gels should be continued [32]. Predialysis serum phosphorous concentrations should be maintained between 4.5 and 5.0 mg/dl by these measures [23].

*Vitamin D*    Small amounts of 1,25-dihydroxycholecalciferol correct the abnormal calcium and phosphorus metabolism [34] and ameliorate secondary hyperparathyroidism [35] related to the failure of the diseased kidney to manufacture this metabolically active form of vitamin D. Specifically, 1,25-dihydroxycholecalciferol has a calcemic effect in chronic dialysis, decreases levels of immunoreactive parathyroid hormone, and is associated with histologic improvement in bone disease [35].

*Other vitamins and minerals*    Blood levels of water soluble vitamins are decreased in chronic renal failure because of inadequate intake and altered metabolism. Further reductions occur during dialysis [13,23,35,36]. It is currently recommended that supplements of folic acid, pyridoxine hydrochloride, ascorbic acid, and other water soluble vitamins be given. Uremia causes serum elevations in retinol binding protein and therefore vitamin A levels as well. Supplements of vitamins A, E, and K are not necessary. Zinc supplementation may improve altered taste acuity [37].

**Effects of the diet**    The degree of azotemia may be markedly reduced by protein restriction. Dietary management may permit a patient with a glomerular filtration rate of 10 to 1.5 ml/min to function well and lead a moderately productive life [9]. In fact, the diet can prolong life and eliminate the symptoms of uremia (gastrointestinal upsets, disorientation, and itching) in instances where dialysis or transplantation are not available or possible [2]. If the patient is able to take a diet providing adequate essential amino acids and 1,800–3,500 kcal/day, amelioration of uremic symptoms and positive nitrogen balance often occur [12]. Survival is dependent upon the amount of residual renal function remaining; once the glomerular filtration rate falls below 2 ml/min, the condition of the patient deteriorates rapidly [9].

One study has also attributed preservation of peripheral nerve function in severe uremia to treatment with a low protein, high kilocalorie diet and a surplus of essential amino acids [38].

**Indications for use**    Protein restriction is indicated when the glomerular filtration rate falls below 20–30 ml/min [3,6,29]. For the patient not receiving dialysis severe restrictions are necessary when this rate is below 10 ml/min [29]. Potassium should be reduced to below 40 meq or 1,560 mg/day when serum potassium exceeds 6.0 meq/litre but never reduced to below 30 meq or 1,270 mg/litre or to a level where it is not possible to maintain nitrogen balance.

In children, protein restrictions that may compromise growth requirements should not be initiated until severe renal insufficiency becomes apparent [10,15].

***Possible adverse reactions*** *Negative nitrogen balance and growth failure* Serious consequences to growth and development can occur in children if caloric and nutritional needs are not met by the controlled protein, sodium, and potassium diet [10,39–41]. Serious protein wasting can occur in adults [22].

*Potassium deficiency* In certain renal patients total body potassium stores may be deficient in the presence of a normal serum potassium level and may be corrected by hemodialysis [42]. Thus, potassium should not be routinely restricted in renal disease prior to the demonstration of hyperkalmia.

*Vitamin and calcium deficiency* The diet may be inadequate in certain vitamins and minerals, such as thiamine, riboflavin, and niacin, at lower levels of protein intake. Calcium supplements should be provided to prevent renal osteodystrophy in patients with chronic renal failure [9,32,43].

***Contraindications*** Restrictions of any of the components in the diet prescription may promote adverse reactions if they are not formulated to suit the specific clinical and biochemical profile of the individual patient. Such measurements should be made routinely during the course of the disease and the diet adjusted accordingly.

***Suggestions for the dietitian*** Nutritional management of renal disease presents a formidable challenge that presupposes an understanding of the disease, its manifestations and complications, and recent developments in the field, as well as the principles that govern dietary intervention. In certain instances where traditional forms of diet therapy have not produced the desired results, the oral or intravenous administration of synthetic amino acid diet may be beneficial [44–46].

In the future the use of amino acid precursors such as alpha keto and alpha hydroxy acid analogues may become a realistic alternative to more traditional therapy [44–49]. Although essential amino acid analogues may enable persons with renal disease to manufacture essential amino acids from their own urea nitrogen, it should be understood that their entire mechanism of action cannot be attributed solely to either their transamination to essential amino acids or their action as a nitrogen sponge [45].

Patient counseling sessions should stress the importance of the diet and the risks of lack of adherence, the need to consume sufficient quantities of low electrolyte foods to meet caloric and nutrient needs, as well as the techniques of successful low protein cookery when indicated [50,51].

Dietary adherence and adequate kilocalorie intake are facilitated by specialty products such as Controlyte,\* Polycose,† Hy Cal,‡ Cal

---

\* Doyle Pharmaceutical Co., Minneapolis, MN 55416.
† Ross Laboratories, Columbus, OH 43216.
‡ Beecham-Massingill Pharmaceuticals, Melrose, MA 02176.

Power,§ and Aproten,§ low protein macaroni products. In addition, a synthetic orally administered essential amino acid product is now available. Amin-Aid⊥ may be used as the principal dietary source of nitrogen or as a supplement. It contains the eight essential amino acids plus histidine and nonprotein kilocalories in the form of sucrose and soybean oil.

§ Henkel Corp., Minneapolis, MN 55435.
⊥ McGaw Laboratories, Irvine, CA 92705.

**Recommended Dietary Intake for Uremic Patients With or Without Dialysis**

| Component | No dialysis | Hemodialysis | Peritoneal dialysis |
|---|---|---|---|
| Protein | Men: 40 g/day (0.55–0.60 g/kg/day) (28 g of high biologic value) | 1.0 g/kg/day (50% of high biologic value) | 1.2–1.5 g/kg/day (50% of high biologic value) |
| | Women, small men: 35 g/day (23–25 g of high biologic value) | | |
| Calories | 35 kcal/kg/day unless patient is overweight or grossly malnourished | 35 kcal/kg/day unless patient is overweight or grossly malnourished | 35 kcal/kg/day unless patient is overweight or grossly malnourished |
| Vitamins* | | | |
| Thiamine (mg/day) | 1.5 | 1.5 | 1.5 |
| Riboflavin (mg/day) | 1.8 | 1.8 | 1.8 |
| Pantothenic acid (mg/day) | 5.0 | 5.0 | 5.0 |
| Niacin (mg/day) | 20.0 | 20.0 | 20.0 |
| Pyridoxine hyrochloride (mg/day) | 5.0 | 5.0 | 5.0 |
| Vitamin $B_{12}$ (mg/day) | 3.0 | 3.0 | 3.0 |
| Vitamin C (mg/day) | 70–100 | 100.0 | 100.0 |
| Folic acid (mg/day) | 1.0 | 1.0 | 1.0 |
| Vitamin A | None | None | None |
| Vitamin D | Not estab. | Not estab. | Not estab. |
| Vitamin E (IU/day) | 15.0 | 15.0 | 15.0 |
| Vitamin K | None | None | None |
| Minerals | | | |
| Sodium (mg/day) | 1,000–3,000 | 1,500–2,000 | 1,400–2,000† |
| Potassium (mg/day) | 1,560–2,760 | 1,560–2,760 | 2,925–3,500 |
| Phosphorus (mg/day) | 600–1,200 | 600–1,200 | 600–1,200 |
| Calcium (mg/day) | 1,000–2,000 | 1,000–1,500 | 1,000–2,000‡ |
| Magnesium (mg/day) | 200–300 | 200–300 | 200–300 |
| Trace elements | Unknown | Unknown | Unknown |
| Iron§ | | | |
| Water | Up to 3,000 ml/day as tolerated. Individualized intake should balance output | Individualized to patient tolerance-usually limited to 1 litre | Individualized to patient tolerance-usually limited to 1 litre |

*Sources*:  Adapted from Nutritional management of chronic renal failure [13] and Nutritional management of the adult patient undergoing peritoneal dialysis [23].
* To be provided in the form of supplements.
† Persons undergoing frequent home peritoneal dialysis are often allowed 2–3 g sodium/day [9].
‡ Dietary intake must be supplemented in order to provide these levels.
§ Certain nephrologists recommend routine use of supplemental iron.

**Food Lists for Controlled Protein, Sodium, and Potassium Diets**

MILK LIST
1 cup equals 8 g protein, 335 mg potassium

Buttermilk, unsalted
Evaporated milk, reconstituted
Low-sodium milk
Nonfat dry milk, reconstituted
Skim milk
Whole milk

FOODS TO AVOID
Commercial foods made of milk:
Chocolate milk
Condensed milk
Ice cream
Malted milk
Milkshake
Milk mixes
Sherbet

MEAT OR SUBSTITUTE LIST
1 oz cooked equals 7 g protein, 100 mg potassium

Beef, chicken, duck, lamb, liver, pork, tongue (unsalted), turkey, veal

FOODS TO AVOID
Brains, kidneys
Canned, salted, or smoked meats, as: bacon, bologna, chipped beef, corned beef, frankfurters, ham, kosher meats, luncheon meats, salt pork, sausage, smoked tongue

Cod, flatfish (flounder and sole), kingfish (whiting), haddock, perch; canned salmon and tuna (omit on sodium-restricted diet)
Clams, crab, lobster, oysters, scallops, shrimp (all omitted on sodium-restricted diet)
Egg (1 egg equals 7 g protein, 65 mg potassium)
Cheese (1 oz equals 7 g protein, 25 mg potassium), cheddar, cottage, American, Swiss

Frozen fish fillets
Canned, salted, or smoked fish: anchovies, caviar, cod (dried and salted), herring, halibut, sardines, salmon, tuna

Omit on sodium-restricted diets

VEGETABLE LIST, GROUP 1
1 g protein, 110 mg potassium per serving

½-cup servings of raw cabbage, cucumber, lettuce, onion, tomato

1 g protein, 125 mg potassium per serving

½-cup servings of canned green or wax beans, carrots (+), spinach (+); fresh cooked cabbage, eggplant, mustard greens, onion, summer squash

*The following may be used for diets with liberal potassium allowance:*
1 g protein, 190 mg potassium per serving
½-cup servings of canned beets (+), rutabagas, tomatoes; fresh cooked carrots (+), turnips (+); frozen summer squash, winter squash

FOODS TO AVOID
All items marked (+) if diet is sodium restricted
Artichokes
Beans, baked
Beans, dried
Beans, lima
Beet greens
Broccoli, fresh
Brussels sprouts
Carrot, raw
Celery, raw
Chard
Endive, raw
Parsnips
Peas
Potato in skin, or frozen
Sauerkraut
Spinach, fresh or frozen
Squash, baked

### Vegetable List, Group 2
2 g protein, 160 mg potassium per serving

½-cup servings of canned asparagus; fresh or frozen green or wax beans, okra

*The following may be used for diets with liberal potassium allowance:*
2 g protein, 245 mg potassium per serving

½-cup servings of fresh or frozen cauliflower; cooked dandelion greens (+); potato, boiled (pared before cooking), or mashed

### Vegetable List, Group 3
3 g protein, 210 mg potassium per serving

½-cup servings of kale (+); frozen asparagus, broccoli, collards (+), mixed vegetables (+), whole kernel corn

### Fruit List, Group 1
Less than 0.5 g protein, 85 mg potassium per serving

| | |
|---|---|
| Apple, raw | 1 small |
| Grapes, European | 12 |

½-cup servings of canned applesauce, pears, pineapple; watermelon (diced)
½ cup of these juices: apple, grape, peach nectar, pear nectar, orange-apricot, pineapple-grapefruit, pineapple-orange

*The following may be used for diets with liberal potassium allowance:*
Less than 0.5 g protein, 145 mg potassium per serving

½-cup servings of apricot nectar, pineapple juice; canned fruit cocktail, peaches, purple plums

### Fruit List, Group 2
1 g protein, 135 mg potassium per serving

| | |
|---|---|
| Pear, raw | 1 small |
| Tangerine | 1 small |

½-cup servings of fresh or frozen blackberries, blueberries, boysenberries; canned cherries, figs; canned or fresh grapefruit; frozen red raspberries

*The following may be used for diets with liberal potassium allowance:*
1 g protein, 200 mg potassium per serving

| | |
|---|---|
| Orange | 1 small |
| Peach, raw | 1 small |
| Plums, fresh | 2 medium |
| Strawberries, fresh | ⅔ cup |

### Foods to Avoid
All dried and frozen fruits with sodium sulfite added
Apricots, fresh
Avocado
Bananas
Glazed fruits
Maraschino cherries
Nectarines
Prunes
Raisins

½-cup servings of cantaloupe, honeydew, frozen melon balls, fresh or frozen rhubarb

½ cup of these juices: grapefruit, grapefruit-orange, orange, tomato

Avoid tomato juice if diet is sodium restricted

BREADS AND SUBSTITUTES
2 g protein, 30 mg potassium per serving

| | |
|---|---|
| Bread | 1 slice |
| Cereals, dry | 1 cup |
|    Cornflakes, Puffed Rice, Puffed Wheat, shredded wheat | |
| Cereals, cooked | ½ cup |
|    cornmeal, farina, oatmeal, rice, rolled wheat | |
| Crackers, soda | 3 squares |
| Flour | 2 tbsp |
| Grits | 1 cup |
| Macaroni, noodles, or spaghetti | ¼ cup |
| Rice | ½ cup |

FOODS TO AVOID
Yeast breads or rolls or melba toast made with salt or from commercial mixes
Quick breads made with baking powder, baking soda, or salt, or made from commercial mixes
Commercial baked products
Dry cereals except as listed
Self-rising cornmeal
Graham or other crackers except low-sodium dietetic
Self-rising flour
Salted popcorn
Potato chips
Pretzels
Waffles containing salt, baking powder, baking soda, or egg white

FATS
Negligible protein and potassium

Butter
Cream, light or heavy (1 oz contains 35 mg potassium)
Fat or cooking oil
Margarine
Salad dressings: French or mayonnaise

FOODS TO AVOID
Salted fats on sodium-restricted diets
Avocado
Bacon, bacon fat
Olives
Nuts
Salt pork

MISCELLANEOUS
Cornstarch
Flavoring extracts
Ginger ale
Hard candies
Herbs
Honey
Jam or jelly
Jellybeans
Rice starch
Spices
Sugar, white, confectioners'
Syrup
Tapioca, granulated
Vinegar
Wheat starch

FOODS TO AVOID
Antacids, laxatives
Bouillon, broth
Canned, dried, frozen soups
Chocolate
Cocoa, instant cocoa mixes
Coconut
Consommé
Fruit-flavored powders and prepared beverage mixes
Fountain beverages
Commercial candies except as listed
Commercial gelatin desserts
Regular baking powder and soda
Rennet tablets
Molasses
Pudding mixes
Peanut butter
Most carbonated beverages

SEASONINGS TO AVOID
Catsup, celery leaves, celery salt, chili sauce, garlic salt, prepared horseradish, meat extracts, meat sauces, meat tenderizers, monosodium glutamate, prepared mustard, onion salt, pickles, relishes, salt and salt substitutes, soy sauce, Worcestershire sauce

**Sample Menu**

Controlled protein, sodium, and potassium diet (approximately 60 g protein)

A.M.

1 cup pineapple–grapefruit juice
½ cup farina with ½ cup milk and 1 tsp sugar
1 slice whole wheat bread with 1 tsp fortified margarine
Coffee*

NOON

2 oz sliced turkey on 2 slices enriched bread with 2 tsp fortified margarine
1 sliced tomato salad with 1 tsp French dressing
1 small tangerine
½ cup milk

P.M.

3 oz pot roast of beef
½ cup frozen green beans
½ cup summer squash
1 raw pear
1 slice whole wheat bread with 1 tsp fortified margarine
Coffee or tea*

*Source·* Adapted from *Manual of Diets,* Departments of Dietetics, Hospital of St. Raphael, Veterans Administration Hospital, and Yale-New Haven Medical Center, New Haven, CT, 1972. Diet in Normal and Therapeutic Nutrition [3] revised by Marilyn R. Lawler, 1976.

* Depending on fluid allowance.

**References**

1. Jones, W. O.: Diet Guide for Patients on Chronic Dialysis. New York: National Institute of Arthritis, Metabolism, and Digestive Diseases, 1975.
2. Burton, B. T.: Current concepts of nutrition and diet in diseases of the kidney. I. General principles of dietary management. J. Am. Diet. Assoc. 65: 623, 1974.
3. Robinson, C. H., and Lawler, M. R.: Normal and Therapeutic Nutrition. 15th ed. New York: Macmillan, 1977.
4. Blackburn, G. L.; Etter, G. B. A.; and MacKenzie, B. S.: Criteria for choosing amino acid therapy in acute renal failure. Am. J. Clin. Nutr. 31: 1841, 1978.
5. Yium, J. J.: Determination of diet orders by analysis of lab values. Tex. Med. 69: 71, 1973.
6. Cost, J. S.: Diet in chronic renal disease: a focus on calories. J. Am. Diet. Assoc. 74: 186, 1974.
7. Munro, H. N.: Energy and protein intakes as determinants of nitrogen balance. Kid. Int. 14: 313, 1978.
8. Lee, H. A.; Down, P. F.; Fowell, E.; and Hyne, B. E. H.: Amino acid tablet substituted diets in the management of chronic renal failure. Nutr. Metab. 17: 154, 1974.
9. Burton, B. T.: Current concepts of nutrition and diet in diseases of the kidney. II. Dietary regimen in specific kidney disorders. J. Am. Diet. Assoc. 65: 627, 1975.
10. Chan, J. C. M.: Dietary management of renal failure in infants and children. Clin. Pediatr. 12: 707, 1973.
11. Halliday, M. A.; Wassner, S.; and Ramirez, J.: Intravenous nutrition in uremic children with protein calorie nutrition. Am. J. Clin. Nutr. 31: 1854, 1978.
12. Blumenkrantz, M. J.; Kopple, J. D.; Koffler, A.; Kamdar, A. K.; Healfy, M. D.; Feinstein, E. I.; and Massry, S. G.: Total parenteral nutrition in the management of acute renal failure. Am. J. Clin. Nutr. 31: 1831, 1978.
13. Kopple, J. D.: Nutritional management of chronic renal failure. Postgrad. Med. 64: 135, Nov. 1978.
14. Ritz, E.; Mehls, O.; Gilli, G.; and Heuck, C. C.: Protein restriction in the conservative management of uremia. Am. J. Clin. Nutr. 31: 1703, 1978.
15. Lewy, P. R., and Hurley, J. K.: Chronic renal insufficiency. Pediatr. Clin. N. Am. 23: 829, 1976.
16. Varcal, A. R.; Halliday, D.; Carson, E. R.; Richards, P.; and Tavill, A.S.: Anabolic role of urea in renal failure. Am. J. Clin. Nutr. 31: 1601, 1978.
17. Kopple, J. D.; Jones, M.; Fukuda, S.; and Swendseid, M. E.: Amino acid and protein metabolism in renal failure. Am. J. Clin. Nutr. 31: 1532, 1978.

18. Giordano, C.; DeSanto, N. G.; and Pluvio, M.: Nitrogen balance in uremic patients on different amino acid and keto acid formulations—a proposed reference pattern. Am. J. Clin. Nutr. 31: 1797, 1978.
19. Jones, M. R.; Kopple, J. D.; and Swendseid, M. E.: Phenylalanine metabolism in uremic and normal man. Kid. Int. 14: 169, 1978.
20. Furst, P.; Allberg, M.; Alvestrand, A.; and Bergstrom, J.: Principles of essential amino acid therapy in uremia. Am. J. Clin. Nutr. 31: 1744, 1978.
21. Kopple, J. D., and Swendseid, M. E.: Evidence that histidine is an essential amino acid in normal and chronically uremic man. J. Clin. Invest. 55: 881, 1975.
22. Robinson, L. F., and Pauhbitski, A. H.: Diet therapy and educational program for patients with chronic renal failure. J. Am. Diet. Assoc. 61: 581, 1972.
23. Blumenkrantz, M. J.; Roberts, R. E.; Card, B.; Coburn, J. W.; and Kopple, J.D.: Nutritional management of the adult patient undergoing peritoneal dialysis. J. Am. Diet. Assoc. 73: 251, 1978.
24. Norbeck, E. E.; Oro, L.; and Carlson, L. A.: Serum lipoprotein concentrations in chronic uremia. Am. J. Clin. Nutr. 31: 1881, 1978.
25. ElBishiti, M.; Co-unahan, R.; Jarrett, R. J.; Stimmler, L.; Wass, V.; and Chantlr, C.: Hyperlipidemia in children on regular hemodialysis. Arch. Dis. Child. 52: 932, 1977.
26. Sanfellippo, M. L.; Swenson, R. S.; and Reaven, G. M.: Reduction of plasma triglycerides by diet in subjects with chronic renal failure. Kid. Int. 11: 54, 1977.
27. Sanfellippo, M. L.; Swenson, R. S.; and Reaven, G. M.: Response of plasma triglycerides to dietary change in patients on hemodialysis. Kid. Int. 14: 180, 1978.
28. Gokal, R.; Mann, J. I.; Oliver, D. O.; and Ledingham, J. G. G.: Dietary treatment of hyperlipidemia in chronic hemodialysis patients. Am. J. Clin. Nutr. 31: 1915, 1978.
29. Anderson, C. F.; Nelson, R. A.; Margie, J. D.; Johnson, W. J.; and Hunt, J.C.: Nutritional therapy for adults with renal disease. JAMA 223: 68, 1973.
30. Mitchell, H. G.; Rynbergen, H. J.; Anderson. L.; and Dibble, M. V.: Nutrition in Health and Disease 16th ed. New York; J. B. Lippincott, 1976.
31. Beale, M. G.; Salcedo, T. R.; Ellis, D.; and Rao, D. D.: Renal osteodystrophy. Pediatr. Clin. N. Am. 23: 873, 1976.
32. Schoolwerth, A. C., and Engle, J. E.: Calcium and phosphorus in diet therapy of uremia. J. Am. Diet. Assoc. 66: 460, 1975.
33. Slatopolosky, E., and Bricker, N. S.: The role of phosphorus restriction in the prevention of secondary hyperparathyroidism in chronic renal disease. Kid. Int. 4: 141, 1973.
34. Henderson, R. G.; Ledinghan, J. G.; Oliver, D. O.; Small, D. G.; Russell, R. G.; Smith, R.; Walton, R. J.; Preston, C.; and Warner, G. T.: Effects of 1,25-dihydroxycholecalciferol on calcium absorption, muscle weakness, and bone disease in chronic renal failure. Lancet 1: 379, 1974.
35. Berl, T.; Berns, A. S.; Huffer, W. E.; Hamill, K.; Alfrey, N. C.; Arnaud, C. D.; and Schrier, R. W.: 1,25-dihydroxycholecalciferol effects in chronic dialysis. Ann. Intern. Med. 88: 774, 1978.
36. Teehan, B. P.; Smith, L. J.; Sigler, M. H.; Gilgore, G. S.; and Schleifer, C.R.: Plasma pyridoxal-5'-phosphate levels and clinical correlations in chronic hemodialysis patients. Am. J. Clin. Nutr. 31: 1932, 1978.
37. Atkin-Thor, E.; Goddard, B. W.; O'Neon, J.; Stephen, R.; and Kalff, W.J.: Hypogeusion and zinz depletion in chronic dialysis patients. Am. J. Clin. Nutr. 31: 1148, 1978.
38. Bergstrom, J.; Lindblom, T.; and Noree, L. O.: Preservation of peripheral nerve function in severe uremia during treatment with low protein, high calorie diet and surplus of essential amino acids. Acta Neurol. Scand. 51: 99, 1975.
39. Stickler, G. B.: Growth failure in renal disease. Pediatr. Clin. N. Am. 23: 885, 1976.
40. Berger, M.: Dietary management of children with uremia. J. Am. Diet. Assoc. 70: 498, 1977.
41. Spinozzi, N. S., and Grupe, W. E.: Nutritional implications of renal disease. IV. Nutritional aspects of chronic renal insufficiency in childhood. J. Am. Diet. Assoc. 70: 493, 1977.
42. Bilbrey, G. L.; Carter, N. W.; White, M. G.; Schilling, J. F.; and Knockel, J.P.: Potassium deficiency in chronic renal failure. Kid. Int. 4: 423, 1973.

43. Burton, B. J.: Nutritional implications of renal disease. I. Current overview and general principles. J. Am. Diet. Assoc. 70: 479, 1977.

44. Close, J. H.: The use of amino acid precursors in nitrogen accumulation diseases. N. Engl. J. Med. 290: 663, 1974.

45. Richards, P.: The metabolism and clinical relevance of the keto acid analogues of essential amino acids. Clin. Sci. Mol. Med. 54: 589, 1978.

46. Abel, R. M.; Shih, V. E.; Abbott, W. J.; Beck, C. H.; and Fischer, J. E.: Amino acid metabolism in acute renal failure. Ann. Surg. 180: 350, 1974.

47. Burns, J.; Creswell, E.; Ell, S.; Flynn, M.; Jackson, M. A.; Lee, H. A.; Richards, P.; Rowlands, A.; and Talbot, S.: Comparison of the effects of keto acid analogues and essential amino acids on nitrogen homeostasis in uremic patients on moderately protein restricted diets. Am. J. Clin. Nutr. 31: 1767, 1978.

48. Heidland, A.; Kult, J.; Rockel, A.; and Heidbreder, E.: Evaluation of essential amino acids and keto acids in uremic patients on a low protein diet. Am. J. Clin. Nutr.: 31, 1784, 1978.

49. Young, G. A.; Chem, C.; Oli, H. L.; Davidson, A. M.; and Parsons, F.M.: The effects of calorie and essential amino acid supplementation on plasma proteins in patients with chronic renal failure. Am. J. Clin. Nutr. 31: 1802, 1978.

50. Margie, J. D.; Anderson, C. F.; Nelson, R. A.; and Hunt, J. C.: The Mayo Clinic Renal Diet Cookbook. New York: Western Publishing, 1974.

51. Cost, J. S.: Dietary Management of Renal Disease. Thorofare, NJ. Charles S. Black, 1975.

# Gluten Restricted, Gliadin Free Diet

*Definition*    A diet that is free of toxic glutens such as those in wheat, rye, oat, and barley protein, or their derivatives, e.g., malt from barley [1].

*Characteristics of the diet*    Foods containing glutens that produce no ill effects in patients with celiac disease are not restricted. The vegetable proteins found in rice, corn, potatoes, and beans, as well as fish and meat proteins, are well tolerated. Some of these foods also contain glutens, but they appear to be different from those in wheat, rye, oats, and barley [2].

The toxicity of the latter glutens may be related to their amide and bound glutamine and/or proline content [3,4]. Unrestricted foods usually contain 11% or less of the nitrogen as amide nitrogen [5], whereas the percentage of amide nitrogen content of wheat gliadin has been reported to be 24.2; that of wheat glutenin, 18; that of wheat flour, 20.1; that of rye flour, 20.9; and that of oatmeal, 14.4 [4].

*Purpose of the diet*    To eliminate toxic glutens in order to ameliorate symptoms of retarded growth, jejunal mucosal and immunogical abnormalities, secondary steatorrhea, sterility, and possibly osteomalacia in patients with celiac disease [5–10]. Each cereal grain has a characteristic gluten. Wheat, rye, barley, and often oat glutens cause characteristic symptoms and interfere with the absorption of food in these patients [11]. Wheat gluten includes the proteins glutenin and gliadin [2], the latter being most toxic. Its toxicity appears to be caused by two of its low molecular weight polypeptides, which as yet have not been identified [12,13]. The amino acid composition of a typical gliadin protein is about 40% glutamine and 15% proline [14].

*Effects of the diet*    Dramatic improvement of the symptoms of the disease follows the institution of a gluten restricted diet, although recovery may take up to 6 months in some patients. Patients with celiac sprue have a characteristic if not specific lesion of the jejunal mucosa, and may have altered but reversible disaccharide enzyme activity secondary to the lesion [15,16]. Long-term adherence to the diet will produce at least partial restoration of the normal mucosal surface [17–19]. According to a new theory, the disease is caused by an unidentified substance in gluten that binds to receptor sites on intestinal epithelial cells, acting as a lectin and rendering them vulnerable to attack by lymphocytes [19].

Controversy exists as to whether celiac sprue is an inborn error of metabolism due to an intestinal enzyme defect or an immunological disease [8,19,20–23]. The fact that a large percentage of persons with celiac disease have a specific marker, the histocompatibility antigen HLA-8 on the surface of their cells [21], supports the immunological theory.

In young children, dietary treatment may also permit catch-up growth, with eventual restoration of normal height, weight, and bone age [24]. Elevated blood levels of 5-hydroxytryptamine and its urinary metabolite 5-hydroxyindoleacetic acid have been reported in adults and children with untreated disease [25,26]. Clinical recovery after dietary treatment is accompanied by a decrease in the blood levels of the substances [26].

*Indications for use*    For control of symptoms of celiac sprue or secondary gluten induced enteropathy [1–17], and as part of the treatment of the skin lesions of dermatitis herpetiformis [9]. A definitive diagnosis of celiac disease requires a jejunal biopsy in which flattened mucosal villi and other characteristic changes are noted [27]. Response to gluten restriction and gluten challenge also aid in formulating the diagnosis [19,22]. Patients may also have abnormal responses to clinical tests for malabsorption, e.g., xylose tolerance test [28,29]. Skin testing is a useful adjunct to other means of diagnosing and treating the disease [30]. Temporary gluten restriction may be indicated in the treatment of transitory gluten intolerance secondary to any disorder that results in intestinal damage, e.g., in certain instances of gastrointestinal milk allergy of infancy [29].

*Duration of dietary treatment*    Primary celiac sprue is a permanent condition requiring lifelong gluten restriction. When the disease is untreated or neglected, growth is retarded [31]. One study has suggested that the extent of jejunal mucosal recovery is directly proportional to the degree of adherence to the diet; an intake of as little as 0.5 g gluten daily has been found to interfere with recovery in patients with celiac disease [17]. Children who have been rechallenged with gluten after a period of time responded with decreased growth rates and changes in duodenal biopsies [32]. Even in symptomless patients with sprue, the diet is needed for life.

*Possible adverse reactions*    None reported.

*Contraindications*    None reported.

*Suggestions for dietitians*    Gluten restriction represents a lifelong commitment for the patient with celiac disease. A carefully taken dietary history, when used in combination with a gluten antibody test, is a useful way of detecting the inadvertent ingestion of small amounts of gluten from less obvious sources [33,34]. A history of intolerance to sucrose and lactose as well as gluten is not uncommon; some of these patients have low levels of the enzymes sucrase and lactase, which return to normal after treatment. Patient instruction that includes principles of gluten free cookery may facilitate adherence to the diet and improve variety. Arrowroot, corn, potato, rice, soybean, and low gluten wheat starch flours may be used in place of wheat flour in many recipes. Their substitution for wheat will not produce satisfactory results, however, without other adjustments in ingredients and baking techniques. Hints for using wheat flour substitutes, as well as special recipes, have been published [35–38].

**Foods allowed**

*Beverages*

Carbonated drinks, cocoa (no wheat flour added), coffee, decaffeinated coffee to which no wheat flour has been added, fruit juices and drinks, milk (at least 2 cups a day), tea

*Breads and flour products*

Bread products made only from arrowroot, buckwheat, cornmeal, wheat starch, soybean flour, or gluten free wheat starch; cornbread, muffins, and pone with no wheat flour; cornstarch; gluten free macaroni products; gluten free porridge; rice wafers; soybean wafers, pure; rice, sago, and tapioca

**Foods excluded**

*Beverages*

Ale, beer, cereal beverages such as Postum and Ovaltine, commercial chocolate milk with cereal additive, instant coffee containing wheat, root beer

*Breads and flour products*

Breaded foods, breads, rolls, crackers, etc., made from wheat, rye, oats, or barley; commercial gluten bread; commercially prepared mixes for biscuits, cornbread, muffins, pancakes, buckwheat pancakes, waffles, etc.
The following list of foods to be avoided is not all-inclusive (read labels):

| | |
|---|---|
| All-purpose flour | Pancakes |
| Baking powder | Pastry flour |
| biscuits | Pretzels |
| Barley flour | Rye flour |
| Bran | Rye krisp |
| Bread crumbs | Spaghetti flour |
| Bread flour | Self-rising flour |
| Cake mixes | Vermicelli |
| Cookie mixes | Waffles |
| Cracker meal | Wheat, cracked |
| Graham flour | wheat, and |
| Macaroni | whole |
| Malt | wheat flours |
| Matzoth | Wheat germ |
| Noodles | Zwieback |

*Cereals*

Corn or rice cereals such as (read labels):
    Cornmeal
    Cornflakes
    Cream of Rice
    Hominy
    Puffed rice
    Rice flakes

*Cereals*

All cereals containing malt, bran, or wheat germ or made of rye, wheat, oats, or barley
The following is not an all-inclusive list:

| | |
|---|---|
| All Bran | Pep |
| Barley | Pettijohns |
| Branflakes | Puffed wheat |
| Cream of Wheat | Ralston |
| Farina | Ralston Bits |
| Grapenuts | Shredded |
| Grapenuts | Ralston |
| Flakes | Shredded wheat |
| Instant Cream of | Super farina |
| Wheat | Wheatena |
| Kaska | Wheat flakes |
| Krumbles | Wheaties |
| Oatmeal | Wheat Oata |
| Pablum | Whole Bran |

| Foods allowed | Foods excluded |
|---|---|
| *Desserts* | *Desserts* |
| Cakes, cookies, pastries, etc., prepared with permitted low gluten flours or instant potato granules; custard; gelatin desserts; homemade cornstarch and rice puddings; ice cream and sherbet if they do not contain gluten stabilizers; tapioca pudding | Cakes, cookies, commercial ice cream with gluten stabilizers, doughnuts, ice cream cones, pie, prepared mixes, prepared pudding thickened with wheat flour |
| *Fats* | *Fats* |
| Butter; corn oil; French dressing, pure; margarine, fortified; mayonnaise, pure; olive oil, other animal and vegetable fats and oils | Commercial salad dressings that contain gluten stabilizers, homemade cooked salad dressings if thickened with flour |
| *Miscellaneous* | |
| Pepper, pickles, popcorn, potato chips, sugars and syrups, vinegar, molasses | |
| *Soups* | *Soups* |
| Broth, bouillon, clear meat and vegetable soups, cream soups thickened with cream or allowed starches or flours | All soups thickened with wheat products or containing barley, noodles, or other wheat, rye, and oat products in any form |

References

1. Sleisenger, M. H.; Rynbergen, H. J.; Pert, J. H.; and Almy, T. P.: Wheat-rye and oat free diet. J. Am. Diet. Assoc. 33: 1137, 1957.
2. Hjortland, M.; Abowd, M. M.; Birk, A.; Hinshaw, D.; and French, A. B.: Low Gluten Diet with Tested Recipes. Ann Arbor: University of Michigan Medical Center, 1969.
3. Cornell, H. J., and Townley, R. R. W.: The toxicity of certain cereal proteins in coeliac disease. Gut 15: 862, 1974.
4. Van de Kamer, J. H., and Weijers, H. A.: Coeliac disease. V. Some experiments on the cause of the harmful effect of wheat gliadin. Acta Paediatr. Scand. 44: 465, 1955.
5. Holmes, G. K. T.; Asquith, P.; Stokes, P. L.; and Cooke, W. T.: Cellular infiltrate of jejunal biopsies in adult coeliac disease in relation to gluten withdrawal. Gut 15: 278, 1974.
6. Baker, P. G., and Read, A. E.: Reversible infertility in male coeliac patients. Br. Med. J. 2: 316, 1975.
7. Hajjar, E. T.; Vincenti, F.; and Salti, I. S.: Gluten-induced enteropathy: osteomalacia as its principal manifestation. Arch. Intern. Med. 134: 565, 1974.
8 Strober, W.; Falchuk, Z. M.; Rogentine, G. N.; Nelson, D. L.; and Klaevman, H. L.: The pathogenesis of gluten-sensitive enteropathy. Ann. Intern. Med. 83: 242, 1975.
9. Reunala, T.; Blomquist, K.; Tarpila, S.; Halme, H.; and Kangas, K.: Gluten-free diet in dermatitis herpetiformis. Br. J. Derm. 97: 473, 1977.
10. Ratnaike, R. N., and Wangel, A. G.: Immunological abnormalities in coeliac disease and their response to dietary restriction. I. Serum immunoglobulins, antibodies and complement. Aust. N.Z. J. Med. 7: 349, 1977.
11. Baker, P. G., and Read, A. E.: Oats and barley toxicity in coeliac patients. Postgrad. Med. J. 52: 264, 1976.
12. Dissanayake, A. S.; Truelove, S. C.; Oxford, R. E.; and Whitehead, R.: Nature of toxic component of wheat gluten in coeliac disease. Lancet 2: 709, 1973.
13. Hudson, A. A.; Purdham, D. R.; Cornell, H. J.; and Rolles, C. J.: Non-specific cytotoxicity of wheat gliadin components towards cultured human cells. Lancet 1: 339, 1976.
14. Patey, A. L.: Gliadin: the protein mixture toxic to coeliac patients. Lancet 1: 722, 1974.
15. Beck, I. T.; Dinda, P. K.; DaCosta, L. R.; and Beck, M.: Sugar absorption by small bowel biopsy sample from patients with primary lactase deficiency and with adult celiac disease. Am. J. Dig. Dis. 21: 946, 1976.

16. Mitchell, H. S.; Rynbergen, H. J.; Anderson. L.; and Dibble, M. V.: Nutrition in Health and Disease. 16th ed. New York: J. B. Lippincott, 1976.
17. Dissanayake, A. S.; Truelove, S. C.; and Whitehead, R.: Jejunal mucosal recovery in coeliac disease in relation to the degree of adherence to a gluten-free diet. Q. J. Med. 43: 161, 1974.
18. McNicholl, B.; Egan-Mitchell, B.; Stevens, F.; Keane, R.; Baker, S.; McCarthy, C. F.; and Fottrell, P. F.: Mucosal recovery in treated childhood celiac disease (gluten-sensitive enteropathy). J. Pediatr. 89: 418, 1976.
19. Bradsher, R. W.: Celiac disease. Johns Hopkins Med. J.: 142: 128, 1978.
20. Cornell, H. J., and Rolles, C. J.: Further evidence of a primary mucosal defect in coeliac disease. Gut 19: 253, 1978.
21. Stokes, P. L.; Ferguson, R.; Holmes, G. T.; and Cooke, W. T.: Familiar aspects of coeliac disease. Am. J. Med. 45: 567, 1976.
22. Townley, R. W.: Celiac disease—an inborn error of metabolism. Am. J. Dig. Dis. 18: 797, 1973.
23. Katz, A. J., and Falchuk, Z. M.: Current concepts in gluten sensitive enteropathy (celiac sprue). Pediatr. Clin. N. Am. 22: 767, 1975.
24. Barr, D. G. D.; Shmerling, D. H.; and Prader, A.: Catchup growth in malnutrition, studied in celiac disease after institution of gluten-free diet. Pediatr. Res. 6: 521, 1972.
25. Challacombe, D. N.; Goodall, M.; Gaze, H.; and Brown, G. A.: Urinary 5-hydroxyindoleacetic acid in 8-hour collections as an aid in diagnosis of celiac disease. Arch. Dis. Child. 50: 779, 1975.
26. Challacombe, D. L.; Dawkins, P. D.; and Baker, P.: Duodenal tissue concentrations of 5-hydroxytryptamine in celiac disease. Lancet 2: 522, 1977.
27. Hamilton, J. D.; Chambers, R. A.; and Wynn-Williams, A.: Role of gluten, prednisone and azathioprine in nonresponsive celiac disease. Lancet 1: 1213, 1976.
28. Donaldson, R. M., and Gryboski, J. D.: Carbohydrate intolerance. Sleisenger, M. H., and Fordtran, J. S., eds. Gastrointestinal Disease. Philadelphia: W. B. Saunders, 1973.
29. Wallach, J. B.: Interpretation of Diagnostic Tests. A Handbook Synopsis of Laboratory Medicine. 2d ed. Boston: Little, Brown, 1974.
30. Baker, P. G., and Read, A. E.: Positive skin reactions to gluten in coeliac disease. Q. J. Med. 45: 567, 1976.
31. McCrae, W. M.; Martin, M. R.; Eastwood, M. A.; and Sircus, W.: Neglected coeliac disease. Lancet 1: 187, 1975.
32. Hamilton, J. R., and McNeil, L. K.: How long should a celiac child stay on a gluten free diet? Lancet 1: 175, 1973.
33. Baker, P. G., Barry, R. E.; and Read, A. E.: Detection of continuing gluten ingestion in treated coeliac patients. Br. Med. J. 1: 486, 1975.
34. Carswell, F., and Ferguson, A.: Plasma food antibodies during withdrawal and reintroduction of dietary gluten in coeliac disease. Arch. Dis. Child. 48: 583, 1973.
35. Baking for People with Food Allergies. Home and Garden Bulletin No. 146. Rev. Washington, DC: U. S. Department of Agriculture, 1975.
36. Allergy Recipes. Chicago: American Dietetic Association, 1969.
37. Sheedy, C. H., and Keifetz, N.: Cooking for Your Celiac Child. New York: Dial, 1969.
38. Wood, M. N.: Gourmet Food on a Wheat Free Diet. Springfield: Charles C. Thomas, 1972.

# Phenylalanine Restricted Diet

***Definition***    A diet in which the intake of the amino acid phenylalanine is limited to a prescribed level governed by patient tolerances. In cases of "classic" phenylketonuria, tolerances usually range from 250–500 mg phenylalanine/day [1].

***Characteristics of the diet***    Natural foods low in phenylalanine and a casein hydrolysate, Lofenalac,* from which over 95% of the phenylalanine has been removed, form the basis for the diet. Lofenalac contains unsaturated fat, carbohydrate, vitamins, and minerals and in addition to other amino acids is supplemented with tyrosine, which is an essential amino acid for these patients [2]. A certain amount of phenylalanine is-necessary, usually at least 40 mg/kg/day [3], even in the diet of infants with phenylketonuria, to meet needs for growth. Otherwise, phenylalanine deficiency can occur [4]. Levels as low as 15 mg/kg/day may be prescribed for children 6 years of age [5]. The newborn infant may receive small amounts of milk, or in some instances other formula, mixed into the Lofenalac. Fruits, vegetables, and cereals are added to the diet at age appropriate times. Daily menus are planned by the use of food lists that indicate the phenylalanine, protein, and kilocalorie content of foods.

***Purpose of the diet***    (1) To provide protein, phenylalanine, tyrosine, energy, and other essential nutrients in amounts sufficient to permit normal growth and development and adequate nutritional status [4], and (2) to prevent mental retardation and allow the fullest development of intellectual potential by controlling the excessive accumulation of phenylalanine and its metabolites in the plasma. Serum phenylalanine levels should be maintained at a range of 5–10 mg/100 ml plasma by dietary management [3,6].

Control of serum phenylalanine levels, according to one author, becomes more difficult as the child grows older and his growth rate and protein and phenylalanine requirements decrease in relation to his body weight [7]. The latter report recommends a more liberal approach with maintenance of serum phenylalanine levels at between 4 and 8 mg/100 ml during the first year; between 6 and 14 mg/100 ml from 1 to 4 years of age; and from 10 to 20 mg/100 ml above 4 years of age [8].

In classical phenylketonuria there is absence or inactivity of the enzyme phenylalanine hydroxylase, which catalyzes hydroxylation of the essential amino acid phenylalanine to tyrosine [5]. Consequently, phenylalanine is not converted to tyrosine, and a number of alternate metabolites, such as phenylpyruvic acid, phenylacetic acid, and phenyllactic acid, are formed and excreted in the urine [9]. Untreated children are severely mentally retarded. Because tyrosine formation is blocked, affected children lack the pigment melanin and are often blond with blue eyes and fair skin.

Excess phenylalanine and pyruvate in the untreated or poorly

* Mead Johnson and Co., Evansville, IN 47721.

controlled patient with phenylketonuria produce metabolic alterations that may have far-reaching consequences [10]. The exact cause of brain damage in the disorder is still unknown.

***Effects of the diet***    The benefits to be derived from early diagnosis and *appropriate* dietary treatment have been well documented [1,2,11,12]. Comparisons of intelligence quotients of early-treated patients and older siblings who were treated later in life clearly illustrate the value of the diet in preventing mental retardation [11]. Long exposure to treatment may be required to observe improvement in the hyperactive and aggressive behavior of retarded phenylketonuric patients [1].

The effects of the diet on serum lipids in phenylketonuria have been recently investigated. Total and free serum cholesterol values were significantly lower in untreated and treated PKU subjects than in normal subjects; however, total serum lipids did not differ significantly in any of the groups [13].

***Indications for use***    The diet is clearly indicated and is the cornerstone of treatment in "classic" phenylketonuria as diagnosed by the following:

1. Evidence of sustained hyperphenylalaninemia (greater than 16 mg/100 ml) when the dietary intake of phenylalanine is normal [1]
2. Failure of plasma tyrosine to rise after a challenge with phenylalanine [1]
3. Formation of phenylpyruvate and its derivates when activity of phenylalanine aminotransferase enzyme is adequate [13]
4. A fall in plasma phenylalanine concentration to near normal values when phenylalanine intake is restricted to 250–500 mg/day. Dietary tolerance to this level of phenylalanine should remain in this range throughout infancy and early childhood [1].

The question of the optimal age to terminate the diet is controversial and has not been completely resolved [1,7,8,14,15]. A middle-of-the-road approach has been advocated, which permits a gradual liberalization of the diet in children who are at least 4½ years old. In place of the very restricted phenylalanine diet, a transitional diet is instituted, which includes adequate but not excessively large amounts of protein from milk, meat, eggs, beans, and cheese in place of Lofenalac* [16]. However, visual-perceptual difficulties that seemed to hamper the acquiring of academic skills have been noted in one group of children in whom the diet was discontinued at school age [14], while decreases in the rate of mental development have been described in others [17].

Less stringent restrictions in dietary phenylalanine intake are necessary in the "mild" variant of phenylketonuria and in the "transient" variant. In yet another variant in which plasma phenylalanine is consistently less than 15 mg/100 ml on a normal diet [1,3], stringent dietary restrictions appear to bring about little improvement and are unjustified [3].

Maternal hyperphenylalaninemia should be treated with low phenylalanine diet therapy to prevent the occurrence of congenital anomalies, mental retardation, and growth retardation in the affected fetus. Adherence to a low phenylalanine diet by the mother can pro-

tect the child from the effects of a hyperphenylalaninemic environment in the uterus [1,18,19]. More detailed information on levels
of phenylalanine in the serum in phenylketonuria and its variants
is available [20]. A blood test for elevated concentrations of phenylalanine performed no sooner than 24 hours after the onset of milk
feeding and prior to discharge has been recommended as a method
of screening all newborns for phenylketonuria [1].

*Possible adverse reactions*     *Phenylalanine deficiency*     Phenylalanine deficiency can be provoked by dietary mismanagement or a
too stringent reduction in dietary phenylalanine intake. Serum
phenylalanine levels of 2 mg/100 ml or lower are an indication that
dietary phenylalanine intake should be increased. Anorexia and
lethargy can occur, succeeded by a rise in serum phenylalanine levels
to 10–15 mg/100 ml, due to catabolism of phenylalanine containing
body tissues [2,4]. Dietary intakes of phenylalanine should be
increased during periods of febrile infection when nutritional needs
are greater than normal; otherwise, tissue catabolism in response to
an inadequate diet will cause serum phenylalanine levels to rise. The
presence of aminoaciduria on a low level of phenylalanine intake,
along with elevated serum phenylalanine levels, is an additional
indication that dietary phenylalanine intake should be increased.

*Growth retardation and generalized
malnutrition*     Deficient growth, anemia, hypoproteinemia, and
roentgenographic bone changes have been noted in children whose
intakes of kilocalories, protein, phenylalanine, and other nutrients
while on the phenylalanine restricted diet were inadequate [1,4]. Each
component of the diet prescription in phenylketonuria should be
carefully titrated to the specific and changing needs and tolerances of
the child in question if adverse nutritional reactions are to be
avoided. Frequent adjustments of the diet prescription may be
necessary in the young infant, and serum phenylalanine should be
checked weekly during the first 3 months of life [2]. If weight gain is
unsatisfactory or if serum levels are persistently below 2 mg/100 ml,
it is necessary to add small measured amounts of milk to the formula.
If the diet is formulated to provide recommended levels of protein
and kilocalories, it will supply amounts of nitrogen and essential
amino acids that are adequate to support growth [21].

*Suggestions for dietitians*     Frequent monitoring of the patient's
clinical status and serum phenylalanine levels must be accompanied
by just as frequent monitoring of the patient's dietary intake, if
adjustments in the diet prescription are to be properly made when
appropriate. Parents should be instructed in the keeping of some
form of diary for this purpose which can be evaluated at each visit
with the dietitian. Many sessions may be necessary in order for the
parents really to understand the principles of dietary management.
They should actually be able to demonstrate their ability to plan
menus and prepare the formula accurately, as well as their ability to
calculate replacements for foods not eaten. The small amounts of
milk used should always be mixed with the Lofenalac so that the
child does not acquire a taste for milk in preference to the Lofenalac.
By the time the child is ready for more solid foods, the parents should

be confident enough to be able to handle the inclusion of special low phenylalanine recipes [22,23] in meal plans. Home visits may be helpful in the early phases of parent education. Causes of elevated serum phenylalanine levels in treated children and appropriate recommendations for diet changes in specific instances have been published elsewhere [5].

Preliminary trials of one formula are promising. A formula based on whey protein concentrate with a low phenylalanine content (3.5%) has been tested as a protein source in an infant with hyperphenylalaninemia. Whey has a higher protein efficiency ratio than casein. The formula appeared to be more palatable than conventional casein hydrolysates and has a high nutritive value and an amino acid composition similar to breast milk [24,25].

Phenylalanine free products have a distinct advantage for the dietary management of older children with phenylketonuria; they permit greater latitude in choosing natural foods containing phenylalanine to meet dietary requirements. For example, PKU-Aid* is a hydrolysate of beef serum from which phenylalanine has been removed. Phenyl Free,† a phenylalanine free formula, is currently available for older children. When reconstituted with water, it provides 1.29 g protein, 0.4 g fat, 4.2 g carbohydrate, and 25.5 kcal/oz. It is specifically designed for the older child with phenylketonuria (2 or more years) who is consuming appreciable amounts of phenylalanine from table foods, as opposed to the infant whose phenylalanine needs are met to a great extent by Lofenalac* [26].

* Milner Scientific and Medical Research Co., Liverpool, England (manufacturer), and Ross Laboratories, Columbus, OH 43216 (U.S.A. distributor).
† Mead Johnson and Co., Evansville, IN 47721.

**Hyperphenylalaninemias**

| *Specific trait* | *Enzyme defect* | *Clinical features* |
| --- | --- | --- |
| 1. "Classic" phenylketonuria | Trace of phenylalanine hydroxylase activity | Mental retardation and other signs; preventable by early treatment (phenylalanine tolerance 250–500 mg/day) |
| 2. "Mild" phenylketonuria (mild variant with relaxed phenylalanine tolerance | Unknown | Mental retardation without early treatment; high tolerance for dietary phenylalanine during treatment (greater than 500 mg/day) |
| 3. "Transient" phenylketonuria | Partial phenylalanine hydroxylase deficiency | Mental retardation without early treatment; changing status affects treatment needed (greater than 500 mg/day to normal tolerance) |
| 4. Hyperphenylalaninemia without phenylketonuria | Partial phenylalanine hydroxylase deficiency | Plasma phenylalanine is consistently below 16 mg/100 ml plasma, asymptomatic trait (dietary treatment not recommended) [3] |
| 5. Neonatal hyperphenylalaninemia | Presumed phenylalanine hydroxylase deficiency | Often associated with hypertyrosinemia; normal adaptive phenomenon predominantly in premature infants (no treatment recommended) [8] |
| 6. Offspring of maternal phenylketonuria | No significant deficiency in heterozygous offspring | Transient falling postnatal hyperphenylalaninemia, congenital malformation, somatic and cognitive development impaired (mother should be treated during pregnancy) [1] |

*Source*: Adapted from Amino Acid Metabolism and Its Disorders [1].

PRESCRIPTION AND CALCULATION

1. *Establish the child's daily requirements for phenylalanine, protein, and kilocalories according to age.* The amount of phenylalanine each child is able to utilize is individual and varies with growth rate, severity of illnesses, time of day, and other factors. Protein content of the phenylalanine restricted diet has traditionally been greater than normal because a casein hydrolysate is the primary source of protein.

**Phenylalanine, Protein, and Energy for Infants and Preschoolers: Recommended Intake and Prescribed Sources**

| Age | Suggested phenylalanine | Suggested protein* | Suggested energy | Percent protein from Lofenalac | Amount of Lofenalac | Evaporated milk‡ |
|---|---|---|---|---|---|---|
| (mo) | (mg/kg/day) | (g/kg/day) | (kcal/kg/day) | | (ms†/kg) | (oz) |
| 0–3 | 58±18§ | 4.4 | 120 | 85 | 2½–3 | 1–3 |
| 4–6 | 40±10§ | 3.3 | 115 | 85 | 2–2½ | ½–2 |
| 7–9 | 32±9§ | 2.5 | 110 | 90 | 1½–2 | ½–1½ |
| 10–12 | 30±8§ | 2.5 | 105 | 90 | 1½–2 | ½–1 |
| | | (total g/day) | (kcal/day) | | (total ms/day) | |
| 13–24 | 25 | 25.0 | 1300 | 90 | 16 | 0–1 |
| 25–36 | 24±8§ | 25.0 | 1300 | 90 | 16 | None |
| 37–48 | 20 | 30.0 | 1300 | 90 | 19 | None |
| 49–72 | 18 | 30.0 | 1800 | 90 | 19 | None |

*Source*: Adapted from Diet Management of PKU for Infants and Preschool Children [27].
* Considerable controversy exists over protein need of both normal and PKU infants particularly when it is provided by a casein hydrolysate. Because of this, recommended protein intake during infancy is the amount found by the Collaborative Study to promote normal growth.
† A measure of Lofenalac equals 10 g, or 1 tbsp.
‡ One ounce of evaporated milk contains 106 mg phenylalanine, 2.2 g protein, and 44 kcal.
§ ±S.D.

2. *Establish in measures (1 measure = 1 tbsp = 7.5 or 8 mg phenylalanine) the amount of Lofenalac to be given.* The amount of Lofenalac to be prescribed is determined by the total protein requirement of the child. From 85 to 90% of the total protein need of the child must be met by the Lofenalac, as natural foods necessary to meet this need would be too high in phenylalanine.

3. *State the amount, if any, of milk or formula to be added.* During the period before the infant can eat solid food, Lofenalac is the primary source of protein. Since Lofenalac does not contain enough phenylalanine to supply the infant's need for growth during this age period, evaporated milk should be added to the Lofenalac, making a mixture which will contain the amount of phenylalanine needed to maintain normal serum levels. Evaporated milk is added to the Lofenalac mixture on the basis of 1 oz of evaporated milk to supply 107 mg phenylalanine, 2.2 g protein, and 44 kcal. The evaporated milk should be mixed with the Lofenalac, so that it will be consumed throughout the day.

4. *State the amount of water to be used to mix the Lofenalac powder.* Infants need 130–200 ml fluid/kg/day [5]. The child's fluid requirement, as based upon age, weight, and hydration status, preference for fluids, and taste for Lofenalac, determines the amount of water to be used. In general, no more than 32 oz/day is provided unless the patient is dehydrated. Older children may demand extra fluid because Lofenalac is a concentrated source of protein and kilocalories which may stimulate thirst mechanisms to a greater extent than milk or certain other formulas.

5. *Determine the amount of solid foods to be given.* Subtract the phenylalanine, protein, and energy that are supplied in the Lofenalac milk mixture from the total prescription and calculate the amount, type, and number of servings of solid foods to be given. Equivalents are generally used for this purpose. However, the food lists do provide information about phenylalanine, protein, and caloric content of each food to permit use of more specific values by physicians and dietitians who prefer this approach and who have been successful in gaining dietary compliance utilizing it.

*Sources*: Adapted from Recent Advances in Therapeutic Diets [28] and Dietary Management of Inherited Metabolic Disease [5].

## Average Nutrient Content of Serving Lists

| List | Phenylalanine (mg) | Protein (g) | Energy (kcal) |
|---|---|---|---|
| Vegetables | | | |
|   Strained and junior | 15 | 0.5 | 20 |
|   Table | 15 | 0.5 | 10 |
| Fruits | | | |
|   Strained and junior | 15 | 0.6 | 150 |
|   Table and juices | 15 | 0.6 | 70 |
| Bread and cereals | 30 | 0.6 | 30 |
| Fats | 5 | 0.1 | 60 |

When analyses were not available, the phenylalanine content was calculated on the following basis:

| | |
|---|---|
| Breads and cereals | Phenylalanine 5% of protein |
| Fat | Phenylalanine 5% of protein |
| Fruits | Phenylalanine 2.6% of protein |
| Vegetables | Phenylalanine 3.3% of protein |

*Source*:   Reprinted from Diet Management of PKU for Infants and Preschool Children [27].

## Serving Lists
### Part A—Strained and Junior Foods

| Food | Grams per tbsp | Amount | Phenylalanine (mg) | Protein (g) | Energy (kcal) |
|---|---|---|---|---|---|
| *Each serving as listed below contains 15 mg phenylalanine* | | | | | |
| VEGETABLES | 14.3 | | | | |
|   Mixed vegetables | | 3 tbsp | 16 | 0.5 | 15 |
|   Garden vegetables | | 2 tbsp | 16 | 0.5 | 8 |
|   Beets | | 6 tbsp | 15 | 1.1 | 33 |
|   Carrots | | 5 tbsp | 15 | 0.5 | 19 |
|   Creamed spinach | | 2 tbsp | 15 | 0.9 | 14 |
|   Green beans | | 2 tbsp | 15 | 0.3 | 7 |
|   Squash | | 3 tbsp | 14 | 0.3 | 13 |
|   Peas | | 1 tbsp | 17 | 0.5 | 6 |
| FRUITS | 14.3 | | | | |
|   Applesauce | | 11 tbsp | 15 | 0.3 | 127 |
|   Applesauce and apricots | | 10 tbsp | 15 | 0.4 | 124 |
|   Applesauce and cherries | | 18 tbsp | 15 | 0.5 | 239 |
|   Applesauce and pineapple | | 10 tbsp | 15 | 0.4 | 169 |
|   Apricots and tapioca | | 12 tbsp | 14 | 0.7 | 138 |
|   Bananas and tapioca | | 8 tbsp | 15 | 0.8 | 137 |
|   Peaches | | 5 tbsp | 16 | 0.4 | 60 |
|   Pears | | 10 tbsp | 15 | 0.6 | 99 |
|   Pears and pineapple | | 11 tbsp | 15 | 0.6 | 111 |
|   Plums and tapioca | | 11 tbsp | 15 | 0.5 | 154 |
|   Prunes and tapioca | | 8 tbsp | 15 | 0.7 | 105 |
|   Bananas with pineapple and tapioca | | 11 tbsp | 15 | 0.6 | 180 |
|   Apples and pears | | 18 tbsp | 15 | 0.5 | 208 |
| NOTE:   FREE FOOD | | | | | |
|   Applesauce and raspberries | | 10 tbsp | 4 | 0.1 | 151 |
|   Applesauce and cherries | | 7 tbsp | 6 | 0.2 | 93 |
|   Apples and cranberries | | 16 tbsp | 5 | 0.2 | 213 |

**Serving Lists**
**Part A—Strained and Junior Foods**  *(Continued)*

| Food | Grams per tbsp | Amount | Phenylalanine (mg) | Protein (g) | Energy (kcal) |
|---|---|---|---|---|---|
| *Each serving as listed below contains 15 mg phenylalanine* | | | | | |
| FRUIT JUICES | 15.0 | | | | |
| Apple | | 16 oz | 14 | 0.5 | 235 |
| Apple-apricot | | 16 oz | 14 | 0.5 | 336 |
| Apple-cherry | | 10 oz | 15 | 0.6 | 135 |
| Apple-grape | | 16 oz | 14 | 0.5 | 312 |
| Apple-pineapple | | 16 oz | 14 | 0.5 | 336 |
| Mixed fruit | | 6 oz | 14 | 0.5 | 106 |
| Orange | | 4 oz | 16 | 0.6 | 60 |
| Orange-apple | | 6 oz | 14 | 0.5 | 97 |
| Orange-apple-banana | | 4 oz | 16 | 0.6 | 78 |
| Orange-apricot | | 3 oz | 14 | 0.5 | 55 |
| Orange-pineapple | | 4 oz | 16 | 0.6 | 71 |
| Pineapple | | 6 oz | 14 | 0.5 | 99 |
| Pineapple-grapefruit drink | | 6 oz | 14 | 0.4 | 70 |
| Prune-orange | | 4 oz | 16 | 0.6 | 90 |
| Apple-prune | | 10 oz | 15 | 0.6 | 204 |
| *Each serving as listed below contains 30 mg phenylalanine* | | | | | |
| BREADS AND CEREALS | | | | | |
| *Dry cereals* | 2.4 | | | | |
| Barley | | 2 tbsp | 28 | 0.5 | 18 |
| Mixed cereal | | 2 tbsp | 28 | 0.6 | 18 |
| Oatmeal | | 2 tbsp | 30 | 0.8 | 15 |
| Rice cereal | | 4 tbsp | 31 | 0.6 | 36 |
| Mixed cereal with bananas | | 2 tbsp | 29 | 0.6 | 21 |
| Oatmeal with bananas | | 2 tbsp | 30 | 0.6 | 19 |
| Rice cereal with strawberries | | 4 tbsp | 30 | 0.6 | 33 |
| Barley with mixed fruit | | 3 tbsp | 31 | 0.6 | information not available |
| *Cereals in jars* | 14.3 | | | | |
| Strained | | | | | |
| Mixed with applesauce and bananas | | 3 tbsp | 30 | 0.6 | 39 |
| Oatmeal with applesauce and bananas | | 4 tbsp | 30 | 0.5 | 47 |
| Rice with applesauce and bananas | | 15 tbsp | 30 | 0.6 | 148 |
| Rice with mixed fruit | | 3 tbsp | 30 | 0.6 | 37 |
| Junior | | | | | |
| Mixed with applesauce and bananas | | 3 tbsp | 30 | 0.6 | 39 |
| Oatmeal with applesauce and bananas | | 4 tbsp | 30 | 0.5 | 47 |
| STRAINED VEGETABLES | 14.3 | | | | |
| Creamed corn | | 3 tbsp | 30 | 0.7 | 30 |
| Sweet potatoes | | 3 tbsp | 29 | 0.6 | 30 |

**Serving Lists**
**Part B—Table Foods**

| Food | Grams per tbsp | Amount | Phenyl-alanine (mg) | Protein (g) | Energy (kcal) |
|---|---|---|---|---|---|
| *Each serving as listed below contains 15 mg phenylalanine* | | | | | |
| VEGETABLES | | | | | |
| Asparagus, cooked | 9 | 3 tbsp or 1½ stalks | 17 | 0.6 | 5 |
| Beans, green, cooked | 8 | 3 tbsp | 14 | 0.4 | 6 |
| Beans, yellow, cooked | 8 | ¼ cup | 16 | 0.4 | 7 |
| Beans, sprouts, | | | | | |
| Mung, cooked | 8 | 1 tbsp | 16 | 0.3 | 3 |
| Beets, cooked | 10 | ⅔ cup | 16 | 1.2 | 34 |
| Beet greens, cooked | 13 | 3 tbsp | 15 | 0.6 | 6 |
| Broccoli, cooked, | | | | | |
| chopped | 10 | 1 tbsp | 14 | 0.4 | 3 |
| Brussels sprouts, | | | | | |
| cooked | — | 1 medium | 13 | 0.4 | 4 |
| Cabbage, raw, shredded | 6 | ½ cup | 15 | 0.6 | 12 |
| Cabbage, cooked | 10 | ⅓ cup | 14 | 0.6 | 11 |
| Carrots, raw | — | ½ large or 1 small | 18 | 0.6 | 21 |
| Carrots, cooked | — | ⅓ cup | 15 | 0.5 | 16 |
| Cauliflower, cooked | 7 | 3 tbsp | 17 | 0.5 | 5 |
| Celery, raw | 6 | 6 tbsp or 2 stalks | 15 | 0.3 | 6 |
| Celery, cooked, diced | 8 | 6 tbsp | 18 | 0.4 | 7 |
| Chard leaves, cooked | 10 | 3 tbsp | 14 | 0.5 | 5 |
| Collards, cooked | 11 | 1 tbsp | 13 | 0.4 | 4 |
| Cucumber, pared, raw | — | 1 whole | 14 | 0.6 | 14 |
| Eggplant, diced, raw | 13 | 2 tbsp | 13 | 0.3 | 7 |
| Eggplant, cooked | 13 | 3 tbsp | 17 | 0.4 | 7 |
| Kale, cooked | 7 | 2 tbsp | 18 | 0.4 | 4 |
| Lettuce | — | 2 leaves | 14 | 0.4 | 5 |
| Mushroom, raw | 4 | 3 small | 17 | 0.8 | 8 |
| Mushroom, canned | 13 | 3 tbsp | 16 | 0.7 | 7 |
| Mushroom, sauteed | 17 | ½ large | 13 | 0.2 | 10 |
| Mustard greens, cooked | 13 | 2 tbsp | 16 | 0.5 | 5 |
| Okra, cooked | — | 3 tbsp | 17 | 0.7 | 10 |
| Onion, raw, chopped | 10 | ¼ cup | 15 | 0.6 | 15 |
| Onion, cooked | 13 | ¼ cup | 16 | 0.6 | 15 |
| Onion, young, scallion | — | 2 whole | 15 | 0.6 | 14 |
| Parsley, raw, chopped | 3 | 4 tbsp | 17 | 0.4 | 5 |
| Parsnips, cooked, diced | 13 | 3 tbsp | 18 | 0.6 | 26 |
| Peppers, raw, chopped | 10 | 3 tbsp | 17 | 0.4 | 7 |
| Pickles, dill | — | 1 large | 16 | 0.7 | 11 |
| Pickles, sweet | 13 | 1 large | 16 | 0.7 | 146 |
| Pickles, sweet relish | 13 | 8 tbsp | 14 | 0.5 | 144 |
| Pumpkin, cooked | 14 | 4 tbsp | 16 | 0.6 | 18 |
| Radishes, raw | — | 3 small | 13 | 0.3 | 5 |
| Sauerkraut | 15 | ¼ cup | 15 | 0.6 | 11 |
| Spinach, cooked | 11 | 1 tbsp | 15 | 0.3 | 3 |
| Squash, summer, | | | | | |
| cooked | 13 | 5 tbsp | 16 | 0.6 | 9 |
| Squash, winter, | | | | | |
| cooked | 13 | ¼ cup | 16 | 0.6 | 20 |
| Tomato, raw | 17 | ½ small | 14 | 0.6 | 11 |
| Tomato, canned | 17 | ¼ cup | 17 | 0.7 | 14 |
| Tomato juice | 14 | ¼ cup | 16 | 0.6 | 13 |
| Tomato catsup | 17 | 2 tbsp | 17 | 0.7 | 36 |
| Tomato puree | 6 | 6 tbsp | 15 | 0.6 | 14 |
| Tomato sauce | 18 | 3 tbsp | 18 | 0.7 | 52 |
| Turnip greens, cooked | 9 | 2 tbsp | 18 | 0.4 | 4 |
| Turnips, diced, cooked | 10 | 9 tbsp | 15 | 0.7 | 21 |

**Serving Lists**
**Part B—Table Foods**  *(Continued)*

| Food | Grams per tbsp | Amount | Phenyl-alanine (mg) | Protein (g) | Energy (kcal) |
|---|---|---|---|---|---|
| *Each serving as listed below contains 15 mg phenylalanine* | | | | | |
| SOUPS (prepared with equal volume of water) | | | | | |
| Asparagus (Campbell's condensed) | | 3 tbsp | 15 | 0.5 | 12 |
| Beef broth (Campbell's condensed) | | 2 tbsp | 17 | 0.6 | 4 |
| Celery (Campbell's condensed) | | 3 tbsp | 15 | 0.3 | 16 |
| Minestrone (Campbell's condensed) | | 3 tbsp | 18 | 0.8 | 17 |
| Mushroom (Campbell's condensed) | | 2 tbsp | 15 | 0.3 | 17 |
| Onion (Campbell's condensed) | | 3 tbsp | 19 | 0.9 | 11 |
| Tomato (Campbell's (condensed) | | 3 tbsp | 17 | 0.4 | 16 |
| Vegetarian vegetable (Campbell's condensed) | | 3 tbsp | 14 | 0.3 | 12 |
| Vegetable and beef broth (Campbell's condensed) | | 4 tbsp | 16 | 0.5 | 15 |
| Clam chowder and tomato (Campbell's condensed) | | 3 tbsp | 14 | 0.4 | 15 |
| Chicken gumbo (Campbell's condensed) | | 2 tbsp | 14 | 0.4 | 7 |
| Cream of chicken (Campbell's condensed) | | 2 tbsp | 15 | 0.4 | 12 |
| Beef noodle (Campbell's condensed) | | 2 tbsp | 19 | 0.5 | 8 |
| *Each serving as listed below contains 30 mg phenylalanine* | | | | | |
| FRUITS | | | | | |
| Apple, raw | | 2½ small | 15 | 0.5 | 145 |
| Applesauce | 19 | ¾ cup | 14 | 0.5 | 207 |
| Apricots, raw | | 1½ medium | 14 | 0.6 | 31 |
| Apricots, canned | | 3 halves | 14 | 0.6 | 86 |
| Apricots, dried | | 2 halves | 14 | 0.6 | 31 |
| Avocado, cubed or mashed | 9.5 | 3 tbsp | 14 | 0.6 | 48 |
| Banana, raw sliced | | ½ small or ⅓ C sliced | 17 | 0.6 | 43 |
| Blackberries, canned, syrup | 15.6 | 5 tbsp | 16 | 0.6 | 71 |
| Blackberries, raw | 9 | 6 tbsp | 17 | 0.6 | 31 |
| Blueberries, raw | 8.8 | 10 tbsp | 16 | 0.6 | 55 |
| Blueberries, frozen, unsweetened | 10 | 9 tbsp | 16 | 0.6 | 50 |
| Blueberries, canned, syrup | 15 | 10 tbsp | 15 | 0.6 | 151 |
| Cantaloupe, raw, diced | 15 | 5 tbsp | 16 | 0.5 | 23 |
| Sour cherries | 13 | 4 tbsp | 16 | 0.6 | 30 |
| Sweet cherries, canned, syrup | 13 | 5 tbsp | 15 | 0.6 | 53 |
| Cranberries, raw | 6 | 1½ cups | 14 | 0.6 | 66 |
| Cranberry sauce | 20 | 1⅔ cups | 16 | 0.5 | 780 |
| Cranberry, sweetened, cooked | 13 | 1½ cups | 16 | 0.6 | 555 |
| Dates | 11 | 2 tbsp | 15 | 0.6 | 69 |
| Figs, raw | — | 1 large | 15 | 0.6 | 40 |
| Figs, canned, syrup | — | 4 small | 16 | 0.6 | 105 |

**Serving Lists**
**Part B—Table Foods** *(Continued)*

| Food | Grams per tbsp | Amount | Phenyl- alanine (mg) | Protein (g) | Energy (kcal) |
|---|---|---|---|---|---|
| *Each serving as listed below contains 30 mg phenylalanine* | | | | | |
| Figs, dried | — | 1 small | 16 | 0.6 | 41 |
| Fruit cocktail | 13 | ¾ cup | 16 | 0.6 | 119 |
| Grapefruit, raw | 12 | ¾ cup or ½ large | 14 | 0.7 | 59 |
| Grapes, Thompson, seedless | 10 | ½ cup (12 grapes) | 14 | 0.5 | 54 |
| Guava, raw | — | 1 small | 16 | 0.6 | 47 |
| Honeydew, raw, diced | 13 | 5 tbsp | 16 | 0.5 | 21 |
| Mango, raw | — | ½ medium | 18 | 0.7 | 66 |
| Nectarines, raw | — | 2 large | 15 | 0.8 | 80 |
| Oranges, raw | — | 1 medium (3″ diam) | 18 | 1.5 | 74 |
| Papaya, raw | 16 | ⅓ medium or 6 tbsp | 16 | 0.6 | 39 |
| Peaches, raw | 11 | 1 lrg or ¾ C sliced | 16 | 0.8 | 50 |
| Peaches, canned, syrup | 16 | 4 medium halves | 16 | 0.8 | 156 |
| Peaches, dried | 10 | 2½ tbsp | 16 | 0.8 | 66 |
| Pears, raw | — | ½ medium (3×2½″) | 17 | 0.7 | 61 |
| Pears, canned, syrup | 16 | 5 small halves | 15 | 0.5 | 190 |
| Pears, dried | — | ½ pear | 12 | 0.4 | 35 |
| Pineapple, raw | 8 | 1 cup diced | 14 | 0.5 | 67 |
| Pineapple, canned, syrup | 16 | 2 large slices | 16 | 0.6 | 148 |
| Plums, Damson, raw | 13 | 2 whole | 13 | 0.5 | 66 |
| Plums, prune-type, raw | 13 | 1½ whole | 17 | 0.4 | 38 |
| Plums, canned, syrup | 14 | 4 whole | 13 | 0.5 | 110 |
| Prunes dried medium | — | 3 whole | 18 | 0.4 | 54 |
| Raisins, dried, seedless | 10 | 2 tbsp | 15 | 0.5 | 58 |
| Raspberries, black, raw | 11 | ¼ cup | 17 | 0.7 | 32 |
| Raspberries, red, raw | 8 | 6 tbsp | 15 | 0.6 | 27 |
| Raspberries, black, canned, syrup | 13 | 4 tbsp | 15 | 0.6 | 27 |
| Raspberries, red, canned, syrup | 13 | 7 tbsp | 16 | 0.6 | 32 |
| Rhubarb, cooked, added sugar | 15 | 6 tbsp | 15 | 0.5 | 141 |
| Strawberries, raw | 9 | 10 large | 17 | 0.7 | 37 |
| Strawberries, frozen, whole | 15 | 15 large | 15 | 0.6 | 138 |
| Tangerine | — | 1 small or ½ large | 12 | 0.4 | 23 |
| Watermelon, ball or cubes | 12.5 | ⅔ cup | 17 | 0.7 | 36 |

BREADS AND CEREALS
*Prepared cereals*

| Food | Grams per tbsp | Amount | Phenyl- alanine (mg) | Protein (g) | Energy (kcal) |
|---|---|---|---|---|---|
| Alpha Bits | | 3 tbsp | 27 | 0.6 | 23 |
| Apple Jacks | | 6 tbsp | 32 | 0.7 | 47 |
| Cap'n Crunch | | 5 tbsp | 29 | 0.7 | 65 |
| Cheerios | | 2 tbsp | 27 | 0.5 | 15 |
| Corn Chex | | ½ cup | 29 | 0.6 | 30 |
| Cornflakes | | ¼ cup | 28 | 0.6 | 31 |
| Froot Loops | | 5 tbsp | 36 | 0.6 | 40 |
| Kix | | ½ cup | 28 | 0.6 | 32 |
| Lucky Charms | | 3 tbsp | 29 | 0.5 | 23 |
| Puffed Rice | | 10 tbsp | 31 | 0.6 | 40 |
| Puffed Wheat | | ¼ cup | 32 | 0.9 | 12 |
| Cap'n Crunchberries | | ¼ cup | 31 | 0.5 | 47 |
| Cap'n Crunch Peanut Butter Cereal | | 3 tbsp | 32 | 0.6 | 38 |
| Rice Chex | | 6 tbsp | 31 | 0.6 | 44 |
| Rice Krinkles | | ½ cup | 28 | 0.5 | 63 |
| Rice Krispies | | ¼ cup | 28 | 0.5 | 30 |
| Quisp | | ½ cup | 31 | 0.8 | 68 |

| Food | Grams per tbsp | Amount | Phenyl-alanine (mg) | Protein (g) | Energy (kcal) |
|---|---|---|---|---|---|
| *Each serving as listed below contains 30 mg phenylalanine* | | | | | |
| Shredded Wheat | | ¼ biscuit | 29 | 0.6 | 21 |
| Sugar Frosted Flakes | | ½ cup | 30 | 0.6 | 62 |
| Sugar Pops | | ½ cup | 30 | 0.6 | 43 |
| Sugar Smacks | | 7 tbsp | 31 | 0.7 | 55 |
| Trix | | 6 tbsp | 30 | 0.7 | 47 |
| Wheaties | | ¼ cup | 31 | 0.7 | 25 |
| Wheat Chex | | 7 biscuits | 31 | 0.7 | 25 |
| Cocoa Krispies | | ½ cup | 29 | 0.5 | 48 |
| Team Flakes | | 10 tbsp | 30 | 0.6 | 39 |
| Quaker Life | | 1 tbsp | 30 | 0.6 | 12 |
| King Vitamin | | ½ cup | 32 | 0.6 | 63 |
| Special K | | 2 tbsp | 29 | 0.6 | 11 |
| Franken Berry | | 7 tbsp | 30 | 0.6 | 50 |
| Count Chocula | | 6 tbsp | 28 | 0.6 | 42 |
| Sir Grapefellow | | 5 tbsp | 27 | 0.5 | 39 |
| Boo Berry | | 5 tbsp | 27 | 0.5 | 39 |
| Granola | | 1 tbsp | 32 | 0.6 | 19 |
| Grapenuts | | 1 tbsp | 27 | 0.6 | 26 |
| Grapenut Flakes | | 3 tbsp | 29 | 0.7 | 30 |
| *Cooked cereals* | | | | | |
| Cornmeal | | 4 tbsp | 29 | 0.7 | 30 |
| Cream of Rice | | 5 tbsp | 31 | 0.6 | 38 |
| Cream of Wheat | | 2 tbsp | 28 | 0.6 | 17 |
| Farina | | 3 tbsp | 31 | 0.6 | 19 |
| Malt-O-Meal | | 2 tbsp | 30 | 0.6 | 20 |
| Oatmeal | | 2 tbsp | 33 | 0.6 | 17 |
| Pettijohns | | 2 tbsp | 32 | 0.7 | 23 |
| Ralston | | 2 tbsp | 31 | 0.6 | 16 |
| Rice, white | | 3 tbsp | 28 | 0.5 | 29 |
| Rice, brown | | 2 tbsp | 28 | 0.5 | 25 |
| Wheatena | | 2 tbsp | 31 | 0.6 | 22 |
| Wheat Hearts | | 2 tbsp | 31 | 0.7 | 17 |
| *Crackers* | | | | | |
| Animal Crackers | | 5 | 33 | 0.7 | 43 |
| Arrowroot Cookies | | 2 | 30 | 0.6 | 45 |
| Graham Crackers | | 1 | 28 | 0.6 | 21 |
| Ritz Crackers | | 3 | 35 | 0.7 | 45 |
| Saltines | | 2 | 27 | 0.5 | 26 |
| Tortilla, corn | | ¼ (6″ D) | 33 | 0.7 | 27 |
| Wheat Thins | | 4 | 34 | 0.7 | 32 |
| Meal Mates | | 1 | 25 | 0.5 | 24 |
| MISCELLANEOUS | | | | | |
| Corn, cooked | | 2 tbsp | 29 | 0.5 | 17 |
| Hominy grits, cooked | | 6 tbsp | 32 | 0.7 | 31 |
| Macaroni, cooked | | 2 tbsp | 32 | 0.6 | 20 |
| Noodles, cooked | | 2 tbsp | 32 | 0.7 | 20 |
| Potato chips | | 6 (2″ D) | 29 | 0.6 | 68 |
| Potato, Irish, cooked | | ⅓ potato (2¼″ D) | 29 | 0.6 | 21 |
| Potatoes, French fried | | 3 (½×½×2″) | 30 | 0.6 | 41 |
| Instant potatoes (dry) without milk | | 5 tbsp | 33 | 0.7 | 36 |
| Popcorn, popped, plain | | 5 tbsp | 29 | 0.6 | 19 |
| Spaghetti, cooked | | 2 tbsp | 32 | 0.6 | 20 |
| Sweet potatoes, cooked | | 3 tbsp | 28 | 0.6 | 38 |
| Instant sweet potatoes, dry without milk | | 2 tbsp | 29 | 0.6 | 53 |

| Food | Grams per tbsp | Amount | Phenyl-alanine (mg) | Protein (g) | Energy (kcal) |
|---|---|---|---|---|---|
| *Each serving as listed below contains 5 mg phenylalanine* | | | | | |
| FATS | | | | | |
| Butter | | 1 tbsp | 4 | 0.1 | 100 |
| French Dressing, commercial | | 5 tbsp | 5 | 0.2 | 442 |
| Margarine | | 1 tbsp | 5 | 0.1 | 108 |
| Miracle Whip | | 1 tbsp | 5 | 0.1 | 68 |
| Olives, green | | 2 tbsp | 5 | 0.2 | 16 |
| Olives, ripe | | 2 tbsp | 5 | 0.2 | 18 |
| Mayonnaise | | 2 tbsp | 5 | 0.1 | 72 |
| DESSERTS—Comstock | | | | | |
| Apple pie filling | | ¼ cup | 1 | * | 89 |
| Apricot pie filling | | ¼ cup | 8 | 0.4 | 79 |
| Blackberry pie filling | | ¼ cup | 1 | * | 109 |
| Blueberry pie filling | | ¼ cup | 6 | 0.2 | 83 |
| Boysenberry pie filling | | ¼ cup | 11 | 0.4 | 93 |
| Cherry pie filling | | ¼ cup | 11 | 0.4 | 83 |
| Peach pie filling | | ¼ cup | 4 | 0.2 | 78 |
| Pineapple pie filling | | ¼ cup | 4 | 0.1 | 70 |
| Raspberry pie filling | | ¼ cup | 8 | 0.3 | 106 |
| Strawberry pie filling | | ¼ cup | 5 | 0.2 | 79 |

* Less than 0.5

*These foods contain little or no phenylalanine. May be used as desired.*

| Food | Grams per tbsp | Amount | Phenyl-alanine (mg) | Protein (g) | Energy (kcal) |
|---|---|---|---|---|---|
| FREE FOODS | | | | | |
| Apple juice | | 6 oz | | | 85 |
| Candies: | | | | | |
| Butterscotch | | 1 piece | | | 20 |
| Cream mints | | 1 piece | | | 7 |
| Fondant, patties or mint | | 1 piece | | | 40 |
| Gum drops | | 1 large | | | 35 |
| Hard candy | | 2 pieces | | | 39 |
| Jelly beans | | 10 | | | 110 |
| Lollipops | | 1 medium (2½″ diam) | | | 108 |
| Carbonated beverages | | 6 oz | | | 78 |
| Corn syrup | | 1 tbsp | | | 58 |
| Danish dessert | | ½ cup | | | 123 |
| Diet margarine | | 1 tbsp | | | 50 |
| Fruit butter | | 1 tbsp | | | 37 |
| Fruit ices | | ½ cup | | | 69 |
| Jellies | | 1 tbsp | | | 55 |
| Kool Aid | | 4 oz | | | 48 |
| Lemonade | | 4 oz | | | 53 |
| Maple syrup | | 1 tbsp | | | 50 |
| Molasses | | 1 tbsp | | | 46 |
| Popsicle | | 1 twin bar | | | 95 |
| Shortening | | 1 tbsp | | | 123 |
| Start liquid | | 4 oz | | | 60 |
| Sugar, brown | | 1 tbsp | | | 46 |
| Sugar, granulated | | 1 tbsp | | | 43 |
| Sugar, white, powdered | | 1 tbsp | | | 59 |
| Tang liquid | | 4 oz | | | 59 |
| MISCELLANEOUS | | | | | |
| Cake flour | | 1 tbsp | 29 | 0.6 | 29 |
| Corn starch | | 1 tbsp | 1 | trace | 29 |
| Tapioca, granulated | | 1 tbsp | 2 | 0.1 | 35 |
| Wheat starch | | 1 tbsp | 1 | trace | 25 |
| NONDAIRY CREAMS | | | | | |
| Coffee Rich | | 1 tbsp | 3 | trace | 23 |
| Cool Whip | | 1 tbsp | 2 | trace | 14 |

| Food | Grams per tbsp | Amount | Phenyl-alanine (mg) | Protein (g) | Energy (kcal) |
|---|---|---|---|---|---|

*These foods contain little or no phenylalanine. May be used as desired.*

| Food | | Amount | Phenyl-alanine (mg) | Protein (g) | Energy (kcal) |
|---|---|---|---|---|---|
| Dzert Whip, liquid | | 1 tbsp | 9 | 0.2 | 44 |
| Rich's Topping | | 1 tbsp | — | — | 43 |
| Mocha Mix | | 1 tbsp | 2 | trace | 13 |

Less than 0.04 g protein = trace

*Source*: Adapted from Diet Management of PKU for Infants and Preschool Children [27].

**Phenylalanine—Restricted Diet Meal Guide**

Date _____ Age _____ Name _____
Wt _____ Ht _____

Approximate total milligrams phenylalanine daily _____
Approximate total grams protein daily _____
Approximate total energy (kcal) daily _____

_____

| | Phenylalanine (mg) | Protein (g) | Energy (kcal) |
|---|---|---|---|
| _____ measures packed dry Lofenalac | _____ | _____ | _____ |
| Add _____ oz evaporated milk | _____ | _____ | _____ |
| Add water to make _____ oz/oz | _____ | _____ | _____ |
| **A.M.** | | | |
| _____ Lofenalac | | | |
| _____ Servings fruit | _____ | _____ | _____ |
| _____ Servings bread/cereal | _____ | _____ | _____ |
| _____ Servings fat | _____ | _____ | _____ |
| _____ Servings free foods | _____ | _____ | _____ |
| Between meals | | | |
| _____ Servings | _____ | _____ | _____ |
| Noon | | | |
| _____ Lofenalac | | | |
| _____ Servings fruit | _____ | _____ | _____ |
| _____ Servings vegetable | _____ | _____ | _____ |
| _____ Servings bread | _____ | _____ | _____ |
| _____ Servings dessert | _____ | _____ | _____ |
| _____ Servings fat | _____ | _____ | _____ |
| _____ Servings free foods | _____ | _____ | _____ |
| Between meals | | | |
| _____ Servings | _____ | _____ | _____ |
| **P.M.** | | | |
| _____ Lofenalac | | | |
| _____ Servings fruit | _____ | _____ | _____ |
| _____ Servings vegetable | _____ | _____ | _____ |
| _____ Servings bread | _____ | _____ | _____ |
| _____ Servings dessert | _____ | _____ | _____ |
| _____ Servings fat | _____ | _____ | _____ |
| _____ Servings free foods | _____ | _____ | _____ |
| Bedtime | | | |
| _____ Servings | _____ | _____ | _____ |
| Total | _____ | _____ | _____ |
| Per kg | _____ | _____ | _____ |

Comments:

*Source*: Adapted from Diet Management of PKU for Infants and Preschool Children [27].

**Sample Calculation**

<small>INFANT—NEWBORN</small>

Date _____ Age _____ Name _____
Wt _____3 kg_____ Ht _____

Approximate total milligrams phenylalanine daily <u>264</u> (3 kg × 88 mg phenylalanine)
Approximate total grams protein daily      <u>13.2</u> (3 kg × 4.4 g protein)
Approximate total energy (kcal) daily     <u>360</u> (3 kg × 120 kcal)
Total fluid      <u>20 oz</u> (3 kg × 200 ml)

| | *Phenylalanine (mg)* | *Protein (g)* | *Energy (kcal)* |
|---|---|---|---|
| <u>7 scoops</u> packed dry Lofenalac | 56 | 10.50 | 315 |
| Add <u>2 oz</u> evaporated milk | 214 | 4.40 | 88 |
| Add water to make <u>20 oz</u>: | 1 oz = 13.5 | 0.72 | 20 |

<u>Amount of protein from Lofenalac</u> = 85% of 13.2 g protein
     13.2 × .85 = 11.22 g
<u>Amount of Lofenalac to give:</u>
     11.22 g ÷ 1.5 g/measure = 7 measures Lofenalac
<u>Amount of evaporated milk to use:</u>
     total phenylalanine per day − phenylalanine in Lofenalac = amount in milk
     264 mg phenylalanine − 56 mg phenylalanine = 208 mg phenylalanine
     (1 oz evaporated milk = 107 mg phenylalanine)
     208 mg phenylalanine ÷ 107 mg phenylalanine/oz evaporated milk = 2 oz

**Sample Menu**

TODDLER

Date _____ Age __3 yr__ Name _____
Wt _____16 kg_____ Ht _____

| | Phenylalanine (mg) | Protein (g) | Energy (kcal) |
|---|---|---|---|
| Approximate total milligrams phenylalanine daily | 384 | | |
| Approximate total grams protein daily | 25 | | |
| Approximate total energy (kcal) daily | 1300 | | |
| 16 scoops packed dry Lofenalac | 128 | 24 | 720 |
| Add 0 oz evaporated milk | 0 | 0 | 0 |
| Add water to make 32 oz: | 1 oz = 4 | 0.75 | 22.5 |
| **A.M.** | | | |
| ½ grapefruit | 14 | 0.7 | 59 |
| ½ cup Sugar Pops | 30 | 0.6 | 43 |
| 8 oz Lofenalac | 32 | 6.0 | 180 |
| **BETWEEN MEALS** | | | |
| 4 oz orange juice | 16 | 0.6 | 60 |
| **NOON** | | | |
| ½ cup grapes (13) | 14 | 0.5 | 54 |
| 4 tbsp beef broth | 16 | 0.5 | 15 |
| 4 wheat thins | 34 | 0.7 | 32 |
| 1½ tsp butter or fortified margarine | 2 | 0.1 | 50 |
| 8 oz Lofenalac | 32 | 6.0 | 180 |
| **BETWEEN MEALS** | | | |
| 2 tbsp raisins | 15 | 0.5 | 58 |
| 4 oz Lofenalac | 16 | 3.0 | 90 |
| **P.M.** | | | |
| 2 tbsp raisins | 15 | 0.5 | 58 |
| 2 tbsp broccoli | 14 | 0.4 | 3 |
| 2 tbsp mushroom soup | 15 | 0.3 | 17 |
| ⅓ Irish potato | 29 | 0.6 | 21 |
| 1½ tsp butter or fortified margarine | 2 | 0.1 | 50 |
| 2 tbsp cherry pie filling | 6 | 0.2 | 42 |
| 8 oz Lofenalac | 32 | 6.0 | 180 |
| **BEDTIME** | | | |
| 5 animal crackers | 33 | 0.7 | 43 |
| 4 oz Lofenalac | 16 | 3.0 | 90 |
| **TOTALS** | 383 | 31.0 | 1,325 |

References

1. Rosenberg, L. E., and Scriver, C. R.:  Amino Acid Metabolism and Its Disorders. Philadelphia:  W. B. Saunders, 1973.
2. Wong, P. W. K., and Hsia, D. Y.:  Inborn errors of metabolism. Goodhart, R. S., and Shils, M. E., eds.  Modern Nutrition in Health and Disease.  5th ed. Philadelphia:  Lea & Febiger, 1973.
3. Lines, D. R., and Swanson, M.:  Dietary requirement of phenylalanine in infants with hyperphenylalaninemia.  Arch. Dis. Child. 48: 648, 1973.
4. Hanley, W. B.; Linsao, L.; Davidson, W.; and Moes, C. A. F.:  Malnutrition with early treatment of phenylketonuria.  Pediatr. Res. 4: 318, 1970.
5. Acosta, P. B., and Elsas, L. J.:  Dietary Management of Inherited Metabolic Disease:  Phenylketonuria, Galactosemia, Tyrosinemia, Homocystinuria, Maple Syrup Urine Disease. Atlanta:  ACELMU Publishers, 1975.
6. Dr. D. Y. Hsia, Yale School of Medicine:  Personal communication.
7. Robertson, E. F.; Hill, G. N.; Cashel, K.; Rooney, J.; Brummitt, R.; and Pollard, A. C.:  Management of phenylketonuria:  South Australian experience of 13 cases.  Med. J. Aust. 1: 647, 1976.

8. Clayton, B. E.: The principles of treatment by dietary restriction as illustrated by phenylketonuria. Raine, D. N., ed. The Treatment of Inherited Metabolic Disease. New York: American Elsevier, 1974.

9. Justice, P., and Smith, G. F.: PKU-phenylketonuria. Am. J. Nurs. 75: 1303, 1975.

10. Patel, M. S., and Arinze, I. J.: Phenylketonuria: metabolic alterations induced by phenylalanine and pyruvate. Am. J. Clin. Nutr. 28: 183, 1975.

11. Smith, I., and Wolff, O. H.: Natural history of phenylketonuria and influence of early treatment. Lancet 2: 540, 1974.

12. Hanley, W. B.; Linsao, L. S.; and Netley, C.: The efficacy of dietary therapy for phenylketonuria. Can. Med. Assoc. J. 104: 1089, 1971.

13. Acosta, P. B.; Alfin-Slater, R.; and Koch, R.: Serum lipids in children with phenylketonuria. J. Am. Diet. Assoc. 63: 631, 1973.

14. Johnson, C. F.: What is the best age to discontinue the low phenylalanine diet in phenylketonuria? Clin. Pediatr. 11: 148, 1972.

15. Holtzman, N. A.; Welcher, D. W.; and Mellits, E. D.: Termination of restricted diet in children with phenylketonuria: a randomized controlled study. N. Engl. J. Med. 292: 737, 1975.

16. Beckner, A. S.; Centerwall, W. R.; and Holt, L.: Effects of rapid increase of phenylalanine intake in older PKU children. J. Am. Diet. Assoc. 69: 148, 1976.

17. Brown, E. S., and Wainer, R.: Mental development of phenylketonuric children on or off diet after age of six. Psychol. Med. 6: 287, 1976.

18. Arthur, L. J. H., and Hulme, J. D.: Intelligent small for dates baby born to oligophrenic phenylketonuria mother after low phenylalanine diet during pregnancy. Pediatrics 46: 235, 1970.

19. Pueschel, S. M.; Hum, C.; and Andrews, M.: Nutritional management of the female with phenylketonuria during pregnancy. Am. J. Clin. Nutr. 30: 1153, 1977.

20. Blaskonics, M. E.; Schaeffler, G. E.; and Hack, S. P.: Phenylalaninemia, differential diagnosis. Arch. Dis. Child. 49: 835, 1974.

21. Acosta, P. B.; Wenz, E.; and Williamson, M.: Nutrient intake of treated infants with phenylketonuria. Am. J. Clin. Nutr. 30: 198, 1977.

22. Beto, J. A., and Holli, B. B.: Cookie for a low phenylalanine diet. J. Am. Diet. Assoc. 64: 288, 1974.

23. Connecticut State Department of Health: Phenylketonuria Booklet, 1971.

24. Forsum, E., and Hambraeus, L.: Biological evaluation of a whey protein fraction with special reference to its use as a phenylalanine-low protein source in the dietary treatment of PKU. Nutr. Metab. 14: 48, 1972.

25. Hambraeus, L.; Hardell, L. I.; Forsum, E.; and Lorentsson, R.: Use of a formula based on a whey protein concentrate in the feeding of an infant with hyperphenylalaninemia. Nutr. Metab. 17: 84, 1974.

26. Committee on Nutrition, American Academy of Pediatrics: Special diets for infants with inborn errors of amino acid metabolism. Pediatrics 57: 783, 1976.

27. Acosta, P. B., and Wenz, E.: Diet Management of PKU for Infants and Preschool Children. Washington, DC: U.S. Government Printing Office, 1977.

28. University of Iowa Hospitals and Clinics: Recent Advances in Therapeutic Diets. 2d ed. Ames: Iowa State University Press, 1973.

# Gout and the Purine Restricted Diet

*Definition*     A restricted purine diet is one in which uric acid and its precursors, specifically, sources of purines such as glandular meats, dried legumes, lentils, and meat extractives, are eliminated. Other meats and fish are restricted to 4 oz weekly, thus reducing the daily intake of uric acid equivalent to approximately 35 mg/day [1]. The diet has been prescribed with the aim of lowering serum uric acid levels in the treatment of gout [2].

Questions for Consideration     *1.   Is there a biochemical basis for the rigid restriction of dietary purines in patients with gout or uric acid calculi?* Drug therapy has largely replaced the less effective purine restricted diet in the medical management of gout. By inhibition of the enzyme xanthine oxidase the drug allopurinol interferes with uric acid synthesis in patients with hyperuricemia [3–5]. The metabolic effects of the disease have been reviewed in detail elsewhere [6]. The diet decreases only exogenous sources of nucleoproteins, which account for less than half the uric acid found in the blood [7]. It does not appreciably affect the endogenous production of uric acid. For example, simple available compounds, such as carbon dioxide, ammonia, and glycine, may also be synthesized into uric acid [8].

Serum uric acid levels generally decrease from 0.5 to 1.5 mg/100 ml in patients on purine restricted diets [9–11], although one author has reported decreases of greater than 1.5 mg/100 ml serum on a diet that permitted up to 1 g protein/kg of *ideal* body weight [12]. In general, diets severely limited in protein and purine content are unnecessary and of little value. They decrease serum uric acid levels only slightly (less than 0.5 to 1.5 mg/100 ml) [7–9,11].

Drastic reductions in protein or purine intakes are also ineffective in treating uric acid calculi. Stone formation in some but not all cases may be the result of a persistently acid urine due to a defect in ammonium excretion [10,13]; in these instances, treatment includes agents that alkalinize the urine and the ingestion of large volumes of fluids. However, there are certain individuals in whom excessive uric acid excretion appears to play a causal role in calcium oxalate stone formation. Excessive dietary purine intake, i.e., up to 425 mg/day or a daily maximum of 260 mg, was noted to be a major factor in producing hyperuricosuria in a group of 10 such patients [14].

A more rational alternative to a very low purine diet is to limit only foods extremely high in purines in order to avoid any unnecessary metabolic stress on the body [6,9,10] and to identify persons prone to huge excesses of dietary intakes of protein or purine [14]. Such restrictions may be particularly useful in patients managed on drugs other than allopurinol, which increases uric acid excretion [11,15].

Foods high in deoxyribonucleic acid related purines (DNA) have recently been shown to have much less effect on serum uric acid levels than those which are high in ribonucleic acid content (RNA) [16].

Oral administration of the purines hypoxanthine, adenine, adenosine-5′-monophosphate (AMP), guanosine-5′-monophosphate (GMP), and inosine-5′-monophosphate (IMP) to patients with hyperuricemia has been shown to produce elevations in serum uric acid. Conversely, guanine and xanthine had no effect [16]. Although a limited number of foods have recently been analyzed for their RNA and specific purine content [17], the lack of more comprehensive tables makes it impossible to take greater advantage of these findings in planning diets.

2. *Is the elimination of coffee, tea, and cocoa necessary?* Patients with gout were formerly advised to eliminate coffee, tea, and cocoa from their diets because they contain the methylxanthines theobromine, theophylline, and caffeine. This recommendation was based on early reports that the methylxanthines were converted to uric acid in man.

Studies using dogs and rabbits have been cited as providing additional evidence for this exclusion. The validity of implications for human purine metabolism drawn from dog and rabbit studies has been questioned; unlike man, these animals excrete allantoin and not uric acid [18]. The development of more sensitive enzymatic methods of analysis and the use of uric acid excreting animals, such as birds, have led other investigators to the following conclusions: theobromine, theophylline, and caffeine are metabolized in man to methyl urates, not urates, and are not deposited in the gouty tophus. Therefore, there is no scientific basis to support the elimination of coffee, tea, and cocoa on a purine restricted diet [18,19].

**Dietary Recommendations for Patients with Gout, Based on Available Scientific Evidence**

FLUID INTAKE

The patient should be encouraged to increase his intake of fluids to a minimum of 2 qt/day. A large fluid intake is helpful in eliminating uric acid, preventing renal calculi, and retarding progressive involvement of the kidney [4]. The volume of fluid ingested should be sufficient to keep the patient from experiencing thirst at any time and also enough to necessitate voiding at least once during the night [20]. A treatment plan that includes increased fluid intake, urinary alkalanizing agents, and allopurinol has proven to be very effective in the management of uric acid calculi [21].

WEIGHT REDUCTION

Obesity is often associated with gout and may be a contributory factor in the onset of the disease. In such cases, weight reduction by the obese patient may have a beneficial effect on urate metabolism [22]. The reduction in weight should be gradual; fasting or drastic dieting will increase serum uric acid levels. The mechanism by which serum uric acid levels are increased may involve the production of ketones, which inhibit uric acid secretion [20,23].

PURINE AND PROTEIN RESTRICTION

Those foods high in purines or those which contain more than 150 mg/100 g should be eliminated from the diet. Specifically, sweetbreads, anchovies, sardines, shrimp, mackerel, liver, kidney, meat extracts, and dried legumes (high in adenine [17]) should be excluded in order to avoid any additional metabolic stress on the body. In addition, it has been recommended that daily protein intake should not exceed 1 g/kg of ideal body weight [12] or 80 g/day [24].

## RESTRICTION OF ALCOHOLIC BEVERAGES

Overconsumption of alcoholic beverages may precipitate attacks of gout. Excessive intakes of alcohol result in the accumulation in the body of lactic acid, which inhibits the renal secretion of urates [9,25]. In addition, the combined effects of alcohol and fasting are mutually potentiating. On the other hand, when alcohol in amounts less than 100 g/day is taken with food, only minor changes in uric acid metabolism occur [23]. On this basis, alcohol is best taken in a diluted form, e.g., in highballs, and in moderation, by the patient with gout. Complete abstinence is not necessary [8,10].

## OTHER RESTRICTIONS

Appropriate dietary measures should be undertaken for any associated disorders, such as renal insufficiency, hypertension, cardiovascular disease, or hyperlipoproteinemia. Preliminary reports indicate that a diet high in carbohydrate may do more harm than good if a large portion of that carbohydrate is in the form of fructose, as fructose appears to increase uric acid production and excretion [26,27]. Dietary diaries kept for 3 or more days by individuals with hyperuricosuria and analyzed for their kilocalorie, protein, purine, and oxalate content are very useful tools. They help to identify those who need more stringent dietary measures.

References

1. Turner, D.: Handbook of Diet Therapy. 5th ed. Chicago: University of Chicago Press, 1970.
2. Bartels, E. C.: Successful treatment of gout. Ann. Intern. Med. 18: 21, 1943.
3. Rodnan, G. P.: Gout and other crystalline forms of arthritis. Postgrad. Med. 58: 6, Oct. 1975.
4. Rodnan, G. P.; Robin, J. A.; Tolchin, S. F.; and Elion, G. B.: Allopurinol and gouty hyperuricemia, efficacy of a single dose. JAMA 231: 1143, 1975.
5. Fox, I. H.: Purine ribonucleotide catabolism: clinical and biochemical significance. Nutr. Metab. 16: 65, 1974.
6. Wyngaarden, J. B.: Metabolic defects of primary hyperuricemia and gout. Am. J. Med. 56: 651, 1974.
7. Mayer, J.: Nutrition and gout. Postgrad. Med. 45: 277, May 1969.
8. Bayles, T. B.: Nutrition in diseases of the bones and joints. Goodhart, R. S., and Shils, M. E., eds. Modern Nutrition in Health and Disease. 5th ed. Philadelphia: Lea & Febiger, 1973.
9. Salmon, S. E.; Schrier, R. W.; and Smith, L. H.: Hyperuricemia pathogenesis and treatment. Calif. Med. 116: 38, June 1972.
10. Mikkelsen, W. M., and Robinson, W. D.: Physiologic and biochemical basis for the treatment of gout and hyperuricemia. Med. Clin. N. Am. 53: 1331, 1969.
11. Thier, S. O.: An approach to disorders of uric acid metabolism. Arch. Intern. Med. 134: 579, 1974.
12. Talbott, J. H., and Yu, T. F.: Gout and Uric Acid Metabolism. New York: Stratton Intercontinental Medical Book Corp., 1976.
13. Wyngaarden, J. B., and Kelly, W. N.: Gout. Stanbury, J. B.; Wyngaarden, J. B.; and Frederickson, D. S. eds. The Metabolic Basis of Inherited Disease. 3d ed. New York: McGraw-Hill, 1972.
14. Coe, F. L.; Moran, E.; and Kavalich, A. G.: The contribution of dietary purine over-consumption to hyperuricosuria in calcium oxalate stone formers. J. Chron. Dis. 29: 793, 1976.

15. Zollner, N., and Griebsch, A.: Diet and gout. DeVries, A.; Sperling, O.; and Wyngaarden, J. B., eds. Purine Metabolism in Man. Advances in Experimental Medicine and Biology. New York: Plenum, 1973.

16. Clifford, A. J.; Riumallo, J. A.; Young, V. R.; and Scrimshaw, N. S.: Effect of oral purines on serum and urinary uric acid of normal hyperuricemic and gouty humans. J. Nutr. 106: 428, 1976.

17. Clifford, A. J., and Story, D. L.: Levels of purines in foods and their metabolic effects in rats. J. Nutr. 106: 435, 1976.

18. Buchanan, O. H.; Christman, A. A.; and Block, W. D.: The metabolism of the methylated purines. II. Uric acid excretion following the ingestion of caffeine, theophylline and theobromine. J. Biol. Chem. 157: 189, 1945.

19. Wolfson, W. Q.; Huddlestun, B.; and Levine, R.: The transport and excretion of uric acid in man. II. The endogenous uric acid-like chromogen of biological fluids. J. Clin. Invest. 26: 995, 1947.

20. Thier, S. O., M.D., Yale School of Medicine: Personal communication.

21. Smith, L. H.; Van Den Berg, C. J.; and Wilson, D. M.: Nutrition and urolithiasis. N. Engl. J. Med. 298: 87, 1978.

22. Emmerson, B. T.: Alteration of urate metabolism by weight reduction. Aust. N.Z. J. Med. 3: 410, 1973.

23. Maclachlan, M. J., and Rodnan, G. P.: Effects of food, fast and alcohol on serum uric acid and acute attacks of gout. Am. J. Med. 42: 38, 1967.

24. Yu, T. F.: Nephrolithiasis in patients with gout. Postgrad. Med. 63: 166, May 1978.

25. Lieber, C. S.; Jones, D. P.; Losowsky, M. S.; and Davidson, C. S.: Interrelation of uric acid and ethanol metabolism in man. J. Clin. Invest. 41: 1863, 1962.

26. Emmerson, B. T.: Effect of oral fructose on urate production. Ann. Rheum. Dis. 33: 276, 1974.

27. Raivio, K. O.; Becker, M. A.; Meyer, L. J.; Greene, M. L.; Nuki, G.; and Seegmiller, J. E.: Stimulation of human purine synthesis de novo by fructose infusion. Metabolism 24: 861, 1975.

# Tyramine and Dopamine Restricted Diet: Two Milligram Tyramine, Dopamine Free Diet

***Definition***    A diet that eliminates all known major sources of tyramine and dopamine, in particular those foods containing bacteria with enzymes capable of decarboxylating the amino acid tyrosine to tyramine. The diet provides less than 2 mg tyramine daily from minor sources.

***Characteristics of the diet***    Foods that have been fermented or aged or in which protein breakdown is used to increase flavor are not permitted on the diet; they contain bacteria that are capable of forming amines from amino acid precursors [1]. Most cheeses are especially high in tyramine because the organisms they contain (such as coliforms and group D streptococci) have a very active tyrosine decarboxylase [1,2]. Broad bean pods, avocados, and bananas are contraindicated because of their dopamine content [1,2]. Although yogurt is a fermented product, it is not excluded from the diet; no harmful reactions have been reported following its ingestion, and one analysis of its composition failed to detect any appreciable amount of tyramine [3].

***Purpose of the diet***    To prevent the occurrence of serious side effects from the ingestion of monoamines in patients taking drugs that are monoamine oxidase (MAO) inhibitors [2,4].

Monoamines are potentially hazardous pressor substances found in certain foods which cause constriction of blood vessels and an abnormal elevation of blood pressure [5,6]. Normally, they pose no threat to the individual, since the body is endowed with enzyme systems that efficiently and rapidly detoxify them. The enzyme MAO converts ingested monoamines such as tyramine to their harmless metabolites [5–7]; in the presence of a normally active enzyme, tyramine is converted to the nontoxic parahydroxyphenylacetic acid [4].

However, persons ingesting the MAO inhibitor class of antidepressant drugs are bereft of this protection. Drugs that inhibit the action of monoamine oxidase remove the body's first line of defense against toxicity from monoamines [3,5]; those which are not enzymatically deactivated are free to enter the general circulation and may produce serious clinical reactions [8]. The pressor effect of tyramine may be enhanced 100-fold by medications that interfere with its normal metabolism [2,4]. The most important adverse reaction reported in patients taking MAO inhibitors is a hypertensive crisis that may be accompanied by excruciating headaches, tachycardia, or even fatal intracranial hemorrhages [5]. In such instances, as little as 6 mg tyramine by mouth (the amount present in 20 g cheddar cheese) has proven to be enough to cause blood pressure elevations [3]. Whenever MAO inhibitors are prescribed, simultaneous restriction of dopamine and tyramine intake is essential to the prevention of adverse reactions.

***Indications for use*** The tyramine and dopamine restricted diet is indicated whenever one of the following MAO inhibitors is prescribed [9]:

| Generic name | Trademark |
| --- | --- |
| Tranylcypromine sulfate | Parnate (Smith, Kline and French Laboratories) |
| Furazolidone* | Furozone (Eaton Laboratories) |
| Isocarboxazid | Marplan (Roche Laboratories) |
| Pargyline hydrochloride | Eutonyl (Abbott Laboratories) |
| Phenelzine sulfate | Nardil (Warner-Chilcott Laboratories) |
| Nialamide | Niamid (Pfizer Laboratories) |
| Procarbazine | Natulane (Roche Laboratories) |

***Possible adverse reactions*** The diet is a nutritionally adequate one, and there have been no untoward reactions directly attributable to its use; conversely, it is intended to protect the body against the side effects of drug therapy.

***Contraindications*** None that are known.

***Suggestions for dietitians*** *Patient counseling tips* Although most cheeses are prohibited on this diet, patients should be especially warned that the portion of cheese closer to the rind has a much higher tyramine content than portions farthest from the rind. This finding may account for the variations in the magnitude of the adverse responses to cheese in patients taking MAO inhibitors [11]. Dietitians who have patients adhering to the diet may have to add other foods to the list of foods to be avoided as more specific information becomes available on the amine content of foods. Chocolate has been implicated in one hypertensive crisis involving pargyline, but no definite identification of a responsible pressor amine was made [12]. Patients should be advised that there is some uncertainty concerning the use of chocolate on the diet.

*Restricting other amines* At the present time, tyramine is the major offender among the vasoactive amines that have precipitated hypertensive crisis. However, more study is needed to determine the effect of enzyme inhibiting drugs on the way the body metabolizes and disposes of other potentially harmful amines, such as serotonin, norepinephrine, and histamine [1,4,8]. It has been suggested that aminoguanidine, a potent inhibitor of histaminase, a diamine oxidase, may have therapeutic value. If this drug is prescribed, it may become necessary to restrict the intake of histamine in the diet. Beer, wine, and yeast are all examples of foods that are high in histamine as well as tyramine [1]. Implementation of a histamine restricted diet would necessitate the exclusion of fermented foods, such as sauerkraut, as well as chocolate; contaminated fish should be especially avoided [1].

*Restricting coffee, tea, and cocoa* Rat studies on the interaction of caffeine, theophylline, and theobro-

---

* Interactions with furazolidone are not of the same magnitude as those occurring with other MAO drugs, although such interactions are potentially clinically significant [10].

mine (found in coffee, tea, and cocoa) with MAO inhibitors indicate an adverse reaction at least in the rat [12]. If it is deemed desirable by the physician for the patient receiving monoamine oxidase inhibiting drugs to avoid caffeine, theophylline, and theobromine, the patient should be advised to eliminate coffee, tea, cocoa, and cola beverages from the diet. In general, only fresh food or freshly prepared frozen or canned food should be eaten [14].

**Tyramine and Dopamine Modified Diet**

| Foods allowed | Foods excluded [1–13,15–20] |
|---|---|
| *Beverages* | *Beverages* |
| All except those specifically to be avoided; decaffeinated coffee, coffee, tea | Alcoholic beverages, wines, ale, beer |
| *Breads and bread substitutes* | *Breads and bread substitutes* |
| All not specifically excluded, including commercial bread | Homemade yeast breads with substantial quantities of yeast, breads or crackers containing cheese |
| *Fats* | *Fats* |
| All except those excluded | Soured cream |
| *Fruits* | *Fruits* |
| Orange (limit to 1 small orange daily, 2½ in. diameter, which provides 1 mg tyramine); any other fruits not specifically excluded | Bananas<br>Red plums, avocado, figs, raisins (permitted on diets not restricted in dopamine) |
| *Meats and meat substitutes* | *Meats and meat substitutes* |
| Cottage cheese and meats not specifically to be avoided, eggs | Aged game, liver, and canned meats; yeast extracts; commercial meat extracts; stored beef liver; chicken livers; salami; sausage; aged cheese: blue, Boursault, brick, Brie, Camembert, cheddar, colby, Emmentaler, Gouda, mozzarella, Parmesan, provolone, Romano, Roquefort, Stilton; salted dried fish such as herring, cod, or camlin; pickled herring |
| *Vegetables* | *Vegetables* |
| Tomato (limit to ½ cup daily), all other vegetables not specifically excluded | Italian broad beans (pods contain tyramine), green bean pods, eggplant |
| *Miscellaneous* | *Miscellaneous* |
| Fresh homemade gravies; all not specifically excluded | Yeast concentrates, marmite, soup cubes, products made with concentrated yeasts, commercial gravies or meat extracts, soups containing items that must be avoided, soy sauce,* any protein containing food that has been stored improperly or that may have been spoiled or putrid, i.e., all except those that have been freshly prepared |

* Contains 1.7 meq/g of tyramine.

**Sample menu**

A.M.

½ cup grapefruit juice
½ cup farina
1 soft cooked egg
1 slice bread
1 tsp butter or fortified margarine
1 cup coffee
1 tsp sugar
1 cup milk

Noon

3/4 cup creamed chicken on toast
½ cup asparagus
½ sliced tomato on lettuce
2 tsp mayonnaise
1 slice bread
1 tsp butter or fortified margarine
½ cup milk
1 fresh apple
1 cup tea
1 tsp sugar

P.M.

6 oz roast sirloin tip
½ cup mashed potato
½ cup carrots
3/4 cup tossed salad
1 tbsp French dressing
1 slice white bread
½ cup fruit cocktail
1 tsp butter or fortified margarine
1 cup tea
1 tsp sugar
½ cup milk

Between meals

6 oz orange juice

References

1. Lovenberg, W.: Some vaso-and psychoactive substances in food: amines, stimulants, depressants, and hallucinogens. Committee on Food Protection, Food and Nutrition Board, National Academy of Sciences: Toxicants Occurring Naturally in Foods. 2d ed. Washington, DC: National Academy of Sciences, 1973.
2. Hodge, J. V.; Nye, E. R.; and Emerson, G. W.: Monoamine oxidase inhibitors, broad beans, and hypertension. Lancet 1: 1108, 1964.
3. Horwitz, D.; Lovenberg, W.; Engelman, K.; and Sjoerdsma, A.: Monoamine oxidase inhibitors, tyramine, and cheese. JAMA 188: 1108, 1964.
4. Editorial staff: Headache, tyramine, serotonin and migraine. Nutr. Rev. 26: 40, 1968.
5. Boulton, A. A.; Cookson, B.; and Paulton, R.: Hypertensive crisis in a patient on MAOI antidepressants following a meal of beef liver. Can. Med. Assoc. J. 102: 1394, 1970.
6. Blackwell, B.; Marley, E.; Price, J.; and Taylor, D.: Hypertensive interactions between monoamine oxidase inhibitors and foodstuffs. Br. J. Psychiatry 113: 349, 1967.
7. Villiers, J. C.: Intracranial haemorrhage in patients treated with monoamine oxidase inhibitors. Br. J. Psychiatry 112: 109, 1966.
8. Christakis, G., and Miridjanian, A.: Diets, drugs, and their interrelationships. J. Am. Diet. Assoc. 52: 21, 1968.
9. Physician's Desk Reference, s.v. "Parnate," 1975.
10. Arthur Lipman, Pharm.D., University of Utah, Personal communication.

11. Price, K., and Smith, S. E.: Cheese reaction and tyramine. Lancet 1: 130, 1971.
12. Krikler, D. M., and Lewis, B.: Dangers of natural foodstuffs. Lancet 1: 1166, 1965.
13. Sapeika, N.: Food Pharmacology. Springfield: Charles C. Thomas, 1969.
14. Lieb, J.: Degraded protein containing food and monoamine oxidase inhibitors. Am. J. Psychiatry 134: 1444, 1977.
15. Council on Drugs: Paradoxical hypertension from tranylcypromine sulfate. JAMA 186: 854, 1963.
16. Nuessle, W. F.; Norman, F. C.; and Miller, H. E.: Pickled herring and tranylcypromine reaction. JAMA 192: 142, 1965.
17. Hedberg, D. L.; Gordon, M. W.; and Glueck, B. C.: Six cases of hypertensive crisis in patients on tranylcypromine after eating chicken livers. Am. J. Psychiatry 122: 933, 1966.
18. Sen, N. P.: Analysis and significance of tyramine in foods. J. Food Sci. 34: 22, 1969.
19. Berkowitz, B.; Spector, S.; and Pool, W.: The interaction of caffeine, theophylline and theobromine with monoamine oxidase inhibitors. Eur. J. Pharmacol. 16: 315, 1971.
20. Rice, S.; Eitenmiller, R. R.; and Koehler, P. E.: Histamine and tyramine content of meat products. J. Milk and Food Tech. 38: 256, 1974.

# PART D　　　Modifications in Carbohydrate Content

# Carbohydrate Restricted Diet for Management of the Dumping Syndrome

***Definition*** A diet used in the medical management of the dumping syndrome, which provides small, frequent, dry meals containing less than 140 g carbohydrate daily, and in which protein and fat are usually increased in order to meet caloric needs.

***Characteristics of the diet*** Carbohydrate containing foods are restricted because they are more rapidly hydrolyzed to osmotically active substances than are proteins and fats [1–4]. Thus, sugar, alcohol, cookies, pies, pastries, and other concentrated sweets are eliminated, while fruits, breads, cereals, and certain vegetables are restricted. Small, frequent feedings are provided in order to accommodate the reduced capacity of the stomach as a reservoir. Liquids are initially permitted only ½ to 1 hour after meals in order to retard the transit of food from the stomach to the jejunum. Unless weight reduction is indicated for the patient, the intake of protein and fat containing foods is increased in order to provide an adequate caloric intake.

Caffeine is a central nervous system stimulant and like the hormone bradykinin is a vasodilator [5]. However, in the absence of any direct evidence implicating caffeine in the dumping syndrome, coffee and tea are not eliminated from the diet.

***Purpose of the diet*** To prevent the occurrence of the dumping syndrome, a triad of symptoms that may occur after partial gastrectomy [1,2,6].

Symptoms occur following the rapid emptying from the stomach of easily hydrolyzed foods such as carbohydrates and the resulting formation of a hyperosmolar solution in the jejunum [7–9]. Three phases of the disorder have been described: (1) 15–30 minutes after a meal the patient experiences vasomotor symptoms of weakness, dizziness, flushing, sweating, tachycardia, and lightheadedness; (2) gastrointestinal symptoms of nausea, vomiting, or diarrhea often follow; and (3) some patients experience hypoglycemic symptoms due to a rapid fall in blood sugar that occurs 2–3 hours after the meal [10, 11]. These symptoms may be mediated by the augmented secretion of three intestinal hormones, although absolute proof of this theory is lacking [12–14]. However, the hormones bradykinin, a vasodilator; serotonin, a vasoconstrictor; and enteroglucagon, which may have a hypoglycemic effect, have been shown to be released in response to a high carbohydrate load in patients with the disorder [15–17]. Augmented release of a gastric inhibitory polypeptide has been implicated in these patients as the cause of excess insulin release and hypoglycemia [18]. Several of the vasomotor symptoms have been ascribed to augmented release of the hormone bradykinin [19]. Finally, yet another theory has been recently proposed, which relates the occurrence of symptoms to a decrease in hydrogen ion concentration of the stomach contents [20].

*Indications for use*     The diet may be indicated following partial gastrectomy or other operations that either interfere with the pyloric sphincter or compromise the stomach as a reservoir [21].

*Possible adverse reactions*     Care should be taken in susceptible individuals not to increase further the protein or fat content of the diet. The diet is high in cholesterol and saturated fat and may adversely affect serum lipid levels when used over a long period of time. The diet is high in protein and will not be tolerated by patients with seriously impaired renal glomerular filtration rates.

*Contraindications*     The diet as presented is contraindicated in the presence of any accompanying condition in which increases in protein or fat intake may be harmful, e.g., certain forms of cardiovascular or renal disease such as familial hypercholesterolemia or uremia. There is virtually no need for the diet following operative procedures that preserve the pyloric sphincter [22].

*Suggestions for dietitians*     Especially in the initial stages, the diet should be individualized to specific patient tolerances and caloric needs. In the postsurgical state, the diet is usually offered in two stages. Once dumping symptoms have stopped after a day or two on stage I, the patient may progress to stage II of the diet.

In certain patients, eating while reclining may help retard the transit of food, especially liquids [23]. On the other hand, little or no difference was noted in emptying time in other patients after the ingestion of a solid meal, whether they were sitting or reclining [24].

Adaptive changes occurring over a period of time will permit gradual liberalization of the diet. However, additional carbohydrate containing foods should be added slowly and with caution. Milk, in particular, may not be tolerated at all by some patients [25].

For the patient whose nutritional stores are depleted and who may require additional protein and kilocalories, a special high protein food supplement has been developed [26].

A small group of patients are afflicted with what has been termed the late postprandial dumping syndrome; that is, no symptoms are experienced until 1½ to 3 hours after a meal. This form of dumping syndrome is both less common and more responsive to dietary treatment than the early postprandial dumping syndrome. Carbohydrate restriction is necessary in patients with the late dumping syndrome, even though symptoms are not evident immediately and carbohydrate containing foods may appear to relieve temporarily the sensations of hunger that these patients are prone to experience [27].

## Carbohydrate Restricted Diet for Management of the Dumping Syndrome

| Foods allowed | Foods excluded |
|---|---|
| *Beverages* | *Beverages* |
| Milk (whole or skim) or buttermilk if well tolerated by patient, coffee, tea, dietetic carbonated beverages | Alcohol, carbonated beverages, sweetened cereal beverages, sweetened cocoa, sweetened milk products, sweetened fruit drinks |
| *Breads and cereals* | *Breads and cereals* |
| Unsweetened or diet frosted cereals; plain breads, crackers, and rolls; starchy vegetables such as corn, lima beans, parsnips, peas, potato, pumpkin, winter, acorn or butternut squash, yam or sweet potato; rice; pasta; limit to 5 bread exchanges daily* | Sugar frosted or sweetened cereals, or those packaged with dates, raisins, and brown sugar, etc.; "natural" cereals (e.g., Granola or any others of that type) |
| *Desserts* | *Desserts* |
| Initially fruit only | Cakes, cookies, ice cream, and sherbet |
| *Fats* | *Fats* |
| All | None |
| *Fruits* | *Fruits* |
| Unsweetened fruits and fruit juices; limit to 3 fruit exchanges daily* | Sweetened canned fruits and juices |
| *Meat and meat substitutes* | *Meat and meat substitutes* |
| Any type in prepared foods | None |
| *Vegetables* | *Vegetables* |
| Chicory, Chinese cabbage, endive, escarole, lettuce, parsley, radishes, watercress as desired; 1 serving daily from list 2—Vegetable Exchanges.* (Limit to 2 vegetable exchanges) | Any to which sugar has been added |
| *Miscellaneous* | *Miscellaneous* |
| Soups made from allowed foods, broth, nuts, spices, condiments | Gravies thickened with cornstarch or flour, honey, jams, jellies, marmalade, syrups |

\* See exchange lists, pp. F20–F25.

**Daily Food Plan for Stage I** (approximately 95 g carbohydrate, 80 g protein, 90 g fat, and 1,500 kcal)

| Suggested meal plan | Sample menu |
|---|---|
| *Food exchanges** | |

A.M.

| | |
|---|---|
| 1 medium fat meat exchange | 1 egg scrambled in |
| 1 fat exchange | 1 tsp fortified margarine or butter |
| 1 bread exchange | 1 slice toast with |
| 1 fat exchange | 1 tsp fortified margarine or butter |
| ½ whole milk exchange | ½ cup whole milk to be taken 30–60 min after the meal |

BETWEEN MEALS

| | |
|---|---|
| 1 medium fat meat exchange | 1 oz Neufchâtel cheese |
| ½ bread exchange | ½ slice bread |

NOON

| | |
|---|---|
| 2 high fat meat exchanges | 2 oz cooked beef patty (ground chuck 20% fat) |
| ½ bread exchange | ¼ cup rice with |
| 1 fat exchange | 1 tsp fortified margarine or butter |
| 1 fruit exchange | 2 drained, canned, unsweetened peach halves |
| ½ whole milk exchange | ½ cup whole milk to be taken 30–60 min after the meal |

BETWEEN MEALS

| | |
|---|---|
| 1 high fat meat exchange | 1 oz deviled ham with |
| ½ bread exchange | 2 saltines |

P.M.

| | |
|---|---|
| 2 medium fat meat exchanges | 2 oz baked pork loin |
| ½ bread exchange | ½ slice bread with |
| 1 fat exchange | 1 tsp fortified margarine or butter |
| 1 vegetable exchange | ½ cup broccoli with |
| 1 fat exchange | 1 tsp fortified margarine or butter |
| ½ fruit exchange | ¼ cup drained, unsweetened pineapple |
| ½ whole milk exchange | ½ cup whole milk to be taken 30–60 min after the meal |

BEDTIME

| | |
|---|---|
| 1 lean meat exchange | Sandwich: |
| 1 bread exchange | 1 oz sliced chicken on |
| 1 fat exchange | 1 slice bread with |
| | 1 tsp fortified margarine or butter |

* See exchange lists, pp. F20–25.

**Daily Food Plan for Stage II** (approximately 130 g protein, 125 g carbohydrate, 105 g fat, and 1,950 kcal)

| Suggested meal plan | Sample menu |
|---|---|
| *Food exchanges** | |

**A.M.**

| | |
|---|---|
| 1 medium fat meat exchange | 1 egg fried in |
| 1 fat exchange | 1 tsp fortified margarine or butter |
| 1 bread exchange | 1 slice toast with |
| 1 fat exchange | 1 tsp fortified margarine or butter |
| ½ fruit exchange | 2 unsweetened apricot halves |
| 1 milk exchange | 1 cup skimmed milk to be taken 30–60 min after the meal |

**BETWEEN MEALS**

Sandwich:

| | |
|---|---|
| 1 medium fat meat exchange | 1 oz boiled ham with mustard on |
| ½ bread exchange | ½ slice bread |

**NOON**

| | |
|---|---|
| 4 high fat meat exchanges | 4 oz cooked beef patty (ground chuck 20% fat) |
| 1 bread exchange | ½ cup mashed potato |
| 1 fat exchange | 1 tsp fortified margarine or butter |
| 1 vegetable exchange | ½ cup carrots with |
| 1 fat exchange | 1 tsp fortified margarine or butter |
| ½ fruit exchange | 1 small unsweetened drained pear half |
| ½ milk exchange | ½ cup skimmed milk to be taken 30–60 min after the meal |

**BETWEEN MEALS**

| | |
|---|---|
| 1 medium fat meat exchange | 2 tbsp peanut butter on |
| ½ bread exchange | ½ slice bread |

**P.M.**

| | |
|---|---|
| 5 lean meat exchanges | 5 oz baked haddock |
| ½ bread exchange | ½ small baked potato with |
| 1 fat exchange | 1 tsp fortified margarine or butter |
| 1 vegetable exchange | 1 serving green string beans with |
| 1 fat exchange | 1 tsp fortified margarine or butter |
| 1 fruit exchange | 1 small apple |
| ½ milk exchange | ½ cup skimmed milk to be taken 30–60 min after the meal |

**BEDTIME**

| | |
|---|---|
| 2 high fat meat exchanges | 2 oz cheddar cheese on |
| 1 bread exchange | 4 saltines |
| ½ fruit exchange | 5 large drained unsweetened cherries |

* See exchange lists, pp. F20–25.

**References**

1. Pittman, A. C., and Robinson, F. W.: Dumping syndrome—control by diet. J. Am. Diet. Assoc. 34: 596, 1958.
2. Pittman, A. C., and Robinson, F. W.: Dietary management of the dumping syndrome. J. Am. Diet. Assoc. 40: 108, 1962.
3. Randall, H. T.: Enteric feeding. Ballinger, W. F.; Collins, J. A.; Drucker, W. R.; Dudrick, S. J.; and Zeppa, R. Manual of Surgical Nutrition. Philadelphia: W. B. Saunders, 1975.
4. Johansson, C.: Studies in gastrointestinal interactions. IV. Gastric emptying of a composite meal in man. The influence of glucose. Scand. J. Gastroenterol. 8: 533, 1973.
5. Ritchie, J. M.: Central nervous system stimulants. II. Xanthines. Goodman, L. S., and Gilman, A. eds. The Pharmacological Basis of Therapeutics. 5th ed. London: Macmillan, 1975.
6. Wright, H. K., and Tilson, M. D.: Postoperative Disorders of the Gastrointestinal Tract. New York: Grune & Stratton, 1973.
7. Smith, F. W., and Jeffries, G. H.: Late and persistent postgastrectomy problems. Sleisinger, M. H., and Fordtran, J. S. eds. Gastrointestinal Disease. Philadelphia: W. B. Saunders, 1973.
8. French, A. B.; Cook, H. B.; and Pollard, H. M.: Nutritional problems after gastrointestinal surgery. Med. Clin. N. Am. 53: 1389, 1969.
9. Welch, C. E.: Late effects of gastrectomy. JAMA 228: 1287, 1974.
10. Davis, R. L.; Girard, D. L.; and Eaton, R. P.: Hormonal basis for the dumping syndrome. Rocky Mt. Med. J. 71: 94, 1974.
11. Sweeting, J.: The post-gastrectomy syndrome. Med. Times 102: 49, June 1974.
12. Macdonald, J. M.; Webster, M. M.; Tennyson, C. H.; Drapanas, T.: Serotonin and bradykinin in the dumping syndrome. Am. J. Surg. 117: 204, 1969.
13. Stahlgren, L. H.: The dumping syndrome: a study of its hemodynamics. Hosp. Prac. 5: 59, December 1970.
14. Shultz, K. T.; Neelon, F. A.; Nilsen, L. B.; and Lebovitz, H. E.: Mechanism of postgastrectomy hypoglycemia. Arch. Intern. Med. 128: 240, 1971.
15. Zeitlin, I. J., and Smith, A. N.: 5-Hydroxyindoles and kinins in the carcinoid and dumping syndromes. Lancet 2: 986, 1966.
16. Cuschieri, A., and Onabanjo, O. A.: Kinin release after gastric surgery. Br. Med. J. 3: 565, 1971.
17. Bloom, S. R.; Royston, C. M.; and Thomson, J. P. S.: Enteroglucagon release in the dumping syndrome. Lancet 2: 789, 1972.
18. Thomford, N. R.; Sirinek, K. R.; Crockett, S. E.; Mazzaferri, E. L.; and Cataland, S.: Gastric inhibitory polypeptide: response to oral glucose after vagotomy and pyloroplasty. Arch. Surg. 109: 177, 1974.
19. Wong, P. Y.; Talamo, R. C.; Babior, B. M.; Raymond, G. G.; and Colman, R. W.: Kallikrein-kinin system in postgastrectomy dumping syndrome. Ann. Intern. Med. 80: 577, 1974.
20. Thomson, J. P. S.; Russell, R. C. G.; Hobsley, R. M.; and LeQuesne, L. P.: The dumping syndrome and the hydrogen ion concentration of the gastric contents. Gut 15: 200, 1974.
21. Berk, J. L.: The dumping syndrome. Arch. Surg. 102: 88, 1971.
22. Hennessy, T. P. J.; Whelton, M. M.; and Brady, M, P.: The place of pylorus-preserving gastrectomy in the treatment of duodenal ulcer. Br. J. Surg. 61: 844, 1974.
23. McKelvie, S. T. D.: Gastric incontinence and post vagotomy diarrhea. Br. J. Surg. 57: 741, 1970.
24. Kalbasi, H.; Hudson, F. R.; Herring, A.; Moss, S.; Glass, H. I.; and Spencer, J.: Gastric emptying following vagotomy and antrectomy and proximal gastric vagotomy. Gut 16: 509, 1975.
25. Pirk, F.; Skala, I.; and Vulterinova, M.: Milk intolerance after gastrectomy. Digestion 9: 130, 1973.
26. Alexander, C.: A protein dietary supplement for the severe dumping syndrome. Surg. Gynecol. Obstet. 141: 863, 1975.
27. Woodward, E. R., and Neustein, C. L.: The late postprandial dumping syndrome. Buskin, F. L., and Woodward, E. R., eds. Postgastrectomy Syndromes. Vol. 20. Major Problems in Clinical Surgery. Philadelphia: W. B. Saunders, 1976.

# Galactose Free Diet

*Definition*    A diet free of all sources of the monosaccharide galactose. The diet is also lactose free, since galactose is a component of the disaccharide lactose.

*Characteristics of the diet*    The composition of the galactose free diet is similar to that of the lactose free diet. In infancy, a special galactose free formula may be used. All foods excluded on a lactose free diet are also eliminated from the galactose free diet, as well as organ meats such as liver, pancreas, and brain and monosodium glutamate, which contain galactose. Peas, lima beans, and soybeans contain the oligosaccharides raffinose and stachyose, which may release galactose upon digestion. Current studies have suggested, however, that human beings lack the enzymes necessary for the hydrolysis of raffinose and stachyose [1,2]. Therefore, peas, lima beans, and soybeans are not excluded from the galactose free diet. Any vegetable to which lactose may have been added during processing, such as peas, should be excluded.

*Purpose of the diet*    Control of galactosemia and the prevention of severe mental retardation, cataracts, and other symptoms. The goal of dietary treatment is the maintenance of the erythrocyte level of galactose-1-phosphate at less than 3 mg/100 ml and the reduction of urinary galactose below 10 mg/100 ml [3–5].

Galactosemia is a hereditary disorder caused by a deficiency of one of four enzymes essential to the normal conversion of galactose into glucose in the body [6]. The classic form of the disorder involves a severe deficiency of the enzyme galactose-1-phosphate uridyl transferase. In the absence of the necessary enzyme, galactose metabolites such as galactose-1-phosphate accumulate abnormally in the body and cause characteristic tissue damage [7,8]. A constellation of symptoms, including acute brain and liver damage, chronic nutritional failure, cirrhosis, cataracts, and mental retardation, results. In the lens of the eye the conversion of galactose to its alcohol galactitol causes osmotic changes that result in cataracts [5]. Since the missing enzyme cannot be replaced, treatment is based on exclusion of dietary galactose.

*Effects of the diet*    In galactose-1-phosphate uridyl transferase deficiency, cirrhosis, cataract formation, and severe mental retardation may be avoided by prompt dietary management. If the diet is not instituted soon after birth, affected infants may exhibit vomiting, hepatomegaly, jaundice, brain damage, or death [4]. A transient increase in mannitol excretion after the institution of the diet persists until the body has been depleted of its abnormally stored galactitol [9]. Some degree of brain damage may occur before birth, which could explain the fact that despite prompt dietary treatment a number of affected children have demonstrated visual perceptual learning handicaps [10].

Persons who are deficient in the galactokinase enzyme have a much less severe form of galactosemia than those afflicted with a lack of galactose-1-phosphate uridyl transferase. The major symptom exhibited is cataract formation [11–13]. Prompt institution of a galactose free diet within the first 4–6 weeks of life will prevent or at least partially reverse cataract formation [8]. Dietary treatment that is delayed until cataracts have become dense produces less satisfactory results [8].

*Indications for use*    Several variants of galactose-1-phosphate uridyl transferase deficiency have been recognized, as well as a milder form of galactosemia involving a deficiency of the enzyme galactokinase [13–15]. The diet is clearly indicated in the classic form of galactose-1-phosphate uridyl transferase deficiency and in galactokinase deficiency [3–5,11,12]. Carriers of the galactokinase deficient gene have an increased risk of cataracts in adulthood and may benefit from galactose restriction [8,12].

Patients with the Duarte variant of transferase deficient galactosemia are asymptomatic and require no dietary treatment [16]. Prenatal testing for galactosemia is now possible by amniocentesis and culture of amniotic cells. Since cataracts may develop in utero, maternal galactose restriction has been recommended by some investigators when an affected fetus is diagnosed or suspected [5]. Until recently, there were no known cases of galactosemia as a result of a deficiency of the enzyme uridine diphosphate-4-epimerase. A two-year clinical follow-up of the first known human being to be described with a deficiency of epimerase has led the investigators to conclude that this form of galactosemia is benign and does not benefit from dietary galactose restrictions [17].

*Possible adverse reactions*    See lactose free diet.

*Contraindications*    None reported.

*Duration and scope of diet therapy*    Patients diagnosed and treated from birth do better than those who have been exposed to galactose for varying lengths of time. Further studies are needed to determine conclusively the effect of galactose restriction by pregnant mothers who are carriers of the galactosemia gene. The specific role of alternate pathways for galactose metabolism in patients with galactosemia is not clear, although it has been speculated that older school-age children may be able to utilize these pathways. There is some evidence at least in animals, however, that alternate enzymes are not present in large enough amounts to permit normalization of the diet to include liberal intake of galactose [18]. In addition, little is known as to whether there is progressive tissue damage in older children with galactosemia [18]. Therefore, it has been recommended that any liberalization of the diet in older children be undertaken with the greatest of care and be accompanied by biochemical monitoring of its effects [9] and periodic appraisal for cataracts and brain damage.

*Suggestions for dietitians*    Soybean milks are generally well accepted if started at birth. Nutramigen,* a casein hydrolysate, may contain small amounts of lactose because it is prepared from milk; these minute amounts appear not to affect the efficacy of this formu-

* Mead Johnson and Co., Evansville, IN 47721.

la in infants with galactosemia [19,20].

Successful dietary management is related to the caretaker's understanding of the disorder, to the diet, and to the caretaker's ability not only to discipline the child effectively but to develop in him methods of self-discipline. By 3 years of age the child should begin to develop a sense of responsibility for his own diet [5]. Satisfactory erythrocyte galactose-1-phosphate levels do not necessarily indicate an adequate dietary intake. A 3-day dietary recall should be kept by the parents prior to each clinic visit and should be used by the dietitian to assess dietary intake [5]. More detailed suggestions have been published elsewhere [5].

**Basic Four Food Guide (Modified)**

| *Milk substitute group* | *Meat group* |
|---|---|
| 24–32 oz for infants<br>16–24 oz for children | 4–6 oz meat, fish, poultry, eggs, peanut butter, nuts, or legumes |

| *Vegetable–fruit group* | *Bread–cereal group* |
|---|---|
| 4 servings including:<br>1 citrus, tomatoes, pineapple, or green peppers; 1 deep yellow or dark green leafy vegetable | 4 sl or servings whole grain or enriched bread, without milk |

Other foods to be added as desired to satisfy caloric requirements:
1. Margarines—without milk, oils, and salad dressing.
2. Soy milk ice creams may be used to insure an adequate intake of milk substitutes.

*Source:* Adapted from Galactosemia [21].
*Note:* Food exchange lists are as given in Exchange Lists, pp. F20–F25.

References

1. Donnell, G. N.; Bergen, W. R.; and Ng, W. G.: Galactosemia. Biochem. Med. 1: 29, 1967.
2. Gitzelmann, R., and Auricchio, S.: The handling of soya alpha-galactosides by a normal and a galactosemic child. Pediatrics 36: 231, 1965.
3. Cohn, R.M., and Segal, S.: Galactose metabolism and its regulation. Metabolism 22: 627, 1973.
4. Wong, P. K., and Hsia, D. Y.: Inborn errors of metabolism. Goodhart, R. S., and Shils, M. E., eds. Modern Nutrition in Health and Disease. 5th ed. Philadelphia: Lea & Febiger, 1973.
5. Acosta, P. B., and Elsas, L. J.: Dietary Management of Inherited Metabolic Disease: Phenylketonuria, Galactosemia, Tyrosinemia, Homocystinuria, Maple Syrup Urine Disease. Atlanta: ACELMU Publishers, 1976.
6. Koch, R.; Acosta, P.; Ragsdale, M.; and Donnell, G. N.: Nutrition in the treatment of galactosemia. J. Am. Diet. Assoc. 43: 216, 1963.
7. Koch, R.; Acosta, P.; Donnell, G.; and Lieberman, E.: Nutritional therapy of galactosemia. Clin. Pediatr. 4: 571, 1965.
8. Donnell, G. N., and Bergen, W. R.: The galactosemias. Raine, D. N. Treatment of Inherited Metabolic Disease. New York: American Elsevier, 1974.
9. Blau, K.: Increased mannitol excretion in controlled hereditary galactosemia. Clin. Chim. Acta 38: 441, 1972.
10. Donnell, G. N.; Koch, R.; and Bergen, W. R.: Observations on results of management of galactosemic patients. Hsia, D. Y., ed. Galactosemia. Springfield: Charles O. Thomas, 1969.
11. Thalhammer, O.; Gitzelmann, R.; and Pantlitscho, M.: Hypergalactosemia and galactosuria due to galactokinase deficiency in a newborn. Pediatrics 42: 441, 1968.
12. Beutler, E.; Matsumotu, F.; Kuhl, W.; Krill, A.; Levy, N.; Sparkes, R.; and Degnan, M.: Galactokinase deficiency as a cause of cataracts. N. Engl. J. Med. 288: 1203, 1973.

13. Cornblath, M., and Schwartz, R.: Disorders of Carbohydrate Metabolism in Infancy. 2d ed. Philadelphia: W. B. Saunders, 1976.
14. Olambiwonnu, N. O.; McVie, R.; Ng, W. G.; Frasier, S. D.; and Donnell, G. N.: Galactokinase deficiency in twins: clinical and biochemical studies. Pediatrics 53: 314, 1974.
15. Chacko, C. M.; Christian, J. O.; and Nadler, H. L.: Unstable galactose I phosphate uridyl transferase: a new variant of galactosemia. J. Pediatr. 78: 454, 1971.
16. Hansen, R. G.: Hereditary galactosemia. JAMA 208: 2077, 1969.
17. Gitzelmann, R., and Steinmann, B.: Uridine diphosphate galactose 4 epimerase deficiency. II. Clinical follow-up, biochemical studies and family investigation. Helv. Pediatr. Acta 28: 497, 1973.
18. Cohn, R. M., and Segal, S.: Galactose metabolism and its regulation. Metabolism 22: 627, 1973.
19. Segal, S.: Disorders of galactose metabolism. Stanbury, J. B.; Wyngaarden, J. B.; and Fredrickson, D. S., eds. The Metabolic Basis of Inherited Disease. 3d ed. New York: McGraw-Hill, 1972.
20. Yudkoff, M.; Cohn, R. M.; and Segal, S.: Errors of carbohydrate metabolism in infants and children. Clin. Pediatr. 17: 820, 1978.
21. Wenz, E., and Mitchell, M.: Galactosemia. Palmer, S., and Ekvall, S., eds. Pediatric Nutrition in Developmental Disorders. Springfield, IL: C. C. Thomas, 1978.

# Lactose Free Diet

*Definition*  A diet that eliminates virtually all known sources of the disaccharide lactose.

*Characteristics of the diet*  Milk and milk products are excluded as well as other foods that either naturally contain small amounts of lactose or have small amounts added in processing. Lactate, lactic acid, and lactalbumin do not contain lactose and are not eliminated.

*Purpose and effects of the diet*  Total exclusion of dietary lactose may be necessary in the treatment of severely affected individuals in whom the intestinal enzyme lactase is almost completely absent [1,2]. The absence of lactase results in the inability to hydrolyze lactose to glucose and galactose. Undigested lactose, because it cannot be absorbed, remains in the intestinal lumen; there it ferments and causes abdominal cramps, increased motility, distension, and an irritating osmotic diarrhea [3]. Some of these patients become symptomatic after the ingestion of as little as 3 g lactose (the amount found in ¼ cup of milk [4]). Withdrawal of lactose is accompanied by the relief of symptoms.

*Indications for use*  Dietary management with a lactose free diet may be indicated in primary or secondary lactase deficiencies. Primary lactase deficiency occurs as a congenital abnormality in the intestinal mucosa. The Holzel syndrome and the Durand syndrome are both rare primary disorders of infancy that are managed with lactose free diet therapy [2]. Secondary lactose intolerance may result from damage to the intestinal mucosa produced by such diseases as celiac disease [5,6], kwashiorkor, malnutrition [2], gastrointestinal milk protein allergy [7], the irritable bowel syndrome, regional enteritis, and ulcerative colitis [8]. Transient lactose intolerance may also occur after viral enteritis [9]. Intolerance even to the amount of lactose contained in 1 cup of milk (12 g) is a widespread clinically relevant problem [10].

Sensitivity to milk protein as opposed to milk sugar should be considered in forming the diagnosis [11], as dietary treatment would differ slightly. The diet should be prescribed in the presence of a flat lactose tolerance test (an increase in blood sugar of less than 20 mg/100 ml subsequent to an intake of 50 g lactose or approximately 1 g/kg of body weight) followed by gastrointestinal symptoms [12]. In children, an acidic fecal pH of less than 5 or 6, the presence of lactose in the stool greater than 10 mg/100 ml, and a therapeutic response to lactose withdrawal may also be helpful clues in establishing the need for the diet [11,13]. The diagnosis has also been made using a barium-lactose roentgenographic study; 25 g lactose is added to the barium contrast medium and an abdominal film is taken 1 hour later. In lactase deficiency, the small bowel is dilated, the barium is diluted, and there is rapid transit [12,14].

*Possible adverse reactions*  Prolonged adherence to a milk free diet may result in a calcium deficiency unless there is a marked increase in intake of other calcium containing foods [15], e.g., green leafy vegetables, carrots, dates, and prunes. Calcium gluconate supplements are usually needed to ensure adequate calcium intake.

Results of one study suggests that long-term lactose restrictions may lead to osteoporosis as a result of inadequate calcium intake and absorption [16]. Others have noted that increased calcium utilization and retention may compensate for impaired absorption [17] except in patients with limited compensatory mechanisms, e.g., those who have just had gastrectomies [18]. One interesting theory speculates that if there is any benefit to be derived from the concomitant ingestion of calcium and lactose containing foods, it may be dependent upon the hydrolysis of lactose to glucose and galactose; both stimulate intestinal calcium absorption [15].

*Contraindications*    Wide variations exist among lactose intolerant persons in their degree of lactose intolerance. Totally lactose free diets are not indicated for all lactose intolerant individuals and may be counterproductive in persons who can handle small amounts of dietary lactose. Prior to the institution of a lactose free diet, a diet history should be taken in order to determine the approximate amount of lactose ingested daily. In many symptomatic patients who have a large daily intake of lactose, the elimination of milk, and milk products from the diet may relieve symptoms [19].

*Suggestions for dietitians*    Manufacturers of many foods will send upon request lists of ingredients used in their products. This information can be utilized to prepare a shopping guide that is useful in counseling patients who must adhere to a completely lactose free diet. As breads and other locally prepared products may have milk added to them, the guide should include a list of local products that are safe to use. Patients should be advised to scrutinize labels for the presence of whey and casein in addition to nonfat milk solids; one analysis of the composition of casein has reported the existence of small amounts of lactose [20].

Lactose may be added to foods and drugs in a variety of ways. It is often found in drug tablets as a filler or sweetening agent without being properly identified on the label [21,22]. Recipes for foods permitted on the galactose free diet may also be used for lactose free or restricted diets. However, recipes intended for patients with milk protein allergies may not also be lactose free.

Preliminary studies using a milk in which part or all of the lactose has been hydrolyzed have been very encouraging. Although, sweeter and higher in osmolality than ordinary milk, lactose free milk appears to be palatable and well tolerated by lactose intolerant persons; it may prove useful in improving the variety of the diet and the quality of nutritional care for the lactose intolerant patient [12,23–26]. Lactase enzyme is now available commercially* and will hydrolyze a large proportion of the lactose in milk if mixed according to directions.

* Lact-Aid, Sugarlo Co., Atlantic City, NJ 08404.

Lactose Free Diet

| Foods allowed | Foods excluded |
|---|---|

### Beverages

Isomil,* Prosobee,† Pregestimil,† Mocha Mix,‡ meat base formulas used as milk substitutes, carbonated drinks, coffee, freeze dried coffee, fruit drinks, some instant coffees (check labels), Lidalac§ and other lactose free milks or those treated with lactase enzymes; lactose free products such as Ensure,* Ensure Plus Citrotein,* Nutramigen,† Nutri 1000 LF⊥

### Beverages

All untreated milk of any species and all products containing milk, except lactose free milk, such as skim, dried, evaporated, or condensed milk; yogurt; cheese; ice cream; sherbet; malted milk; Ovaltine;° hot chocolate; some cocoas and instant coffees (read labels); powdered soft drinks with lactose curds; whey and casein milk that has been treated with lactobacillus/acidophilus culture rather than lactase, such as Nu-trish•

### Breads and cereals

Breads and rolls made without milk, Italian bread, some cooked cereals and prepared cereals (read labels), macaroni, spaghetti, soda crackers

### Breads and cereals

Prepared mixes, such as muffins, biscuits, waffles, pancakes; some dry cereals such as Total,†† Special K,‡‡ and Cocoa Krispies‡‡ (read labels carefully); Instant Cream of Wheat;§§ commercial breads and rolls to which milk solids have been added; zwieback; French toast made with milk

### Desserts

Water and fruit ices; gelatin; angel food cake; homemade cakes, pies, cookies made from allowed ingredients; puddings made with water

### Desserts

Commercial cakes and cookies and mixes, custard, puddings, sherbets, ice cream made with milk; any containing chocolate, pie crust made with butter or margarine, gelatin made with carrageen

### Eggs

All

### Eggs

Omelets and soufflés containing milk

### Fats

Margarines and dressings that do not contain milk or milk products, oils, shortening, bacon, Rich's Whip Topping,** some nondairy creamers (read labels), nut butters, nuts

### Fats

Margarines and dressings containing milk or milk products, butter, cream, cream cheese, peanut butter with milk solids fillers, salad dressings containing lactose

### Fruits

All fresh, canned, or frozen that are not processed with lactose

### Fruits

Any canned or frozen processed with lactose

### Meat, fish, poultry, etc.

Plain beef, chicken, fish, turkey, lamb, veal, pork, and ham; strained or junior meats and vegetables and meat combinations that do not contain milk or milk products; kosher frankfurters

### Meat, fish, poultry, etc.

Creamed or breaded meat, fish, or fowl; sausage products, such as weiners, liver sausage, cold cuts containing nonfat milk solids; cheese

### Soups

Clear soups, vegetable soups, consommés, cream soups made with Mocha Mix‡ or nondairy creamers

### Soups

Cream soups unless made with allowed ingredients, chowders, commercially prepared soups containing lactose

* Ross Laboratories, Columbus, OH 43216.
† Mead Johnson and Co., Evansville, IN 47721.
‡ Presto Food Products, Los Angeles, CA 90021.
§ Lidano Co., Kalunborg, Denmark.
⊥ Cutter Laboratories, Berkeley, CA 94710.
° Ovaltine Products, Villa Park, IL 60181.

• Knudsen Bros., North Haven, CT 06473.
** Rich Products Corp., Buffalo, NY 14212.
†† General Mills, Minneapolis, MN 55435.
‡‡ Kellogg Co., Battle Creek, MI 49016.
§§ Nabisco, Inc., East Hanover, NJ 07936.

**Foods allowed**

*Vegetables*

Fresh, canned, or frozen: artichokes, asparagus, broccoli, cabbage, carrots, cauliflower, celery, chard, corn, cucumber, eggplant, green beans, kale, lettuce, mustard, okra, onions, parsley, parsnips, pumpkin, rutabagas, spinach, squash, tomatoes, white and sweet potatoes, yams, lima beans, beets

*Miscellaneous*

Soy sauce, carob powder, popcorn, olives, pure sugar candy, jelly or marmalade, sugar, corn syrup, carbonated beverages, gravy made with water, baker's cocoa, pickles, pure seasonings and spices, wine, molasses (beet sugar), pure monosodium glutamate, instant coffees that do not contain lactose

**Foods excluded**

*Vegetables*

Any to which lactose is added during processing; peas; creamed, breaded, or buttered vegetables; instant potatoes, corn curls, and frozen French fries if processed with lactose

*Miscellaneous*

Chewing gum; chocolate; some cocoas; toffee; peppermint; butterscotch; caramels; some instant coffees, dietetic preparations (read labels); certain antibiotics and vitamin and mineral preparations; spice blends if they contain milk products; monosodium glutamate extender; artificial sweeteners containing lactose, such as Equa,⊥⊥ Sweet n' Low,°° Wee Cal;*** some nondairy creamers (read labels)

⊥⊥ G. D. Searle and Co., Skokie, IL 60076.
°° NIFDA (National Institutional Food Distributor Associates, Inc.), Atlanta, GA 30325.
***Domino Amstar Corporation, New York, NY 10020.

## Lactose Free Diet

**Sample Menu**

A.M.
½ cup orange juice
1 egg, soft cooked
2 slices Vienna bread, toasted
2 tsp milk free margarine
1 tbsp grape jelly
2 tsp sugar
Coffee or tea

NOON

3 oz roast beef
½ cup rice
½ cup green beans
1 pear
2 slices Vienna bread
2 tsp milk free margarine
1 tsp sugar
Coffee or tea

BETWEEN MEALS

1 slice angel cake with sliced peaches

P.M.

4 oz round steak
1 small baked potato
2 tsp milk free margarine
½ cup spinach
2 slices Vienna bread, toasted
½ cup fruit cocktail
1 tsp sugar
Coffee or tea

BEDTIME

½ cup apricot nectar

**References**

1. Lindquist, B., and Meeuwisse, G.: Diets in disaccharidase deficiency and defective monosaccharide absorption. J. Am. Diet. Assoc. 48: 307, 1966.
2. Herber, R.: Disaccharidase deficiency in health and disease. Calif. Med. 116: 23, June 1972.
3. Bayless, T. M.: Disaccharidase deficiency. J. Am. Diet. Assoc. 60: 478, 1972.
4. Bedine, M. S., and Bayless, T. M.: Intolerance of small amounts of lactose by individuals with low lactase levels. Gastroenterology 65: 735, 1973.
5. Welsh, J. D.; Zschiesche, O. M.; Anderson, J.; and Walker, A.: Intestinal disaccharidase activity in celiac sprue (gluten-sensitive enteropathy). Arch. Intern. Med. 123: 33, 1969.
6. Beck, J. T.; Dinda, D. K.; DaCosta, L. R.; and Beck, M.: Sugar absorption by small bowel biopsy samples from patients with primary lactose deficiency and with adult celiac disease. Am. J. Dig. Dis. 21: 946, 1976.
7. Matsumura, T.; Kuroume, T.; and Amada, K.: Close relationship between lactose intolerance and allergy to milk protein. J. Asthma Res. 9: 13, 1971.
8. Zamcheck, N., and Broitman, S. A.: Nutrition in diseases of the intestines. Goodhart, R. S., and Shils, M. E., eds. Modern Nutrition in Health and Disease. 5th ed. Philadelphia: Lea & Febiger, 1973.
9. Chandrasekaran, R.; Kumar, V.; Walia, N. S.; and Moorthy, B.: Carbohydrate intolerance in infants with acute diarrhea and its complications. Acta Paediatr. Scand. 64: 483, 1975.
10. Bayless, T. M.; Rothfield, B.; Massa, C.; Wise, L.; Paige, D.; and Bedine, M. S.: Lactose and milk intolerance: clinical implications. N. Engl. J. Med. 292: 1156, 1975.
11. Cornblath, M., and Schwartz, R.: Disorders of Carbohydrate Metabolism in Infancy. 2d ed. Philadelphia: W. B. Saunders, 1976.
12. Newcomer, A. D.: Disaccharidase deficiencies. Mayo Clin. Proc. 48: 648, 1973.
13. Bartrop, R. W., and Hull, D.: Transient lactose intolerance in infancy. Arch. Dis. Child. 48: 963, 1973.
14. Morrison, W. J.; Christopher, N. L.; Bayless, T. M.; and Dana, E. A.: Low lactase levels: evaluation of the radiologic diagnosis. Radiology 111: 513, 1974.
15. Hadley, R. A.: Calcium and hypo-allergenic diets. Ann. Allergy 30: 36, 1972.
16. Birge, S. J.; Keutmann, H. T.; Cuatrecasas, P.; and Whedon, G. D.: Osteoporosis, intestinal lactase deficiency on low dietary calcium intake. N. Engl. J. Med. 276: 445, 1967.
17. Kocian, J.; Skala, I.; and Bakos, K.: Calcium absorption from milk and lactose free milk in healthy subjects and patients with lactose intolerance. Digestion 9: 317, 1973.
18. Kocian, J.; Vulterinova, M.; Bejblova, O.; and Skala, I.: Influence of lactose intolerance on the bones of patients after partial gastrectomy. Digestion 8: 324, 1973.
19. Welsh, J. D.: Diet therapy in adult lactose malabsorption: present practices. Am. J. Clin. Nutr. 31: 592, 1978.
20. Hardinge, M. G.; Swarner, J. B.; and Crooks, H.: Carbohydrates in foods. J. Am. Diet. Assoc. 46: 197, 1965.
21. Allergy Recipes. Chicago: American Dietetic Association, 1969.
22. Baking for People with Food Allergies. Home and Garden Bulletin No. 146. Rev. Washington, DC: U.S. Department of Agriculture, 1975.
23. Skala, I.; Lamacova, V.; and Pirk, F.: Lactose free milk as a solution of problems associated with dietetic treatment of lactose intolerance. Digestion 4: 326, 1971.
24. Paige, D. M.; Bayless, T. M.; Huang, S. S.; and Wexler, R.: Lactose hydrolyzed milk. Am. J. Clin. Nutr. 28: 818, 1975.
25. Turner, S. V.; Daly, T.; Haurigen, J. A.; Rand, A. G.; and Thayer, W. R.: Utilization of a low lactose milk. Am. J. Clin. Nutr. 29: 739, 1976.
26. Payne-Bose, D.; Welsh, J. D.; Gearhart, H. L.; and Morrison, R. D.: Milk and lactose hydrolyzed milk. Am. J. Clin. Nutr. 30: 695, 1977.

# Lactose Restricted Diet

*Definition*     A diet limited in its content of the disaccharide lactose. It provides an amount of lactose small enough not to cause recurrence of symptoms in mild forms of lactose intolerance, usually less than 8–10 g lactose daily.

*Characteristics of the diet*     Wide variations exist among lactase deficient persons as to the amount of lactose tolerated. Some persons with adult onset lactose deficiency may be asymptomatic except when they consume large quantities of milk, while others cannot tolerate any at all. Therefore, the lactose restricted diet should be specialized to accommodate individual tolerance levels [1–3]. Milk beverages, creamed foods, and ice cream may have to be avoided. Fermented forms of milk, such as cheese, in which the lactose has been converted to lactic acid are not restricted [2,3]. Yogurt and buttermilk are fermented forms of milk in which only small amounts of the lactose have been converted to lactic acid [3,4]. For some as yet unexplained reason, certain patients tolerate these well [2,3]. Some individuals may tolerate chocolate milk better than whole milk because of its increased osmolality, which results in a delayed emptying time [5].

*Purpose of the diet*     To prevent the occurrence of symptoms in patients with less severe forms of lactose intolerance or with primary late onset lactose deficiency or adult hypolactosis [6].

*Indications for use*     Current evidence indicates that adult hypolactosis or low intestinal lactase levels are probably present in the majority of adults in most population groups in the world, except Northern European Caucasians. Manifestations of late onset lactose deficiency are in general milder than other forms of lactose intolerance [6]. Restriction of dietary lactose rather than its complete exclusion is usually indicated in these less severely affected patients [2,3].

*Duration and scope of diet therapy*     Treatment of severe manifestations of congenital lactose intolerance, such as the Durand syndrome, may require adherence to a lactose free diet indefinitely [7]. On the other hand, clinical response to the diet may permit progression to a lactose restricted diet in certain patients with other forms of the disease. Finally, lactose intolerance may occur secondary to diseases that produce intestinal damage, such as celiac sprue, etc. In these instances, rigorous therapy of the underlying disorder may bring about sufficient restoration of mucosal surfaces to permit elimination of all lactose restrictions [8].

References     1. Bayless, T. M.:   Disaccharidase deficiency.   J. Am. Diet. Assoc. 60: 478, 1972.
2. Bayless, T. M.:   Lactase deficiency in milk intolerance.   Med. Counterpoint 3: 29, 1971.
3. Gallagher, C. R.; Molleson, A. L.; and Caldwell, J. H.:   Lactose intolerance and fermented dairy products.   J. Am. Diet. Assoc. 65: 418, 1974.
4. Newcomer, A. D.:   Disaccharidase deficiencies.   Mayo Clin. Proc. 48: 648, 1973.

5. Welsh, J. D., and Hall, W. H.:  Gastric emptying time of lactose and milk in subjects with malabsorption.  Am. J. Dig. Dis. 22: 1060, 1977.
6. Lebenthal, E.:  Small intestinal disaccharidase deficiencies.  Pediatr. Clin. N. Am. 20: 757, 1975.
7. Holzel, A.:  Sugar malabsorption and sugar intolerance in childhood.  Proc. R. Soc. Med. 61: 1095, 1968.
8. Welsh, J. D.; Zschiesche, O. M.; Anderson, J.; and Walker, A.:  Intestinal disaccharidase activity in celiac sprue (gluten-sensitive enteropathy).  Arch. Intern. Med. 123: 33, 1969.

# The Practical Significance of Lactose Intolerance in Children

COMMITTEE ON NUTRITION, AMERICAN ACADEMY OF PEDIATRICS

Lactose intolerance has been reviewed in published statements by the Protein Advisory Group of the United Nations System [1], the Food and Nutrition Board of the National Research Council [2], and the American Academy of Pediatrics, Committee on Nutrition [3]. Each of these statements deals principally with the advisability of encouraging population groups with a high rate of lactose intolerance to consume nutritionally beneficial quantities of milk. All three statements conclude that it is inappropriate to discourage the use of milk on the basis of lactose intolerance. Nevertheless, controversy over the practical significance of the widespread prevalence [4,5] of lactose intolerance has continued.

Definitions

Lactose *intolerance* is defined [1] as a clinical syndrome of abdominal pain, diarrhea, flatulence, and bloating after the ingestion of a standard lactose tolerance test dose (2 g of lactose per kilogram of body weight or 50 g/m² of body surface area, maximum 50 g in a 20% water solution). If a maximum increase in blood glucose level of less than 26 mg/dl is observed after a lactose tolerance test dose, lactose *malabsorption* is diagnosed [1]. Lactose intolerance is classified as primary, secondary, or congenital. Lactose intolerance is classified as primary when it is observed with no history or signs of underlying intestinal disease. If there is gastrointestinal disease, it is usually classified as secondary. Primary and secondary lactose intolerance are not uncommon; however, congenital lactose intolerance is rare. This form is present at birth, the histologic features of the gastrointestinal mucosa are normal, and brush-border lactase activity is low or completely absent [6,7]. The three forms of lactose intolerance must be considered separately to avoid confusion.

Primary Lactose Intolerance

Major areas of concern in reviewing the practical implications of primary lactose intolerance are (1) the prevalence at specific ages in particular population groups, (2) the relationship between primary lactose intolerance and intolerance to quantities of milk usually consumed, (3) response to hydrolyzed lactose milk, and (4) the absorption of other nutrients in the presence of amounts of lactose that surpass digestive capacity but do not produce symptoms.

STUDIES ON LACTOSE INTOLERANCE

The widespread prevalence of lactose malabsorption and intolerance in children is well documented in a review by Jones and Latham [4]. Prevalence at specific ages in a particular population group varies. In some groups, 90% prevalence is observed by age 4 years; in others it remains much lower throughout life. Similar information on children of American ethnic groups has been published recently [8–17].

Paige and co-workers [8] studied 116 black children 13 to 59 months old. Twenty-nine percent of these children had lactose malabsorption, and 18% had signs of intolerance. Black children 4 to 9 years old were studied by Garza and Schrimshaw [9]. They reported lactose intolerance in 11% of those 4 to 5 years old, 50% of those 6 to 7 years old, and 72% of those 8 to 9 years old. Paige and co-workers [10] studied another group of children 6 to 13 years old. Fifty-four percent had lactose malabsorption and 65% had symptoms of intolerance. Haverberg et al. [11] and Kwon et al. [12] studied black patients 14 to 19 years old and reported lactose malabsorption prevalence rates of 83% and 81%, respectively.

Studies of Mexican-American children have also been reported. Woteki et al. [13] studied 28 Mexican-American children who were 2 to 14 years old. Eighteen percent of the 2- to 5-year-old children were intolerant to lactose. This prevalence increased to 56% in the 10- to 14-year-old children. Sowers and Winterfeldt [14] found a similar prevalence (50%) in 9- to 21-year-old Mexican-American children. In a study of 301 adolescents and young adults [15] in rural Mexico, 222 of them were classified as having lactose malabsorption, but only 86 of these reported symptoms.

American Indians have been studied by Casky and co-workers [16]. Using hydrogen breath analysis, lactose malabsorption was found in 20% of 3- to 5-year-old children, in 10% of those 6 to 12 years old, and in 70% of those 13 to 19 years old. Newcomer et al. [17] reported a similar study in American Indians in which 104 subjects 5 to 17 years old were studied. Lactose malabsorption was diagnosed in 63% to 74% of the groups stratified by age (5 to 6 years, 7 to 8 years, and so forth). Symptoms were reported in 76% of the children with lactose malabsorption. Prevalence of lactose intolerance at specific ages was not reported.

Prevalence of lactose malabsorption in white children tends to be much lower than in these other groups. Persons classified as white in this country tend to be heterogeneous; therefore, data are difficult to compare with studies published in countries with more homogeneous populations. Data presented by Woteki et al. [13] and Garza and Scrimshaw [9] are representative. Lactose intolerance is rarely observed in 2- to 6-year-old children, and increases to about 30% among adolescents. Lebenthal et al. [18] have reported lactase levels from 172 to 1,077 biopsy specimens. The groups studied were white and were healthy siblings and parents of patients with cystic fibrosis, children with failure to thrive without diarrhea, and patients with "irritable colon syndrome." No low lactase activity was encountered in children less than 5 years old.

Comparable data on the prevalence of lactose intolerance in American children from other ethnic backgrounds who were expected to have a high prevalence of lactose intolerance (e.g., Chinese, Japanese, and Greek) are not available.

Assessing the relationship between lactose and milk consumption is also important in determining the practical significance of lactose intolerance in children. Comparison of the standard lactose tolerance test dose with quantities of milk normally consumed shows that the test dose is representative of the amount of milk consumed by young infants but not of that consumed by weaned children. The 200 to 250 ml of milk usually consumed at one sitting by the latter children contains 12 g of lactose. This is substantially less than the 2 g/kg usually provided in the lactose tolerance test.

Paige et al. [19] reported that lactose intolerance in elementary school children adversely influenced their acceptance of moderate amounts of milk. Milk's significant role in publicly sponsored, supplemental feeding programs led Paige and other investigators to study lactose intolerance further. Paige et al. [8] found no differences in milk consumption between lactose-tolerant and lactose-intolerant black children 13 to 59 months old. Garza and Schrimshaw [9] found no differences in milk consumption between lactose-tolerant and lactose-intolerant black children 6 to 7 and 8 to 9 years old, although the 8- to 9-year-old black children consumed less milk regardless of lactose tolerance status than a comparable group of white children. Woteki et al. [13] reported no difference in milk consumption by the lactose-tolerant and lactose-intolerant Mexican-American children they studied. In a study in rural Mexico, [15] conflicting results were obtained and do not help to determine whether lactose malabsorption interferes with milk consumption.

Stephenson and Latham [20] studied slightly older children with lactose malabsorption; no difference in milk consumption was observed between the lactose-tolerant and lactose-intolerant subjects in this study. In Newcomer and co-workers' study [17] of American Indians, two thirds of the 156 subjects studied were less than 18 years old, and those with lactose malabsorption had mean daily lactose intakes of 19 g compared to 25 g in those with lactose absorption. Woteki et al. [13] reported no differences in milk intakes between those with lactose absorption and malabsorption, but children classified as Anglo-American drank more milk than the Mexican-American children. In contrast, Paige et al. [21] reported that 50% of 6- to 12-year-old children with lactose malabsorption consumed less than one-half pint of milk offered in school feeding programs. They found that children with lactose malabsorption who were classified as milk-drinkers had higher increases in blood glucose level than those classified as non-milk-drinkers. Lebenthal et al. [18] have also reported greater milk consumption (>960 ml/day) in individuals with high intestinal lactase levels and their families than in patients and families with low lactase levels (<250 ml/day).

The question of tolerance to various lactose intake levels in intolerant subjects and those with lactose malabsorption has also been examined. Garza and Schrimshaw [9] report that, despite the significant prevalence of lactose intolerance they observed in 4- to 9-year-old black children, no child was intolerant to 240 ml of milk. In contrast, Mitchell et al. [22], who studied 11- to 18-year-old black adolescents, found that 21% had symptoms after consuming 240 ml of milk. In double-blind studies, Haverberg et al. [11] and Kwon et al. [12] report, respectively, that 28% and 9% of adolescents with lactose malabsorption had symptoms after drinking 240 ml of milk, as did 16% and 19% of those with lactose absorption. In a slightly older age group studied by Stephenson and Latham [20], all those with lactose malabsorption could tolerate 240 ml of whole milk without any or only mild symptoms. In studies of native American Indians, Newcomer et al. [23] report that all of the subjects they studied who had malabsorption (6 to 62 years old) tolerated amounts of lactose equivalent to 240 to 300 ml of milk taken with a meal with no intestinal symptoms attributable to lactose. In contrast, lower tolerance levels are reported in older adults by Bayless et al. [24] and in Peruvian children by Paige et al. [25]. Studies from other countries have reported a lack of symptoms in lactose-intolerant children comparable to those reported here [26,27].

A possible solution for circumventing intolerance to normal intakes of milk is to hydrolyze the lactose. Although studies such as those of Jones et al. [28] report that lactose hydrolysis substantially increases milk tolerance in adults, other studies cast doubt on the efficacy of lactose hydrolysis in children. Paige and co-workers [29] tested whole milk, 50% hydrolyzed lactose milk, and 90% hydrolyzed lactose milk in 22 black 13- to 18-year-old subjects with lactose malabsorption. Three of these teenagers reported symptoms to untreated whole milk and to 80% hydrolyzed lactose milk. None reported symptoms to 50% hydrolyzed lactose milk. Similarly, Kwon et al. [12] reported that 28 to 45 teenagers with lactose malabsorption did not experience symptoms to 240 ml of whole milk or lactose-free milk. Ten of the others had inconsistent symptoms; some had symptoms to lactose-free milk only, some to both lactose-free milk and whole milk, and others to 240 ml but not 480 ml of whole milk. Seven subjects had consistent symptoms, but none had symptoms to 240 ml of milk, with or without lactose.

MILK IN THE DIET

The importance of milk in the American diet rests on its high nutrient content. The U.S. Department of Agriculture [30] estimates that dairy products, excluding butter, contribute only 11% of the available food energy; however, they provide 75% of the calcium, 39% of the riboflavin, 35% of the phosphorus, 22% of the magnesium, 20% of the vitamin $B_{12}$, and substantial proportions of other nutrients. The question of the bioavailability of these nutrients in the presence of lactose malabsorption without symptoms of intolerance is, therefore, important. Unfortunately, little data are available. Significant malabsorption is unlikely if there are no symptoms; however, the chronic effects of subtle differences in bioavailability of various nutrients might be significant, especially under conditions of marginal intakes. There are substantial data on the "malabsorption of lactose," but there are no studies estimating metabolizable energy in lactose-containing diets of children with lactose malabsorption. Less increase in blood glucose levels has been demonstrated [29] in those with lactose malabsorption than in those with lactose absorption after milk ingestion. The possibility that slower but sustained digestion of lactose is responsible for these smaller increases remains unknown.

A metabolic study in which milk provided all dietary protein was designed by Calloway and Chenoweth [31] and was conducted in lactose-tolerant and -intolerant adults. After adjustments for metabolizable energy were made, no effect on nitrogen balance was demonstrated. Unpublished results from this study indicate that calcium, phosphorus, and magnesium absorption also were not influenced by the presence of lactose.

Leichter and Tolensky [32], in a study on weaned rats that were fed lactose-containing diets, obtained suggestive evidence that lactose may reduce protein and fat absorption in animals with low lactase activity. Bowie [33] reported the effects of lactose-induced diarrhea on nitrogen and fat absorption. Nitrogen absorption was depressed in those with lactose malabsorption who were fed milk compared to a disaccharide-free diet, but nitrogen retentions were similar with both diets. No differences in fat absorption were noticed. In a separate study by Bowie et al. [34], absorption was studied by using xylose. No difference in xylose excretion was observed when malnourished, lactose-intolerant subjects were fed whole milk or a disaccharide-free formula. A recent study [35] conducted in 2- to 8-month-old infants compared calcium and magnesium absorption when untreated milk, milk treated with lactase ten minutes before feeding, and a lactose-free milk were fed. Calcium and magnesium absorption was best (72% and 81%, respectively) with lactase-treated milk and poorest (calcium 37% and magnesium 39%) with lactose-free milk. The infants were presumably lactose tolerant.

SUMMARY

Lactose intolerance is observed in black and Mexican-American children by age 3 years, and it probably occurs in other non-northern European ethnic groups at a similar age. However, intolerance to the consumption of 250 ml of milk apparently is rarely seen in preadolescents. Current research on the response of adolescents to hydrolyzed lactose milk suggests that the symptoms observed in lactose-intolerant subjects after milk ingestion may be unrelated to lactose or may be mild enough to be of little practical significance. The effect of undigested lactose on nutrient absorption has received little attention, but preliminary data suggest that this is not a problem, except perhaps when overall intakes are marginally adequate.

Secondary Lactose Intolerance

The predominant view at present is that primary lactose intolerance is genetically predetermined. The following observations support this view: its prevalence among apparently healthy populations, its absence among specific groups [36–38], the inevitable decrease with age in lactase activity in most mammalian species [38], and the apparently noninducible nature of the enzyme in humans [26,40]. However, the environment's role in accelerating the age of lactose intolerance, determining the severity of its expression, and increasing the prevalence within population groups has not been assessed. Few studies have been directed at a basic understanding of the physiology of the intestinal mucosal cells as it relates to lactose intolerance and malabsorption. Yet the importance of the environment is repeatedly demonstrated by the apparently transient decrease in lactase activity and intolerance to lactose commonly associated with gastrointestinal disease or significant malnutrition. This condition is classified as secondary lactose intolerance. Areas of concern in assessing its practical implications are (1) its significance in the treatment of malnutrition, which is common to gastrointestinal disease; and (2) the "reversibility" of this condition and its effects on the expression of a presumably genetically determined decrease in lactase.

Lactose intolerance in malnutrition has been well described [34, 41–43]; however, the relevance of this intolerance to milk feeding is controversial. Reddy and Pershad [26], in a study evaluating a milk-based diet in refeeding programs, conclude that this is a self-limiting problem and of little practical importance. An ongoing evaluation [43] of a supplemental milk feeding program serving 32,000 rural Haitians and an accompanying program refeeding the severest cases of malnutrition (301 subjects) make the same conclusions. A favorable outcome was reported for 93% of the subjects in a refeeding program. Milk intolerance could not be excluded as a possible cause of failure in only 1% of the subjects. In a study reported by Prinsloo et al. [42], children refed on cow's milk did not have more diarrhea than those fed formulas with glucose, sucrose, or D-maltose, although lactic acid excretion was high in children fed cow's milk.

In the study by Bowie [33] referred to earlier, lactose-induced diarrhea had no effect on nitrogen retention or fat absorption. He concluded that, as long as milk is the most widely available and cheapest source of good protein, it should be used. However, he does caution that children with severe diarrhea will require a lactose-free formula for a variable period of time. Mason et al. [44] reported similar tolerances.

Mitchell et al. [45] reported results of blind-controlled feeding trials evaluating prehydrolyzed lactose milk and a reconstituted whole milk. Thirty-five slightly undernourished Australian aboriginal infants were studied. No complications were seen in children fed either milk, but five of those fed whole milk failed to gain weight compared to only one in the hydrolyzed lactose milk group. Children fed the hydrolyzed lactose milk had a mean 70% larger weight gain than those fed the whole milk. Children with diarrhea or weights less than 90% of expected weight for age who were fed hydrolyzed lactose milk had statistically significant higher weight gains than comparable groups of children fed whole milk.

The effect of previous malnutrition or gastrointestinal disease on the prevalence of primary lactose intolerance is difficult to evaluate because few studies have attempted to quantitate the severity of observed intolerance or malabsorption. Paige and co-workers [25] report no differences in prevalence between previously malnourished children and their siblings who had no history of significant malnutrition, although tolerance levels in both groups appear lower than observed in children in this country. Woteki et al. [13] found the prevalence of lactose intolerance of Mexican-Americans similar to that reported by Sowers and Winterfeldt [14] from rural Mexico. Stoopler et al. [27] restudied children with lactose malabsorption seven months after an initial evaluation and found that 21% had normal lactose tolerance curves on retesting. In Britain, no correlation was found among continuing lactose intolerance, maximal increase in blood glucose level after a standard lactose test dose, intestinal lactase levels, and small intestinal morphology on reevaluation [46] of 30 children 2 to 38 months old with a previous diagnosis of presumably secondary lactose intolerance.

SUMMARY

Individuals using milk-based diets in refeeding programs occasionally report initial problems with diarrhea aggravated or precipitated by lactose. In this early phase, a hydrolyzed lactose or lactose-free milk may be optimal. Apparently, however, whole milk is successfully used for refeeding, unless there is severe diarrhea. This suggests that the milder cases seen out of the hospital may present less significant problems. The report by Mitchell et al. [45], however, suggests that the effect of lactose may be more subtle. Although unavailable lactose may not present major problems to fat and nitrogen absorption, the decrease in metabolizable energy may be enough to decrease the rate of weight gain, lengthen hospital stays, and therefore decrease the effectiveness of lactose in refeeding programs, unless compensated for in the total diet. Comparable studies should be repeated in hospital and supplementary feeding programs to determine whether or not potential effects on nutrient bioavailability are as significant as this study suggests.

Congenital Lactose Intolerance    The extremely low or absent activity of brush-border lactase [6,7] in congenital lactose intolerance can be life-threatening because of the accompanying severe diarrhea and dehydration when lactose is fed. The condition is rare, but it is not unusual for secondary lactose intolerance to be misdiagnosed during the newborn period as congenital lactose intolerance. A definite diagnosis requires intestinal biopsy for histology and enzyme assay. Nontheless, it is imperative that a lactose-free formula be provided as soon as the diagnosis is suspected because of the seriousness of the condition.

Recommendations and Conclusions    The committee's position remains unchanged. On the basis of present evidence it would be inappropriate to discourage supplemental milk feeding programs targeted at children on the basis of primary lactose intolerance. The committee continues to encourage the development of nutritious and acceptable supplementary foods in areas with inefficient and uneconomical milk production. The use of milk should not be discouraged in the refeeding of malnourished children—except if they have severe diarrhea—as long as milk continues to provide the best and cheapest source of high-quality protein. However, the committee cautions that some of these children will require lactose-free diets if recovery is to be achieved with minimal complications. It also urges that studies such as those of Mitchell et al. [45] be continued in inpatient and outpatient facilities for reasons outlined here; that more attention be given to studies of environmental effects on enterocyte function, thereby increasing our understanding of the development of low lactase levels; and that efforts to provide effective, low-cost, supplemental foods to children be continued as part of comprehensive health planning for decreasing morbidity in children.

References

1. PAG *ad hoc* working group on milk intolerance: Nutritional implication. PAG Bull. 2: 7, 1972.
2. Food and Nutrition Board, National Academy of Sciences: Background Information on Lactose and Milk Intolerance. Washington, DC: National Research Council, May 1972.
3. Committee on Nutrition: Should milk drinking by children be discouraged& Pediatrics 53: 576, 1974.
4. Jones, D. V., and Latham, M. C.: The implications of lactose intolerance in children. J. Trop. Pediatr. 20: 262, 1974.
5. Simoons, F. J.; Johnson, J. D.; and Kretchmer, N.: Perspective on milk-drinking and malabsorption of lactose. Pediatrics 59: 98, 1977.
6. Asp, N. G.; Dahlqvist, A.; Kuitunen, P.; et al.: Complete deficiency of brush-border lactase in congenital lactose malabsorption. Lancet 2: 329, 1973.
7. Freiburghaus, A. U.; Schmitz, J.; Schindler, M.; et al.: Protein patterns of brush border fragments in congenital lactose malabsorption and in specific hypolactasia of the adult. N. Engl. J. Med. 294: 1030, 1976.
8. Paige, D. M.; Bayless, T. M.; Mellitis, E. D.; and Davis, L.: Lactose malabsorption in preschool black children. Am. J. Clin. Nutr. 30: 1018, 1977.
9. Garza, C., and Scrimshaw, N. S.: Relationship of lactose intolerance to milk intolerance in young children. Am. J. Clin. Nutr. 29: 192, 1976.
10. Paige, D. M.; Bayless, T. M.; and Dellinger, W. S., Jr.: Relationship of milk consumption to blood glucose rise in lactose intolerant individuals. Am. J. Clin. Nutr. 28: 677, 1975.
11. Haverberg, L.; Kwon, P. H.; and Scrimshaw, N. S.: Comparative tolerance of adolescents of differing ethnic backgrounds to lactose containing and lactose-hydrolyzed milk: I. Initial experience with a double blind procedure. Unpublished manuscript.
12. Kwon, P. H.; Rorick, M.; and Scrimshaw, N. S.: Comparative tolerance of adolescents of differing ethnic backgrounds to lactose containing and lactose-hydrolyzed milk: II. Experience with improved double blind procedure. Unpublished manuscript.
13. Woteki, C. E.; Weser, E.; and Young, E. A.: Lactose malabsorption in Mexican-American children. Am. J. Clin. Nutr. 29: 19, 1976.
14. Sowers, M. F., and Winterfeldt, E.: Lactose intolerance among Mexican-Americans. Am. J. Clin. Nutr. 28: 704, 1975.
15. Lisker, R.; Lopez-Habib, G.; Daltabuit, M.; et al.: Lactose deficiency in a rural area of Mexico. Am. J. Clin. Nutr. 27: 756, 1974.
16. Casky, D. A.; Payne-Bose, D.; Welsh, J. D.; et al.: Effects of age on lactose malabsorption in Oklahoma Native Americans as determined by breath $H_2$ analysis. Am. J. Dig. Dis. 22: 113, 1977.
17. Newcomer, A. D.; Thomas, P. J.; McGill, D. B.; and Hoffman, A. F.: Lactase deficiency: a common genetic trait of the American Indian. Gastroenterology 72: 234, 1977.
18. Lebenthal, E.; Antonowicz, I.; and Schwachman, H.: Correlation of lactase activity, lactose intolerance, and milk consumption in different age groups. Am. J. Clin. Nutr. 28: 595, 1976.
19. Paige, D. M.; Bayless, T. M.; Ferry, G. D.; and Graham, G. G. Lactose malabsorption and milk rejection in Negro children. Johns Hopkins Med. J. 129: 163, 1971.

20. Stephenson, L. S., and Latham, M. C.: Lactose intolerance and milk consumption: the relation of tolerance to symptoms. Am. J. Clin. Nutr. 27: 296, 1974.
21. Paige, D. M.; Bayless, T. M., and Dellinger, W. S., Jr.: Relationship of milk consumption to blood glucose rise in lactose intolerant individuals. Am. J. Clin. Nutr. 28: 677, 1975.
22. Mitchell, K. J.; Bayless, T. M.; Paige, D. M.; et al.: Intolerance of eight ounces of milk in healthy lactose intolerant teen-agers. Pediatrics 56: 718, 1975.
23. Newcomer, A. D.; McGill, D. B.; Thomas, P. J.; and Hoffman, A. F.: Tolerance to lactose among lactose deficient American Indians. Unpublished manuscript.
24. Bayless, T. M.; Rothfeld, B.; Massa, C.; et al.: Lactose and milk intolerance: clinical implications. N. Engl. J. Med. 292: 1156, 1975.
25. Paige, D. M.; Leonardo, E.; Nakashima, J.; et al.: Response of lactose intolerant children to different lactose levels. Am. J. Clin. Nutr. 25: 467, 1972.
26. Reddy, V., and Pershad, J.: Lactase deficiency in Indians. Am. J. Clin. Nutr. 25: 114, 1972.
27. Stoopler, M.; Frayer, W.; and Alderman, M. H.: Prevalence and persistence of lactose malabsorption among young Jamaican children. Am. J. Clin. Nutr. 27: 728, 1974.
28. Jones, D. V.; Latham, M. C.; Kosikowski, F. V.; and Woodward, G.: Symptom response to lactose-reduced milk in lactose-intolerant adults. Am. J. Clin. Nutr. 29: 633, 1976.
29. Paige, D. M.; Bayless, T. M.; Huang, S. S.; and Wexler, R.: Lactose hydrolyzed milk. Am. J. Clin. Nutr. 28: 818, 1975.
30. Marston, R., and Friend, B.: Nutritional Review, National Food Situation. Publ. NFS-158. Economic Research Service, U.S. Department of Agriculture, November 1976: 25.
31. Calloway, D. H., and Chenoweth, W. L.: Utilization of nutrients in milk and wheat-based diets by men with adequate and reduced abilities to absorb lactose: I. Energy and nitrogen. Am. J. Clin. Nutr. 26: 939, 1973.
32. Leichter, J., and Tolensky, A. F.: Effect of dietary lactose on the absorption of protein, fat, and calcium in the postweaning rat. Am. J. Clin. Nutr. 28: 238, 1975.
33. Bowie, M. D.: Effect of lactose-induced diarrhea on absorption of nitrogen and fat. Arch. Dis. Child. 50: 363, 1975.
34. Bowie, M. D.; Barbezat, G. O.; and Hansen, J. D. L.: Carbohydrate absorption in malnourished children. Am. J. Clin. Nutr. 20: 89, 1967.
35. Kabayashi, A.; Kawai, S.; Ohbe, Y.; and Nagashima, Y.: Effects of dietary lactose and a lactase preparation on the intestinal absorption of calcium and magnesium in normal infants. Am. J. Clin. Nutr. 28: 681, 1975.
36. Cook, G. C., and Al-Torki, M. T.: High intestinal lactase concentrations in adult Arabs in Saudi Arabia. Br. Med. J. 3: 135, 1975.
37. Cook, G. C., and Kajubi, S. K.: Tribal incidence of lactase deficiency in Uganda. Lancet 1: 725, 1966.
38. Kretchmer, N.; Ransome-Kuti, O.; Hurwitz, R.; et al.: Intestinal absorption of lactose in Nigerian ethnic groups. Lancet 2: 392, 1971.
39. Kretchmer, N.: Lactose and lactase. Sci. Am. 227: 71, October 1972.
40. Keusch, G.; Troncale, F. J.; Thavaramara, B.; et al.: Lactase deficiency in Thailand: effect of prolonged lactose feeding. Am. J. Clin. Nutr. 22: 638, 1969.
41. Bowie, M. D.; Brinkman, G. L.; and Hansen, J. D. L.: Acquired disaccharide intolerance in malnutrition. J. Pediatr. 66: 1083, 1965.
42. Prinsloo, J. G.; Wittmann, W.; Pretorius, P. J.; et al.: Effect of different sugars on diarrhea of acute kwashiorkor. Arch. Dis. Child. 44: 593, 1969.
43. Marshall, F. N.; Hilaire, J. A.; and Garnier, M. J.: Personal communications.
44. Mason, J. B.; Hay, R. W.; Leresche, J.; et al.: Treatment of severe malnutrition in relief. Lancet 1: 332, 1974.
45. Mitchell, J. D.; Brand, J.; and Halbisch, J.: Weight-gain inhibition by lactose in Australian Aboriginal children: a controlled trial of normal and lactose hydrolysed milk. Lancet 1: 500, 1977.
46. Harrison, M., and Walker-Smith, J. A.: Reinvestigation of lactose intolerant children: lack of correlation between continuing lactose intolerance and small intestinal morphology, disaccharidase activity and lactose tolerance tests. Gut 18: 48, 1977.

# Sucrose Restricted Diets

*Sucrose free diet*    One that eliminates all known sources of dietary sucrose.

*Sucrose restricted diet*    One that excludes all foods containing more than 2% sucrose and limits the intake of those containing less. In general, the diet provides between 5 and 15 g sucrose daily, depending upon the food choices.

*Characteristics of the diet*    All foods that naturally contain sucrose or to which it has been added in processing are either eliminated or restricted. Cakes, cookies, pastries, and pies prepared with sucrose are prohibited. Glucose, lactose, or preferably fructose are used as substitute sweetening agents. Because of the high sucrose concentration of many fruits and vegetables, only a limited variety is permitted in the diet. In instances when total abstinence from all dietary sucrose is indicated, virtual exclusion of all fruits and vegetables becomes a necessity. Iron, thiamine, and niacin intake may be low.

*Purpose of the diet*    To ameliorate or prevent symptoms of primary or secondary sucrase-isomaltase deficiency [1,2].

In the absence of adequate enzyme activity, isomaltose is not changed to glucose, and sucrose is not changed to glucose and fructose. The osmotic action of the undigested and thus unabsorbed sucrose causes fluid to pour into the intestine of the untreated patient. Abdominal distension, cramps, and increased gastrointestinal motility result. In the colon, the undigested sucrose is fermented by bacteria to short chain fatty acids such as lactic and acetic acids that raise the osmolarity, lower the pH, interfere with the reabsorption of fluid, and have a sour odor [3]. The carbon dioxide and hydrogen produced by this fermentation probably also contribute to the bloating and frothy diarrhea [3]. The disorder appears much like and is often misdiagnosed as celiac disease. Intolerance to isomaltose is less of a problem in these patients than is intolerance to sucrose [1,4,5], although starches that contain appreciable amounts of amylopectin may not be well tolerated by certain patients [6,7]. Starches such as those derived from corn and rice contain mainly amylose and are well tolerated because amylose yields only small amounts of isomaltose upon hydrolysis [6].

*Effects of the diet*    Symptoms of sucrase-isomaltase deficiency disappear within 24 hr after the diet is instituted [1,2]. Substitution of foods high in fructose for those high in sucrose may have a beneficial effect upon sucrase enzyme activity. Specifically, it has been reported that high fructose diets result in small increases in enzyme activity of certain patients with sucrase-isomaltase deficiency [8–10].

*Indications for use*    In congenital or acquired sucrase-isomaltase deficiency. The diet should be prescribed in the presence of a low stool pH (normal is 6.3 or higher [2]) and a flat sucrose tolerance test followed within hours by gastrointestinal symptoms and watery, acid diarrhea [1]. The presumptive diagnosis may be confirmed by analysis of intestinal biopsy specimens that reveal deficient enzyme activity [1].

The diet may also be indicated in any disease that involves damage to the small intestinal mucosa in such a way as to decrease or interfere with the activity of the sucrase-isomaltase enzymes [11]. For example, the disorder has been reported as a postoperative complication in Hirschsprung's disease and severe gastroenteritis.

An enzyme substitute is now available that may augment the effect of sucrose restriction [7]. When taken before major meals, the enzyme glucomylase permits most patients to progress to the more liberal sucrose restricted diet, rather than continuing to rely on total sucrose abstinence.

***Possible adverse reactions***   Continued use of an *unsupplemented* sucrose free diet may provoke deficiencies of ascorbic acid and folic acid, as the diet is inadequate in these nutrients. Iron, thamine, and niacin intakes may also be low.

***Contraindications***   None that have been described among patients with proven sucrase-isomaltase deficiency.

***Suggestions for dietitians***   Except for those individuals in whom it is desirable to achieve weight loss, sucrose derived kilocalories should be replaced by the inclusion in the diet of other sources of carbohydrate.

It has been reported that young infants with the disorder should be placed on a sucrose free diet initially and gradually advanced to one that is sucrose restricted after a week or so [1]. Sucrose containing foods should be added gradually, particularly in patients not receiving an oral enzyme substitute.

A specially prepared infant formula (CHO Free*) is now available, which contains no added carbohydrate and to which glucose or preferably fructose may be added.

When rigid adherence to a sucrose free diet necessitates the omission of all fruits and vegetables, ascorbic acid supplements should be provided. Even when certain fruits and vegetables are permitted, menus must be carefully planned to include each day sources of ascorbic acid and folic acid, such as tomatoes, strawberries, potato, liver, beef, eggs, etc.

Sucrose is now added to many different commercially prepared baby foods, especially pureed fruits. Mothers of sucrose intolerant children should be instructed to read labels carefully so as to seek out less obvious sources of sucrose in the diet. Where appropriate substitutes are not available, it may be necessary to instruct the mother in the homemade preparation of certain blenderized foods suitable for infant feeding.

Symptoms evoked by dietary indiscretions vary depending upon the degree of enzyme deficiency, the amount of ingested sucrose, and the age of the patient. Dietary compliance is particularly important in the young infant: symptoms evoked by dietary noncompliance are more pronounced in infants and younger children than in older children [12].

---

* Syntex Laboratories, Palo Alto, CA 94304.

**Sucrose Free Diet**

| Foods allowed | Foods excluded |
|---|---|

*Beverages*

CHO Free infant formula, milk (whole or skim), evaporated milk, buttermilk, plain yogurt, diet sodas not sweetened with sucrose

*Beverages*

Chocolate milk and drink, condensed milk, flavored yogurt or any made with sweetened fruit, milk shakes, ice cream, sherbet, regularly sweetened carbonated beverages

*Desserts*

Custard and vanilla pudding made with allowed ingredients, without sugar or sucrose containing beverages

*Desserts*

Commercially prepared gelatin desserts sweetened with sucrose; cakes, cookies, pies, pastries, and puddings containing sucrose or wheat germ

*Fats*

Butter, margarine, vegetable oils, sour cream, cream cheese, cream

*Fats*

Mayonnaise, salad dressings, peanut butter

*Fruits*

None

*Fruits*

All

*Meat and meat substitutes*

Beef, pork, lamb, veal, chicken, turkey, and other meats and poultry prepared without the addition of sugar, such as sucrose or corn syrup, etc.; eggs; cream cheese, cottage cheese, other plain cheeses unprocessed; fish

*Meat and meat substitutes*

Frankfurters, cold cuts to which sucrose may be added as a filler, commercially prepared infant meat and vegetable dinners to which sucrose may be added, some processed cheese spreads

*Vegetables*

None

*Vegetables*

All

*Miscellaneous*

Saccharin, sugars, and artificial sweeteners that are free of sucrose, such as Sweet n' Low, Sugar Twin, Sucaryl; pure spices and herbs

*Miscellaneous*

Allspice; cane sugar, molasses, honey; most pickles, catsup, carob powder; almonds, chestnuts, coconut and coconut milk, macadamia nuts, pecans; jams, jellies, preserves made with sucrose, corn syrup, invert sugar

**Sucrose Restricted Diet**

**In Addition to All Foods Permitted on the Sucrose Free Diet, the Following Foods Should Be Added to the Diet:**

*Fruits and fruit juices containing 1% or less sucrose [10,11,13,14]:* gooseberries, loganberries, blackberries, cranberries, currants, lemons, rhubarb, pomegranates

Limit to 3–4 one-half cup servings daily

*Fruits and fruit juices containing more than 1% but less than 2% sucrose:* boysenberries, bing cherries, figs, Tokay or Thompson seedless grapes, guava, lime juice, pears, raspberries, strawberries

Limit to 1 one-half cup serving daily

*Vegetables containing 1% or less sucrose:* snap, string, or green beans; cabbage; cauliflower; celery; corn; eggplant; lettuce; potato (white); pumpkin; radishes; hubbard, butternut, or crookneck squash; tomatoes; tomato juice

Limit to 3–4 one-half cup servings daily

*Grains, cereals, nuts, miscellaneous, etc. containing 1% or less sucrose:* corn meal, puffed rice, whole wheat cereals and crackers, patent wheat flour, rice (brown or white), macaroni, spaghetti, Kraft Mayonnaise, Kraft Salad Bowl Mayonnaise, commercial salad dressings, pecans, honey

As desired

*Source:* Adapted from Sucrase-isomaltase deficiency—a frequently misdiagnosed disease [1].

**Sample Menu**

A.M.

4 oz cranberry juice
1 cup milk
Egg scrambled in fortified margarine
½ cup puffed rice with 2 tsp fructose
Toast with fortified margarine

Noon

Hamburger on a bun with 1 sliced tomato
French fried potatoes
½ cup corn
½ cup fresh strawberries or frozen unsweetened with 1 tsp fructose
1 cup milk
1 tsp fortified margarine

P.M.

3 oz pot roast
½ cup mashed potato
½ cup butternut squash
1 slice bread
2 tsp fortified margarine
1 cup milk
½ cup raw bing cherries

Between meals

Custard made with fructose

**References**

1. Ament, M. E.; Perera, D. R.; and Esther, L. J.: Sucrase-isomaltase deficiency—a frequently misdiagnosed disease. J. Pediatr. 83: 721, 1973.
2. Ament, M. E., and Bill, A. H.: Persistent diarrhea due to sucrase-isomaltase deficiency in a postoperative child with Hirschsprung's disease. J. Pediatr. Surg. 8: 543, 1973.
3. Bayless, T. M.: Disaccharidase deficiency. J. Am. Diet. Assoc. 60: 478, 1972.
4. Newcomer, A. D.: Disaccharidase deficiencies. Mayo Clin. Proc. 48: 648, 1973.
5. Prader, A.: Inborn errors of metabolism. Bibl. Nutr. Dieta. 18: 179, 1973.
6. Lindquist, B., and Meeuwise, G.: Diets in disaccharidase deficiency and defective monosaccharide absorption. J. Am. Diet. Assoc. 48: 307, 1966.
7. Fomon, S. J.: Infant Nutrition. 2d ed. Philadelphia: W. B. Saunders, 1974.
8. Greene, H. L.; Stifel, F. B.; and Herman, R. H.: Dietary stimulation of sucrase in a patient with sucrase-isomaltase deficiency. Lancet 1: 651, 1971.
9. Greene, H. L.; Stifel, F. B.; and Herman, R. H.: Dietary stimulation of sucrase in a patient with sucrase-isomaltase deficiency. Biochem. Med. 6: 409, 1972.
10. Rosensweig, N. S.: Diet and intestinal enzyme adaptation. Am. J. Clin. Nutr. 28: 648, 1975.
11. Herber, R.: Disaccharidase deficiency in health and disease. Calif. Med. 116: 23, 1972.
12. Cornblath, M., and Schwartz, R.: Disorders of Carbohydrate Metabolism in Infancy. 2d ed. 3. Major Problems in Clinical Pediatrics. Philadelphia: W. B. Saunders, 1976.
13. Hardinge, M. G.; Swarner, J. B.; and Crooks, H.: Carbohydrates in foods. J. Am. Diet. Assoc. 46: 197, 1965.
14. Eheart, J. F., and Mason, B. S.: Sugar and acid in the edible portion of fruits. J. Am. Diet. Assoc. 50: 130, 1967.

PART E          Modifications in Fat Content

# Fat Restricted Diet

***Moderately fat restricted diet*** One that limits all types of fat ingested, regardless of the source, to less than 25% of total kilocalories [1].

***Severely fat restricted diet*** One that limits all types of fat ingested, regardless of the source, to less than 10%–15% of the total kilocalories [1].

***Mildly fat restricted diet*** One that limits all types of fat ingested, regardless of the source, to less than 35%–40% of the total kilocalories [1].

***Characteristics of the diet*** All forms of fat are restricted; no attempt is made to differentiate among various forms.

***Purpose of the diet*** The amelioration of symptoms of steatorrhea in disorders in which the hydrolysis, absorption, and transport of fat is abnormal.

***Indications for use*** *In chronic pancreatitis* As an adjunct to enzyme replacement in controlling pancreatic steatorrhea and its accompanying fat and fat soluble vitamin losses. Pancreatic enzyme replacement remains the primary treatment for steatorrhea associated with chronic pancreatitis; however, alterations in dietary fat intake may bring additional benefit [2]. In order to promote weight gain and maximum nutrient intake, the patient should be given the greatest amount of fat that he can tolerate without an increase in steatorrhea or pain [3,4]. Fat intake should be reduced to 50 g/day or less and gradually increased until the patient reaches the limit of his level of tolerance [2]. Substitution of medium chain triglycerides for a portion of the long chain triglycerides may bring further improvement in fat absorption [2,5].

*In other disorders involving fat malabsorption* Fat malabsorption may occur as a complication of cirrhosis [6,7], intestinal bypass surgery [8,9], gastrectomy [9], and the short gut syndrome [10]. Treatment of the short gut syndrome has been categorized into three stages, the first two of which involve very rigid fat restrictions [9]. In many of these patients, the steatorrhea in response to fat ingestion diminishes markedly after 4 to 12 months [9]. Finally, in instances in which substitution of medium chain trigylcerides for a portion of the long chain triglycerides in the diet is either contraindicated or proven to be of no value, restricting the total amount of fat may be the only dietary alternative. In some patients, steatorrhea occurs subsequent to bypass surgery and massive ileal resections that contribute to oxalate renal stone formation. A low fat, low oxalate diet is helpful in these instances [11].

*In gallbladder disease* A fat restricted diet is believed by some physicians to be of benefit in the symptomatic patient with gallbladder disease [12–15]. The purpose of the diet is to prevent biliary colic by lessening fat-induced gall bladder contractions [14]. In these instances, moderate restriction of dietary fat to 25% of total kilocalories [1] or 45–75 g/day [13] is usually deemed sufficient. *Note:* The rationale for the use of drastic fat reductions in gallbladder disease has been questioned [16,17]. Although fatty acids stimulate the gallbladder to contract by liberating cholecystokinin, amino acids have the same effect [16]. In addition, the hypothesis that symptoms of cholecystitis are precipitated by the ingestion of fatty foods may be invalid [17]. It has been suggested that patients with gallbladder disease were no less tolerant of fried foods than normal persons [18].

At the present time, surgery and not medical treatment is the therapy of choice for gallstones [16]. Preliminary studies using chenodeoxycholic acid to dissolve gallstones have been encouraging [19–21]. In addition, there is little reason in the postoperative period to restrict the patient's fat intake in any way [22].

***Diagnostic clues to the need for fat restriction***     Positive results from a Sudan stain of stool for fat and a serum carotene level of less than 60 ug/100 ml are suggestive of fat malabsorption [9]. The fecal excretion of more than 5–6 g fat per 24 hours over a 3-day period in patients receiving a diet containing 100 g dietary fat daily is considered to be evidence of fat malabsorption in most laboratories [9,23]. A description including cost effectiveness of a number of different tests for malabsorption has been published elsewhere [24].

***Possible adverse reactions***     Providing kilocalories are adequate, and adequate fat is included to preclude essential fatty acid deficiency, none.

***Contraindications***     Restriction of fat in certain liver diseases such as uncomplicated hepatitis has been found to be based on fallacious assumptions [25–27].

***Suggestions for dietitians***     When a severely fat restricted diet is indicated, the diet may be modified to approximately 20 g by eliminating the fat choices.

Fat Restricted Diet

| **Foods allowed** | **Foods excluded** |
|---|---|
| *Beverages* | *Beverages* |
| Skim milk or buttermilk made with skim milk, coffee, tea, Postum, fruit juice, soft drinks, cocoa made with cocoa powder and skim milk | Whole milk, buttermilk made with whole milk, chocolate milk, cream in excess of amounts allowed under fats |
| *Bread and cereal products* | *Bread and cereal products* |
| Plain, nonfat cereals, spaghetti, noodles, rice, macaroni; plain whole grain or enriched bread | Biscuits, breads, egg or cheese bread, sweet rolls made with fat, pancakes, doughnuts, waffles, fritters, popcorn prepared with fat, muffins, natural cereals and breads to which extra fat is added. |
| *Cheese* | *Cheese* |
| Cottage, ¼ cup to be used as substitute for an ounce of cheese, or specially processed American cheese containing less than 5% butterfat | Whole milk cheeses |

| **Foods allowed** | **Foods excluded** |
|---|---|
| *Desserts* | *Desserts* |
| Sherbet made with skim milk; fruit ice; gelatin; rice, bread, cornstarch, tapioca, or Junket pudding made with skim milk; fruit whips with gelatin, sugar, and egg white; fruit; angel food cake; meringues | Cake, pie, pastry, ice cream, or any dessert containing shortening, chocolate, or fats of any kind, unless especially prepared using part of fat allowance |
| *Eggs* | *Eggs* |
| 3 per week prepared only with fat from fat allowance; egg whites as desired; low fat egg substitutes | More than 1/day unless substituted for part of the meat allowed |
| *Fats* | *Fats* |
| Choose up to the limit allowed on diet among the following (1 serving in the amount listed equals 1 fat choice):<br>1 tsp butter or fortified margarine<br>1 tsp shortening or oil<br>1 tsp mayonnaise<br>1 tbsp Italian or French dressing<br>1 strip crisp bacon<br>⅛ avocado (4'' diameter)<br>2 tbsp light cream<br>1 tbsp heavy cream<br>6 small nuts<br>5 small olives | Any in excess of amount prescribed on diet; all others |
| *Fruits* | *Fruits* |
| As desired | Avocado in excess of amount allowed on fat list |
| *Lean meat, fish, poultry* | *Meat, fish, poultry* |
| Choose up to the limit allowed on diet among the following: poultry without skin, fish, veal (all cuts), liver, lean beef, pork, and lamb, with all visible fat removed—1 oz cooked weight equals 1 equivalent; ¼ cup water packed tuna or salmon equals 1 equivalent | Fried or fatty meats, sausage, scrapple, frankfurters, poultry skins, stewing hens, spareribs, salt pork, beef unless lean, duck, goose, ham hocks, pig's feet, luncheon meats, gravies unless fat free, tuna and salmon packed in oil, peanut butter |
| *Milk* | *Milk* |
| Skim, buttermilk or yogurt made from skim milk | Whole, chocolate, buttermilk made with whole milk |
| *Seasonings* | *Seasonings* |
| As desired | None |
| *Soups* | *Soups* |
| Bouillon, clear broth, fat free vegetable soup, cream soup made with skimmed milk, packaged dehydrated soups | All others |
| *Sweets* | *Sweets* |
| Jelly, jam, marmalade, honey, syrup, molasses, sugar, hard sugar candies, fondant, gumdrops, jelly beans, marshmallows | Any candy made with chocolate, nuts, butter, cream, or fat of any kind |
| *Vegetables* | *Vegetables* |
| All plainly prepared vegetables | Potato chips; buttered, au gratin, creamed, or fried vegetables unless made with allowed fat; commercially frozen vegetables, casseroles, or frozen vegetables in butter sauce |

**Daily Food Allowances for 50 g Fat Diet**

| Food | Amount | Approximate fat content (g) |
|---|---|---|
| Skim milk | 2 cups or more | 0 |
| Lean meat, fish, poultry | 6 oz | 18 |
| Whole egg or egg yolks | 3 per week | 3 |
| Vegetables | 3 servings or more, at least 1 or more dark green or deep yellow | 0 |
| Fruits | 3 or more servings, at least 1 citrus | 0 |
| Breads, cereals | As desired | 0 |
| Fat exchanges* | 5–6 exchanges daily | 25–30 |
| Desserts and sweets | As desired from permitted list | 0 |
| | Total fat | 46–51 |

**Sample Menu**

A.M.

Stewed apricots
Cornflakes with skim milk and sugar
1 poached egg
2 slices whole wheat toast with 2 tsp fortified margarine
Coffee with skim milk and sugar

Noon

Sandwich with lettuce and 3 oz sliced chicken and 1 tsp fortified margarine
Celery sticks and green pepper rings
Angel cake with sliced peaches
Coffee with skim milk and sugar
1 cup skim milk

P.M.

Fresh fruit cup
3 oz broiled round steak
1 baked potato
Carrots
Romaine, spinach, and cherry tomato salad
2 plain rolls with 2 tsp fortified margarine
1 banana
1 cup skim milk
Coffee with skim milk and sugar

Between meals

1 serving sherbet
Skim milk or juice

* See exchange lists, p. F25.

References

1. Council on Foods and Nutrition: The regulation of dietary fat. JAMA 181: 139, 1962.
2. Taubin, H. L., and Spiro, H. M.: Nutritional aspects of chronic pancreatitis. Am. J. Clin. Nutr. 26: 367, 1973.
3. Losowsky, M. S.; Walker, B. E.; and Kelleher, J.: Malabsorption in Clinical Practice. Edinburgh: Livingstone Churchill, 1974.
4. Iber, F. L.: Treatment of pancreatic insufficiency. Johns Hopkins Med. J. 122: 172, 1968.
5. Katka, E. C., and Kalser, M. H.: Pancreatic disease. Postgrad. Med. 57: 140, January 1975.
6. Gabuzda, G. J.: Nutrition and liver disease. Med. Clin. N. Am. 54: 6, 1970.

7. Linscheer, W. G.: Malabsorption in cirrhosis. Am. J. Clin. Nutr. 23: 488, 1970.
8. Swenson, S. A., and Oberst, B.: Pre- and postoperative care of the patient with intestinal bypass for obesity. Am. J. Surg. 129: 224, 1975.
9. Wright, H. K. and Tilson, M. D.: Postoperative Disorders of the Gastrointestinal Tract. New York: Grune & Stratton, 1973.
10. Andersson, H.: Treatment of steatorrhea with fat-reduced diet in small bowel disease. Bibl. Nutr. Dieta 19: 64, 1973.
11. Stauffer, J. Q.: Hyperoxaluria and calcium oxalate nephrolithiasis after jejunoileal bypass. Am. J. Clin. Nutr. 30: 64, 1977.
12. Morrissey, K., and Eisenmenger, W.: Medical aspects of diseases of the gallbladder and biliary tree. Am. J. Med. 51: 642, 1971.
13. Robins, R. E., and Trueman, G. E.: The gallbladder and extra-hepatic bile ducts. Boguch, A. ed. Gastroenterology. New York: McGraw-Hill, 1973.
14. Snodgrass, P., and Abbruzzese, A.: Diseases of the gallbladder and bile ducts. Wintrobe, M. M.; Thorn, G. W.; Adams, R. D.; Braunwald, E.; Isselbacker, K. J.; and Petersdorf, R. D., eds. Harrison's Principles of Internal Medicine. 7th ed. New York: McGraw-Hill, 1974.
15. Gray, R.: Disappearing gallstones: report of 2 cases. Br. J. Surg. 61: 101, 1974.
16. Williams, C. N.: Diet and diseases of the gastrointestinal tract. N.S. Med. Bull. 52: 211, 1973.
17. Manier, J. W.: Diet and cholelithiasis. Halpern, S.; Lukby, A. L.; and Berensen, G. eds. Nutrition and Metabolism in Medical Practice. New York: Futura, 1973.
18. Price, W. H.; Gallbladder dyspepsia. Br. Med. J. 2: 138, 1963.
19. Bell, G. D.; Mok, H. Y. I.; Thwe, M.; Murphy, G. M.; Henry, K.; and Dowling, R. H.: Liver structure and function in cholelithiasis; effect of chenodeoxycholic acid. Gut 15: 165, 1974.
20. Mok, H. Y. I.; Bell, G. D.; and Dowling, R. H.: Effect of different doses of chenodeoxycholic acid on bile-lipid composition and on frequency of side-effects in patients with gallstones. Lancet 2: 253, 1974.
21. Lahana, D. A., and Schoenfield, L. J.: Progress in medical therapy of gallstones. Surg. Clin. N. Am. 53: 1053, 1973.
22. Spiro, H. M.: Clinical Gastroenterology. New York: Macmillan, 1970.
23. Westergaard, H., and Dietscht, J. M.: Normal mechanisms of fat absorption and derangements induced by various gastrointestinal diseases. Med. Clin. N. Am. 58: 1513, 1974.
24. Steinberg, W. M., and Toskes, P. P.: A practical approach to evaluating maldigestion and malabsorption. Geriatrics 2: 73, 1978.
25. Crews, R. H., and Faloon, W. W.: The fallacy of a low fat diet in liver disease. JAMA 181: 754, 1962.
26. Sherlock, S.: Progress report. Chronic hepatitis. Gut 15: 581, 1974.
27. Davidson, C.: Diseases of the liver. Goodhart, R. S., and Shils, M. E., eds. Modern Nutrition in Health and Disease. Philadelphia: Lea & Febiger, 1973.

# Fat Controlled Diet: Cholesterol and Fat Restricted, Increased Polyunsaturated Fat, and Decreased Saturated Fat Content

*Definition*     A diet in which both the amount and the type of fat are limited to a prescribed level, or one that is designed to provide a certain percentage of fat derived kilocalories or certain percentages or ratios of fatty acids [1,2]. Fat controlled diets developed by the American Heart Association provide a maximum of 300 mg cholesterol daily, 35% of the kilocalories in the form of fat, a maximum of 10% of the kilocalories in the form of saturated fats, and 10% of the kilocalories in the form of polyunsaturated fats [2,3].

*Characteristics of the diet*     Beef, lamb, and pork are restricted to three 3 oz portions/week, and only skim milk and lean meats may be used. No more than 3 egg yolks/week are permitted; liver may be used, but only as a substitute for eggs. Shellfish, except shrimp, are allowed in accordance with 1972 data on cholesterol content of foods published by the U.S. Department of Agriculture [4]. Butter, cream, and whole milk cheeses are excluded in favor of skim milk cheeses and special margarines that contain adequate amounts of polyunsaturated liquid vegetable oils. Oils such as safflower, corn, soy, or cottonseed are the main vehicles by which the polyunsaturated fat in the diet is increased; commercial mayonnaise and French dressings that contain a certain amount of these oils may also be used to a limited degree [2,5].

*Purpose of the diet*     The American Heart Association fat controlled diets are designed to lower elevated levels of serum cholesterol and other lipids in an effort to reduce the risk of heart disease [2–14]. The most effective nutritional mechanisms for lowering elevated levels combine decreases in saturated fat and dietary cholesterol intake with increased intakes of polyunsaturated fat [6–10,14]. Critical limits of dietary fat composition for effective serum cholesterol reduction have been established [7]. Claims have been made that the serum cholesterol lowering effects of decreased dietary cholesterol intake and increased polyunsaturated fat intake may be independent of each other [15]. However, the specific manner in which increased polyunsaturated fats reduce serum cholesterol has yet to be elucidated [16]. In the obese individual, reduction of serum cholesterol is also dependent upon the normalization of body weight [8].

*Effects of the diet*     Significant and sustained reductions in serum cholesterol and plasma lipids have been demonstrated in persons adhering to the diet. Low density lipoprotein (LDL) serum cholesterol levels are decreased. High density lipoprotein (HDL) serum cholesterol levels are not decreased nor adversely affected by the diet but may actually be increased [17]. The extent of the reductions varies somewhat with the condition of the dietary intervention; average decreases of serum cholesterol of approximately 9.6% [11], 9.2%

to 11.4% [18], and 13% [19] are among those that have been reported. Maintenance of reduced serum cholesterol levels is difficult to achieve without vigorous long-term counseling.

The diet produces changes in adipose tissue; the proportion of polyunsaturated fatty acids is increased at the expense of saturated fatty acids [11].

Although encouraging reports have been published [20–22], particularly for young survivors of acute myocardial infarctions [21], final assessment of the effect of the diet in reducing the actual incidence and complications of heart disease must await the results of long-term dietary intervention trials in free living populations [23].

Changes in lactate dehydrogenase, lactate dehydrogenase isoenzymes, lactate, and pyruvate have been demonstrated as a result of feeding low fat diets to healthy men and women [24]. An increase in glycolytic activity occurred as a consequence of increased carbohydrate intake, particularly on a diet providing 25% of the kilocalories in the form of fat. Results are suggestive of a dynamic change in carbohydrate metabolism on such a diet [24].

Changes in platelets have been noted in healthy volunteers fed large meals of unsaturated fats, which warrant further study to explore their possible relevance to diets high in polyunsaturated fats. Antithrombin activity was observed to increase and heparin clotting time was prolonged after feeding large meals of unsaturated fats, as opposed to saturated fats [25].

*Indications for use*    To lower serum cholesterol levels in those persons who exhibit elevated levels and who are otherwise at risk of developing heart disease.

*Possible adverse reactions*    One study has reported an increase in serum urate in patients while on the diet [11]. Further research is needed to confirm that this effect was really attributable to the diet.

Adherence to the diet requires substitution of polyunsaturated fats and some carbohydrates for saturated fats, and, frequently, higher carbohydrate intakes are the result. Although not a consistent finding, increases in carbohydrate intake from mono- and disaccharides may provoke concomitant rises in serum triglyceride levels in some individuals [10,26–28].

It has been suggested that there is an increased incidence of gallstones occurring in patients as a consequence of the increased polyunsaturated fat intake of fat controlled diets [29], although others have disputed this finding [30]. At the present time, however, the risk of heart disease far outweighs such a *possible* adverse reaction of the diet [31].

The long-term effects of the diet when initiated in early childhood are not known, and its use is controversial [32]. Infants fed skim milk formulas from birth have frequently been noted to develop less lean body mass than infants fed traditional formulas from birth [33]. Some investigators have claimed that dietary manipulations resulting in decreased cholesterol and saturated fat intakes may be detrimental in early life; dietary cholesterol may be essential for the myelination of the brain as well as for the regulation of cholesterol metabolism later in life [32,34]. On the other hand, one study of children from birth until the age of 3 has reported no ill effects in children fed a low saturated fat, low cholesterol diet since birth [35]. Furthermore, children with the very low plasma cholesterol levels of familial lipoproteinenemia show normal neurologic development [36]. At present, the prudent course seems to be to identify and treat the 5–7% of the young children in the United States genetically predisposed to atherosclerosis [37]. The American Heart Association has taken the following position [36]: "that children with elevated plasma cholesterol or triglyceride levels should be placed on an appropriate diet and . . . although the evidence does not yet support the recommendation that cholesterol and saturated fat should be reduced in the diets of all children, the public should be advised that such modifications appear to be safe."

*Contraindications*    Unless modified to provide for a decreased carbohydrate intake [38], the diet may be contraindicated in type IV hyperlipidemia or hypertriglyceridemia [39]. Whenever possible, it is advisable to determine the levels of all serum lipoproteins in persons with hyperlipidemia, so that nutritional management may be tailored to the specific lipoprotein abnormality [38].

*Suggestions for dietitians*    Acceptable margarines and solid shortenings should contain at least 25% linoleic acid and no more than 25% saturated fatty acids [40, 41], or a P/S (polyunsaturated to saturated fat) value of 1.0 to 1.5 or greater [42] and preferentially 2.0 or more. The nutrient composition of the American Heart Association Fat Controlled Diet Meal Plans, as well as other background information [2,5], may be helpful to the dietitian in adjusting the diet to suit the patient's needs. Compliance with the principles of the diet may involve drastic changes in dietary habits. However, there are now several fat controlled cookbooks available with recipes that in many instances are as tasty as, or even preferable to, others that contain large amounts of saturated fat [43–46].

### Fatty Acid Composition of Commercial and Salad Oils (g per 100 g)

| Oil | Saturated fatty acids | Mono-unsaturated fatty acids | Poly-unsaturated fatty acids |
|---|---|---|---|
| **Salad oil** | | | |
| Corn | 13 | 25 | 58 |
| Cottonseed | 26 | 19 | 51 |
| Olive | 14 | 72 | 9 |
| Peanut | 19 | 46 | 30 |
| Safflower | 9 | 12 | 74 |
| Soybean, unhyd.* | 15 | 23 | 58 |
| Soybean, hyd.† | 13 | 47 | 40 |
| Sunflower | 10 | 21 | 64 |
| Blend, 10% cottonseed, 90% soybean | 16 | 23 | 57 |
| Sesame | 15 | 40 | 40 |
| Walnut | 11 | 15 | 66 |
| Wheat germ | 17 | 16 | 61 |
| **Commercial oil** | | | |
| Coconut | 86 | 6 | 2 |
| Palm | 48 | 38 | 9 |
| Palm kernel | 81 | 11 | 1 |
| Vegetable P/S>1 | 15 | 47 | 34 |
| Blend, 50% cottonseed, 50% hyd. soya | 20 | 33 | 45 |

(From Nutrition Coding Center, University of Minnesota: Food Table Information Listing Fat and Fatty Acid Fields. Minneapolis, MN, Dec. 1976).
* Unhyd. = unhydrogenated.
† hyd. = partially hydrogenated, specially processed.

### Composition of Fat Controlled Diets Recommended by the American Heart Association

| Nutrient and dietary pattern | Preventive diet* | Therapeutic diets | | | |
|---|---|---|---|---|---|
| | | 1,200 kcal | 1,800 kcal | 2,000–2,200 kcal | 2,400–2,600 kcal |
| **Nutrients** | | | | | |
| Carbohydrate (g) | 273 | 120 | 200 | 270 | 335 |
| Protein (g) | 114 | 75 | 85 | 95 | 110 |
| Fat (g) | 83 | 42 | 68 | 70 | 84 |
| Saturated fatty acids (g) | 18 | 7 | 10 | 11 | 12 |
| Linoleic acid (g) | 26 | 14 | 26 | 26 | 33 |
| Cholesterol (mg) | 356 | 258 | 258 | 279 | 286 |
| Iron (mg) | 21.6 | 12 | 14 | 17 | 19 |
| **Dietary patterns** | | | | | |
| % kcal from carbohydrate | 47 | 41 | 45 | 51 | 52 |
| % kcal from protein | 20 | 26 | 20 | 18 | 17 |
| % kcal from fat | 33 | 32 | 35 | 30 | 30 |
| % kcal from saturated fatty acids | 7 | 5 | 5 | 4 | 4 |
| % kcal from linoleic acid | 10 | 10 | 13 | 11 | 11 |
| P:S ratio† | 1.4:1 | 2:1 | 2.6:1 | 2.4:1 | 2.8:1 |

*Source*: Adapted from A dietary approach to coronary artery disease [48].
* 2,300 kcal.
† Ratio of linoleic acid to saturated fatty acids.

**Approximate Nutrient Composition of Food Groups for Fat-Controlled and Hyperlipoproteinemia Diets**

| Food group | Amount | Weight (g) | Protein (g) | Total fat (g) | Saturated fatty acids (g) | Linoleic fatty acid (g) | Cholesterol* (mg) | Carbohydrate (g) |
|---|---|---|---|---|---|---|---|---|
| Milk, skim | ½ pt (8 oz) | 240 | 8 | tr. | 0 | 0 | 5 | 12 |
| Vegetables | ½ cup | 100 | 2 | 0 | 0 | 0 | 0 | 5 |
| Fruit, unsweetened | varies | 0 | 0 | 0 | 0 | 0 | 0 | 10 |
| Bread and cereal | varies | 0 | 2 | 0 | 0 | 0 | 0 | 15 |
| Meat, fish, poultry, lean (weighted average)† | 1 oz | 30 | 8 | 2 | 0.6 | 0.1 | 21 | 0 |
| Meat, lean only | 1 oz | 30 | 8 | 3 | 0.6 | 0.1 | 21 | 0 |
| Egg (3/week) | 3/7 | 21 | 3 | 3 | 0.9 | 0.2 | 108 | 0 |
| Fat | | | | | | | | |
|   Vegetable oil‡ | 1 tbsp | 14 | 0 | 14 | 2.0 | 8.0 | 0 | 0 |
|   Margarine, soft§ | 1 tbsp | 14 | 0 | 11 | 2.0 | 4.0 | 0 | 0 |
| Sugar and desserts | varies | 0 | 0 | 0 | 0 | 0 | 0 | 12 |

*Source*:  Adapted from Nutrition in Health and Disease [49].
* Feeley [50].
† Weighted average assumes weekly consumption to be: beef, lamb, pork, ham—3 servings; poultry, veal—2 servings; fish—5 servings.
‡ Corn, cottonseed, safflower, soybean oils.
§ Nutrition Label, Chiffon Margarine, 1973.

**Foods allowed**

**Foods excluded**

*Breads and cereals*

*Breads and cereals*

One serving contains 2 g protein, 15 g carbohydrate, and 70 kcal.
See exchange lists, pp. F22–F23, for complete list

Commercial biscuits, muffins, corn-breads, waffles, griddle cakes, cookies, popovers, crackers; mixes for biscuits, muffins, and cakes; coffee cakes; cakes (except angel food and those made from low fat recipes); pies; sweet rolls; pastries; potato chips; French fried potatoes; spoon bread, cereals containing saturated fat or coconut

*Desserts, sugars, and sweets*

*Desserts, sugars, and sweets*

One serving contains about 12 g carbohydrate and 50 kcal
1 tbsp each of the following:
White, brown, or maple sugar; corn syrup or maple syrup; honey; molasses; jelly, jam, or marmalade

Desserts
(all desserts except sugar cookies are fat free):

¼ cup tapioca or cornstarch pudding made with fruit and fruit juice or with skim milk
¼ cup fruit whip, such as prune or apricot, made from egg whites, no cream
⅓ cup gelatin dessert
¼ cup sherbet, preferably water ice
⅓ cup sweetened canned or frozen fruit (equals 1 portion fruit plus 1 tbsp sugar)
1 small slice angel food cake
2 sugar cookies
3 nut meringues
¾ cup (6 oz) carbonated beverage
⅔ cup cocoa (not chocolate) made with skim milk from allowance
Candies—3 medium or 14 small gum drops; 3 marshmallows; 4 hard fruit drops; or 2 mint patties without chocolate

Puddings, custards, and ice creams unless made with skim milk or nonfat dry milk; whipped cream desserts; cookies unless made with allowed fat or oil or egg; candies made with chocolate, butter, cream, or coconut

If kilocalories are not restricted and if these items are allowed, skim milk, fat, and eggs are used in the preparation of sugar cookies, chiffon cake, quick yellow cake, white cake, and fruit pies

*Eggs*

*Eggs*

One serving 3 times a week or 3/7 egg contains 3 g protein, 3 g fat, 108 mg cholesterol, 0.9 g saturated fatty acids, 0.2 g linoleic acid, and 35 kcal

Two ounces of the following may be substituted for one egg: shrimp, liver, sweetbreads

Any shrimp, liver, sweetbreads in excess of that allowed

Egg whites as desired

| Foods allowed | Foods excluded |
|---|---|
| *Fats* | *Fats* |
| One serving or 1 tbsp contains 14 g fat, 2 g saturated fatty acid, 8 g linoleic acid, and 125 kcal* | |
| 50% polyunsaturated: corn oil; cottonseed oil; safflower oil; sesame seed oil; soybean oil; sunflower oil; mayonnaise made with any oils listed above (1 tsp mayonnaise equals 1 tsp oil); French dressing made with allowed oil (1½ tbsp dressing equals 1 tbsp oil); special soft margarines†; olive oil—P/S value of 0.6—use on a very limited basis only | Butter, ordinary margarines, ordinary solid shortenings, lard, salt pork, chicken fat, coconut oil |
| *Fruit* | *Fruit* |
| One serving contains 10 g carbohydrate and 40 kcal | |
| See exchange lists, pp. F21–F22, for complete list. | Avocado, olives |
| *Meat, fish, poultry, etc.* | *Meat, fish, poultry, etc.* |
| One serving or 1 oz contains 8 g protein, 2 g fat, 0.6 g saturated fat, 1 g linoleic acid, 21 mg cholesterol, and 75 kcal‡ | |
| Make selections from this group for 11 of the 14 meals: poultry without skin—chicken, turkey, Cornish hens, squab; fish—any kind except shrimp§; veal—any lean cut; cottage cheese—preferably uncreamed; sapsago cheese—ricotta from skim; mozzarella cheese—made from skim milk; specially prepared cheese high in polyunsaturated fat; dried beans or peas; peanut butter; nuts, especially walnuts | Skin of chicken or turkey; duck or goose; fish roe; caviar; fish canned in olive oil; shrimp other than that used as an egg substitute; cheese made from whole milk or cream, pasteurized process cheese, cheese foods and mixed dishes prepared with them, American, bleu, Roquefort, Camembert, cheddar, Edam, Gouda, Neufchâtel, Parmesan, full cream ricotta, Swiss, full cream mozzarella; beef high in fat or marbled; lamb high in fat; pork high in fat content, bacon, salt pork, spareribs, frankfurters, sausage, cold cuts; canned meats and meat mixtures; stew, hash; organ meats such as kidney, brain; liver, sweetbreads, and heart other than that being used as a substitute for an egg; any visible fat on meat; commercially fried meats, chicken, or fish; frozen or packaged casseroles or dinners |
| Make selections from this group for 3 of the 14 main meals: | |
| Beef: hamburger—ground or chuck; roasts, pot roasts, stew meats, sirloin tip, round rump, chuck, arm; steaks—flank, sirloin, T-bone, porterhouse, tenderloin, round, cube; soup meats—shank or loin; other—dried chipped beef | |
| Lamb: roast or steak-leg; chops, loin, rib, shoulder | |
| Pork: roast—loin, center cut ham; chops, loin; tenderloin | |
| Ham: baked, center cut steaks, picnic, butt, Canadian bacon | |
| Liver, sweetbreads, heart (may only be used as a substitute for an egg, e.g., 2 oz liver, sweetbreads, or heart may be used in place of one egg) | |

\* For NIH diets 1–5, 1 serving = 1 tsp oil or 4.6 g; also include the following on diets 2, 3, 4, and 5 as 1 serving each: 1 tbsp commercial salad dressing containing no sour cream, avocado (1/8 of 4″), nuts (except coconut, cashews, macadamia nuts), 5 small olives, 2 tsp peanut butter.

† Approximately 11 g fat, 2 g saturated fat, 4 g linoleic acid, and 100 kcal per serving.

‡ If number of servings of beef, lamb, and pork is not restricted, calculate as 8 g protein, 3 g fat, per ounce.

§ Shrimp (2 oz) may be substituted for 1 egg.

| **Foods allowed** | **Foods excluded** |
|---|---|
| *Milk* | *Milk* |
| One serving contains 8 g protein, 12 g carbohydrate, 5 mg cholesterol, and 80 kcal | |
| 1 cup skim milk, ¼ cup nonfat dried milk <br> 1 cup buttermilk (made from skim milk) <br> ½ cup yogurt (made from skim milk) | Whole milk, canned whole milk, cream, powdered cream, sweet cream, commercial ice cream, sour cream, whole milk buttermilk and whole milk yogurt, cheese made from whole milk, chocolate drinks, eggnog, malted milk |
| *Vegetables* | *Vegetables* |
| One serving contains 2 g protein, 5 g carbohydrate, and 25 kcal | |
| See exchange lists, p. F21, for complete list. | Vegetables packaged with butter or cream sauces |
| *Miscellaneous* | *Miscellaneous* |
| Coffee, coffee substitutes, tea, unsweetened carbonated beverages, artificial sweeteners, unsweetened gelatin, lemons and lemon juice, fat free consommé and bouillon, pickles, relishes, catsup, vinegar, prepared mustard, herbs, spices, commercial egg substitutes | Coconut, chocolate, macadamia nuts, sauces and gravies unless made with allowed fat or oil or made with skimmed milk, cream soups, creamed dishes (unless prepared with skim milk and allowed oil), foods containing egg yolk except from day's allowance, commercial popcorn, substitutes for coffee cream |

*Sources:*  Adapted from Planning Fat Controlled Meals for Approximately 2000–2600 Calories, Revised, 1967 [41]; Nutrition in Health and Disease [49]; The Dietary Management of Hyperlipoproteinemia: A Handbook for Physicians and Dietitians [51].

## Fat Controlled Diet

**Sample Menu for 1,800 Kcal Diet**

A.M.

1 half grapefruit
3/4 cup dry cereal
1 cup skim milk
1 soft-cooked egg (optional)
1 slice toast
1 tsp special margarine
1 tsp marmalade
2 tsp sugar for cereal, fruit, or beverage
Coffee or tea

Noon

Tomato stuffed with chicken salad (use 1 tomato; ½ cup diced chicken; 2 tbsp mayonnaise; capers; parsley; celery; lettuce)
1 large hard roll
1 tsp special margarine
1 cup skim milk
1 small banana
Coffee or tea

P.M.

Baked fish fillet (4 oz)
   (use 1 tsp oil and ¼ cup bread crumbs)
Broccoli with 1½ tsp special Hollandaise sauce*
Scalloped tomatoes (use ½ cup canned tomatoes; 1 slice diced bread; 1 tsp oil; salt; pepper; basil)
1 slice brown bread
1 tsp special margarine
1 canned pear, sweetened, with syrup
Coffee or tea

*Source:*  Adapted from Planning Fat Controlled Meals for 1200 and 1800 Calories, 1966 [40].
* Use recipe given in source.

**References**

1. Turner, D.: Handbook of Diet Therapy. 5th ed. Chicago: University of Chicago Press, 1970.
2. Zukel, M. C.: Revising booklets on fat-controlled meals. J. Am. Diet. Assoc. 54: 20, 1969.
3. Nutrition Committee of the Steering Committee for Medical and Community Programs: Diet and Coronary Heart Disease. American Heart Association, 1978.
4. Seeley, R. M.; Crinear, P. E.; and Watt, B. K.: Cholesterol content of foods. J. Am. Diet. Assoc. 61: 134, 1972.
5. Zukel, M. C.: Appraising and revising educational health materials. J. Am. Diet. Assoc. 54: 25, 1969.
6. Council on Foods and Nutrition: The regulation of dietary fat. JAMA 181: 139, 1962.
7. Brown, H. B., and Farrand, M. E.: Pitfalls in constructing a fat-controlled diet. J. Am. Diet. Assoc. 49: 303, 1966.
8. Bortz, W. M.: The pathogenesis of hypercholesterolemia. Ann. Intern. Med. 80: 738, 1974.
9. Nestel, P. J.; Havenstein, Y. H.; Scott, T. W.; and Cook, L. J.: Increased sterol excretion with polyunsaturated fat-high cholesterol diets. Metabolism 24: 189, 1975.
10. Dietschy, J. M.: Biosynthesis and metabolism of cholesterol. Halpern, S.; Lukby, A. L.; and Berensen, G. eds. Nutrition and Metabolism in Medical Practice. New York: Futura, 1973.
11. Wilson, W. S.; Hulley, S. B.; Burrows, M. I.; and Nichaman, M. Z.: Serial lipid and lipoprotein responses to the American Heart Association fat controlled diet. Am. J. Med. 51: 491, 1971.
12. North, A. F.: Should pediatricians be concerned about children's cholesterol levels? Clin. Pediatr. 14: 439, 1975.
13. Brown, H. B.: The national diet—heart study: implications for dietitians and nutritionists. J. Am. Diet. Assoc. 52: 279, 1968.
14. Whyte, H. M., and Havenstein, N.: A perspective view of dieting to lower the blood cholesterol. Am. J. Clin. Nutr. 29: 784, 1976.
15. Anderson, J. T., and Grande, F.: Independence of the effects of cholesterol and degree of saturation of the fat in the diet on serum cholesterol in man. Am. J. Clin. Nutr. 29: 1184, 1976.
16. Myant, N. B.: The influence of some dietary factors on cholesterol metabolism. Proc. Nutr. Soc. 34: 271, 1975.
17. Hulley, S.; Cohen, R.; and Widdowson, G.: Plasma high density lipoprotein cholesterol level. Influence of risk factor intervention. JAMA 238: 2269, 1977.
18. Remmell, P. S.; Casey, M. P.; McGandy, R. B.; and Stare, F. J.: A dietary program to lower serum cholesterol. J. Am. Diet. Assoc. 54: 13, 1969.
19. Buchwald, H.; Moore, R. B.; and Varco, R. L.: Surgical treatment of hyperlipidemia. Circulation 49: 1, 1974.
20. Karvonen, M. J.: Diet and cardiovascular disease. Practitioner 212: 518, 1974.
21. Leren, P.: Prevention of coronary heart disease by diet. Postgrad. Med. J. 51: 44, 1975.
22. Miettinen, M.: Prevention of coronary heart disease by cholesterol lowering diet. Postgrad. Med. J. 51: 47, 1975.
23. Podell, R. N.: Current status of the cholesterol hypothesis. Am. Fam. Phys. 9: 145, Jan. 1974.
24. Marshall, M. W.; Iacono, J. M.; Wheeler, M. A.; Mackin, J. F.; and Canary, J. J.: Changes in lactate dehydrogenase, LDH isoenzymes, lactate, and pyruvate as a result of feeding low fat diets to healthy men and women. Metabolism 25: 169, 1976.
25. O'Brien, J. R.; Etherington, M. D.; and Jamieson, S.: Acute platelet changes after large meals of saturated and unsaturated fats. Lancet 1: 878, 1976.
26. Mirkin, G.: Carbohydrate loading: a dangerous practice. JAMA 223: 1511, 1973.
27. Fry, M. M.; Spector, A. A.; Connor, S. L.; and Connor, W. E.: Intensification of hypertriglyceridemia by either alcohol or carbohydrate. Am. J. Clin. Nutr. 26: 798, 1973.
28. Ginsberg, H.; Olefsky, J. M.; Kimmerling, G.; Crapo, P.; and Reaven, G. M.: Induction of hypertriglyceridemia by a low fat diet. J. Clin. Endocrinol. Metab. 42: 729, 1976.

29. Sturdevant, R. A. L.; Pearce, M. L.; and Dayton, S.: Increased prevalence of cholelithiasis in men ingesting a serum cholesterol-lowering diet. N. Engl. J. Med. 288: 24, 1973.
30. Miettinen, M.; Turpeinen, O.; Karvonen, M. J.; Paavilainen, E.; and Elosuo, R.: Prevalence of cholelithiasis in men and women ingesting a serum-cholesterol-lowering diet. Ann. Clin. Res. 8: 111, 1976.
31. Hoffman, A. F.; Northfield, T. C.; and Thistle, J. L.: Can a cholesterol-lowering diet cause gallstones? N. Engl. J. Med. 288: 46, 1973.
32. Laird, W. P.: Childhood and diet as related to atherosclerosis. Can the pediatrician help protect against adult coronary artery disease? Clin. Pediatr. 14: 485, 1975.
33. Fomon, S. J., Filer, L. J. Jr., Ziegler, E. E., Bergmann, K. E. and Bergmann, R. L.: Skim Milk in infant feeding. Acta Paediatr. Scand. 66: 17–30, 1977.
34. McBean, L. D., and Speckman, E. W.: An interpretive review: diet in early life and the prevention of atherosclerosis. Pediatr. Res. 8: 837, 1974.
35. Friedman, G., and Goldberg, S. J.: An evaluation of the safety of a low saturated fat, low cholesterol diet beginning in infancy. Pediatrics 58: 655, 1976.
36. Steering Committee for Medical Care Community Programs, American Heart Association: The value and safety of diet modification to control hyperlipidemia. Circulation 58: 381A, 1978.
37. Pennock Laird, W.: Childhood and diet as related to atherosclerosis. Clin. Pediatr. 14: 485, 1975.
38. Hulley, S. B.; Burrows, M. I.; Wilson, W. S.; and Nichaman, M. Z.: Lipid and lipoprotein responses of hypertriglyceridemic outpatients to a low carbohydrate modification of the A.H.A. fat controlled diet. Lancet 2: 7777, 1972.
39. Albrink, M. J.: Serum lipids, diet and cardiovascular disease. Postgrad. Med. 55: 87, Apr. 1974.
40. American Heart Association: Planning Fat Controlled Meals for 1200 and 1800 Calories, 1966.
41. American Heart Association: Planning Fat Controlled Meals for approximately 2000–2600 Calories, Revised 1967.
42. The Subcommittee on Diet and Hyperlipidemia, American Heart Association: A Maximal Approach to the Dietary Treatment of the Hyperlipidemias. Diet C: The Low Cholesterol, High Polyunsaturated Fat Diet. New York: American Heart Association, 1973.
43. Eshelman, R., and Winston, M.: The American Heart Association Cookbook. New York: David McKay, 1973.
44. Bickel, J., and Gray, J.: A Low Cholesterol Diet Manual. Iowa City: University of Iowa Press, 1968.
45. Jones, J.: Diet for a Happy Heart. San Francisco: 101 Productions, 1975.
46. Payne, A. S., and Callahan, D.: The Fat and Sodium Control Cookbook. 4th ed. Boston: Little, Brown, 1975.
47. Brown, H. B.: Current focus on fat in the diet. White paper, American Dietetic Association, Chicago, 1977.
48. Mueller, J. F.: A dietary approach to coronary artery disease. J. Am. Diet. Assoc. 62: 613, 1973.
49. Mitchell, H. S.; Rynbergen, H. J.; Anderson, L.; and Dibble, M. V.: Nutrition in Health and Disease. 16th ed. New York: J. B. Lippincott, 1976.
50. Feeley, R. M.; Criner, P. E.; and Watt, B. K.: Cholesterol content of foods. J. Am. Diet. Assoc. 61: 134, 1972.
51. Frederickson, D. S.; Levy, R. I.; Jones, E.; Bonnell, M.; and Ernst, M.: The Dietary Management of Hyperlipoproteinemia: A Handbook for Physicians and Dietitians. Washington, DC: Government Printing Office, 1973.

# Diet and Coronary Heart Disease

COUNCIL ON FOODS AND NUTRITION

Coronary heart disease is the major public health problem in the United States and in many other countries. In 1970, for example, some 666,000 Americans, of whom about 171,000 were under the age of 65, died of coronary heart disease (CHD) and many more were disabled by the same disorder. It is particularly disturbing that many relatively young Americans in their most productive years are killed or incapacitated by this disease.

Epidemiologic, experimental, and clinical investigations have identified a number of "risk factors" associated with susceptibility to CHD that can be manipulated. These include an elevation in plasma lipids, especially plasma cholesterol, high blood pressure (hypertension), heavy cigarette smoking, obesity, and physical inactivity. The evidence is not sufficient to quantitate the benefits that may be expected to come from modifying these various risk factors, but the seriousness of the situation demands that all reasonable means be used to reduce the conditions that contribute to risk of CHD.

There is abundant evidence that the risk of developing CHD is positively correlated with the level of cholesterol in the plasma. This risk, independent of other risk factors mentioned above, is relatively small at levels less than 220 mg/100 ml but increases progressively with each increment in plasma cholesterol above this level. Approximately one-third of American men, and a less definitely known proportion of women, consuming their usual diets maintain plasma cholesterol levels at or below 220 mg/100 ml. There is extensive evidence that the level of cholesterol in the plasma of most people can be lowered by appropriate dietary modification. Generally, such lowering can be achieved most practicably by partial replacement of the dietary sources of saturated fat with sources of unsaturated fat, especially those rich in polyunsaturated fatty acids, and by a reduction in the consumption of foods rich in cholesterol. Preliminary evidence suggests that faithful and continued consumption of a cholesterol-lowering diet over a period of years can reduce the coronary attack rate in middle-aged men. As would be expected in dealing with a chronic disease of this kind, early intervention appears to be more effective than intervention after the disease is evident.

Elevation of other plasma lipids (plasma triglycerides) also imposes an increased risk of CHD. The elevation of plasma triglycerides is often, but not always, associated with an elevation of plasma cholesterol. Plasma triglycerides can also be modified by dietary intervention. Although there are as yet no satisfactory epidemiologic data to support the conclusion that triglyceride-lowering diets can reduce the occurrence of CHD in persons with hypertriglyceridemia,

Reprinted from JAMA 222: 1647, Dec. 1972. This is a joint policy statement of the AMA Council on Foods and Nutrition and the Food and Nutrition Board of the National Academy of Sciences—National Research Council. Copyright 1972, American Medical Association.

the inference from clinical studies that such a reduction can be anticipated is strong.

In summary, the average level of plasma lipids in most American men and women is undesirably elevated. The importance of lowering the plasma cholesterol in any individual depends in large part upon his usual plasma cholesterol concentration.

The evidence now available is sufficient to discourage further temporizing with this major national health problem. Therefore the Food and Nutrition Board and the Council on Foods and Nutrition recommend that:

(1) Measurement of the plasma lipid profile, particularly plasma cholesterol, become a routine part of all health maintenance physical examinations. Such measurements should be made in early adulthood, when coronary heart disease is still rare, and repeated at appropriate intervals. The potential impact of other risk factors should also be periodically assessed.

(2) Persons falling into "risk categories" on the basis of their plasma lipid levels be made aware of this and receive appropriate dietary advice. Such advice may vary somewhat with the nature of the blood lipid profile [1–4]. As indicated above, Americans should be advised to maintain a desirable body weight by an appropriate combination of physical activity and kilocalorie intake. In "risk categories" it is important to decrease substantially the intake of saturated fat and to lower cholesterol consumption. In practice, this entails substituting polyunsaturated vegetable oils for part of the saturated fat in the diet.

(3) Care be taken to assure that the dietary advice given does not compromise the intake of essential nutrients. Desirable intakes of nutrients are indicated in the Recommended Dietary Allowances found in the National Academy of Sciences publication 1694 (1968).

(4) Since the foregoing recommendations will be effective only if they can be accomplished with relative ease, modified and ordinary foods useful for this purpose be readily available on the market, reasonably priced, and easily identified by appropriate labeling. Any existing legal and regulatory barriers to the marketing of such foods should be removed.

(5) High priority be given to the conduct of studies that will determine reliably the extent to which the modification of plasma lipids, by dietary or other means, as well as modification of other risk factors, can reduce the risk of developing coronary artery disease.

References

1. Frederickson, D. S.; Levy, R. I.; and Lees, R. S.: Fat transport in lipoproteins—an integrated approach to mechanisms and disorders. New Engl. J. Med. 276: 34–44, 1967.
2. Lees, R. S.; Wilson, D. E.: The treatment of hyperlipidemia. New Engl. J. Med. 284: 186–195, 1971.
3. Report of the Inter-Society Commission for Heart Disease Resources: Primary prevention of the atherosclerotic diseases. Circulation 42: A55–A95, 1970.
4. American Health Foundation: Position statement on diet and coronary heart disease. Prev. Med. 1: 255–286, 1972.

# Desirable Amounts and Proportions of Dietary Fat and Carbohydrate

COMMITTEE ON DIETARY ALLOWANCES, FOOD AND NUTRITION BOARD, NATIONAL RESEARCH COUNCIL

Many nutritionists and physicians believe that the health of a significant proportion of the United States population could be improved by changes in life style, including dietary modifications. Although some of the proposed changes in diet are currently controversial, there is sufficient evidence to support some recommendations for dietary changes that would be consonant with better health. It should be emphasized that most chronic or degenerative diseases have a number of contributing factors, only one of which may be diet. Changes in diet only, without consideration of measures to alter other risk factors, will probably have minimal desirable effects.

Associated with diet and nutritional practices is the problem of obesity and general overweight. In the Ten State Nutrition Survey, up to 25% of adult males and 42% of females were classified as obese [1]. Reduction in body weight to the desirable level is considered to be one of the most beneficial measures related to diets that the U.S. population could implement. For much of the U.S. population, maintenance of desirable body weight could be achieved most readily by controlling caloric intake and increasing physical activity.

In countries, such as the United States, whose populations consume large amounts of fat, a sizable proportion of the population has relatively high blood concentrations of cholesterol and triglycerides. Although the relative significance of these blood lipids in coronary artery disease is controversial, hypercholesterolemia is generally considered to be one important risk factor among several (including genetic background, smoking, hypertension, and overweight) associated with this disease. In addition to coronary artery disease, other chronic diseases are also considered to have risk factors that include diet.

At this time the Committee on Dietary Allowances does not believe that it is desirable to make a blanket recommendation for dietary change for the entire population; however, some guidelines can be offered for individual consideration, especially by individuals suspected or known to be in the high-risk category for certain diseases. These guidelines are not intended to replace therapeutic or modified diets prescribed by a physician for specific medical conditions.

• Total fat intake, particularly in diets below 2,000 kcal, should be reduced so fat is not more than 35% of dietary energy. Since fat has the highest caloric density of the primary nutrients, a decrease in fat consumption can produce the greatest change in dietary energy.

Reprinted from Recommended Dietary Allowances, 9th Ed., Committee on Dietary Allowances—Food and Nutrition Board, National Research Council, National Academy of Sciences, Washington, DC, 1980.

There should be greater reduction in fats containing predominantly saturated fatty acids, such as those from animal sources, than in vegetable fats containing predominantly unsaturated fatty acids. These simultaneous changes in amount and type of dietary fat would increase the ratio of polyunsaturated to saturated fatty acids. The Committee on Dietary Allowances believes that, in view of the possible hazards of high intakes of polyunsaturated oils [2], an upper limit of 10% of dietary energy as polyunsaturated fatty acids is advisable.

• Intake of refined sugar should be reduced and complex carbohydrates maintained or even increased. Refined sugar (sucrose) confers no nutritional value other than as a source of energy and under some conditions is a contributory factor in dental caries. Dietary sources of complex carbohydrate often provide necessary vitamins and minerals and in addition are considered desirable for proper intestinal function.

• For many individuals a reduction in alcohol consumption would also assist in achieving proper caloric balance.

These recommendations for desirable types and amounts of dietary fat and carbohydrate do not entail radical changes in eating habits and could be accomplished with the United States food supply. Indeed, many individuals normally have dietary practices that follow this pattern. The American Heart Association [3] and the Working Party of the Royal College of Physicians of London [4] believe that these dietary recommendations, in conjunction with measures to decrease other risk factors, have a reasonable hope of being beneficial. Furthermore, an increase in nutrient concentration of the diet or food supply (by decreasing fat, sugar, and alcohol) will increase the possibility that all allowances for nutrients are met for those whose energy needs are less than 2,000 kcal.

References

1. U.S. Department of Health, Education, and Welfare: Ten-State Nutrition Survey, 1968–1970. III. Clinical Anthropometry. Dental. Publ. No. (HSM) 72–8134, Washington, DC: U.S. Dept. Health, Education, and Welfare, 1972.
2. FAO (Food and Agriculture Organization of the United Nations): Dietary fats and oils in human nutrition. Report of a FAO Expert Committee, FAO Food and Nutrition Paper No. 3. Rome, 1977.
3. Glueck, C. J.; McGill, H. C.; Shank, R. E.; and Lauer, R. M.: Value and safety of diet modification to control hyperlipidemia in childhood and adolescence. Circulation 58: 381A, 1978.
4. Anonymous: Prevention of coronary heart disease. Report of a joint working party of the Royal College of Physicians of London and the British Cardiac Society. J. Royal Coll. Physicians London 10: 213, 1976.

# Dietary Treatment of Hyperlipoproteinemia

*Hyperlipidemia*    An elevation of the concentration of one or more of the lipids in the blood [1].

*Hypercholesterolemia*    An elevation of the level of serum cholesterol [1].

*Hypertriglyceridemia*    An elevation in the level of serum triglycerides [1].

*Hyperlipemia*    A lactescent (milky) appearance of blood caused by increased concentration of the triglyceride fraction of either very low density lipoproteins (VLDL) or chylomicrons [1].

*Hyperchylomicronemia*    An elevation in the serum levels of chylomicrons [1].

*Lipoprotein*    A protein found circulating in the blood bound to cholesterol, triglycerides, and phospholipids, which serves as a means of lipid transportation. Five specific lipoproteins have been identified, each containing different concentrations of these lipids [2].

*Hyperlipoproteinemia*    Increased concentrations of one or more of the lipoproteins in the blood. Five distinct types of hyperlipoproteinemia have been identified, based on the characteristics of the specific lipoprotein abnormality [2] (see table 1).

*Indications for classification and treatment*    Both hypercholesterolemia and hypertriglyceridemia have been associated with an increased prevalence of coronary heart disease. However, it is now clear that cholesterol and triglyceride measurements are nonspecific and that hypercholesterolemia is just a sign of a heterogenous group of disorders differing in their symptoms and response to therapy. By identifying the specific lipoprotein abnormality and by interpreting hyperlipidemia in terms of hyperlipoproteinemia, the chances for successful therapy are increased. Eventually, it may help to determine whether the treatment of hyperlipoproteinemia can serve as a tool in the prevention of coronary heart disease [2–5]. A distinction should be made between primary hyperlipoproteinemia and that secondary to other disorders. A finding of primary hyperlipoproteinemia would necessitate a complete family screening, with repeated evaluations as a preventative measure [6]. Effective dietary treatment must be individualized to the manifestations of each of the five hyperlipoproteinemias; specific dietary regimens have been published by the National Institutes of Health for this purpose [7–12] (see table 2).

**Table 1. Five Types of Primary Hyperlipoproteinemia**

| | Type I | Type IIa | Type IIb or III | Type IV | Type V |
|---|---|---|---|---|---|
| Incidence | Very rare | Common | Relatively uncommon | Common | Uncommon |
| Origin; possible mechanism | Genetic recessive; deficiency in lipoprotein lipase | When genetic, dominant, sporadic; decreased catabolism of beta-lipoprotein | When genetic, recessive; sporadic? | When genetic, dominant, sporadic; excessive endogenous glyceride synthesis or deficient glyceride clearance? | Probably genetic, dominant, sporadic |
| Age of detection | Early childhood | Early childhood (in severe cases) | Adulthood (over age 20) | Adulthood | Early adulthood |
| Appearance of plasma (after storage at 4°C) | Cream layer over clear infranatant fluid on standing | Clear | Clear, cloudy or milky | Slightly turbid to cloudy, unchanged with standing | Cream layer over turbid infranatant on standing |
| Cholesterol | Normal or elevated | Elevated | Elevated | Normal or elevated | Elevated or normal |
| Triglyceride | Markedly elevated | Normal or slightly elevated | Usually elevated | Elevated | Elevated to markedly elevated |
| Lipoprotein family | Elevated chylomicrons | Increased LDL | IIb Increased LDL and VLDL III Increased ILDL | Increased VLDL | Increased chylomicrons and VLDL |
| Clinical presentation | Lipemia retinalis, eruptive xanthomas, hepatosplenomegaly, abdominal pain | Xanthelasma, tendon and tuberous xanthomas, juvenilis corneal arcus, accelerated atherosclerosis | Xanthoma planum; tuberoeruptive and tendon xanthomas; accelerated atherosclerosis of coronary and peripheral vessels | Accelerated coronary vessel disease, abnormal glucose tolerance, hyperuricemia | Lipemia retinalis, eruptive xanthomas, hepatosplenomegaly, abdominal pain, hyperglycemia, hyperuricemia |
| Conditions to be excluded* | Dysgammaglobulinemia, insulinopenic diabetes | Dietary cholesterol excess, porphyria, myxedema, myeloma, nephrosis, obstructive liver disease | Myxedema, dysgammaglobulinemia | Diabetes, glycogen storage disease, nephrotic syndrome, pregnancy, Werner's syndrome | Myeloma, dysproteinemias, diabetic acidosis, nephrosis, alcoholism, pancreatitis |

*Source*: Adapted from Nutrition in Health and Disease [1].
* Secondary hyperlipoproteinemias.

**Table 2. Summary of Diets for Types I–V Hyperlipoproteinemia**

| | *Type I* | *Type IIa* | *Type IIb & Type III* | *Type IV* | *Type V* |
|---|---|---|---|---|---|
| Diet prescription | Low fat, 25–35 g | Low cholesterol Polyunsaturated fat increased | Low cholesterol Approximately: 20 % kcal pro. 40% kcal fat 40% kcal CHO | Controlled CHO Approximately 45% of kilocalories Moderately restricted cholesterol | Restricted fat, 30% of kilocalories Controlled CHO, 50% of kilocalories Moderately restricted cholesterol |
| Kilocalories | Not restricted | Not restricted | Achieve and maintain "ideal" weight, i.e., reduction diet if necessary | Achieve and maintain "ideal" weight, i.e., reduction diet if necessary | Achieve and maintain "ideal" weight, i.e., reduction diet if necessary |
| Protein | Total protein intake is not limited | Total protein intake is not limited | High protein | Not limited other than control of patient's weight | High protein |
| Fat | Restricted to 25–35 g Type of fat not important | Saturated fat intake limited Polyunsaturated fat intake increased | Controlled to 40% of kilocalories (polyunsaturated fats recommended in preference to saturated fats) | Not limited other than control of patient's weight (polyunsaturated fats recommended in preference to saturated fats) | Restricted to 30% of kilocalories (polyunsaturated fats recommended in preference to saturated fats) |
| Carbohydrate | Not limited | Not limited | Controlled—concentrated sweets are restricted | Controlled—concentrated sweets are restricted | Controlled—concentrated sweets are restricted |
| Cholesterol | Not restricted | As low as possible; the only source of cholesterol is the meat in the diet | Less than 300 mg—the only source of cholesterol is the meat in the diet | Moderately restricted to 300–500 mg | Moderately restricted to 300–500 mg |
| Alcohol | Not recommended | May be used with discretion | Limited to 2 servings (substituted for carbohydrate) | Limited to 2 servings (substituted for carbohydrate) | Not recommended |

*Source*: Adapted from The Dietary Management of Hyperlipoproteinemia: A Handbook for Physicians and Dietitians [7].

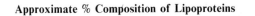

**Approximate % Composition of Lipoproteins**

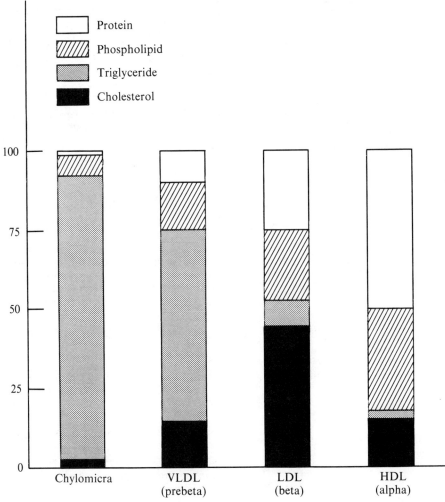

Schematic representation of the four lipoprotein families as defined by paper electrophoresis and analytical ultracentrifugation. Reprinted from Diet, hyperlipidemia and atherosclerosis [2].

**Table 3. Plasma Lipid and Lipoprotein Cholesterol Concentrations: "Normal Limits" Based on Washington Area Population Sample**

| Age of subjects | Plasma cholesterol (mg/100 ml) | Very-low-density lipoproteins (mg/100 ml) | Low-density lipoproteins (mg/100 ml) | High-density lipoproteins (mg/100 ml) | | Plasma triglyceride (mg/100 ml) |
|---|---|---|---|---|---|---|
| | | | | M | F | |
| Newborn "cord blood" | 50–95 | 0–15 | 20–45 | 30–55 | 30–55 | 10–65 |
| 1–9 yr | 120–230 | 5–25 | 50–170 | 30–65 | 30–65 | 10–140 |
| 10–19 | 120–230 | 5–25 | 50–170 | 30–65 | 30–70 | 10–140 |
| 20–29 | 120–240 | 5–25 | 60–170 | 35–70 | 35–75 | 10–140 |
| 30–39 | 140–270 | 5–35 | 70–190 | 30–65 | 35–80 | 10–150 |
| 40–49 | 150–310 | 5–35 | 80–190 | 30–65 | 40–85 | 10–160 |
| 50–59 | 160–330 | 10–40 | 80–210 | 30–65 | 35–85 | 10–190 |

*Source*: Reprinted from Diet, hyperlipidemia and atherosclerosis [2].
*Note*: "Normal limits," as defined here, are not necessarily "safe" or "acceptable" limits. The "normal" ranges exhibited by this population sample do not necessarily hold for other countries or even for other regions of the United States.

**Table 4. Concentrations of Cholesterol, Low Density Lipoproteins, or Triglycerides Which, If Exceeded, Clearly Indicate Hyperlipidemia**

| Age (yr) | Cholesterol (mg/100 ml) | Low-density lipoproteins (mg/100 ml) | Triglycerides |
|---|---|---|---|
| 1–19 | 230 | 170 | 150 |
| 20–29 | 240 | 170 | 200 |
| 30–39 | 270 | 190 | 200 |
| 40–49 | 310 | 190 | 200 |
| 50– | 330 | 210 | 200 |

*Source*: Adapted from The Dietary Management of Hyperlipoproteinemia: A Handbook for Physicians and Dietitians [7].

**Table 5.  Nomogram for Estimation of Plasma Low Density Lipoprotein (LDL) (milligrams LDL per 100 mg cholesterol)**

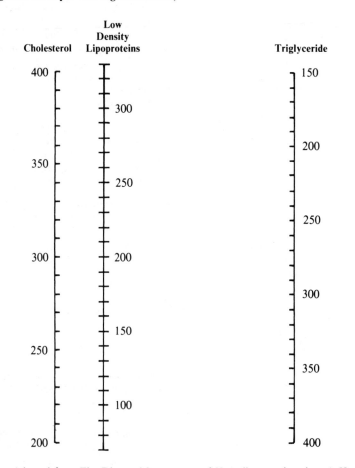

*Source*:  Adapted from The Dietary Management of Hyperlipoproteinemia:  A Handbook for Physicians and Dietitians [7].

*Note*:  A nomogram for estimation of plasma LDL concentration (in terms of mg per 100 ml of cholesterol (C) in this lipoprotein). It is derived from the equation LDL = C − (TG/5 + HDL), where HDL (high density lipoprotein) is assumed to be 45. Lay a straight edge connecting the plasma concentration of cholesterol on line "C" and the triglyceride (TG) concentration on line "TG." Read the LDL concentration where the straight edge crosses line "LDL." As a rough rule, LDL above 180 means type II. (Example:  for a C of 320 and a TG of 250, LDL = 225. This is type II or, more accurately, subtype IIb, because TG is abnormally high.)

**Table 6.  Type of Hyperlipoproteinemia As Suggested by Cholesterol (C) and Triglyceride (TG)**

| | |
|---|---|
| C high;  TG normal | Type IIa |
| C high;  TG 150–400 | Type IIb, III, or IV |
| C high; TG 400–1000 | Type II, IV, or V |
| C high; TG > 1000 | Type I or V |
| C normal; TG high | Type IV (I or V) |

*Source*:  Adapted from The Dietary Management of Hyperlipoproteinemia:  A Handbook for Physicians and Dietitians [7].

**References**

1. Mitchell, H. S.; Rynbergen, H. J.; Anderson, L.; and Dibble, M. V.: Nutrition in Health and Disease. 16th ed. New York: Lippincott, 1976.
2. Levy, R. I., and Ernst, N.: Diet, hyperlipidemia and atherosclerosis. Goodhart, R. S., and Shils, M. E., eds. Modern Nutrition in Health and Disease. Philadelphia: Lea & Febiger, 1973.
3. Levy, R. I.; Bonnell, M.; and Ernst, N. D.: Dietary management of hyperlipoproteinemia. J. Am. Diet. Assoc. 58: 406, 1971.
4. Stone, M. C.: The role of diet in the management of hyperlipoproteinemias. Proc. Nutr. Soc. 31: 311, 1972.
5. Kuo, P. T.: Hyperlipidemia and coronary artery disease—principles of diet and drug treatment. Med. Clin. N. Am. 58: 351, 1974.
6. Berenson, G. S.; Srinivasan, S.; and Frerichs, R. R.: Not-so-hyper hyperlipoproteinemia and coronary artery disease. Postgrad. Med. 58: 173, April 1976.
7. Frederickson, D. S.; Levy, R. I.; Jones, E.; Bonnell, M.; and Ernst, N.: The Dietary Management of Hyperlipoproteinemia: A Handbook for Physicians and Dietitians. Washington, DC: Government Printing Office, 1973.
8. Frederickson, D. S.; Levy, R. I.; Bonnell, M.; and Ernst, N.: Diet 1: For the Dietary Management of Hyperchylomicronemia (Type I Hyperlipoproteinemia). Washington, DC: Government Printing Office, 1973.
9. Frederickson, D. S.; Levy, R. I.; Bonnell, M.; and Ernst, N.: Diet 2: For the Dietary Management of Hypercholesterolemia (Type II Hyperlipoproteinemia). Washington, DC: Government Printing Office, 1973.
10. Frederickson, D. S.; Levy, R. I.; Bonnell, M.; and Ernst, N.: Diet 3: For the Dietary Management of Hypercholesterolemia with Endogenous Hyperglyceridemia (Type IIb or Type III Hyperlipoproteinemia). Washington, DC: Government Printing Office, 1973.
11. Frederickson, D. S.; Levy, R. I.; Bonnell, M.; and Ernst, N.: Diet 4: For the Dietary Management of Endogenous Hyperglyceridemia (Type IV Hyperlipoproteinemia). Washington, DC: Government Printing Office, 1973.
12. Frederickson, D. S.; Levy, R. I.; Bonnell, M.; and Ernst, N.: Diet 5: For the Management of Mixed Hyperglyceridemia (Type V Hyperlipoproteinemia). Washington, DC: Government Printing Office, 1973.

# Fat Restricted Diet for Management of Type I Hyperlipoproteinemia

*Diet for control of hyperchylomicronemia or type I hyperlipoproteinemia*    A very low fat diet containing 25–35 g fat daily, which may also contain medium chain triglycerides (MCT) [1,2].

*Characteristics of the diet*    Unless MCT are used, food must be prepared without the addition of any fats or oils. Cholesterol is not restricted. Because of the extremely low level of fat provided by the diet, the fat content of all food must be considered in its calculation. The 5 oz lean meat included in the diet daily provides the only major source of fat. At intakes of 1,600–2,400 kcal, approximately 10 g basic fat is added to the diet by low fat food items such as bread, skim milk, cereals, and fruit. If MCT are not used as a source of kilocalories, the carbohydrate content of the diet may be high; additional carbohydrate containing kilocalories may be necessary for weight maintenance in the nonobese person [1–3].

*Purpose and effects of the diet*    Type I hyperlipoproteinemia is associated with a tremendous increase in fasting concentration of chylomicrons and an inability to clear the plasma of triglycerides [4]. A low fat diet circumvents the body's lack of the necessary lipase to break down chylomicrons: it reduces the amount of chylomicrons that are formed as vehicles of fat transportation. Beneficial effects of the diet include (1) a dramatic clearing of hyperglyceridemia, (2) reduction of the hyperchylomicronemia, (3) alleviation of abdominal pains [3–5], and (4) eventual resolution of xanthomas and other symptoms [6]. Lack of response to existing forms of drugs increases the importance of the therapeutic role played by the diet in type I hyperlipoproteinemia [7,8]. At the present time dietary modification is the only effective treatment.

*Indications for use*    In type I hyperlipoproteinemia, patients in whom the diet is necessary are usually young and may have lipemia retinalis, hepatosplenomegaly, eruptive xanthomas, and bouts of abdominal pain associated with ingestion of dietary fat. A discrete cream layer forms in the plasma of these patients after it is stored overnight at 4° C. This cream layer is easily discernible, and its identification is of diagnostic significance. The plasma cholesterol may be normal or elevated; triglyceride concentrations are grossly elevated (often above 5,000 mg/100 ml) [1]. A very low fat formula has been recommended as part of the diagnostic procedure in infants [1].

*Possible adverse reactions*    The diet is extremely low in fatty acids and may be inadequate in iron and vitamin E and other fat soluble vitamins [1,2]. In addition, the lack of fat in the diet is a serious detriment to its palatability and acceptance.

*Contraindications*    Not applicable to any other type of hyperlipidemia. If MCT are used in the diet, the diet would be contraindicated in circumstances in which MCT are contraindicated (see article on the LCT restricted MCT diet, pp. E65–E70).

***Suggestions for dietitians***     The meat allowance was calculated using the value of 8 g protein and 3 g fat per ounce. The lists of foods permitted and excluded on the LCT restricted MCT diet (pp. E67–E68) may be used in planning the menus with one exception; all the fat exchanges must be eliminated. Additional information is available from the detailed booklets published by the National Institute of Health describing dietary management of all five forms of hyperlipoproteinemia [1,2].

**Daily Food Plan for the Adult with Type I Hyperlipoproteinemia (1,700–2,000 kcal)**

1 qt skim milk
5 oz cooked poultry, fish, or lean trimmed meat
5 servings of vegetables and fruits
6 or more servings whole grain or enriched bread or cereal
1 or more servings potato, rice, etc.
Allowed desserts
Sugar, sweets

**Sample Menu**

A.M.

6 oz orange juice
3/4 cup cornflakes
1 cup skim milk
2 slices whole wheat bread
1 tbsp jelly or preserves
Coffee or tea
1 tsp sugar

Noon

2 oz baked chicken
½ cup rice
½ cup carrots
1 slice enriched white bread
1 pear
1 cup skim milk
Coffee or tea
1 tsp sugar, if desired

P.M.

3 oz baked haddock
½ cup mashed potato
½ cup peas
2 small dinner rolls
Angel food cake with peach slices
1 cup skim milk
Coffee or tea
1 tsp sugar

Between meals

1 cup skim milk
1 cup fruited gelatin

*Source:* Adapted from The Dietary Management of Hyperlipoproteinemia:  A Handbook for Physicians and Dietitians [1].

**References**

1. Frederickson, D. S.; Levy, R. I.; Jones, E.; Bonnell, M.; and Ernst, N.: The Dietary Management of Hyperlipoproteinemia: A Handbook for Physicians and Dietitians. Washington, DC: Government Printing Office, 1973.
2. Frederickson, D. S.; Levy, R. I.; Bonnell, M.; and Ernst, N.: Diet 1: For the Dietary Management of Hyperchylomicronemia (Type I Hyperlipoproteinemia). Washington, DC: Government Printing Office, 1973.
3. Levy, R. I., and Ernst, N.: Diet, hyperlipidemia and atherosclerosis. Goodhart, R. S., and Shils, M. E., eds. Modern Nutrition in Health and Disease. Philadelphia: Lea & Febiger, 1973.
4. Levy, R. I.; Bonnell, M.; and Ernst, N. D.: Dietary management of hyperlipoproteinemia. J. Am. Diet. Assoc. 58: 406, 1971.
5. Farmer, R. G.; Winkelman, E. I.; Brown, H. B.; and Lewis, L. A.: Hyperlipoproteinemia and pancreatitis. Am. J. Med. 54: 161, 1973.
6. Fleischmajer, R.; Dowlati, Y.; and Reeves, R. T.: Familial hyperlipidemias. Arch. Dermatol. 110: 43, 1974.
7. Berenson, G. S.; Srinivasan, S.; and Frerichs, R. R.: Not-so-hyper hyperlipoproteinemia and coronary artery disease. Postgrad. Med. 58: 173, April 1976.
8. Levy, R.; Morganroth, J.; and Rifkind, B. M.: Treatment of hyperlipidemia. N. Engl. J. Med. 290: 1295, 1975.

# Cholesterol and Fat Restricted, Increased Polyunsaturated Fat, Decreased Saturated Fat Diet for Management of Type IIa Hyperlipoproteinemia

***Diet for control of hypercholesterolemia or type IIa hyperlipoproteinemia (hyperbetalipoproteinemia)***　　A low cholesterol, modified fat, increased polyunsaturated fat diet that provides 300 mg cholesterol or less daily [1,2]. The polyunsaturated fat:saturated fat ratio of the diet varies from 2.8 to a minimum of 1.8 [3,4].

***Dietary management of hypercholesterolemia***　　Therapy is aimed at reducing serum levels of cholesterol by controlling endogenous and exogenous sources of cholesterol. Increasing the level of polyunsaturated fats at the expense of saturated fat and reducing total fat content will reduce endogenous production of cholesterol from these sources in the liver; restricting the amount of cholesterol containing foods consumed reduces the exogenous sources [5]. Specifically designed dietary regimens for treatment of this disorder have been published by the National Institutes of Health [3,4]. The American Heart Association Diet for the control of hypercholesterolemia on pp. E13–E16 may also be used. A recently published adaptation of the basic diet designed for use in young children provides an efficient approach to early dietary intervention [6,7].

***Indications for use***　　Primary type II hyperlipidemia is indicated when the values in table 4 of "Dietary Treatment of Hyperlipoproteinemia" (p. E27) are exceeded or when serum cholesterol, after a 12–14 hr fast, exceeds 220 mg/100 ml in persons under age 55 [3].

***Effects of the diet, possible adverse reactions, and contraindications***　　The diet for control of type IIa hyperlipoproteinemia is similar to the American Heart Association's fat controlled diet but provides for stricter control than the "prudent diet." The effects and reactions listed for the fat controlled diet would conceivably be more pronounced in instances where the type II diet is more rigid.

***Effect of diet and drug therapy on plasma vitamin A and E levels***　　The question of possible adverse reactions from combined diet and drug therapy on plasma vitamin A and E levels has been raised. Vitamins E and A and betalipoprotein levels are highly correlated, and vitamin E is transported in the plasma by betalipoproteins. Therefore, therapy designed to lower cholesterol and betalipoprotein might also reduce plasma vitamin A and E levels. One short-term study has determined that children with type II hyperlipidemia actually have supranormal amounts of these vitamins prior to treatment and that effective lowering of cholesterol and betalipoprotein levels did not present any immediate threat to vitamin A and E status [8].

**Daily Food Plan for the Adult with Type IIa Hyperlipoproteinemia (1,700–2,000 kcal)**

1 pt or more skim milk
6–9 oz cooked poultry, fish, or lean trimmed meat
7 or more servings whole grain or enriched bread or cereal
5 servings of vegetable and fruit, including 1 serving citrus fruit, 1 serving dark green
    or deep yellow vegetable, 1 or more servings of potato, rice, etc.
6–9 tsp allowed fat
Allowed desserts and sweets

**Sample Menu**

A.M.

6 oz orange juice
3/4 cup cornflakes
½ cup skim milk
2 slices whole wheat bread
2 tsp special margarine
1 tbsp jelly or preserves
Coffee or tea
1 tsp sugar

Noon

3 oz baked chicken
½ cup rice
½ cup carrots
2 slices enriched bread
2 tsp special margarine
1 pear
Coffee or tea
1 tsp sugar if desired
½ cup skim milk

P.M.

4 oz baked haddock
½ cup mashed potato
½ cup peas
2 small dinner rolls
3 tsp special margarine
½ cup canned peaches
½ cup skim milk
Coffee or tea
1 tsp sugar if desired

Between meals

½ cup skim milk
1 cup fruited gelatin

*Source:* Adapted from The Dietary Management of Hyperlipoproteinemia: A Handbook
    for Physicians and Dietitians [3].

References    1. Mitchell, H. S.; Rynbergen, H. J.; Anderson, L.; and Dibble, M. V.: Nutrition
    in Health and Disease. 16th ed. New York: Lippincott, 1976.
2. Levy, R. I., and Ernst, N.: Diet, hyperlipidemia and atherosclerosis. Good-
    hart, R. S., and Shils, M. E., eds. Modern Nutrition in Health and Disease.
    Philadelphia: Lea & Febiger, 1973.
3. Frederickson, D. S.; Levy, R. I.; Jones, E.; Bonnell, M.; and Ernst, N.: The
    Dietary Management of Hyperlipoproteinemia: A Handbook for Physicians
    and Dietitians. Washington, DC: Government Printing Office, 1973.
4. Frederickson, D. S.; Levy, R. I.; Bonnell, M.; and Ernst, N.: Diet 2: For the
    Dietary Management of Hypercholesterolemia (Type II Hyperlipoproteinemia).
    Washington, DC: Government Printing Office, 1973.
5. Levy, R. I.; Bonnell, M.; and Ernst, N. D.: Dietary management of hyperlipo-
    proteinemia. J. Am. Diet. Assoc. 58: 406, 1971.
6. Larsen, R.; Glueck, C. J.; and Tsang, R.: Special diet for familial type II
    hyperlipoproteinemia. Am. J. Dis. Child.: 128, 67, 1974.

7. West, R. J.; Fosbrooke, A. S.; and Lloyd, J. K.: Treatment of children with familial hypercholesterolaemia. Postgrad. Med. J. 51: 82, 1975.
8. Glueck, C. J.; Tsang, R. C.; Fallat, R. W.; and Scheel, D.: Plasma vitamin A and E levels in children with familial type II hyperlipoproteinemia during therapy with diet and cholestyramine resin. Pediatrics 54: 51, 1974.

# Carbohydrate Controlled, Fat Modified and Controlled, Low Cholesterol Diet for Management of Type IIb or Type III Hyperlipoproteinemia

***Diet for control of hypercholesterolemia with endogenous hyperglyceridemia or type IIb or type III hyperlipoproteinemia (hyperbetalipoproteinemia with hyperpre-betalipoproteinemia)*** A controlled carbohydrate, controlled and modified fat, low cholesterol diet that includes the following:

1. A reduction diet until the patient achieves ideal weight
2. A maintenance diet, with a caloric level to hold ideal weight, that emphasizes the following:
   a. Controlled carbohydrate intake—approximately 40% of kilocalories
   b. Controlled and modified fat intake—approximately 40% of kilocalories
   c. Cholesterol intake restricted to 300 mg or less, with polyunsaturated fats recommended in preference to saturated fats [1,2].

***Characteristics and composition of the maintenance diet***

Fat
40–43% of total kilocalories or 55–130 g. P/S ratio is not emphasized. It is higher (1:1) than the average American diet (0.3:1) because of the substitution of polyunsaturated fat for saturated fat.

Cholesterol
Cholesterol intake is restricted to 300 mg or less per day. The only source of cholesterol should be the meat in the diet. All high cholesterol foods, such as egg yolk, organ meats, etc., are eliminated.

Protein
18–21% of total kilocalories or 63–125 g. This amount of protein is well above the recommended allowance and classifies the diet as a high protein one.

Alcohol
Alcohol, at the physician's discretion, may be substituted for carbohydrate foods in limited amounts. The total amount of alcohol is limited to 2 servings/day, which are substituted for bread exchanges on pp. F22–F23. Any one of the following in the amount listed is 1 serving: 1 oz gin, rum, vodka, or whiskey, 1½ oz dessert or sweet wine, 2½ oz dry table wine, 5 oz beer.

*Source:* Adapted from The Dietary Management of Hyperlipoproteinemia: A Handbook for Physicians and Dietitians [1].

***Purpose of the diet*** To reduce elevated serum levels of triglycerides and cholesterol. Endogenous hyperglyceridemia can be controlled by caloric restrictions; therefore, the first goal of nutritional therapy is normalization of body weight. Restrictions in the carbohydrate and fat intake are necessary in the second stage of the regimen to prevent the elevation of serum triglycerides that occurs in patients with an excessive intake of these nutrients [1–4].

*Effects of the diet*    The results of dietary management of patients with types IIb and III hyperlipidemia are usually very gratifying. Diet alone will often reduce serum cholesterol and triglyceride concentrations to within normal limits [3,4]. For example, 25 out of 35 patients in a recent study achieved normal lipid levels with diet therapy alone [5]. Patients often present with plantar xanthomas (orange-yellow lipid deposits in the creases of the palms of the hands), as well as tubero-eruptive lesions (over the elbows, knees, and buttocks) and tendon xanthomas [6]. Continued adherence to the diet often produces dramatic resolution of cutaneous xanthomas [6,7] and improvements in the peripheral circulation [8].

*Indications for use*    In types IIb and III hyperlipoproteinemia patients have clear, cloudy, or milky plasma with elevations in both cholesterol and triglyceride concentrations in the range of 350–800 mg/100 ml [9]. Clinical distinctions between mild examples of types II and IV are blurred. They can be separated on the basis of their estimated low density lipoprotein concentrations [9]. The ratio of very low density lipoprotein cholesterol to the plasma triglyceride concentration ($C_{VLDL}/TG = r$) has proven to be a valuable chemical index in making the diagnosis [10]. Although floating betalipoproteins are present in nearly all patients with a high $r$ value, they also appear inconsistently in many other patients. When the plasma triglyceride concentration is between 150 and 1,000 mg/100 ml, an $r$ not less than 0.25 is suggestive of and a value not less than 0.30 is diagnostic of type III hyperlipoproteinemia [11].

*Possible adverse reactions*    The diet for the patient with type III hyperlipoproteinemia may be inadequate in iron [1]. The patient's state of iron nutrition should be periodically assessed, and iron supplements should be provided as needed in order to prevent complications of iron deficiency anemia.

*Contraindications*    None that are known.

**Diet 3 Maintenance Plan: Controlled Carbohydrate, Controlled Modified Fat, Low Cholesterol—Suggested Food Distribution for Diet Plans at Various Caloric Levels**

| Kilocalories | 1,500 | 1,800 | 2,000 | 2,200 | 2,400 | 2,600 | 2,800 |
|---|---|---|---|---|---|---|---|
| Protein (g) | 75 | 80 | 90 | 115 | 120 | 120 | 125 |
| Fat (g) | 70 | 80 | 95 | 100 | 110 | 120 | 130 |
| Carbohydrate (g) | 135 | 180 | 195 | 210 | 225 | 255 | 285 |
| Food groups | | | | | | | |
| Lean cooked meat servings* (3 oz is 1 serving) | 2 | 2 | 2 | 3 | 3 | 3 | 3 |
| Skim milk servings | 2 | 2 | 3 | 3 | 3 | 3 | 3 |
| Bread, cereal, etc., servings | 5 | 8 | 8 | 9 | 10 | 12 | 14 |
| Fat servings | 10 | 12 | 15 | 15 | 17 | 19 | 21 |
| Fruit servings† | 3 | 3 | 3 | 3 | 3 | 3 | 3 |

Vegetables except those grouped with breads and cereals are not limited.

*Source*:  Adapted from The Dietary Management of Hyperlipoproteinemia:  A Handbook for Physicians and Dietitians [1].
* For 1 oz meat, fish, or poultry, 8 g protein and 3 g fat have been calculated.
† For ½ cup of any fresh or unsweetened fruit or juice, 10 g carbohydrate has been calculated.

**Daily Food Plan for the Adult with Type IIb or Type III Hyperlipoproteinemia (1,800 kcal)**

2 cups skim milk
6 oz lean meat, poultry, or fish
7 servings of whole grain or enriched bread and cereals
1 serving potato, rice, etc.
3 servings fruit
2 servings vegetables
12 servings allowed fat

**Sample Menu**

A.M.

4 oz orange juice
¾ cup cornflakes
1 cup skim milk
2 slices whole wheat bread
3 tsp special margarine
Coffee or tea

NOON

3 oz baked chicken
½ cup rice
lettuce/tomato salad with 5 small olives
1 tbsp mayonnaise
1 slice enriched bread
2 tsp special margarine
1 pear
½ cup skim milk
Coffee or tea

P.M.

3 oz baked haddock
½ cup mashed potato
½ cup green beans
2 slices whole wheat bread
3 tsp special margarine
½ cup skim milk
½ cup canned unsweetened peaches
Coffee or tea

*Source:* Adapted from The Dietary Management of Hyperlipoproteinemia: A Handbook for Physicians and Dietitians [1].

References

1. Frederickson, D. S.; Levy, R. I.; Jones, E.; Bonnell, M.; and Ernst, N.: The Dietary Management of Hyperlipoproteinemia: A Handbook for Physicians and Dietitians. Washington, DC: Government Printing Office, 1973.
2. Frederickson, D. S.; Levy, R. I.; Bonnell, M.; and Ernst, N.: Diet 3: For the Dietary Management of Hypercholesterolemia with Endogenous Hyperglyceridemia (Type IIb or Type III Hyperlipoproteinemia). Washington, DC: Government Printing Office, 1973.
3. Levy, R. I., and Ernst, N.: Diet, hyperlipidemia and atherosclerosis. Goodhart, R. S., and Shils, M. E., eds. Modern Nutrition in Health and Disease. Philadelphia: Lea & Febiger, 1973.
4. Levy, R. I.; Bonnell, M.; and Ernst, N. D.: Dietary management of hyperlipoproteinemia. J. Am. Diet. Assoc. 58: 406, 1971.
5. Morganroth, J.; Levy, R. I.; and Frederickson, D. S.: The biochemical, clinical, and genetic features of type III hyperlipoproteinemia. Ann Intern. Med. 82: 158, 1975.
6. Fleischmajer, R.; Dowlati, Y.; and Reeves, R. T.: Familial hyperlipidemias. Arch. Dermatol. 110: 43, 1974.
7. Palmer, A. V., and Blacket, R.: Regression of xanthoma of the eyelids with modified fat diet. Lancet 1: 66, 1972.

8. Zelis, R.; Mason, D. T.; Braunwald, E.; and Levy, R. L.: Effects of hyperlipoproteinemias and their treatment on the peripheral circulation. J. Clin. Invest. 49: 1007, 1970.

9. Berenson, G. S.; Srinivasan, S.; and Frerichs, R. R.: Not-so-hyper hyperlipoproteinemia and coronary artery disease. Postgrad. Med. 58: 173, Apr. 1976.

10. Glueck, C. J.; Tsang, R. C.; Fallat, R. W.; and Scheel, D.: Plasma vitamin A and E levels in children with familial type II hyperlipoproteinemia during therapy with diet and cholestyramine resin. Pediatrics 54: 51, 1974.

11. Frederickson, D. S.; Morganroth, J.; and Levy, R. I.: Type III hyperlipoproteinemia: an analysis of two contemporary definitions. Ann. Intern. Med. 82: 150, 1975.

# Carbohydrate Controlled, Fat Modified, Moderately Restricted Cholesterol Diet for Management of Type IV Hyperlipoproteinemia

***Diet for control of endogenous hyperglyceridemia or type IV hyperlipoproteinemia (hyperpre-betalipoproteinemia)*** A controlled carbohydrate, modified fat, moderately restricted cholesterol diet that includes the following:

1. A reduction diet until the patient achieves ideal weight
2. A maintenance diet with a caloric level designed to hold ideal weight, with the following modifications:
   a. Controlled carbohydrate intake—approximately 45% of kilocalories
   b. A modified fat intake—decreased saturated fat
   c. Cholesterol intake moderately restricted to 300–500 mg/day, with polyunsaturated fats recommended in preference to other fats [1].

***Characteristics of the diet*** Protein and fat intakes are not restricted, but saturated fat is restricted as in the regimen for type III hyperlipoproteinemia. The diet for type IV hyperlipoproteinemia differs from the regimen for type III hyperlipoproteinemia in that it contains more fat and cholesterol [2,3], i.e., 300–500 mg cholesterol daily, with 3 egg yolks/week or the substitution of organ meats, or the choice of an unlimited quantity of meat [4]. Carbohydrate restrictions are still necessary, however, because the serum triglyceride levels of patients with type IV hyperlipoproteinemia are increased by excessive intakes of carbohydrate [5].

***Approximate composition of maintenance diet***

Carbohydrate  44–46% of total kilocalories or 165–315 g. All concentrated sweets and many desserts are eliminated in the diet. The carbohydrate intake should not exceed 4–5 g/kg of body weight daily.

Protein and fat  Protein and fat intake are not limited other than to control the patient's weight. The P/S ratio can vary greatly, depending on the amount of meat eaten and the amount of unsaturated fat.

Cholesterol  Cholesterol intake is moderately restricted to 300–500 mg/day.

Alcohol  Alcohol, at the physician's discretion, may be substituted for carbohydrate foods in limited amounts. The total amount of alcohol is limited to 2 servings/day. Serving sizes are listed on p. E39.

*Source:* Adapted from The Dietary Management of Hyperlipoproteinemia: A Handbook for Physicians and Dietitians [4].

***Purpose and effects of the diet*** The purpose of the diet is to reduce elevated serum levels of triglycerides and pre-betalipoproteins [1–3]. In susceptible subjects, weight gain may be sufficient to induce type IV hyperlipidemia [6,7]. In one series of patients the diet reduced elevated serum triglycerides by 50% [8]. Weight reduction alone will often result in complete normalization of blood lipids [2,9]. If triglycerides are not restored to normal within a few months, a reduction in dietary carbohydrate may be needed [10]. In these patients a high carbohydrate diet leads to hepatic synthesis of triglycerides and therefore to increased serum concentrations [5,10]. In addition, fatty acids synthesized from carbohydrate are highly saturated. Results of one study imply that saturated fats are preferentially incorporated into pre-betalipoproteins and that increasing polyunsaturated fats in the diet may result in decreased serum triglyceride and pre-betalipoprotein levels [11].

Alcohol must be limited, since alcoholic excesses tend to intensify the hypertriglyceridemia [12–14].

***Indications for use*** In type IV hyperlipoproteinemia, an isolated increase in endogenous glycerides or very low density lipoproteins. The plasma may be cloudy or milky depending on the triglyceride concentration. Once triglyceride levels exceed 400 mg/100 ml, most patients either have type IV or type V. Those with a negative chylomicron test probably have type IV [4]. Cholesterol levels may be normal, but as a rule, for each 5 mg/100 ml increase in triglycerides, there will be a 1 mg/100 ml increase in plasma cholesterol [4]. Polyarthritis has been described in a small group of these patients [15]. About 50% of the patients with type IV hyperlipidemia have abnormal glucose tolerance tests, and many will have hyperuricemia [4].

***Possible adverse reactions*** The diet may be inadequate in iron [4] and thiamine. The patient's state of iron nutrition should be periodically assessed and iron supplements provided as indicated to prevent complications of iron deficiency anemia.

The total fat content of the diet is not limited other than initially, during the period of weight reduction. If total fat intake is increased to replace carbohydrate kilocalories, a rise in serum cholesterol may occur. This can be offset by preferential use of polyunsaturated fats over saturated fats [5].

***Contraindications*** None that are known.

**Daily Maintenance Diet Plan for Type IV Hyperlipoproteinemia (1,500 kcal)**

2 cups skim milk
6 oz lean meat, poultry or fish
3 servings whole grain or enriched bread or cereal
2 servings potato or rice
3 servings fruit
10 servings fat
2 servings vegetables

**Sample Menu**

A.M.

4 oz orange juice
1 slice whole wheat toast
2 tsp fortified margarine
1 cup skim milk
Coffee or tea

NOON

3 oz broiled chicken with 1 tsp fortified margarine
½ cup enriched rice with 1 tsp fortified margarine
½ cup carrots with 1 tsp fortified margarine
1 slice enriched bread with 1 tsp fortified margarine
1 pear—fresh or unsweetened
Coffee or tea

P.M.

3 oz baked haddock
½ cup mashed potato with 1 tsp fortified margarine
½ cup green beans with 1 tsp fortified margarine
1 slice whole wheat bread with 2 tsp fortified margarine
½ cup unsweetened fruit cocktail
Coffee or tea

BETWEEN MEALS

1 cup skim milk

References

1. Frederickson, D. S.; Levy, R. I.; Bonnell, M.; and Ernst, N.:   Diet 4:   For the Dietary Management of Endogenous Hyperglyceridemia (Type IV Hyperlipoproteinemia). Washington, DC:   Government Printing Office, 1973.
2. Levy, R. I., and Ernst, N.:   Diet, hyperlipidemia and atherosclerosis. Goodhart, R. S., and Shils, M. E., eds.   Modern Nutrition in Health and Disease. Philadelphia:   Lea & Febiger, 1973.
3. Levy, R. I.; Bonnell, M.; and Ernst, N. D.:   Dietary management of hyperlipoproteinemia.   J. Am. Diet. Assoc. 58: 406, 1971.
4. Frederickson, D. S.; Levy, R. I.; Jones, E.; Bonnell, M.; and Ernst, N.:   The Dietary Management of Hyperlipoproteinemia:   A Handbook for Physicians and Dietitians. Washington, DC:   Government Printing Office, 1973.
5. Quarfordt, S. H.; Frank, A.; Shames, D. M.; Berman, M.; and Steinberg, D.:   Very low density lipoprotein triglyceride transport in type IV hyperlipoproteinemia and the effects of carbohydrate rich diets.   J. Clin. Invest. 49: 2281, 1970.
6. Blacket, R. B.; Leelarthaepin, B.; Woodhill, J. M.; and Palmer, A. J.:   Type IV hyperlipidemia and weight gain after maturity.   Lancet 2: 518, 1975.
7. Blacket, R. B.; Woodhill, J. M.; Palmer, A. J.; and Leelarthaepin, B.:   Type IV hyperlipidemia and weight gain after maturity.   Lancet 2: 517, 1975.
8. Smith, L. K.; Luepker, R. V.; Rothchild, S. S.; Gillis, A.; Kochman, L.; and Warhasse, V. R.:   Management of Type IV hyperlipoproteinemia. Evaluation of practical clinical approaches.   Ann. Intern. Med. 84: 22, 1976.
9. Frederickson, D. S.; Morganroth, J.; and Levy, R. I.:   Type III hyperlipoproteinemia:   an analysis of two contemporary definition.   Ann. Intern. Med. 82: 150, 1975.
10. Albrink, M. A.:   Serum lipids, diet and cardiovascular disease.   Postgrad. Med. 55: 86, Apr. 1974.
11. Chait, A.; Onitiri, A.; Nicoll, A.; Rabaya, E.; Davis, J.; and Lewis, B.:   Reduction of serum triglyceride levels by polyunsaturated fat.   Atherosclerosis 20: 347, 1974.
12. Mendelson, J. H.:   Significance of alcohol-induced hypertriglyceridemia in patients with type IV hyperlipoproteinemia.   Ann. Intern. Med. 80: 270, 1974.
13. Fry, M. M.; Spector, A. A.; Connor, S. L.; and Connor, W. E.:   Intensification of hypertriglyceridemia by either alcohol or carbohydrate.   Am. J. Clin. Nutr. 26: 798, 1973.
14. Ostrander, L. D.; Lamphiear, D. E.; Block, W. D.; Johnson, B. C.; Ravenscroft, C.; and Epstein, F. H.:   Relationship of serum lipid concentrations to alcohol consumption.   Arch. Intern. Med. 134: 451, 1974.
15. Buckingham, R. B.; Bole, C. G.; and Bassett, D. R.:   Polyarthritis associated with type IV hyperlipoproteinemia.   Arch. Intern. Med. 135: 286, 1975.

# Fat Restricted and Modified, Carbohydrate Controlled, Moderately Restricted Cholesterol Diet for Management of Type V Hyperlipoproteinemia

***Diet for control of mixed hyperglyceridemia or type V hyperlipoproteinemia (hyperchylomicronemia associated with hyperpre-betalipoproteinemia)*** A restricted and modified fat, controlled carbohydrate, and moderately restricted cholesterol diet that emphasizes:

1. A reduction diet until the patient achieves ideal weight
2. A maintenance diet with a caloric level to hold ideal body weight, with the following modifications:
   a. Restricted and modified fat intake—approximately 30% of kilocalories with polyunsaturated fats recommended in preference to saturated fats
   b. Controlled carbohydrate intake—approximately 50% of kilocalories
   c. Cholesterol intake moderately restricted to 300–500 mg/day [1,2].

***Characteristics of the diet*** The diet plan is quite rigid. It provides more cholesterol than is permitted on the diet used for control of type III hyperlipoproteinemia and provides for the same substitutions of 3 egg yolks/week, etc., as on the diet used in type IV hyperlipoproteinemia [3,4].

***Approximate composition of maintenance diet***

| | |
|---|---|
| Fat | 25–30% of total kilocalories or 35–85 g. This amount of fat is less than in the average American diet. P/S ratio is not emphasized. It is higher (range 0.5:1 to 1:1) than the average American diet (0.3:1). The ratio will depend on the choice of oil and margarine. The amount of polyunsaturated fat that can be used is limited because of total fat restriction. |
| Cholesterol | Cholesterol intake is moderately restricted to 300–500 mg/day. |
| Carbohydrate | 48–53% or 153–370 g/day. |
| Protein | 21–24% of total kilocalories or 72–145 g. This amount of protein is well above the recommended allowances and classifies the diet as a high protein one. |
| Alcohol | Alcohol is not recommended for the patient with type V hyperlipoproteinemia (it may be associated with a marked exacerbation in plasma triglyceride concentrations). |

*Source:* Adapted from The Dietary Management of Hyperlipoproteinemia: A Handbook for Physicians and Dietitians [1].

***Purpose and effects of the diet*** To reduce elevated serum levels of triglycerides, pre-betalipoproteins, and chylomicrons. Diet therapy stresses caloric restriction and normalization of body weight.

Sometimes, as in type IV hyperlipoproteinemia, weight reduction alone will result in complete normalization of blood lipids. On an unrestricted diet, plasma triglycerides may range from 1,000–1,600 mg/100 ml. Both fat and carbohydrate may contribute to increased triglyceride levels in the patient with type V hyperlipoproteinemia. A fat and carbohydrate restricted diet will usually allow the maintenance of plasma triglyceride concentrations below 300–600 mg/100 ml in the patient who has achieved his ideal weight. The restriction of both fat and carbohydrate is impractical. Since these patients have bouts of abdominal pain after consuming increased amounts of fat, fat restriction rather than carbohydrate restriction is emphasized. If pain persists, it may be necessary to restrict fat intake severely and to follow the very low fat diet used for control of type I hyperlipoproteinemia [3,4].

*Indications for use*    In type V hyperlipoproteinemia, which is characterized by a mixed hyperlipidemia, both exogenous (chylomicrons) and endogenous glycerides (pre-betalipoproteins) accumulate in the plasma [1]. These patients usually have symptoms after age 20 years. They may have all the features of patients with type I hyperlipoproteinemia, e.g., creamy plasma, abdominal pain, and hepatic splenomegaly, but unlike type I patients, they have grossly elevated triglyceride levels of over 1,000 mg/100 ml [1].

*Possible adverse reactions*    The diet may provoke iron deficiency in the patient with marginal iron stores, as it is inadequate in iron [1]. The state of the patient's iron nutrition should be periodically assessed and supplements given as indicated.

*Contraindications*    In the patient with recurrent pancreatitis or in one who is intolerant even to this level of fat, the very low fat diet for type I hyperlipoproteinemia may be more appropriate [1].

**Diet Plan for Type V Hyperlipoproteinemia: Suggested Food Distribution for Diet Plans at Various Caloric Levels**

| Kilocalories | 1,500 | 1,800 | 2,000 | 2,200 | 2,400 | 2,600 | 2,800 |
|---|---|---|---|---|---|---|---|
| Protein (g) | 90 | 100 | 105 | 130 | 135 | 140 | 145 |
| Fat (g) | 50 | 50 | 65 | 70 | 70 | 85 | 85 |
| Carbohydrate (g) | 180 | 235 | 250 | 265 | 310 | 325 | 370 |
| Food groups | | | | | | | |
| Lean cooked meat servings* (3 oz is 1 serving) | 2 | 2 | 2 | 3 | 3 | 3 | 3 |
| Skim milk servings | 3 | 4 | 4 | 4 | 4 | 4 | 4 |
| Bread, cereal, etc., servings | 7 | 10 | 11 | 12 | 15 | 16 | 19 |
| Fat servings | 6 | 6 | 9 | 9 | 9 | 12 | 12 |
| Fruit servings† | 3 | 3 | 3 | 3 | 3 | 3 | 3 |

Vegetables except those grouped with breads and cereals are not limited.

*Source*: Adapted from The Dietary Management of Hyperlipoproteinemia: A Handbook for Physicians and Dietitians [1].
* For 1 oz of meat, fish, or poultry, 8 g protein and 3 g fat have been calculated.
† For ½ cup of any fresh or unsweetened fruit or juice, 10 g carbohydrate has been calculated.

**Sample Menu For 1,500 Kcal Maintenance Diet**

A.M.

4 oz grapefruit juice
2 slices white toast
2 tsp special margarine
1 cup skim milk
Coffee or tea

NOON

½ cup cottage cheese
¼ cup plain tuna on lettuce
½ cup potato salad with 2 tsp mayonnaise
½ cup carrot strips
1 apple
1 cup skim milk
1 fresh roll
Coffee or tea

P.M.

3 oz lean roast lamb, trimmed
1 small boiled potato with parsley and 1 tsp special margarine
½ cup spinach with 1 tsp special margarine
2 slices rye bread
1 orange
1 cup skim milk
Coffee or tea

BETWEEN MEALS

½ cup tomato juice

References
1. Frederickson, D. S.; Levy, R. I.; Jones, E.; Bonnell, M.; and Ernst, N.:   The Dietary Management of Hyperlipoproteinemia:  A Handbook for Physicians and Dietitians. Washington, DC:   Government Printing Office, 1973.
2. Frederickson, D. S.; Levy, R. I.; Bonnell, M.; and Ernst, N.:   Diet 5:  For the Management of Mixed Hyperglyceridemia (Type V Hyperlipoproteinemia). Washington, DC:   Government Printing Office, 1973.
3. Levy, R. I., and Ernst, N.:   Diet, hyperlipidemia and atherosclerosis. Goodhart, R. S., and Shils, M. E., eds.:   Modern Nutrition in Health and Disease. Philadelphia:   Lea & Febiger, 1973.
4. Levy, R. I.; Bonnell, M.; and Ernst, N. D.:   Dietary management of hyperlipoproteinemia.   J. Am. Diet. Assoc. 58: 406, 1971.

# The Composition of the Different Diets Used in the Treatment of Hyperlipidemic States

AMERICAN HEART ASSOCIATION

| Diet designation | | Choles-terol content (mg) | Fat content (% of total kcal) | | | P/S value† | Iodine no.‡ | Carbo-hydrate (% of to-tal kcal) |
|---|---|---|---|---|---|---|---|---|
| | | | Total | Polyun-saturated* | Satu-rated | | | |
| Diet A | Low cholesterol, moderately low fat | 100 | 20 | 8.1 | 5.3 | 1.5 | 96 | 65 |
| Diet B | Low cholesterol, moderately low fat (less restric-tive than Diet A) | 200 | 25 | 8.5 | 6.1 | 1.4 | 92 | 60 |
| Diet C | Low cholesterol, high polyunsatu-rated fat | 200 | 35 | 12.6 | 7.6 | 1.7 | 98 | 48 |
| Diet D | Extremely low fat§ | | 12 | | | | | 68–71 |

*Source:* Adapted from Subcommittee on Diet and Hyperlipidemia, Council on Arterioscle-rosis: A Maximal Approach to the Dietary Treatment of the Hyperlipidemias. Dallas: American Heart Association, 1973.

*Notes:* All diets should be prescribed at the caloric level needed to maintain ideal body weight except as otherwise specified. In all diets the protein content is 15–20% of total kilocalories; the amino acid content more than meets the FAO requirements; the carbohydrate is derived from mixed sources. The diets at eucaloric levels meet the requirements as specified by the National Academy of Sciences—National Research Council: Recommended Dietary Allowances (A Report of the Food and Nutrition Board), 7th ed., Washington, DC, 1968, for all nutrients except that the iron content of all four diets at 2,000 kcal is approximately 4 mg less than the designated 18 mg.

* This is the maximum of polyunsaturated fat that would be included. Unless the use of safflower oil and the most unsaturated margarines is stressed, the patient could select other unsaturated oils and margarines that would lower the polyunsaturated content of the diets.

† The ratio of polyunsaturated to saturated fat in the diet.

‡ The iodine number is similar for all diets because the same fats were used to determine the fatty acid values. The differences in the fat of the diets pertain generally to the amount of fat rather than the kind of fat.

§ The small amount of fat in this diet contains adequate essential fatty acids and also a small quantity of medium chain triglycerides (4% of kilocalories) to enhance palatability. The caloric density of medium chain triglycerides is 8.3 kcal/g.

# Summary: Lipid Lowering Diets

Nutritional intervention is the cornerstone of treatment for primary hyperlipidemia and has met with great success in lowering elevated serum lipid and abnormal serum lipoprotein levels. As a result, a plethora of diets designed to normalize lipid levels and lipoprotein patterns now exists, including (1) The American Heart Association's preventative diet, "The Way to a Man's Heart"; (2) The American Heart Association's therapeutic diets, "Planning Fat Controlled Meals for 1200 and 1800 Calories" and "Planning Fat Controlled Meals for 2000–2600 Calories"; (3) The NIH Heart and Lung Institute's Diets 1 through 5 for the management of types I through V hyperlipoproteinemias; and, finally, (4) The American Heart Association's "A Maximal Approach to the Dietary Management of the Hyperlipidemias, Diets A, B, C and D." The only question that remains is what is the best management and educational vehicle for any particular patient. Despite their similarities in composition and dietary strategies, there are also differences among the diets, which, if left unexplained, may obscure appropriate indications for use and complicate implementation.

The choice of the most appropriate serum lipid lowering diet depends not only upon characteristics of the specific lipid disorder but upon the physician's philosophy, as well as the motivation and learning abilities of the patient. The food lists given on pp. E4–E5 may be used with both the NIH Diets and American Heart Association Fat Controlled Diets. From this base, meal plans and special instructions to the patient can then be individualized by the dietitian to suit differences in diet composition and dietary strategies.

The majority of Americans who are at risk of developing heart disease have milder forms of hyperlipidemia, which are diet induced. For such persons, the initial recommendation might be the American Heart Association's preventative diet. It is the most liberal of all the fat controlled diets, with a P/S ratio of 1.4:1, and is intended for widespread use. In instances where lipid response to this diet is inadequate, classification into one of the five types of hyperlipoproteinemia is in order. An energy restricted diet may also be a frequent first diet prescription, since return to ideal weight of the overweight individual may correct the lipid disorder without further treatment. The NIH diets are strictly therapeutic in nature and not designed for general use as preventative diets.

Among the therapeutic diets the most frequently prescribed are the NIH Diets 2a and 4 and the American Heart Association energy restricted, fat controlled diets. For the person with hypercholesterolemia (type IIa), either the "Planning Fat Controlled Meals" booklets or NIH's Diet 2 is indicated. For the individual with endogenous hypertriglyceridemia (type IV), the NIH Diet 4 is indicated. The Heart Association fat controlled diets cannot be used successfully without further limitations in alcohol and carbohydrate content for persons with types III, IV, or V hyperlipoproteinemia. Sugars must be reduced in the management of patients with these three disorders, as they would otherwise augment the observed elevated serum triglyceride levels.

Hyperchylomicronemia (type I) requires a diet that is low in fat. Since the P/S ratio, or the degree of saturation or unsaturation of the fat, is immaterial here, the American Heart Association fat controlled diets are not appropriate for the management of this disorder. Similarly, persons with mixed hyperglyceridemia (type V) exhibit hyperchylomicronemia or exogenous hypertriglyceridemia (fat induced), as well as endogenous hypertriglyceridemia (carbohydrate induced). They should follow the NIH Diet 5. Individuals with type IIb should begin with NIH Diet 3. If the result is a lessening of triglyceride excess or continued elevation of betalipoproteins, the stricter control of Diet 2 may be indicated.

The most restrictive group in the armamentarium of lipid lowering diets is the American Heart Association's Maximal Approach series of Diets A, B, C, and D. These have not been reproduced here except for a summary of their composition (p. E51). They are designed for a maximal lipid lowering response or for patients who have been unresponsive to other lipid lowering diets. They involve a very restrictive modification of the usual eating habits and are suitable only for highly motivated patients. Diet D is indicated in cases of severe exogenous hypertriglyceridemia or hyperchylomicronemia (type I and type V). It provides only 12% or less of its kilocalories in the form of fat. Diet A contains less than 100 mg cholesterol and a P/S ratio of 1.5. It may be used for highly motivated patients with elevated serum cholesterol levels. Diets B and C contain less than 200 mg cholesterol. The physician may also opt to use these diets if he thinks it advisable to increase polyunsaturated fat to a lesser degree than accompanies the use of other serum cholesterol lowering diets.

**Differences in Diet Composition—American Heart Association Fat Controlled Diets and NIH Diets**

DIETS 1–5 (NIH)

PLANNING FAT CONTROLLED MEALS (AMERICAN HEART ASSOCIATION)

*Fat group*

One serving equals 4.5 g fat
One teaspoon oil equals 1 serving; also, allow the following as 1 serving on only Diets 3, 4, and 5:
1 tbsp commercial salad dressing containing no sour cream
avocado (⅛ of 4″)
1 tsp coarsely chopped nuts
5 small olives
2 tsp peanut butter

*Fat group*

One serving equals 14 g fat
One tablespoon oil equals 1 serving

*Egg yolks*

None permitted on Diets 2 and 3
3 per week allowed on Diet 1 as a substitute for meat
3 per week allowed on Diets 4 and 5, in addition to other meat choices

*Egg yolks*

3 per week permitted in addition to other meal choices

*Meat group*

Calculated using 8 g protein, 3 g fat per ounce of meat, fish, or poultry, except on Diet 2, which uses 8 g protein, 2 g fat for 1 oz meat, fish, or poultry, because of limitation of beef, lamb, and pork to three 3-oz servings weekly

*Meat group*

Calculated using 8 g protein, 2 g fat, because of limitation of beef, lamb, and pork to three 3 oz servings per week

*Bread group*

Calculated using 15 g carbohydrate
2 g protein per serving
1 g fat per serving

*Bread group*

Calculated using 15 g carbohydrate
2 g protein per serving

*Recommended P/S ratio for diets*

1.18:1–2.8:1

*Recommended P/S ratio for diets*

1.4:1 (preventative diets)
2:1–2.8:1 (therapeutic diets) only or 11–13% of kilocalories as polyunsaturated fats, 4–5% of kilocalories as saturated fat

# Diet and Coronary Heart Disease

NUTRITION COMMITTEE, AMERICAN HEART ASSOCIATION

The nature of coronary heart disease is such that prevention is the primary means by which a reduction in morbidity and mortality will be realized. As a consequence, it appears prudent for the American people to follow a diet aimed at lowering serum lipid concentrations. For most individuals, this can be achieved by lowering intake of kilocalories, cholesterol, and saturated fats. There is substantial evidence that the diets recommended in this statement will aid in the control of serum lipid levels in man. Diets similar to those recommended here have been consumed by many persons in the United States for periods of more than 15 years without any evidence of harmful effects. Worldwide population studies have yielded similar findings.

The multifaceted etiology of atherosclerotic coronary heart disease has been amply documented and repeatedly emphasized. The American Heart Association statement on "Risk Factors and Coronary Disease" [1] describes the factors known to be associated with the risk of future coronary disease. The identified risk factors are: hypertension, cigarette smoking, hyperlipidemia, diabetes, obesity, male sex, heredity, advancing age, personality traits and sedentary lifestyle. Many of these risk factors are amenable to change and some (hyperlipidemia, diabetes, obesity) to dietary modification.

In well-documented population studies using standard methods for diet and coronary disease assessment, no population habitually subsisting on a low-fat and cholesterol diet or one that is low in saturated fats and cholesterol has an appreciable amount of coronary disease [2–6]. This evidence suggests that a diet high in saturated fat and/or cholesterol is an important factor for a high incidence of coronary heart disease [2–6]. It is also established that other risk factors such as hypertension and cigarette smoking are contributory causes. These data as well as those from early controlled trials [7–11] provide sufficient evidence to warrant taking prudent action at this time, in the population at large.

This pamphlet addresses the relationship of habitual diet to coronary heart disease and makes appropriate suggestions for dietary modifications. The four previous statements [12] on this subject by the American Heart Association are brought up to date by this report.

A definitive, prospective study of the effect of diet on the prevention of coronary heart disease has not been undertaken although a preliminary feasibility study was completed [13]. In 1971 after thorough study by the National Heart and Lung Institute Task Force on Arteriosclerosis, the decision was made not to conduct a nationwide, controlled diet study because of design and implementation problems. Instead, the National Heart, Lung and Blood Institute is conducting several studies which include dietary alterations. Current knowledge and understanding are based on preliminary reports of these newer studies and on published findings of worldwide epidemiologic studies, studies in selected populations, prolonged treatment of persons who have had myocardial infarctions or elevations in serum cholesterol, and animal studies [2–11,13–24].

It is recognized that the data derived from such investigations do not permit unequivocal conclusions. Nevertheless, the evidence is strong enough to indicate that elevated levels of serum* cholesterol and triglyceride are associated with accelerated rates of atherogenesis. At a serum cholesterol level of 260 mg/100 ml, a level common in American adults, the risk for developing coronary heart disease is about twice that of persons with a serum level of 210 mg/100 ml; at higher serum cholesterol levels, the risk for coronary heart disease is even greater [21,22].

It is urged that determination of fasting serum cholesterol and triglyceride, particularly the former, be made part of all health-maintenance examinations. Abnormalities of serum cholesterol and triglyceride in most individuals can be identified by the analysis of a *fasting* serum sample for these components. If the results indicate either component to be elevated, the test should be repeated before initiating treatment. Lipids are transported in the serum in combination with specific proteins. The triglycerides are present mainly in a very low density lipoprotein fraction (VLDL). Cholesterol is carried mainly in the low density lipoprotein (LDL), with some also present in the high density lipoprotein fraction (HDL). Elevated LDL, and in some cases VLDL, fractions have been associated with an increased incidence of coronary heart disease (CHD). Recent studies suggest that individuals whose HDL cholesterol level is elevated may be less likely to have CHD. Conversely, low HDL cholesterol levels are associated with increased risk of CHD [25,26].

Numerous authoritative scientific nutrition councils stress that the average level of the serum lipids of typical American men and women is undesirably high and that reasonable means should be adopted to modify the conditions that contribute to high serum lipid levels [22,23]. The evidence now available is sufficient to discourage further temporizing with this major national health problem [22,23]. Since dietary modifications do influence serum cholesterol and triglyceride levels, they must be considered important preventive and therapeutic measures [2,3,27]. To be maximally effective for prevention of atherosclerosis, a diet that effects reduction of serum lipids will need to be consumed throughout life, hence it should be palatable, effective, economically feasible, and nutritionally adequate [2,3,27].

Persons who have severe aberrations in serum lipoproteins may require further modification of diet with or without drug therapy [6].

* If analysis is performed on plasma instead of serum, resulting cholesterol measurements will be about 3% lower than the corresponding serum values.

This is a matter for the individual judgment of a physician with the help of a nutritionist or dietitian. Appropriate diets for the management of patients with specific lipoprotein abnormalities based on lipoprotein analysis have been developed and are available from the National Heart, Lung and Blood Institute. However, the majority of blood lipid problems do not require lipoprotein analysis [24]. The American Heart Association [28] and others [29,30] have also recommended further modifications of the basic fat-controlled diet for the management of specific severe problems. The general recommendations given below are intended for the general population and are effective in lowering the lipids of most people [31].

Implementation of these dietary recommendations can be accomplished more easily if suitable food items are readily available. Some food manufacturers and food service establishments have made modifications that are in keeping with these recommendations. However, the effectiveness of these dietary recommendations will be facilitated by the development and distribution of additional foods which have been tested for safety and acceptability. The availability of such foods would make adherence to this diet convenient and attractive.

General Dietary Recommendations

## 1. A Caloric Intake Adjusted to Achieve and Maintain Ideal Body Weight

Obesity, if it occurs in conjunction with hypertension, hyperglycemia, or hypercholesterolemia, significantly increases the risk for coronary heart disease. Correction of obesity often results in reduced serum lipid levels, decreased blood pressure, and improved glucose tolerance [32,33]. Avoidance of obesity, beginning early in life [3,27], or a supervised weight reduction for those above their ideal body weight, is strongly recommended. Moderate exercise often is a useful adjunct in a program for weight control.

## 2. A Reduction in Total Fat Kilocalories Achieved by a Substantial Reduction in Dietary Saturated Fatty Acids

Approximately 40% of the total kilocalories in the American diet are derived from fat. It is desirable to decrease this level to 30%–35%. The proportion of saturated fatty acids in the diet should be brought into proper balance. To this end, the level of saturated fatty acids should be decreased to less than 10% of the total kilocalories [3,22, 23]. This modification is somewhat difficult and usually will require considerable change from the customary dietary pattern. Polyunsaturated fatty acids should supply up to 10% of the total kilocalories, which can be accomplished easily. When these proportions are achieved, the remainder of the ingested fat is derived from monounsaturated sources [34]. The Food and Drug Administration has published regulations allowing manufacturers to state the fat and cholesterol content on the labels of packaged foods [35]. Such labeling is of value to the consumer in making a selection between two products and planning a modification of the total diet. For optimal use of this information better nutrition education is needed.

### 3. A Substantial Reduction in Dietary Cholesterol

Dietary cholesterol is an important contributor to total body cholesterol, although a major portion is endogenously synthesized [36–41]. It is recommended that the average daily intake of cholesterol by adults be less than 300 mg [13,22,23]. For persons with severe hypercholesterolemia, an even greater reduction may be warranted. Since cholesterol is present in most foods from animal sources, care must be taken to assure adequate protein intake if stringent restriction of cholesterol is undertaken. High quality proteins from vegetable sources can be substituted for the reduced animal protein.

### 4. Dietary Carbohydrate

When the proportion of kilocalories from fat in the diet is reduced, the caloric difference will be made up with carbohydrate. Reduction of dietary fat intake to 30–35% of total calories will require a modest increase in carbohydrate which can be derived from vegetables, fruits, and cereals. This substitution may cause a small transient rise in fasting plasma triglyceride of some individuals but it will tend to lower postprandial triglyceride. There are many population groups habitually consuming high carbohydrate diets in whom serum lipids, including triglycerides, are low [5,42–44].

### 5. Dietary Sodium

The increased incidence of coronary heart disease with hypertension is well recognized [45]. A causal relationship in man between sodium intake and hypertension has not been firmly established, but there is increasing evidence that current levels of sodium intake in the U.S. contribute as one of the multiple factors in the etiology of hypertension. Information available to date from human and experimental animal studies suggests that it is prudent to avoid excessive sodium in the diet [46]. In the control of established hypertension, congestive heart failure, or edema, the level of sodium restriction imposed must be determined by the physician and based on the patient's response.

### 6. Other Dietary Factors

Alcoholic beverages can contribute an appreciable quantity of kilocalories to the diet with obesity and hyperlipidemia as possible consequences.

There is great interest in the possible role of other dietary factors (fiber, coffee, trace minerals, hardness of water, vitamins) in the development of coronary heart disease. Available evidence does not permit specific recommendations to be made at this time with regard to these factors. Their role is the subject of continuing review within the American Heart Association and elsewhere.

Conclusion    The development and progression of coronary heart disease is influenced by heredity, environment, and life-style. Among these factors, a diet rich in kilocalories, saturated fat, and cholesterol can contribute to hyperlipidemia and obesity.

There is substantial evidence that the diets recommended here will aid in the control of serum lipid levels in man. Present evidence also suggests that maintaining plasma lipids at reduced levels will lower the incidence of coronary heart disease. Diets similar to those recommended here have been consumed by many persons in the United States for periods of more than 15 years without any evidence of harmful effects. Worldwide population studies have yielded similar findings.

In the application of these recommendations to family groups, any change in the diet must preserve the principles of good nutrition. Although nutritional requirements differ during the various stages of the normal life cycle, the demands for optimal nutrition during periods of growth and development of infants, children, and adolescents, and of pregnancy and lactation, can be met by appropriate modifications of these recommendations. Dietary habits formed during the developing years may continue lifelong and influence the severity of atherosclerosis in later life.

This statement is designed for use by the medical community. A more detailed discussion of this subject is contained in the report of the Inter-Society Commission for Heart Disease Resources [22] and the report of the special Advisory Committee to the National Heart, Lung and Blood Institute [47]. The nature of coronary heart disease is such that prevention is the primary means by which a reduction in morbidity and mortality will be realized. As a consequence, it appears prudent for the American people to follow a diet aimed at lowering serum lipid concentrations. For most individuals, this can be achieved by lowering intake of kilocalories, cholesterol, and saturated fats. Advice by a physician on the importance of diet in coronary heart disease prevention is recommended. This can be augmented by individualized nutrition counseling by a consulting nutritionist (Registered Dietitian). Changes in dietary patterns require education as well as changes in life-style. Opportunity for initial counseling, follow-up guidance, and reinforcement should be provided in order to effect long-term change. The American Heart Association has translated these dietary recommendations into several publications which are available to the general public and to patients through local Heart Associations and the National Office of the American Heart Association.

For patients, on a doctor's prescription only:
"Planning Fat-Controlled Meals for 1200 and 1800 Calories" (50–017–A), "Planning Fat-Controlled Meals for 2000–2600 Calories" (50–017–B), "A Maximal Approach to the Dietary Treatment of the Hyperlipidemias" (70–017–B, C, D, E)

For the general public, no prescription required:
Two companion booklets, "The Way to a Man's Heart" (51–018–A) and "Recipes for Fat-Controlled, Low Cholesterol Meals" (50–020–B)
"Guide for Weight Reduction" (50–034–A)

All of the publications listed above are available to physicians, dietitians, nutritionists, and other related professions.

*This statement was prepared by the Nutrition Committee of the Steer-*

*ing Committee for Medical and Community Program of the American Heart Association. Membership of the Committee at the time this statement was prepared:*

EDWIN L. BIERMAN, M.D. *Chairman*
ROBERT D. CORWIN, M.D.
JOHN W. FARQUHAR, M.D.
JACK C. GEER, M.D.
CHARLES J. GLUECK, M.D.
SCOTT M. GRUNDY, M.D., PH.D.
WILLIAM INSULL, JR., M.D.
LEWIS H. KULLER, M.D.
*Consultants:*
JOHN F. MUELLER, M.D.
ROBERT E. SHANK, M.D.
*Council-Committee Liaison:*
FRED H. MATTSON, PH.D.
CYNTHIA FORD
JOHN D. BRUNZELL, M.D.

References

1. Central Committee for Medical and Community Program, American Heart Association: Risk Factors and Coronary Disease: A Statement for Physicians. New York: American Heart Association, 1968.
2. Connor, W. E., and Connor, S. L.: The key role of nutritional factors in the prevention of coronary heart disease. Prev. Med. 1: 49–83, 1972.
3. Glueck, C. J., and Connor, W. E.: Diet-coronary heart disease relationships reconnoitered. Am. J. Clin. Nutr. 31: 727–737, 1978.
4. Sacks, F. M.; Castelli, W. P.; Donner, A.; et al.: Plasma lipids and lipoproteins in vegetarians and controls. N. Engl. J. Med. 292: 1148–51, 1975.
5. Sinnett, P. F., and Whyte, H. M.: Epidemiological studies in a total highland population, Tukisenta, New Guinea: Cardiovascular disease and relevant clinical, electrocardiographic, radiological, and biochemical findings. J. Chron. Dis. 26: 265–90, 1973.
6. Rifkind, B. M., and Levy, R. I., eds.: Hyperlipidemia: Diagnosis and Therapy. Clinical Cardiology Monographs, New York: Grune & Stratton, 1977.
7. Dayton, S.; Pearce, M. L.; Hashimoto, S.; et al.: A controlled clinical trial of a diet high in unsaturated fat in preventing complications of atherosclerosis. Circulation 40 (Suppl. II): II–I–II–63, 1969.
8. Miettinen, M.; Turpeinen, O.; Karvonen, M. J.; et al.: Effect of cholesterol-lowering diet on mortality from coronary heart disease and other causes: a twelve year clinical trial in men and women. Lancet 2: 835–38, 1972.
9. Leren, P.: The Oslo diet-heart study: eleven-year report. Circulation 42: 935–42, 1970.
10. Bierenbaum, M. L.; Fleischman, A. I.; Green, D. P.; et al.: The 5-year experience of modified fat diets on younger men with coronary heart disease. Circulation 42: 943–52, 1970.
11. Rinzler, S. H.: Primary prevention of coronary heart disease by diet. Bull. NY Acad. Med. 44: 936–49, 1968.
12. Committee on Nutrition, American Heart Association: Diet and Coronary Heart Disease, New York: American Heart Association, 1965, rev. 1968, 1973.
13. The national diet-heart study: final report. National Diet–Heart Study Research Group. Circulation 37 (Suppl. I): I–I–I–428, 1968.
14. Kuller, L. H.: Epidemiology of cardiovascular diseases: current perspectives. Am. J. Epidemiol. 104: 425–56, 1976.
15. Gordon, T., and Kannel, W. B.: Premature mortality from coronary heart disease: the Framingham study. JAMA 215: 1617–25, 1971.
16. Anitschikow, N. N.: A history of experimentation on arterial atherosclerosis in animals. Blumenthal, H. T. ed: Cowdry's Arteriosclerosis: A Survey of the Problem. 2d ed. Springfield: Charles C. Thomas, 1967: 21–44.

17. Zilversmit, D. B.:  Metabolism of arterial lipids. Jones, R. J. ed:  Athero-sclerosis:  Proceedings of the Second International Symposium, New York:  Springer-Verlag, 1970: 35–41.

18. Blankenhorn, D. H.; Brooks, S. H.; Selzer, R. H.; et al.:  The rate of atherosclerosis change during treatment of hyperlipoproteinemia.  Circulation 57: 355–61, 1978.

19. Keys, A., editor:  Coronary heart disease in seven countries.  Circulation 41 (Suppl. I):  I–I–I–211, 1970.

20. Armstrong, M. L.; Warner, E. D.; and Connor, W. E.:  Regression of coronary atheromatosis in rhesus monkeys.  Circ. Res. 27: 59–67, 1970.

21. Kannel, W. B.; Castelli, W. P.; Gordon, T.; et al.:  Serum cholesterol, lipoproteins and the risk of coronary heart disease:  the Framingham study.  Ann. Intern. Med. 74: 1–12, 1971.

22. Primary prevention of the atherosclerotic diseases, Atherosclerosis and Epidemiology study groups of the Inter-society Commission for Heart Disease Resources.  Circulation 42: A55–A95, 1970, rev. 1972.

23. Diet and coronary heart disease:  a council statement. AMA Council on Foods and Nutrition and the Food and Nutrition Board of the National Academy of Sciences—National Research Council.  JAMA 222: 1647, 1972.

24. Levy, R. I.; Fredrickson, D. S.; Shulman, R.; et al.:  Dietary and drug treatment of primary hyperlipoproteinemia.  Ann. Intern. Med. 77: 267–94, 1972.

25. Castelli, W. P.; Doyle, J. T.; Gordon, T.; et al.:  HDL cholesterol and other lipids in coronary heart disease:  the cooperative lipoprotein phenotyping study.  Circulation 55: 767–72, 1977.

26. Glueck, C. J.; Gartside, P.; Fallat, R. W.; et al.:  Longevity syndromes:  familial hypobeta and familial hyperalpha lipoproteinemia.  J. Lab. Clin. Med. 88: 941–57, 1976.

27. Council on Arteriosclerosis, Subcommittee on Diet and Hyperlipidemia, American Heart Association:  A Maximal Approach to the Dietary Treatment of the Hyperlipidemias:  A Manual of Dietary Modifications and Instructions for Patients with Hyperlipidemia as a Prescription from Their Physicians. New York:  American Heart Association, 1973.

28. Glueck, C. J.; McGill, H. C.; Lauer, R. M.; et al.:  The Value and Safety of Diet Modification to Control Hyperlipidemia in Childhood and Adolescence: A Statement for Physicians.  Circulation 58: 381A, 1978.

29. Wilson, W. S.; Hulley, S. B.; Burrows, M. I.; et al.:  Serial lipid and lipoprotein responses to the American Heart Association fat-controlled diet.  Am. J. Med. 51: 491–503, 1971.

30. Hulley, S. B.; Wilson, W. S.; Burrows, M. I.; et al.:  Lipid and lipoprotein responses of hypertriglyceridaemic outpatients to a low-carbohydrate modification of the AHA fat-controlled diet.  Lancet 2: 551–55, 1972.

31. Hall, Y.; Stamler, J.; Cohen, D. B.; et al.:  Effectiveness of a low saturated fat, low cholesterol, weight-reducing diet for the control of hypertriglyceridemia.  Atherosclerosis 16: 389–403, 1972.

32. Bierman, E. L.; Porte, D., Jr.; and Bagdade, J. D.:  Hypertriglyceridemia and glucose intolerance in man. Levine, R., and Pfeiffer, E. F. eds. Hormone and Metabolic Research. Suppl. 2:  Adipose Tissue:  Regulation and Metabolic Functions; B. Jeanrenaud and D. Hepp guest eds. New York:  Academic, 1970: 209–12.

33. Ashley, F. W., and Kannel, W. B.:  Relation of weight change to changes in atherogenic traits: the Framingham study.  J. Chron. Dis. 27: 103–14, 1974.

34. Stamler, J.:  Acute myocardial infarction—progress in primary prevention.  Br. Heart J. 33 (Suppl.):  145–64, 1971.

35. Food and Drug Administration, DHEW:  Regulations for the enforcement of the federal food, drug, and cosmetic act and the fair packaging and labeling act (21 CFR).  Federal Register 38: 2124–37, Jan. 19, 1973.

36. Connor, W. E.:  Dietary sterols: their relationship to atherosclerosis.  J. Am. Diet. Assoc. 52: 202–08, 1968.

37. Frantz, I. D., Jr., and Moore, R. B.:  The sterol hypothesis in atherosclerosis.  Am. J. Med. 46: 684–90, 1969.

38. Borgstrom, B.:  Quantification of cholesterol absorption in man by fecal analysis after the feeding of a single isotope-labeled meal.  J. Lipid Res. 10: 331–37, 1969.

39. Quintao, E.; Grundy, S. M.; and Ahrens, E. H., Jr.:  Effects of dietary cholesterol on the regulation of total body cholesterol in man.  J. Lipid Res. 12: 233–47, 1971.

40. Dietschy, J. M., and Gamel, W. G.: Cholesterol synthesis in the intestine of man: regional differences and control mechanisms. J. Clin. Invest. 50: 872–80, 1971.

41. Mattson, F. H.; Erickson, B. A.; and Kligman, A. M.: Effect of dietary cholesterol on serum cholesterol in man. Am. J. Clin. Nutr. 25: 589–94, 1972.

42. Nestel, P. J.; Carroll, K. F.; and Haverstein, N.: Plasma triglyceride response to carbohydrates, fats, and caloric intake. Metabolism 19: 1–18, 1970.

43. Little, J. A.; Birchwood, B. L.; Simmons, D. A.; et al.: Interrelationship between the kinds of dietary carbohydrate and fat in hyperlipoproteinemic patients. Atherosclerosis 11: 173–81, 1970.

44. Keys, A.: Sucrose in the diet and coronary heart disease. Atherosclerosis 14: 193–202, 1971.

45. Kannel, W. B.; Schwartz, M. J.; and McNamara, P. M.: Blood pressure and risk of coronary heart disease: the Framingham study. Dis. Chest 56: 43–52, 1969.

46. Dahl, L. K.: Salt and hypertension. Am. J. Clin. Nutr. 25: 231–44, 1972.

47. Arteriosclerosis: A Report by the National Heart and Lung Institute Task Force on Arteriosclerosis. Vol. I, DHEW Publ. (NIH) 72–137. U.S. National Institutes of Health, June 1971.

# Long Chain Triglyceride Restricted, Medium Chain Triglyceride Diet

*Medium chain triglycerides (MCT)*    Glycerol esters of medium chain fatty acids or fats composed almost entirely of fatty acids containing eight and ten carbon atoms: i.e., caprylic or octanoic acid ($C_8$) and capric or decanoic acid ($C_{10}$). MCT are liberated from coconut oil by steam hydrolysis and provide 8.3 kcal/g [1].

*Long chain triglycerides (LCT)*    Naturally occurring glycerol esters of long chain fatty acids or fats composed of fatty acids containing twelve or more carbon atoms, mainly lauric ($C_{14}$), palmitic ($C_{16}$), stearic ($C_{18}$), oleic ($C_{18.1}$), and linoleic ($C_{18.2}$) acids.

*LCT restricted, MCT diet*    One based on the use of triglycerides containing mainly octanoic and decanoic acids (MCT), which also limits the intake of fats derived from long chain fatty acids. At least 20% of the total kilocalories and 65% of the fat derived kilocalories are provided in the form of MCT, which are substituted for the long chain fats as a source of kilocalories [2].

*Characteristics of the diet*    No more than 5 oz very lean meat, fish, or poultry is permitted daily. Each ounce of cooked meat is calculated as 8 g protein and 3 g fat. Egg yolks are limited to 3 per week, and 1 egg should be substituted for 1 oz of meat when used. Foods ordinarily prepared with the addition of LCT are prepared using MCT. Skim milk is substituted for whole milk. Supplementary feedings containing MCT may be provided in order that large quantities of MCT need not be consumed at any one meal. The MCT are ingested in the form of an oil that weighs 4.6 g/tsp.

*Purpose of the diet*    Substitution of MCT for a certain amount of LCT has proven to be an effective form of nutritional therapy in a variety of malabsorptive disorders in which long chain fats are poorly digested and absorbed [3]. Fecal fat losses may be reduced while unpleasant symptoms that accompany steatorrhea may be alleviated. In addition, the prompt institution of an LCT restricted MCT diet may also have a beneficial effect on calcium absorption in patients with primary biliary cirrhosis [4].

*Mechanism of effect of MCT*    The nutritional advantages of MCT over LCT in the area of digestion and absorption are related to the following characteristics of MCT as compared to LCT: (1) more soluble in water and in body solutions [2], (2) more easily hydrolyzed despite pancreatic lipase or bile salt deficiencies [5,6], (3) transported without requiring chylomicron formation [5], and (4) transported directly to the liver via the portal vein, bypassing the lymph system [2,5].

*Indications for use*    The LCT restricted MCT diet may be indicated as part of the management of defects in the hydrolysis, absorption, and transport of fat, i.e., disorders involving lymphatic drainage into the abdomen, as well as bile salt and pancreatic lipase deficiencies [3]:

1. MCT may play an integral role in the nutritional care of patients with the following disorders: massive bowel resection [7–9], blind loop syndrome unresponsive to antibiotics [5], abetalipoprotein-emia with steatorrhea [5], chyluria, chylous ascites, intestinal lymphangiectasia [5,10,11], and chylothorax [11,12], hyperchylo-micronemia [3], or type I hyperlipidemia.
2. MCT may be useful as an adjunct to other forms of therapy in: pancreatic deficiency [13], regional enteritis with steatorrhea, ileal disease with steatorrhea [5], primary biliary cirrhosis [4], and, much less frequently, celiac disease, Whipple's disease, and cystic fibrosis [5].
3. MCT feeding may have a beneficial effect on the physiological steatorrhea occurring in certain premature infants, according to one study [14].

***Possible adverse reactions*** There is lack of general agreement on the advisability of using MCT in patients with cirrhosis of the liver. Impaired hepatic clearance of MCT may cause dangerous elevations in serum and cerebrospinal octanoic acid levels that have a narcotic effect [5,14,15]. Caution has been advised in the use of MCT, particularly if the octanoic acid binding capacity has been reduced by hypoproteinemia. However, a more recent study failed to confirm prior observations and suggests that MCT are not clinically contraindicated even in patients with hepatic encephalopathy [15,16].

Ingestion of large amounts of MCT may produce abdominal distension or cramps, nausea, and diarrhea. Symptoms are related to the hyperosmolar load produced by rapid hydrolysis of MCT and possible irritating effects of high levels of free fatty acids in the stomach and intestine [15,17]. Such symptoms are rare at the levels of MCT included in the LCT restricted MCT diet. They can usually be overcome by consuming the MCT containing foods more slowly and by the use of smaller, more frequent meals, which reduce the amount of MCT that must be ingested at any one meal [15,17].

Large amounts of MCT may cause ketosis and caution is advised in the administration of MCT to persons with diabetes, particularly if they are ketosis prone [18]. Such patients may tolerate up to 40 or 50 g MCT daily, but this amount should be given in small, frequent feedings, and the insulin dosage may have to be adjusted [5].

***Contraindications*** An LCT restricted MCT diet may be contra-indicated in cirrhosis of the liver, particularly if associated with hypoproteinemia and shunting, although there is lack of general agreement on this point.

MCT should never be substituted for diagnostic efforts to uncover the underlying cause of the steatorrhea nor for more effective forms of therapy where available, e.g., gluten restriction in celiac disease or antibiotics in Whipple's disease [8,17].

***Suggestions for dietitians*** *Incorporation of MCT into the diet* MCT may be used in the cooking of meats, fish, and poultry in a variety of ways. Although the oil is useful in frying and imparts a golden color to fried foods, it should be used in this manner only if all the oil is removed from the pan and consumed by the patient. It may be utilized as an ingredient in cooking vegetables, seasonings, salad dressings, barbecue sauces, cream sauces made with skim milk, marinades, pie crust, and cakes and cookies made with skim milk and allowed eggs. Considerable time should be allotted while the patient is in the hospital to careful counseling in the principles of the diet and of MCT cookery. Copies of published recipes should be made available to the patient [19–21].

*Use of MCT based supplements and formulas*    Additional MCT may be provided in the form of one or two casein based formulas containing MCT: lactose free Pregestimil,* which contains only monosaccharides as the carbohydrate source, and low lactose Portagen* (less than 0.15% lactose), which contains monosaccharides and disaccharides (see pp. 185–186). Pregestimil is most useful in the nutritional management of infants or those who are intolerant of disaccharides and even minute amounts of lactose.

*Modifications of the basic diet*
The meat allowance can be increased to 7 oz/day if beef, lamb, and pork are restricted to three 3-oz portions weekly. In order to provide for weight maintenance where indicated, kilocalories may be increased by extra servings of such foods as fruits and fat free desserts. If the diet is to be used in treating type I hyperlipidemia, the fat content must be further reduced by eliminating butter and margarine completely.

* Mead Johnson and Co., Evansville, IN 47721.

## Long Chain Triglyceride (LCT) Restricted, Medium Chain Triglyceride (MCT) Diet

| Foods allowed | Foods excluded |
|---|---|
| *Beverages* | *Beverages* |
| Skim milk, cereal beverages, coffee, tea, soft drinks | Whole milk; buttermilk; partially skim milk; light, heavy or sour cream |
| *Breads and bread substitutes* | *Breads and bread substitutes* |
| Hamburger rolls; hard rolls; white, enriched, whole wheat, pumpernickel, or rye bread (bread products contain some LCT but are permitted to add palatability and variety to the diet); cooked or dry cereals; macaroni; noodles; rice; spaghetti | Commercial biscuits, coffeecake, cornbread, crackers, doughnuts, muffins, sweet rolls |
| *Desserts* | *Desserts* |
| Water ices, angel food cake, gelatins, meringues, any made from MCT special recipes, frostings with no fat, fruit whips; mixes only if they contain no LCT | Commercial cakes, pies, cookies, pastries, puddings, and custards |
| *Fats* | *Fats* |
| Butter or margarine in prescribed amounts, gravies made from clear soups and MCT oil | Oils and shortenings of all types, sauces and gravies except those made with MCT oil, commercial salad dressings and mayonnaise, whipped toppings |
| *Fruits* | *Fruits* |
| All except avocado | Avocado |

**Foods allowed**

*Meat and meat substitutes*

Skim milk cottage cheese; egg whites as desired; egg yolks and whole eggs only in prescribed amounts; lean, well trimmed, skinless meat; fish; canned water pack fish; poultry only in prescribed amounts

*Soups*

Fat free broth, bouillon, consommé, fat free vegetable soup, soups made with skim milk

*Vegetables*

All to which no fat is added except MCT

*Miscellaneous*

Pickles, salt, spices, jelly, syrups, sugars; any special recipe for which MCT is substituted for long chain fats; cocoa (limit to 1 tbsp dry cocoa per day)

**Foods excluded**

*Meat and meat substitutes*

Any cheese other than skim milk cottage cheese, fatty meats, fish canned in oil, frankfurters, cold cuts and sausages, whole eggs and egg yolks except as prescribed, goose, duck

*Soups*

Cream soups made from whole milk or soups containing stock from fatty meats

*Vegetables*

Creamed vegetables or those prepared with fats other than MCT added

*Miscellaneous*

Butter, chocolate, coconut, or cream candies; creamed dishes; commercial popcorn; frozen dinners; homemade products containing eggs, whole milk, and fats; mixes for biscuits, muffins, and cake; olives; nuts; commercially fried foods such as potato chips, French fried potatoes, and fried fish

**Daily Food Plan for LCT Restricted, MCT Diet**

APPROXIMATE COMPOSITION

*Kilocalories:* 2,150

*Carbohydrate:* 240 g

*MCT:* 70 g, 68% of fat derived kilocalories
27% of total kilocalories

*LCT:* 30 g, 32% of fat derived kilocalories
12% of total kilocalories

**Sample Menu**

| A.M. | Protein (g) | Fat (g) | Carbohydrate (g) | MCT (g) |
|---|---|---|---|---|
| ½ grapefruit | — | — | 10 | — |
| 1 medium soft cooked egg | 6 | 6 | — | — |
| 2 slices MCT French toast [21] | 13 | 1 | 30 | 28 |
| 2 tbsp maple syrup | — | — | 30 | — |
| Coffee or tea | — | — | — | — |
| 1 tsp sugar | — | — | 5 | — |
| 4 oz skim milk | 4 | — | 6 | — |
| **NOON** | | | | |
| Bouillon with vegetables | 2 | — | 7 | — |
| Turkey sandwich: | | | | |
|   2 oz sliced turkey | 16 | 6 | — | — |
|   2 slices whole wheat bread | 4 | — | 30 | — |
| 1 tsp fortified margarine | — | 4 | — | — |
| Lettuce and tomato salad | — | — | — | — |
| 1 tbsp MCT mayonnaise [21] | — | — | — | 11 |
| 2 MCT drop cookies [19] | 2 | 1 | 18 | 4.3 |
| 1 tsp sugar | — | — | 5 | — |
| Coffee or tea | — | — | — | — |
| 4 oz skim milk | 4 | — | 6 | — |
| **P.M.** | | | | |
| Shrimp creole: | | | | |
|   2 oz shrimp | 16 | 6 | 0 | 0 |
|   1 serving creole sauce | | | | |
|     (½ recipe) [21] | 3 | 1 | 3 | 21 |
| ½ cup steamed rice | 2 | — | 15 | — |
| ½ cup asparagus | — | — | — | — |
| 1 tsp fortified margarine | — | 4 | — | — |
| Green bean and romaine salad | — | — | — | — |
| 1 tbsp MCT celery | | | | |
|   seed dressing [21] | — | — | — | 7 |
| 1 slice enriched white bread | 2 | — | 15 | — |
| 1 medium apple | — | — | 10 | — |
| Coffee or tea | — | — | — | — |
| Sugar | — | — | 5 | — |
| 4 oz skim milk | 4 | — | 6 | — |
| **BETWEEN MEALS** | | | | |
| 4 oz skim milk | 4 | — | 6 | — |
| ⅛ of a 10″ diameter | | | | |
|   angel food cake | 3 | — | 32 | — |
| **Total** | **85** | **29** | **239** | **71** |

**References**

1. Senior, J. R.: Medium Chain Triglycerides. Philadelphia: University of Pennsylvania Press, 1968.
2. Schizas, A. A.; Cremen, J. A.; Larson, E.; and O'Brien, R.: Medium-chain triglycerides—use in food preparation. J. Am. Diet. Assoc. 51: 228, 1967.
3. Hashim, S. A.: Medium-chain triglycerides—clinical and metabolic aspects. J. Am. Diet. Assoc. 51: 221, 1967.
4. Kehayoglou, K.; St. Hadziyannis, S.; Kostamis, P.; and Malamos, B.: The effect of medium chain triglyceride on 47 calcium absorption in patients with primary biliary cirrhosis. Gut 14: 653, 1973.
5. Holt, P.: Medium chain triglycerides. Dis. Month., June 1971.
6. Cohen, M.; Morgan, R. G.; and Hofmann, A. F.: Lipolytic activity of human gastric and duodenal juice against medium and long chain triglycerides. Gastroenterology 60: 1, 1971.
7. Williams, C. N., and Dickson, R. C.: Cholestyramine and medium chain triglyceride in prolonged management of patients subjected to ileal resection or bypass. Can. Med. Assoc. J. 107: 626, 1972.
8. McHardy, G.: Medium chain triglycerides and their applicability to the short bowel syndrome. Halpern, S.; Lukby, A. L.; and Berenson, G. eds. Nutrition and Metabolism in Medical Practice. New York: Futura, 1973.
9. Wright, H. K., and Tilson, M. D.: Postoperative Disorders of the G. I. Tract. New York: Grune & Stratton, 1973.
10. Fried, D.; Gotlieb, A.; and Zaidel, L.: Intractable diarrhea of infancy due to lymphangiectasia. Am. J. Dis. Child. 127: 416, 1974.
11. Tift, W. L., and Lloyd, J. K.: Intestinal lymphangiectasia. Long term results with MCT diet. Arch. Dis. Child. 50: 269, 1975.
12. Gershanik, J. J.; Jonsson, H. T.; Riopek, D. A.; and Packer, R. M.: Dietary management of neonatal chylothorax. Pediatrics 53: 400, 1974.
13. Kosloske, A. M.; Martin, W. W.; and Schubert, W. K.: Management of chylothorax in children by thoracentesis and medium chain triglyceride feedings. J. Pediatr. Surg. 9: 365, 1974.
14. Tantibhedyangkul, P., and Hashin, S. A.: Medium chain triglyceride feeding in premature infants: effects on fat and nitrogen absorption. Pediatrics 55: 359, 1975.
15. Harrison, J. E.; McHattke, J. D.; Ligon, I. R.; Jeejeebhoy, K. N.; and Finlay, J. M.: Effect of medium chain triglyceride on fecal calcium losses in pancreatic insufficiency. Clin. Biochem. 6: 136, 1973.
16. Morgan, M. H.; Bolton, C. H.; Morris, J. S.; and Read, A. E.: Medium chain triglycerides and hepatic encephalopathy. Gut 15: 180, 1974.
17. Greenberger, N. J., and Skilman, T. G.: Medium-chain triglycerides—physiologic considerations and clinical implications. N. Engl. J. Med. 280: 1045, 1969.
18. Gordon, E. E., and Duga, J.: Experimental hyperosmolar response to medium chain triglycerides. Diabetes 24: 301, 1975.
19. Howard, B. D., and Morse, E. H.: Muffins and pastry made with medium chain triglyceride oil. J. Am. Diet. Assoc. 62: 51, 1973.
20. Bowman, F.: MCT cookies, cakes and quick breads; quality and acceptability. J. Am. Diet. Assoc. 62: 180, 1973.
21. Recipes Using MCT Oil and Portagen. Evansville, IN: Mead Johnson, 1970.

# Medium Chain Triglyceride Based Ketogenic Diet

***Definition*** A high fat, low carbohydrate diet that induces ketosis in the body and is based on the use of triglycerides containing mainly octanoic and decanoic acids. It provides approximately 50–70% of the total kilocalories in the form of medium chain triglycerides (MCT), a maximum of 19% from carbohydrate, a maximum of 29% from protein and carbohydrate combined, and a minimum of 11% from fats exclusive of MCT [1].

***Characteristics of the diet*** The use of the American Diabetes Association and American Dietetic Association exchange lists (pp. F20–F25) [2] in the calculating of the meal pattern exclusive of MCT permits greater flexibility and is less time consuming than methods used to calculate traditional ketogenic diets. Accurate weighing of foods served is not necessary, and household measures may be used. The intake of noncaloric fluids need not be restricted.

***Purpose of the diet*** Ketogenic diets have a therapeutic effect on certain epileptic seizures. The aim of the MCT ketogenic diet is to induce and maintain a state of ketosis in the body in order to achieve an anticonvulsant effect. The exact mechanism of the anticonvulsant action of the diet in uncertain [3].

The effectiveness of the diet has been corroborated by more than one group of researchers [3–7]. Complete oxidation of fats is dependent on the presence of a certain amount of glucose precursors. Ketones are produced whenever large amounts of fat are metabolized in the absence of carbohydrate [8–11]. MCT are more ketogenic than equivalent amounts of long chain triglycerides (LCT) [11]. Therefore, a diet based on the use of MCT rather than LCT will maintain ketosis while providing less total fat and more carbohydrate and protein. In addition, somewhat lower levels of serum cholesterol have been reported on the MCT ketogenic diet than on the traditional 3:1 ratio ketogenic diet [1,12].

A ketogenic diet has been recently reported to have been used successfully in the management of pyruvate dehydrogenase deficiency. Higher plasma levels of betahydroxybutyric acid (giving evidence of a greater ketogenic effect) were demonstrated when a ketogenic diet supplemented with MCT was used than when one not so supplemented was used [13]. In another study plasma levels of betahydroxybutyrate and acetoacetate in children maintained on a 3:1 ratio traditional ketogenic diet (87% total fat) were noted to be similar to those in children receiving a 60% MCT diet (72% total fat) [4].

***Indications for use*** The MCT ketogenic diet is prescribed for its anticonvulsant effect. It may be indicated for the control of akinetic and myoclonic seizures in children who are resistant to treatment based on anticonvulsant medications or in whom side effects have developed. The diet is most effective in the young preschool child. Older children respond to the diet with less marked ketonuria [1,3,4] and do not achieve as high levels of serum betahydroxybutyric acid.

*Possible adverse reactions*  Nausea, vomiting, and abdominal cramps are possible side effects of the diet. These effects are probably related to the rapid hydrolysis of MCT and the resulting high concentrations of free fatty acids in the stomach and intestines [14]. Such a hyperosmolar solution can cause an influx of large amounts of fluid, which can be irritating to the bowel. Many of these symptoms can be prevented by eating the MCT containing food slowly. Also, the MCT should never be ingested alone, without the consumption of other foods as well. See LCT restricted MCT diet (pp. E65–E69) for an explanation of other adverse reactions.

*Essential fatty acid deficiency*  Essential fatty acid deficiency has been reported in humans receiving MCT and no source of linoleic acid [15]. Improperly planned MCT ketogenic diets that do not include adequate amounts of food sources of linoleic acid can be expected to have similar effects.

*Effects of the diet*  *Serum lipids*  A slight rise in serum total fatty acids but no elevations of serum cholesterol have been noted [4].

*Effects on blood glucose*  A slight depression in blood glucose levels has been noted, which is not accompanied by clinical hypoglycemia and does not correlate with the anticonvulsant effect.

*A significant anticonvulsant effect*  Clinical evidence of the anticonvulsant effect, including EEG findings, correlates with the degree of elevation of blood levels of the ketone bodies betahydroxybutyrate and acetoacetate [4,6]. A significantly greater proportion of children with mean betahydroxybutyrate levels above 2 mM/litre achieve good to excellent seizure control than do children with mean blood levels of less than 2 mM/litre [4].

*Contraindications*  See LCT restricted MCT diet (pp. E65–E69) for specific contraindications. The diet is of little value in the treatment of grand mal seizures [3].

*Suggestions for dietitians*  MCT can be added to the diet in various ways. They can be utilized in milkshakes and incorporated into casseroles, tomato sauce, pizza, and ice cream with relative ease. They are usually divided into three or four servings, depending on the patient's needs. Some children respond more favorably when a bedtime feeding containing MCT is provided.

*Procedure for calculation of the diet*  The following calculations for a 1–3 year old child weighing 13 kg illustrates the calculation of a typical MCT ketogenic diet:

1. Establish caloric need according to the Recommended Dietary Allowances (pp. I3–I5):
     1,300 kcal

2. Determine amount of MCT oil to be given:  50%–70% of total kilocalories, depending on the amount needed to induce ketosis in the individual child:

   60% of 1,300 = 780 kcal from MCT

   1 g MCT = 8.3 kcal

   780 ÷ 8.3 = approximately 94 g MCT

   15 ml (1 tbsp) MCT = 14 g

   94 ÷ 14 = 6.7 tbsp (6 tbsp +   2 tsp) MCT

3. Determine kilocalories to be provided by foods exclusive of MCT:

   1,300 − 780 = 520 kcal

4. Establish protein intake according to recommended allowance and patient's desires:  at least 23 g protein for a 1–3 year old weighing 13 kg. In this example, protein content was established at 29 g.

   29 × 4 = 116 kcal protein

5. Estimate maximum kilocalories to be given in form of carbohydrate:

   19% of 1,300 = no more than 247 kcal

   247 kcal ÷ 4 = no more than 62 g carbohydrate

   61 × 4 = 244 kcal

6. Estimate maximum kilocalories to be given in form of protein and carbohydrate combined:

   29% of 1,300 = no more than 377 kcal from protein and carbohydrate

   116 + 244 = 360 kcal from protein + carbohydrate

7. Estimate minimum kilocalories to be given in form of fats exclusive of MCT oil:

   11% of 1,300 kcal = at least 143 kcal from other fats

   18 × 9 = 162 kcal fat exclusive of MCT

8. The dietary pattern can be calculated using the exchange lists developed jointly by the American Diabetes Association, the American Dietetic Association, and the U.S. Public Health Service, as shown in table 1.

**Table 1. Diet Exclusive of MCT Oil for a 1–3 Year Old Child**

| Exchange | Amount (exchanges) | *Approximate composition* | | |
|---|---|---|---|---|
| | | Protein | Fat | Carbohydrate |
| Skim milk | 1 ½ | 12 | 0 | 18 |
| Meat, med. fat | 2 | 14 | 10 | 0 |
| Fruit | 1 ½ | 0 | 0 | 15 |
| Bread | 1 ½ | 3 | 0 | 23 |
| Vegetable | 1 | 2 | 0 | 5 |
| Fat | 1 ½ | 0 | 8 | 0 |
| Total | | 31 | 18 | 61 |

*Note*: Kilocalories from foods exclusive of MCT = 530 kcal. Total kilocalories including MCT = 1,302 kcal.

## Suggested Meal Plan and Sample Menu

| *Meal Plan** | *Sample Menu* |
|---|---|
| **A.M.** | |
| ½ medium fat meat exchange | ½ egg scrambled in |
| ½ fat exchange | ½ tsp butter or fortified margarine |
| ½ bread exchange | ¼ cup Cream of Wheat with |
| 1 oz skim milk | 1 oz skim milk |
| 1 fruit exchange | ½ cup orange juice |
| 3 oz skim milk | 3 oz skim milk blenderized with |
| 2 tbsp. (28 g) MCT | 2 tbsp MCT |
| **NOON** | |
| ½ high fat meat exchange | ½ frankfurter |
| ½ bread exchange ⎫ | 4 French fried potato strips |
| ½ fat exchange ⎬ | (½ x ½ x 2 in.) |
| ½ vegetable exchange | Salad with 2 leaves lettuce + ½ tomato + 1 tsp low kilocalorie Italian dressing |
| 3 oz skim milk | 3 oz skim milk blenderized with |
| 2 tbsp (28 g) MCT | 2 tbsp MCT |
| **P.M.** | |
| 1 medium fat meat exchange | 1 oz cooked round steak |
| ½ vegetable exchange | ¼ cup cooked green beans |
| ½ fruit exchange | ½ cup canned unsweetened peaches |
| ½ bread exchange | ½ slice bread |
| ¼ fat exchange | ¼ tsp butter or fortified margarine |
| 3 oz skim milk | 3 oz skim milk blenderized with |
| 2 tbsp (28 g) MCT | 2 tbsp MCT |
| **BEDTIME** | |
| 2 oz skim milk | 2 oz skim milk blenderized with |
| 2 tsp (9.2 g) MCT | 2 tsp MCT |

*Note*: Artificial flavorings, such as strawberry, vanilla, and so forth, may be used if desired. Use a variety that has less than 5 kcal/tsp.
* 1½ medium fat meat exchanges plus ½ high fat meat exchange substituted for 2 medium fat meat exchanges and ¼ tsp butter.

References

1. Signore, J. M.: Ketogenic diet containing medium-chain triglycerides. J. Am. Diet. Assoc. 62: 285, 1973.
2. Meal Planning with Exchange Lists. Chicago: American Dietetic Association, 1976.
3. Huttenlocher, P. R.; Wilbourn, A. J.; and Signore, J. M.: Medium chain triglycerides as a therapy for intractable childhood epilepsy. Neurology 21: 1097, 1971.
4. Huttenlocher, P. R.: Ketonemia and seizures: metabolic and anticonvulsant effects of two ketogenic diets. Pediatr. Res. 10: 536, 1976.
5. Isom, J. B.: Treatment of minor motor seizures. Unpublished paper presented at Annual Meeting, Child Neurology Society, October 10–12, 1974.
6. Stephenson, J. B. P.; House, F. M.; and Stromberg, P.: Medium chain triglycerides in a ketogenic diet. Dev. Med. Child. Neurol. 19: 693, 1977.
7. Berman, W.: Ketogenic diet and clonazepam in the treatment of childhood myoclonic epilepsy. Dev. Med. Child. Neurol. 18: 819, 1976.
8. Aftergood, L., and Alfin-Slater, R. B.: Absorption, digestion and metabolism of lipids. Wohl, M. S., and Goodhart, R. S., eds. Modern Nutrition in Health and Disease. Philadelphia: Lea & Febiger, 1968.
9. Freund, G.: The caloric deficiency hypothesis of ketogenesis tested in man. Metabolism 14: 985, 1965.
10. Freund, G., and Weinsier, R. L.: Standardized ketosis following medium chain triglyceride ingestion. Metabolism 15: 980, 1966.
11. Pi-Sunyer, F. X.; Hashim, S. A.; and Van Itallie, R. B.: Insulin and ketone responses to ingestion of medium and long chain triglycerides in man. Diabetes 18: 96, 1969.
12. Dekaban, A. S.: Plasma lipids in epileptic children treated with the high fat diet. Arch. Neurol. 15: 177, 1966.
13. Falk, R. E.; Cederbaum, S. J.; Blass, J. P.; Gibson, G. E.; Kark, P.; and Carrel, R. E.: Ketonic diet in the management of pyruvate dehydrogenase deficiency. Pediatrics 58: 713, 1976.
14. Greenberger, N. J., and Skillman, T. G.: Medium chain triglycerides—physiologic considerations and clinical implications. N. Engl. J. Med. 280: 1045, 1969.
15. Hirona, H.; Suzuki, H.; Igarashi, Y.; and Koono, T.: Essential fatty acid deficiency induced by total parenteral nutrition and by medium chain triglyceride feeding. Am. J. Clin. Nutr. 30: 1670, 1977.

# Traditional Ketogenic Diet

For those individuals who prefer or are accustomed to a more traditional ketogenic diet or in whom medium chain triglycerides are contraindicated, the following improved ketogenic diet food lists provide another alternative. The diet is initially formulated to provide a ketogenic:antiketogenic ratio of 4:1 and usually liberalized to a 3:1 ratio once ketosis is established [1].

The diet provides no milk and only 65% of the Recommended Dietary Allowance for protein, and it is also inadequate in calcium, B vitamins, and iron.

**Table 1. Equivalent Groups for Traditional Ketogenic Diet**

| Equivalent list | Energy (kcal) | Protein (g) | Fat (g) | Carbohydrate (g) |
|---|---|---|---|---|
| meat | 9 | 1.0 | 0.5 | 0 |
| vegetable A | 5 | 0.2 | 0 | 1.0 |
| vegetable B | 7 | 0.5 | 0 | 1.0 |
| fruit | 4 | 0 | 0 | 1.0 |
| fat | 45 | 0 | 5.0 | 0 |
| whipping cream* | 160 | 1.0 | 17.0 | 1.5 |

*Source*: Reprinted from An improved ketogenic diet for treatment of epilepsy [1].
* At least 32% fat.

**Table 2.   Equivalent Groups of Foods**

| Food | Amount (g) | Food | Amount (g) |
|---|---|---|---|
| MEAT EQUIVALENTS | | Carrots | |
| *One meat equivalent is equal to the weight listed and contains 1 g protein, 0.5 g fat, 9 kcal.* | | Raw | 10 |
| Meat | | Cooked | 15 |
| Lean beef, veal, ham (fresh or smoked), lamb, pork | 3.5 | Celeriac root | 10 |
| Liver—beef, calf, chicken (uncooked) (add 0.5 g fat*) | 5.0 | Celery, raw | 25 |
| Frankfurter (all meat, uncooked) (omit 1.5 g fat*) | 7.5 | Cucumber | 25 |
| Bologna (all meat) (omit 1.0 g fat and 0.3 g carbohydrate*) | 7.5 | Eggplant, cooked | 25 |
| Bacon (omit 1 g fat*) | 3.0 | Green pepper, raw or cooked | 25 |
| Canadian bacon | 3.5 | Kohlrabi, raw or cooked | 15 |
| Beef, dried (uncooked) (add 0.5 g fat*) | 3.0 | Leeks | 10 |
| Poultry | | Okra | |
| Turkey, light or dark meat (add 0.5 g fat*) | 3.0 | Fresh, cooked | 15 |
| Chicken, light or dark meat (add 0.5 g fat*) | 3.5 | Frozen, boiled | 10 |
| Chicken, canned | 4.5 | Onion | |
| Fish | | Raw | 10 |
| Raw | | Cooked | 15 |
| Bass, bluefish, bonito, cod, croaker, flounder, halibut, haddock, lobster, perch, pompano, roe, salmon, shrimp, shad, smelt, snapper, sole, sturgeon, swordfish, tilefish, trout, tuna, whitefish, scallops (add 0.5 g fat*) | 5.0 | Parsnip, cooked | 6 |
| | | Pimiento, canned—solids and liquid | 15 |
| | | Pumpkin | 15 |
| | | Radish | 25 |
| | | Red pepper, raw | 15 |
| Canned | | Rutabagas, raw or cooked | 10 |
| Lobster (add 0.5 g fat*) | 5.0 | Sauerkraut | 25 |
| Salmon | 5.0 | Squash | |
| Tuna, canned in oil, drained | 3.5 | Summer | 25 |
| Crabs, clams (add 0.5 g fat*) | 6.0 | Winter | 10 |
| Shrimp (add 0.5 g fat*) | 4.0 | Tomato | |
| Sardines, canned in brine, mustard or tomato sauce—solids and liquid | 5.0 | Raw, canned, or juice | 25 |
| | | Paste | 6 |
| Smoked | | Puree | 10 |
| Sturgeon (add 0.5 g fat*) | 3.0 | Turnip, boiled | 25 |
| Whitefish (add 0.5 g fat*) | 5.0 | | |
| Salmon | 4.5 | VEGETABLE B EQUIVALENTS | |
| Cheese | | *One vegetable B equivalent is equal to the weight listed and contains 1 g carbohydrate, 0.5 g protein, and 7 kcal.* | |
| American, brick, cheddar, blue, Roquefort, Swiss (omit 0.5 g fat*) | 4.0 | Asparagus—fresh, frozen, or canned, cooked | 25 |
| | | Beet greens, raw or cooked | 25 |
| Cottage cheese, creamed (add 0.5 g fat and omit 0.2 g carbohydrate*) | 7.5 | Broccoli, cooked | 25 |
| Cream cheese (omit 4 g fat and 0.3 g carbohydrate*) | 12.5 | Brussels sprouts | 15 |
| Egg | | Cauliflower | |
| Whole (omit 0.5 g fat*) | 8.0 | Raw | 15 |
| White (add 0.5 g fat*) | 9.0 | Cooked | 25 |
| Yolk (omit 1.5 g fat*) | 6.0 | Endive and escarole | 25 |
| Peanut butter (omit 1.5 g fat and 0.8 g carbohydrate*) | 4.0 | Mustard greens | |
| | | Raw | 15 |
| | | Cooked | 25 |
| VEGETABLE A EQUIVALENTS | | Mushrooms, raw | 25 |
| *One vegetable A equivalent is equal to the weight listed and contains 1 g carbohydrate, 0.2 g protein, and 5 kcal.* | | Mung bean sprouts | 15 |
| | | Spinach, raw or cooked | 25 |
| Beans, green, yellow, or wax—fresh, frozen, or canned, cooked | 15 | Swiss chard | 25 |
| | | Watercress | 25 |
| Beets | | | |
| Canned | 10 | FRUIT EQUIVALENTS | |
| Fresh, cooked | 15 | *One fruit equivalent is equal to the weight listed and contains 1 g carbohydrate and 4 kcal.* | |
| Cabbage | | Acerola | 15 |
| Raw | 15 | Apple | |
| Cooked | 25 | Raw | 6 |

| Food | Amount (g) |
|---|---|
| Apple *(Continued)* | |
|    Juice | 10 |
|    Sauce | 10 |
| Apricots | |
|    Raw | 6 |
|    Canned | 10 |
| Banana, raw | 6 |
| Berries | |
|    Blackberries | |
|       Raw | 6 |
|       Canned | 10 |
|    Blueberries | |
|       Raw | 6 |
|       Canned | 10 |
|    Boysenberries, canned | 10 |
|    Cranberries, raw | 10 |
|    Raspberries | |
|       Raw | 6 |
|       Canned | 10 |
|    Strawberries, raw | 10 |
| Cherries | |
|    Raw | 6 |
|    Canned | 10 |
| Figs, canned | 10 |
| Fruit cocktail, canned | 10 |
| Grapefruit | |
|    Raw | 10 |
|    Juice, canned, fresh, or frozen | 10 |
|    Canned | 15 |
| Grapefruit and orange juice, canned or frozen | 10 |
| Grapes, raw or canned | 6 |
| Guava, raw | 6 |
| Lemon juice, raw or canned | 15 |
| Lime juice, raw or canned | 10 |
| Mango, raw | 6 |
| Melon | |
|    Cantaloupe | 15 |
|    Casaba | 15 |
|    Honeydew | 15 |
|    Watermelon | 15 |
| Nectarine, raw | 6 |
| Orange | |
|    Raw | 10 |
|    Juice, raw, canned, or frozen | 10 |
| Papaya, raw | 10 |
| Peach, raw or canned | 10 |
| Pear | |
|    Raw | 6 |
|    Canned | 10 |
| Pineapple | |
|    Raw | 6 |
|    Canned | 10 |
|    Juice, canned or frozen | 6 |
| Plums | |
|    Raw | 6 |
|    Canned | 10 |
| Prunes, juice | 6 |
| Rhubarb, raw | 25 |
| Tangerine, raw | 10 |

### FAT EQUIVALENTS

*One fat equivalent is equal to the weight listed and contains 5 g fat and 45 kcal.*

| Food | Amount (g) |
|---|---|
| Butter, margarine, cooking fats, chicken fat, lard, salad oils | 5.5 |
| Olives, green (omit 0.5 g protein and 0.5 g carbohydrate*) | 39.5 |
| Olives, mission (omit 1 g carbohydrate*) | 25.0 |
| Avocado (omit 0.5 g protein and 2.0 g carbohydrate*) | 30.5 |
| Almonds, salted, dried, or roasted (omit 1.5 g protein and 1.5 g carbohydrate*) | 9.0 |
| Walnuts (omit 1 g protein and 1 g carbohydrate*) | 8.0 |
| Pecans (omit 0.5 g protein and 1 g carbohydrate*) | 7.0 |

### WHIPPING CREAM EQUIVALENT

*One whipping cream equivalent is equal to 46 g whipping cream and contains 1 g protein, 17 g fat, 1.5 g carbohydrate, and 160 kcal. The whipping cream must contain at least 32% fat.*

### MISCELLANEOUS EQUIVALENTS

*Items in the following list all contain 1 g carbohydrate in the weight listed and varying amounts of protein and fat. If used, they must be calculated in the diet. Kitchen measurements are given as well as weight in grams to determine if a satisfactory amount of food could be used.*

| Food | Amount (g) |
|---|---|
| Quaker Puffed Rice (1 cup = 13 g) | 1.0 |
| Quaker Puffed Wheat (1 cup = 12 g) (0.1 g protein) | 1.0 |
| Cheerios (1 cup = 25 g) (0.1 g protein, 0.1 g fat) | 1.5 |
| Special K Cereal (1 cup = 16 g) (0.2 g protein) | 1.0 |
| Barnum's Animal Crackers (1 cracker = 2 g) (0.1 g fat) | 1.0 |
| Cheese Tid-Bits (10 = 3.5 g) (0.2 g protein, 0.2 g fat) | 2.0 |
| Ritz Cracker (1 = 3.3 g) (0.1 g protein, 0.4 g fat) | 1.5 |
| Pretzels, Veri-Thin (10 = 2.8 g) (0.1 g protein) | 1.0 |
| Popcorn, popped, plain (1 cup = 14 g) (0.1 g protein) | 1.5 |
| Mustard | |
|    Yellow (0.7 g protein, 0.6 g fat) | 15.5 |
|    Brown (1 g protein, 1 g fat) | 19.0 |
| Bran with added sugar and malt extract or added sugar and defatted wheat germ (0.1 g protein) | 1.0 |
| Soybean flour | |
|    Full-fat or high-fat (1 cup = 72 g) (1.0 g protein, 0.5 g fat) | 3.0 |
|    Low-fat or defatted (1.0 g protein) | 2.5 |
| Cocoa (1 level tbsp = 7 g) (0.5 g fat) | 2.0 |
| Catsup | 4.0 |
| Pickles, cucumber—dill or sour (0.3 g protein) | 25.5 |
| Apricot spread, Cellu brand† | 10.0 |
| Blackberry jelly, Cellu brand† | 10.0 |

*Source*: Reprinted from An improved ketogenic diet for treatment of epilepsy [1].
\* For weight of equivalent as listed.

## Table 3. Sample Meal Patterns

| Equivalent list | Number of equivalents | Protein (g) | Fat (g) | Carbohydrate (g) |
|---|---|---|---|---|
| BREAKFAST | | | | |
| Meat | 4 | 4.0 | 2.0 | 0 |
| Fruit | 2 | 0 | 0 | 2.0 |
| Fat | 3 | 0 | 15.0 | 0 |
| Whipping cream | 1 | 1.0 | 17.0 | 1.5 |
| Total | | 5.0 | 34.0 | 3.5 |
| NOON MEAL | | | | |
| Meat | 3 | 3.0 | 1.5 | 0 |
| Vegetable B | 2 | 1.0 | 0 | 2.0 |
| Fat | 2 | 0 | 10.0 | 0 |
| Whipping cream | 1 | 1.0 | 17.0 | 1.5 |
| Total | | 5.0 | 28.5 | 3.5 |
| EVENING MEAL | | | | |
| Meat | 4 | 4.0 | 2.0 | 0 |
| Vegetable A | 1 | 0.2 | 0 | 1.0 |
| Fat | 4 | 0 | 20.0 | 0 |
| Fruit | 1 | 0 | 0 | 1.0 |
| Whipping cream | ¾ | 0.8 | 12.8 | 1.1 |
| Total | | 5.0 | 34.8 | 3.1 |

*Source*: Reprinted from An improved ketogenic diet for treatment of epilepsy [1].

## Table 4. Typical Menus for One Day Using Meal Patterns in Table 3

| Food | Equivalent list | Amount (g) |
|---|---|---|
| BREAKFAST | | |
| Canadian bacon | meat | 14.0 |
| Orange juice | fruit | 20.0 |
| Butter or margarine | fat | 16.5 |
| Whipping cream | whipping cream | 46.0 |
| NOON MEAL | | |
| Frankfurter* | meat | 22.5 |
| Broccoli | vegetable B | 50.0 |
| Butter or margarine | fat | 11.0 |
| Whipping cream | whipping cream | 46.0 |
| EVENING MEAL | | |
| Roast lamb | meat | 14.0 |
| Carrots, cooked | vegetable A | 15.0 |
| Butter | fat | 22.0 |
| Cherries, canned | fruit | 10.0 |
| Whipping cream | whipping cream | 34.5 |

*Source*: An improved ketogenic diet for treatment of epilepsy [1].
* Because frankfurter is used as the meat, fat provided by the fat and whipping cream equivalents is reduced by 4.5 g.

References    1. Lasser, J. L., and Brush, M. K.:  An improved ketogenic diet for treatment of epilepsy.  J. Am. Diet. Assoc. 62: 281, 1973.

# Principles of Nutrition and Dietary Recommendations for Individuals with Diabetes Mellitus: 1979

In 1971, the Committee on Food and Nutrition of the American Diabetes Association published a special report entitled "Principles of Nutrition and Dietary Recommendations for Patients with Diabetes Mellitus." Publication of the report was prompted by new and emerging information regarding the effects of diet on blood glucose concentration in diabetic persons and by information relating aberrations of blood lipid levels, particularly cholesterol, with atherosclerosis in the general population. The present report updates these original principles and recommendations and is based on information accumulated since 1971.*

Principles

(a) For all healthy individuals, nutritional requirements are fundamentally the same, varying primarily in amounts during the various stages of the life cycle. The dietary recommendations for diabetic persons are, in most respects, the same as for non-diabetic persons and are based on sound principles of nutrition [1]. Ordinarily, the nutrient needs of diabetic persons may be met without the use of special "dietetic" or "diabetic" foods.

(b) In insulin-dependent diabetic persons and in some non-insulin dependent persons treated with oral glucose-lowering agents, special precautions regarding amount, distribution, and timing of food intake are required to avoid inordinate swings in blood glucose and potentially dangerous episodes of hypoglycemia.

(c) In non-insulin-dependent, obese, diabetic individuals, a professionally supervised weight control and exercise program with strong reinforcement by qualified health care professionals is of primary importance if long-term change in life style is to be maintained. Maintenance of a normal amount of body fat is the best method of treating this type of diabetes and may help to control the hypertension and hyperlipidemia commonly found in these individuals.

(d) Education of diabetic persons regarding basic nutrition, food selection and preparation, daily food plans, and the nutrient composition of food is the key to achieving an effective meal plan. Each diabetic person should have the opportunity to discuss the reasons for the diet and to set dietary goals with a professional diet counselor working closely with a physician and other health care professionals. This must be a continuing educational process conducted in an understanding and non-judgmental manner, in which psychologic, physical, and socioeconomic factors are considered in developing each individual's daily food plan. The use of "pre-printed handout" diet plans will not achieve these objectives and is strongly discouraged.

Reprinted from J. Am. Diet. Assoc. 75: 527, 1979.

* Prepared by Frank Q. Nuttall, M.D., PH.D., and John D. Brunzell, M.D. This report has been reviewed and approved by the American Diabetes Association's Committee on Food and Nutrition.

(e) Dietary recommendations should be as flexible as possible. The widest possible options in food choices and distribution of food intake should be given, consistent with fundamentals of good nutrition and with the approval of the attending physician. The personality, life style, and physical conditioning of the diabetic person should be considered. A flexible meal plan may be more practical and more acceptable for less compulsive persons, while a rigid dietary regimen may be suitable for compulsive persons. It is imperative that an appropriate family member also understand and be able to implement the diabetic person's daily meal plan, should this be necessary. Every effort should also be made to work with family members so that the meal plan neither creates conflicts within the family nor disrupts usual family activities.

(f) Insulin-dependent diabetic persons may find it easier to adapt their insulin regimens than to change basic eating habits. A suitable meal plan acceptable to these individuals should be identified and the insulin treatment integrated with the dietary program.

## Goals of Diet Therapy for Individuals with Diabetes Mellitus

(a) Improve the overall health of the patient by attaining and maintaining optimum nutrition.

(b) Attain and/or maintain an ideal body weight.

(c) Provide for normal physical growth in the child; provide for adequate nutrition for the pregnant woman and hence for her fetus; provide adequate nutrition for lactation needs if she chooses to breast-feed her infant.

(d) Maintain plasma glucose as near the normal physiologic range as possible.

(e) Prevent and/or delay the development and/or progression of cardiovascular, renal, retinal, neurologic, and other complications associated with diabetes, insofar as these are related to metabolic control.

(f) Modify the diet as necessary for complications of diabetes and for associated diseases.

(g) Make the dietary prescription as attractive and realistic as possible. Provide each patient with an individualized educational and follow-up program. Repeat visits serve to extend and clarify the instruction, to provide assurance, and to check progress.

Diabetes now appears to represent a number of different diseases, all of which are characterized by an abnormally high circulating blood glucose concentration. The two principal clinical categories of diabetes are the insulin-dependent (usually thin or normal weight, ketosis-prone) and the non-insulin-dependent, obese subtype† (usually ketosis-resistant).

In each category, dietary management plays a primary role in control of the blood glucose concentration.

In the discussion that follows, dietary management in general is considered as well as the special requirements of persons within these two major categories of diabetes.

† In the proposed classification of idiopathic diabetes recommended by the National Diabetes Data Group, National Institutes of Health, this type of diabetes would be Class IIb.

General Considerations    (a) Although it is not certain that restriction of dietary saturated fat and cholesterol and replacement with unsaturated fat will slow the progression of atherosclerosis, it is a reasonable expectation. Therefore, dietary sources of fat that are high in saturated fatty acids and foods containing cholesterol should be restricted.

(b) There is evidence suggesting that dietary fiber may be important in preventing some colon abnormalities and, possibly, colon carcinoma. It has also been reported to lower post-meal plasma glucose in diabetic persons. Although the long-term effects of dietary fiber in diabetic persons are unknown, it seems reasonable to estimate the amount of food fiber in any given diet. Wherever acceptable to the patient, natural foods containing unrefined carbohydrate with fiber should be substituted for highly refined carbohydrates which are low in fiber. Changes in fiber content of the diet should be brought to the physician's attention, since they may change insulin requirements.

(c) All nutritionally imbalanced ("fad") diets should be avoided. In particular, commercially available, high-protein mixtures that contain low quality protein for use in modified starvation diets should be avoided. Prolonged use of these products has been associated with death from cardiac arrhythmias.

(d) Lacto and lacto-ovo vegetarian diets can be nutritionally adequate. But if one or both of these food groups is also omitted, nutritional adequacy is jeopardized. It may be necessary to provide iron, calcium, zinc, iodine, and vitamin D. Pure vegetarian diets will need to be supplemented with vitamin $B_{12}$ and perhaps iron and calcium.

(e) In general, the average American eats more salt (NaCl) than is necessary or desirable. In some cases, prolonged use of excessive amounts may lead to hypertension. Modest restriction of salt intake should be considered in well controlled, diabetic persons without other medical problems. It should also be considered in the treatment of diabetic persons with hypertension. However, this decision should be made only by the attending physician and only after a thorough consideration of the individual's needs. For example, in poorly controlled persons or in those with renin-angiotensin-aldosterone insufficiency, sodium restriction could be harmful.

(f) The amounts of fructose, xylitol, sorbitol, and mannitol acceptable in a food plan for diabetic persons is uncertain at present. In normal individuals, they induce only a modest rise in plasma glucose concentration. However, their long-term effects on plasma glucose control and on metabolism in diabetic individuals have not been well studied. At present, there is not enough evidence either to accept or to reject the use of these nutritive sweeteners by diabetic persons. This is also the status of available non-nutritive sweeteners.

(g) With the approval of the responsible physician, alcoholic beverages in prescribed amounts may be consumed by diabetic persons. The type and quantity of calories present should be counted and included in the dietary plan, as with other foods. The caloric value of alcohol is approximately 7 kcal/g, but it has no other nutritional value. Its metabolic fate is similar to fats.

Special Dietary Considerations in Insulin-Dependent Diabetic Persons

Diet is important in control of plasma glucose abnormalities and prevention of hypoglycemia. Whether it plays a role in preventing or delaying the development of neuropathy, microvascular disease, or atherosclerosis in these patients is uncertain. Nevertheless, effective insulin treatment requires a standardized daily regimen of food intake. The following variables must be considered when planning a diet for these individuals: (a) the timing of meals, (b) diet composition, (c) energy content of the diet, and (d) level of physical activity.

### REGULARITY OF MEALS

The time of day at which meals are taken and the number of meals eaten each day should be dictated by individual needs, i.e., life style, physical activity, and administered insulin. In persons taking insulin, regularity of food intake is particularly important in maintaining good metabolic management. The need for maintenance of a regular eating and exercise pattern should be strongly emphasized in all diabetic persons receiving insulin or oral glucose-lowering agents. Vigorous exercise is seldom contraindicated in these individuals. With improved use of glucose by the exercising muscles and a more rapid rate of insulin release into the blood, an increase in food or a decrease in insulin dosage may be indicated. If vigorous physical activity is known to induce hypoglycemia, ingestion of a carbohydrate-rich snack just prior to the exercise period often is the simplest means of avoiding a hypoglycemic reaction.

### DIET COMPOSITION

For most insulin-dependent diabetic persons, a nutritionally adequate diet is satisfactory, with the exception that the amounts of glucose and glucose-containing disaccharides (sucrose, lactose) are restricted, particularly when added to the usual caloric intake. Protein of appropriately good quality should account for 12 to 20% of total energy intake. Carbohydrate should usually account for 50 to 60% of total energy intake, and fat should make up the difference. The level of saturated fatty acids in the diet should be decreased to less than 10% of total calories; polyunsaturated fatty acids should supply up to 10% of total calories, and the remainder of ingested fat is derived from monounsaturated sources.

The above percentages are general recommendations and not rigid requirements. It is more appropriate to adapt the dietary plan to the individual's usual diet, provided it meets the nutritional needs of that individual. Day-to-day consistency in amounts and distribution of carbohydrates, fat, and protein should be a major goal. If the only diet acceptable to the patient is unusual in content or daily caloric distribution or if dietary consistency is not possible, communication among the patient, diet counselor, and physician is imperative.

### ENERGY CONTENT

Since the majority of insulin-dependent diabetic persons are thin when first diagnosed, a diet adequate in energy for normal growth and development in children and for attainment of a desirable body weight in adults should be a major goal. Special attention should be given to the nutritional needs of the pregnant diabetic woman to insure normal growth and development of the fetus.

Standardization of total daily energy intake for each meal should be emphasized to the patient and reinforced with each visit to the diet counselor. If the patient is taking two to three injections of short-acting insulin daily, or using short-acting insulin as a supplement to the longer-acting insulins, greater flexibility in meals may be allowed by adjustment of insulin dosage. However, this decision must be made by the patient's physician. Variations in exercise patterns that require adjustments in food intake also should be brought to the attention of the physician and should be thoroughly explained to the patient.

Special Dietary Considerations in Obese, Non-Insulin-Dependent Diabetic Persons

In epidemiologic studies, obesity is almost invariably associated with the expression of diabetes in a variety of populations. It has long been known that weight reduction in obese persons reduces hyperglycemia, hyperlipidemia, and elevated blood pressure, factors associated with an increased risk for atherosclerosis. Therefore, the single most important objective in dietary management of the obese, non-insulin-dependent diabetic person is to achieve and maintain a desirable body weight. This can be accomplished only by a reduction in total energy intake to levels below energy expenditure. With weight loss and successful maintenance of that weight loss, glucose tolerance in many patients returns to or toward normal, and they no longer need to be treated with insulin or oral glucose-lowering agents. This often occurs even before achievement of desirable weight and is frequently an encouragement to the patient. A supervised weight reducing program with on-going support by health care professionals functioning as a team is of primary importance. However, the results of attempted weight control in this manner are not necessarily better in the diabetic than in the non-diabetic obese population. Therefore, the pragmatic physician will not delay introducing other modalities of treatment, if deemed necessary.

DIET COMPOSITION

The macronutrient composition of the diet of the non-insulin-dependent, obese diabetic person is less important than in the insulin-dependent diabetic person. The diet should provide adequate nutrients. For weight reduction, the diet should be nutritionally adequate for that individual, but calories should be restricted. During a severe weight reduction regimen, vitamin and mineral supplements may be required. Such supplements may be appropriate for adults consuming fewer than 1,000 to 1,200 kcal/day. Diets below 1,500 kcal should be evaluated for nutritional adequacy.

REGULARITY OF MEALS

In the obese, non-insulin-dependent diabetic person treated with insulin or oral glucose-lowering agents, regularity of meals and the relationship of meals to physical activity may be important, just as it is in the ketosis-prone diabetic individual. In the obese diabetic person not receiving insulin or oral glucose-lowering agents, this requirement is less important than decreased caloric, but an otherwise nutritionally adequate, intake.

Individualization of the Meal Plan

The above recommendations are generalizations applicable to most persons with diabetes. However, individualization of treatment in relation to the ethnic background, previous dietary habits, and specific metabolic abnormalities and complications associated with the diabetic state of each patient must be emphasized. An appropriate dietary recommendation also presupposes prior diagnostic evaluation by a physician for conditions that may influence diet.

Summary

The need for essential basic nutrients is the same for all persons of equivalent age, sex, and size, whether diabetic or not. For persons with diabetes treated with insulin or oral glucose-lowering agents, special precautions regarding kinds, amounts, distribution, and timing of food intake are required. In general, some liberalization in carbohydrate intake is recommended, preferably as complex carbohydrate (starch associated with fiber) and as a replacement for some of the fat. This does not imply that unlimited ingestion of carbohydrate, particularly as sugars, is advocated. A regimen of insulin, diet, and exercise should be designed that takes into consideration, when feasible, the food preferences and eating habits of that individual.

Therapy for the obese, non-insulin-dependent diabetic person is based primarily on weight control. Although compliance with such regimens may be difficult, special attention on the part of health care professionals working as a team can yield encouraging results.

It is recognized that the field of nutrition is a dynamic science. As new facts emerge and concepts change, the nutritional recommendations for diabetic and non-diabetic persons will continue to undergo evolution and modification. However, with the information now available, it is possible to make the diet for individuals with diabetes more flexible and compatible with usual American life styles. It is hoped it will also lead to improved health and life expectancy.

COMMITTEE ON FOOD AND NUTRITION OF THE AMERICAN DIABETES ASSOCIATION

RONALD A. ARKY, M.D., *Co-Chairman*
FRANK Q. NUTTALL, M.D., PH.D., *Co-Chairman*
BURNESS G. WENBERG, R.D., *Vice-Chairman*
MARIA ALOGNA, R.N.
JAMES W. ANDERSON, M.D.
DOLLY AUSTIN, R.D.
DIANA CAMACHO, R.D.
BETTY ANN CLAMP, R.D.
PHYLLIS CRAPO, R.D.
ALBERT B. EISENSTEIN, M.D.
STEVEN G. GABBE, M.D.
MILDRED KAUFMAN, R.D.

ERROLL B. MARLISS, M.D.
WENDY R. MIDGLEY, R.D.
JERROLD N. OLEFSKY, M.D.
BARBARA PRATER, R.D.
DOROTHEA F. TURNER, R.D.
BETTY WEDMAN, R.D.

References    1. Food and Nutrition Board:  Recommended Dietary Allowances. 8th rev. ed. Washington, DC:  National Academy of Sciences, 1974.

# Kilocalorie, Protein, Fat, and Carbohydrate Controlled Diets

***Definition*** A diet in which the dietary intake is carefully controlled from day to day; it implies assurance that total amounts do not increase caloric consumption above the optimum level, as well as appropriate consistency in the timing, division amounts, and characteristics of carbohydrate (sugar vs. starch) consumed [1].

***Characteristics of the diet*** The diet includes a variety of many different foods from the normal diet that have been incorporated into the current lists by the American Diabetes Association, the American Dietetic Association, and the National Institutes of Health [2]. The foods within each group in the amounts listed are approximately equal in their protein, fat, and carbohydrate content. In general, diets for persons with diabetes need not be disproportionately restricted in carbohydrate [3]. The daily carbohydrate intake should approximate the average consumption in the United States (50% of total kilocalories) and may be even higher without provoking ill effects [3–7]. Concentrated sugars and sweets that are rapidly absorbed, such as candies, frostings, syrups, sugar, jellies, etc., should be avoided because they result in a greater and more immediate glucose response than calorically equivalent amounts of certain complex starches [8,9].

***Purpose of the diet*** (1) To attain and maintain ideal body weight [10]; (2) to meet individual nutritional needs for essential nutrients; (3) to facilitate normal growth and development in the juvenile patient with diabetes [11] and in the developing fetus of a pregnant woman with diabetes [12]; (4) to minimize glycosuria [13] and maintain serum glucose levels as close to physiological levels as possible, in order to avoid metabolic derangements such as ketoacidosis, severe hyperglycemia, severe glycosuria, or hypoglycemia [4,14,15]; and (5) to reduce elevated serum lipid levels that are associated with glucose intolerance [10] and cardiovascular complications of diabetes [3]. In the pregnant woman with diabetes, the diet should provide additional protein for growth and development of the fetus. It should be carefully controlled and designed to avoid even mild degrees of hyperglycemia, which are associated with an increased risk of fetal complications [12].

Diabetes is a genetic disease involving either a relative lack or an absolute lack of functioning insulin secretion by the beta cells of the pancreas; hyperglycemia and a specific form of microangiopathy, which entails a thickening of the basement membranes of almost every capillary in the body, ultimately results [16]. Insulin deficiency causes a secondary defect—the inability to inhibit release of the hormone glucagon, which also contributes to diabetic hyperglycemia [17–20] and worsens the consequences of insulin lack [21,22]. Symptomology, pathology, complications, treatment, theories of etiology, and promising new approaches to treatment, such as the artificial pancreas and islet cell transplants, have been outlined in detail in other publications [23–58].

Increase of dietary carbohydrate, even to extremes, without increase of total kilocalories, does not appear to increase insulin requirements in the insulin treated patient with diabetes [3,4]. Under certain conditions, in mild diabetes, a high carbohydrate diet may actually improve glucose tolerance [1,5,52,53,59]. In addition, a liberalized carbohydrate intake may facilitate a decreased intake of fat and cholesterol and permit lowering of elevated serum lipid levels [60].

***Effects of the diet*** A large percentage of persons with maturity onset of diabetes are obese [15]. Weight reduction has a very beneficial effect and may be all that is required to achieve control in mild cases of the adult onset type [15,46–48].

Dietary treatment alone may improve glucose tolerance in certain patients with mild cases of the disorder [46]. According to one point of view, a combination of certain oral hypoglycemic agents and dietary treatment is no more effective in prolonging the life of a diabetic than effective dietary therapy alone [1,23,47,49,50]. Oral hypoglycemic agents are contraindicated in certain situations such as coronary artery disease or liver or kidney disease. Their use is controversial in all persons with diabetes, and one of them, Fenformin, has been banned by the Food and Drug Administration [61].

Plasma lipids are often elevated in diabetes. Strict control of blood sugar is also very important in managing hyperlipidemia [62]. A fat controlled diet has been shown to reduce significantly the incidence of hyperlipoproteinemia more effectively than control of blood sugar levels alone [63]. The effectiveness of diet in altering the incidence of cardiovascular complications of diabetes has yet to be determined [51].

The normal hemoglobin variant $A_{1c}$ is increased in hyperglycemia, and its concentration in persons with diabetes is correlated with the degree of control of the disease. It can be expected, therefore, that dietary noncompliance will be associated with a rise in serum levels of hemoglobin $A_{1c}$, while dietary adherence is associated with a decrease in serum triglyceride levels as well as a decrease in serum hemoglobin $A_{1c}$ levels [64,65].

Additional research needs to be done on the specific effects of individual carbohydrates on glucose tolerance. Preliminary studies indicate that diets high in guar or pectin have a beneficial effect on carbohydrate tolerance [66].

***Indications for use*** Diet therapy is indicated as soon as a diagnosis of diabetes mellitus has been made by (1) fasting hyperglycemia (whole venous blood glucose levels above 120 mg/100 ml) [67], or (2) an abnormal response to the glucose tolerance test. In the latter, glucose levels as determined 1 hour after a glucose load should not be higher than the following age adjusted levels, according to one author [16]:

Age 30–39 years—261 mg/100 ml
Age 40–49 years—274 mg/100 ml
Age 50–59 years—288 mg/100 ml
Age 60–69 years—300 mg/100 ml

Yet another interpretation of an abnormal response as determined 2 hours after a glucose load is as follows [68]:

Age 30–39 years—140 mg/100 ml
Age 40–49 years—150 mg/100 ml
Age 50–59 years—160 mg/100 ml
Age 60–69 years—300 mg/100 ml

In the severely obese patient in whom clinical determinations are borderline or in whom results are equivocal, weight reduction through kilocalorie control should not await positive confirmation of the diagnosis.

***Possible adverse reactions*** The value of a fixed caloric intake and a food exchange system for achieving it has been questioned for young persons with diabetes on a fixed dose of insulin. It is argued that externally imposed rigid diabetic diets have adverse emotional and physical effects in certain patients. The combination of an inflexible insulin dose and a fixed kilocalorie intake may provoke hypoglycemic episodes in response to variations in work, play, and exercise in the young person with diabetes. Prolonged hypoglycemia may lead to permanent neuromotor deficits in children [51]. A liberalized version of the diet is thought by some to be a more rational alternative to traditionally rigid diets for the young with diabetes [37,51].

Such a diet should be designed to meet the specific nutritional needs of the patient, avoid concentrated sweets, and achieve regularity and day to day consistency in meals, without unduly sacrificing the flexibility to respond to sudden changes in needs. It should also aid in the achievement of metabolic control and prevent obesity and hyperlipidemia [65]. A recent statement by the American Diabetes Association, which reviewed the evidence linking poor diabetic control to the incidence of diabetic complications, concluded that control of blood glucose should be aimed for even in children, and thus the burden of proof should be on those who advocate a more liberal approach [69].

***Contraindications*** As noted previously, although overall nutritional management should be part of the program of therapy for the young person with diabetes, once good control is established, and the patient has attained ideal body weight and is growing and developing satisfactorily, a normal diet that allows some flexibility may be more beneficial than one that is dependent on inflexible and absolute daily intakes of protein, fat, carbohydrate, and kilocalories [37,51].

***Suggestions for dietitians*** Spacing of meals should reflect the type and action of insulin used [70]. For example, a person receiving NPH insulin before breakfast should receive an afternoon and evening snack, each providing approximately $1/10$ of the day's carbohydrate and caloric intake, in order to avoid hypoglycemia during the peak periods of insulin activity.

Liquid medicinals often have sugar added to them and when prescribed in large amounts may contribute significantly to the intake of carbohydrates. An excellent table of sugar content of liquid medicinals has been published, which is useful in assessing the patient's true carbohydrate intake [71].

Despite the obvious benefits to be derived from dietary management in many patients with diabetes, attempts at achieving dietary adherence and regulation are associated with a high degree of failure [1]. Confusion as to the dietary goals, strategies, and priorities is listed as among one of several deterrents to successful nutritional management in one excellent paper [1]. Among other problems in persons with diabetes that make dietary treatment a formidable challenge are the tendency for the disease to manifest itself at emotionally critical periods of puberty and middle age and the psychological meaning of various foods for certain patients [72]. Several new teaching aids and techniques have recently emerged that may be useful in promoting dietary compliance, such as simplified meal planning charts [73], interdisciplinary group classes [74,75], expanded exchange lists for commercial and convenience foods, and specialized cookbooks [76,77].

The composition of certain foods differs from one locale to the next. The exchange lists should be supplemented by regional lists of ethnic and convenience foods compiled by groups of dietitians working within their own areas.

Limited use of sorbitol and fructose as sweeteners is acceptable and may be advantageous in certain persons with diabetes, as they produce a lessened postprandial hyperglycemia [78]. The American Diabetes Association has concluded that there is insufficient evidence to warrant a ban on saccharin use but recommends it be used in prudent amounts by pregnant women and children [79]. Overall, however, users of artificial sweeteners as a group have little or no excess risk of cancer of the lower urinary tract [80].

Educational programs for persons with diabetes should incorporate the latest techniques of nutritional care planning and should be formulated with provisions for periodic evaluations of patient compliance and degree of learning achieved. Guidelines for evaluation of patient education programs have been published [81,82].

**Checklist for Diabetic Dietary Prescription**

1. *In order of priority*, what are the main general purposes (not strategies or methods) of this patient's prescription?
2. How much does the patient weigh? How much do the doctor, dietitian, and patient think he (she) should weigh? How much would the patient *like* to weigh?
3. What is the appropriate level of caloric consumption for this patient?
4. Does the patient require insulin? If so, is the blood glucose level relatively stable, moderately labile, or severely labile? What kind of insulin is to be given? At what time? In what amount?
5. What and when and how much would the patient *like* to eat if he (she) did not have diabetes? Are there any special considerations relating to economic factors or to family or cultural dietary propensities?
6. Is the level of carbohydrate to be limited? To what level or range? To what extent and under what conditions, if any, are concentrated carbohydrates to be used?
7. Are there any special requirements concerning levels of protein?
8. Are there any specific or general requirements with respect to levels of dietary fat, either saturated or unsaturated?
9. How much alcohol is to be permitted? Under what conditions? Should alcohol be exchanged for food? If so, what kind and in what amount?
10. If time distribution of food is of any importance, are there specific requirements concerning (a) the relative size and timing of each of the three main meals or (b) the timing, size, and characteristics of any extra feedings?
11. To what degree is day-to-day consistency required in (a) total kilocalories and (b) size and characteristics of specific feedings such as lunch?

12. Are dietary adjustments to be made for exercise or marked glycosuria? Of what nature?
13. Are there any special conditions unrelated to diabetes requiring special diet (e.g., gout, hyperlipidemia, renal or cardiac failure)?
14. Can all elements of the prescription be reconciled, and how should this be done? (For example, it is usually not feasible to construct a palatable diet for a lean diabetic if the prescription restricts both carbohydrate and fat.)
15. What kinds and degrees of changes are to be made subsequently by the dietitian without consulting the physician?
16. What should this patient do if he (she) finds it necessary to postpone or modify a meal (e.g., when attending a dinner meeting or social affair)? How should he (she) adjust diet if appetite fails (e.g., during illness)?
17. Tactical questions: (a) How much precision is required in the various elements of this prescription? (b) What foods can be freely allowed? (c) What foods, if any, are to be weighed or measured? (d) Are any modifications of the standard exchange system appropriate, such as simplification? (e) In general, is food to be unmeasured, estimated, measured, or weighed? (f) Is it necessary or desirable to teach this patient the carbohydrate, protein, and fat content of the common foods? (g) Under what circumstances are artificial sweeteners and diet drinks to be used?
18. Has this patient's understanding of dietary principles and methods been systematically evaluated?

*Source*:    Adapted from Diet and diabetes [79].

**Dietary Strategies for Patients with the Two Main Types of Diabetes**

| *Strategy* | *Obese diabetics who do not require insulin* | *Nonobese, insulin-dependent diabetics* |
|---|---|---|
| 1. Decrease number of kilocalories | Yes | No |
| 2. Protect or improve pancreatic beta-cell function | Very urgent priority | Seldom important because beta cells are usually extinct |
| 3. Increase frequency and number of feedings | Usually no* | Yes |
| 4. Maintain day-to-day consistency of intake of kilocalories, carbohydrate, protein, and fat | Not crucial if average caloric intake remains in low range | Very important |
| 5. Maintain day-to-day consistency of ratios of carbohydrate, protein and fat for each of the feedings† | Not crucial | Desirable |
| 6. Time meals consistently | Not crucial | Very important |
| 7. Allow extra food for unusual exercise | Not usually appropriate | Usually appropriate |
| 8. Use food to treat, abort, or prevent hypoglycemia | Not necessary | Important |
| 9. During complicating illness, provide small frequent feedings or give carbohydrate intravenously to prevent starvation ketosis | Often not necessary because of resistance to ketosis | Important |

*(See following page for source and notes)*

**Dietary Strategies for Patients with Two Main Types of Diabetes** *(Continued)*

*Source*: Adapted from Diet and diabetes [79].

\* There are some theoretical advantages in dividing the diet into four or five feedings even in mild diabetes *if* this can be done without increasing caloric consumption. However, because limitation of kilocalories has highest priority in obese diabetics, there are some potential disadvantages in providing extra feedings. Giving fat people an opportunity to eat at bedtime is particularly risky if weight reduction is the prime goal.

† The total daily insulin requirement is not much affected when the dietary constituents are changed *under isocaloric conditions*. But insulin requirement *immediately* after a high-carbohydrate meal is higher than it is immediately after a low-carbohydrate meal, even if the meal is isocaloric.

## Insulin Preparations Commercially Available in the United States, Classified According to Approximate Duration of Action

| Classification | Insulin preparation* | | Action | | |
|---|---|---|---|---|---|
| | | | *Onset* | *Peak* | *Duration* |
| Rapid | Regular (neutral) | IV:† | immediate | 15–30 min | 1–2 hr |
| | | IM: | 5–30 min | 30–60 min | 2–4 hr |
| | | SC: | 30 min | 1–2 hr | 5–10 hr |
| | Semilente (insulin zinc suspension prompt) | SC: | 1 hr | 3–4 hr | 10–16 hr |
| Intermediate | Globin zinc insulin | SC: | 2 hr | 6–8 hr | 12–18 hr |
| | NPH (isophane insulin suspension) | SC: | 2 hr | 8–14 hr | 18–24 hr |
| | Lente (insulin zinc suspension) | SC: | 2 hr | 8–14 hr | 18–24 hr |
| Slow | Protamine zinc insulin suspension | SC: | 6 hr | 16–20 hr | 24–30 hr |
| | Ultralente (insulin zinc suspension extended) | SC: | 6 hr | 18–29 hr | 30–36 hr |
| Combinations | Regular + NPH | SC: | 30 min | 2–10 hr | 18–24 hr |
| | Regular + Lente | SC: | 1 hr | 2–10 hr | 18–24 hr |
| | Semilente + Lente | SC: | 1 hr | 4–10 hr | 18–24 hr |
| | Semilente + Ultralente | SC: | 1 hr | 2–24 hr | 30–36 hr |

*Source*: Reprinted from Managing insulin dependent diabetic patients [70].

\* Preparations are available in concentrations of 40, 80, and 100 units/ml in 10-ml vials. Regular (Concentrated) Iletin is also available in a concentration of 500 units/ml in 20-ml vials. Regular, NPH, and Lente insulins are available as beef-pork insulin mixtures and as special monospecies insulins made exclusively from beef or pork pancreas.

† IV, IM, and SC denote intravenous, intramuscular, and subcutaneous routes of administration.

## Distribution of Major Nutrients in Normal and Diabetic Diets (United States)

| Diet | Nutrients (% of total kcal) | | | | | |
|---|---|---|---|---|---|---|
| | *Starch and other polysaccharides** | *Sugars and dextrins†* | *Total carbohydrate* | *Fat* | *Protein* | *Alcohol* |
| Typical diet | 25–35 | 20–30 | 45–50 | 35–45 (two thirds saturated) | 12–19 | 0–10 |
| Traditional diabetic diets | 25–30 | 10–15‡ | 35–40 | 40–45 | 16–21 | 0 |
| Newer diabetic diets | 30–45 | 5–15‡ | 45–55§ | 25–35§ (half saturated) | 12–24 | 0–6 |

*Source*: Adapted from Diet and diabetes [79].

\* A very substantial majority of these kilocalories are starch, but complex carbohydrates also include cellulose, hemicellulose, pentosans, and pectin.

† These are monosaccharides and disaccharides, mainly sucrose, but also include fructose, glucose, lactose, maltose, and both refined and natural sugars.

‡ These are almost exclusively natural sugars, mainly in fruit and milk (lactose).

§ Even higher levels of starch and lower levels of fat would be desirable but are seldom possible in Western societies because they differ too much from traditional diets of those cultures.


**Determining the Diet Prescription: How to Approximate the Individual Dietary Needs**

Factors to consider:

   I.   Weight and height

  II.   Caloric needs

 III.   Division into protein, carbohydrate and fat

 IV.   Division into meals and snacks

  V.   Limitations (Modifications for special conditions)

 VI.   Need for insulin

VII.   Individual food habits

VIII.   Family food budget

*Source:* Reprinted from A Guide for Professionals: The Effective Application of "Exchange Lists for Meal Planning" [13].


**Factors to Consider in Determining the Individual Diet Prescription**

   I.  WEIGHT AND HEIGHT

| *Build* | *Women* | *Men* | *Children* |
|---------|---------|-------|------------|
| Medium | Allow 100 lb for first 5 ft of height, plus 5 lb for each additional inch | Allow 106 lb for first 5 ft of height, plus 6 lb for each additional inch | Chart growth pattern on graph (Wetzel, Iowa, or Stuart) every 3–6 months |
| Small | Subtract 10% | Subtract 10% | |
| Large | Add 10% | Add 10% | |

  II.  DETERMINATION OF CALORIC NEEDS

     a. For Adults
       1. Basal kilocalories equals desirable body weight (lb) × 10
       2. Add activity kilocalories
         a. Sedentary equals desirable body weight (lb) × 3
         b. Moderate equals desirable body weight (lb) × 5
         c. Strenuous equals desirable body weight (lb) × 10
       3. Add kilocalories for indicated weight gain, growth (pregnant women), or lactation
       4. Subtract kilocalories for indicated weight loss.
     b. For Children
       1. Children vary markedly in their caloric needs depending on rate of growth and level of activity.
       2. Estimate caloric requirement from chart of Recommended Daily Dietary Allowances (pp. I3–I5).
       3. Adjust caloric intake as needed to maintain normal rate of growth.

 III.  DETERMINATION OF GRAMS OF PROTEIN, CARBOHYDRATE, AND FAT

     a. Protein: 20% of total kilocalories for growing children and pregnant women, minimum of 0.5 g per lb desirable body weight for other adults
     b. Carbohydrate: from 50–70% of nonprotein kilocalories
     c. Fat: from 30–50% of nonprotein kilocalories.

IV. SUGGESTED DIVISION INTO MEALS AND SNACKS

    a. Meals usually contain $^2/_{10}$ to $^4/_{10}$ of the kilocalories and carbohydrate, and snacks usually contain $^1/_{10}$ of the kilocalories and carbohydrate.

    b. In the non-insulin dependent individual, food is usually divided into three meals per day; in the insulin dependent individual, food is usually divided into three meals and a bedtime snack and occasionally a midafternoon and/or midmorning snack, depending on plasma glucose levels.

V. LIMITATIONS (MODIFICATIONS FOR SPECIAL CONDITIONS)
    a. Protein
    b. Saturated fat and/or cholesterol
    c. Sodium
    d. Potassium
    e. Other

*Source*: Reprinted from A Guide for Professionals: The Effective Application of "Exchange Lists for Meal Planning" [13].


**Calculation of a Specific Diet**

STEP I. DETERMINE TOTAL KILOCALORIES

a. For adults:
  1. Basal kilocalories: desirable body weight × 10     = _____
  2. Activity kilocalories
    a. Sedentary: desirable body weight × 3     = + _____
    b. Moderate: desirable body weight × 5     = + _____
    c. Strenuous: desirable body weight × 10     = + _____
  3. Growth kilocalories
    a. Pregnancy: add 300 kcal/day to gain 23 lb in 9 months   = + _____
      Add calcium to provide 1.5 g/day and supplemental vitamins if needed.
    b. Lactation: add 500 kcal/day     = + _____
    c. To gain 1 lb/week, add 500 kcal/day     = + _____
  4. To lose 1 lb/week, subtract 500 kcal/day     = − _____

                Total kilocalories needed  = [ _____ ]

b. For children: see Recommended Daily Dietary Allowances Chart on pp. I3–I5.

STEP II. DIVIDE KILOCALORIES INTO GRAMS OF PROTEIN, CARBOHYDRATE, AND FAT. The following is an example of the division of 1,800 kcal into 20% protein, 50% carbohydrate, and 30% fat. The same procedure can be used to develop any ratio desired.

a. Determine grams of protein
   20% of total kilocalories = 360 kcal ÷ 4 = [90] g protein (to nearest 5)
b. Determine grams of carbohydrate
   50% of total kilocalories = 900 kcal ÷ 4 = [225] g carbohydrate (to nearest 5)
c. Determine grams of fat
   30% of total kilocalories = 540 kcal ÷ 9 = [60] g fat (to nearest 5)

STEP III. CALCULATE MEAL PLAN IN EXCHANGES

STEP IV. USING TENTHS, DIVIDE KILOCALORIES AND CARBOHYDRATE INTO MEALS AND SNACKS

*Source*: Adapted from A Guide for Professionals: The Effective Application of "Exchange Lists for Meal Planning" [13].

## One Example of How to Calculate a Meal Plan

*Example*   Prescription:   Kilocalories per day 1,800

Protein (grams) <u>90</u>          Carbohydrate (grams) <u>225</u>          Fat (grams) <u>60</u>

| List | Exchange group | No. of exchanges | CHO (g) | | Protein (g) | | Fat (g) | |
|---|---|---|---|---|---|---|---|---|
| | | | | *per* | | *per* | | *per* |
| 1 | Milk, non-fat | 2 | 24 | 12 | 16 | 8 | | Tr. |
| 1 | Milk, 1% fat | | | 12 | | 8 | | 2.5 |
| 1 | Milk, 2% fat | | | 12 | | 8 | | 5 |
| 1 | Milk, whole | | | 12 | | 8 | | 10 |
| 2 | Vegetable | 2 | 10 | 5 | 4 | 2 | | — |
| 3 | Fruit | 7 | 70 | 10 | | — | | — |
| | Total carbohydrates from sources other than Bread Exchanges | | 104 | | | | | |

<u>225</u> g carbohydrate in prescription

<u>−104</u> g carbohydrate from sources other than Bread Exchange

<u>121</u> g carbohydrate ÷ 15 = no. of Bread Exchanges <u>8</u>

   (15 g carbohydrates/1 Bread Exchange)

| List | Exchange group | No. of exchanges | CHO (g) | | Protein (g) | | Fat (g) | |
|---|---|---|---|---|---|---|---|---|
| 4 | Bread | 8 | 120 | 15 | 16 | 2 | | — |
| 4 | Prepared food | | | 15 | | 2 | | 5 |
| 4 | Prepared food | | | 15 | | 2 | | 10 |
| | Total protein from sources other than Meat Exchange | | | | 36 | | | |

<u>90</u> g protein in prescription

<u>−36</u> g protein from sources other than Meat Exchange

<u>54</u> g protein ÷ 7 = no. of Meat Exchanges <u>8</u>
   (7 g protein/1 Meat Exchange)

| List | Exchange group | No. of exchanges | CHO (g) | | Protein (g) | | Fat (g) | |
|---|---|---|---|---|---|---|---|---|
| 5 | Meat, lean | 6 | | — | 42 | 7 | 18 | 3 |
| 5 | Meat, medium-fat | 2 | | — | 14 | 7 | 11 | 5.5 |
| 5 | Meat, high-fat | | | — | | 7 | | 8 |
| | Total fat from sources other then Fat Exchange | | | | | | 29 | |

<u>60</u> g fat in prescription

<u>−29</u> g fat from sources other than Fat Exchange

<u>31</u> g fat ÷ 5 = no. of Fat Exchanges <u>6</u>
   (5 g fat/1 Fat Exchange)

| List | Exchange group | No. of exchanges | CHO (g) | | Protein (g) | | Fat (g) | |
|---|---|---|---|---|---|---|---|---|
| 6 | Fat | 6 | | — | | — | 30 | 5 |

**Resolution**

| | | | CHO | Protein | Fat |
|---|---|---|---|---|---|
| | Total grams: carbohydrates, protein, and fat | | 224 | 92 | 59 |
| | Determine kilocalories: 4 kcal/1 g carbohydrate 4 kcal/1 g protein 9 kcal/1 g fat | | × 4 = 896 | × 4 = 368 | × 9 = 531 |
| | Total calories per Meal Plan | | 1,795 | | |

Adapted from A Guide for Professionals:   The Effective Application of "Exchange Lists for Meal Planning" [13].

**An 1,800 Kcal Diet: 90 g protein, 60 g fat, 225 g carbohydrate**
**Translation into Food Exchanges**

| Food | Total for day | Carbohydrate (g) | Protein (g) | Fat (g) |
|---|---|---|---|---|
| Milk, skim | 2 | 24 | 16 | 0 |
| Vegetables | 2 | 10 | 4 | 0 |
| Fruit | 7 | 70 | 0 | 0 |
| Bread | 8 | 120 | 16 | 0 |
| Meat, lean | 6 | 0 | 42 | 18 |
| Meat, medium fat | 2 | 0 | 14 | 11 |
| Fat | 6 | 0 | 0 | 30 |
| Total distribution | | 224 | 92 | 59 |

**Example of Caloric Distribution by Meals/Snacks**

| | A.M. | Noon | P.M. | Between meals |
|---|---|---|---|---|
| Milk, skim | ½ cup | ½ cup | ½ cup | ½ cup |
| Vegetables | 0 | 1 | 1 | 0 |
| Fruit | 3 | 3 | 1 | 0 |
| Bread | 2 | 2 | 3 | 1 |
| Meat, lean | 0 | 3 | 3 | 0 |
| Meat, medium fat | 1 | 0 | 0 | 1 |
| Fat | 3 | 2 | 1 | 0 |
| Total carbohydrate | 66 | 71 | 66 | 21 |
| Total kilocalories | 513 | 580 | 520 | 218 |
| Fractional Distribution | $^3/_{10}$ | $^3/_{10}$ | $^3/_{10}$ | $^1/_{10}$ |

*Note*: There are many possible variations, depending on the individual's needs and preferences and the dosage and type of insulin administered.

## Exchange Lists

### List 1—Nonfat Milk Exchanges

One Exchange of nonfat milk contains 12 grams of carbohydrate, 8 grams of protein, a trace of fat and 80 kilocalories.

Milk is the leading source of calcium. It is a good source of phosphorus, protein, some of the B complex vitamins, including folacin and vitamin $B_{12}$, and vitamins A and D. Magnesium is also found in milk.

Whole milk contains 12 grams of carbohydrate, 8 grams of protein, 9 grams of fat and 160 kilocalories.

The milk shown on your meal plan can be used to drink, to add to cereal, in coffee or tea, or with other foods.

**This list shows the kinds and amounts of milk or milk products to use for one nonfat exchange:**

| Nonfat fortified milks | Amount to use |
|---|---|
| **Skim or nonfat milk** | 1 cup |
| **Powdered (nonfat dry)** | ⅓ cup |
| **Canned, evaporated—skim** | ½ cup |
| **Buttermilk made from skim milk** | 1 cup |
| **Yogurt made from skim milk (plain, unflavored)** | 1 cup |
| **1% skim** | 1 cup |

*2% fortified skim* (omit 1 Fat Exchange) — 1 cup

*Whole milks:* (omit 2 Fat Exchanges)

| | |
|---|---|
| Whole milk | 1 cup |
| Canned, evaporated | ½ cup |
| Buttermilk made from whole milk | 1 cup |
| Yogurt made from whole milk (plain, unflavored) | 1 cup |

**List 2—Vegetable Exchanges**

One Exchange of most vegetables on this list is ½ cup and contains about 5 grams of carbohydrate, 2 grams of protein, and 25 kilocalories.

Dark green and deep yellow vegetables are leading sources of vitamin A. Some vegetables such as asparagus, broccoli, brussels sprouts, cauliflower, cabbage, green peppers, greens, and tomatoes contain vitamin C. Green leafy vegetables contain folacin; and broccoli, cabbage, carrots, spinach, and tomatoes are good sources of vitamin $B_6$. Brussels sprouts, greens, tomatoes, and broccoli contain potassium. Spinach is a source of zinc, and magnesium is found in green beans, broccoli, and tomatoes. Vegetables are good sources of fiber.

Serve vegetables cooked or raw. If fat is added in preparation, omit the equivalent number of fat exchanges.

| | |
|---|---|
| **Asparagus** | **Greens:** |
| **Bean sprouts** | **Mustard** |
| **Beets** | **Spinach** |
| **Broccoli** | **Turnip** |
| **Brussels sprouts** | **Mushrooms** |
| **Cabbage** | **Okra** |
| **Carrots** | **Onions** |
| **Cauliflower** | **Radishes** |
| **Celery** | **Rhubarb** |
| **Cucumbers** | **Rutabaga** |
| **Eggplant** | **Sauerkraut** |
| **Green pepper** | **String beans, green or yellow** |
| **Greens:** | **Summer squash** |
|   **Beet** | **Tomatoes** |
|   **Chards** | **Tomato juice** |
|   **Collards** | **Turnips** |
|   **Dandelion** | **Vegetable juice cocktail** |
|   **Kale** | **Zucchini** |

*Raw* celery, chicory, chinese cabbage, cucumbers, endive, escarole, lettuce, and watercress can be used, as desired.

Starch vegetables are found in the **Bread Exchanges**

**List 3—Fruit Exchanges**

One Exchange of fruit contains 10 grams of carbohydrate and 40 kilocalories.

Fruits are valuable for vitamins and minerals and fiber. Oranges, tangerines, grapefruit, strawberries, cantaloupe, and honeydew melon are good sources of vitamin C. Apricots and peaches contain vitamin A. Mangoes and papaya contain both vitamin A and vitamin C. Bananas, nectarines, oranges, plums, and dried fruits are sources of potassium. Canteloupe, oranges, and strawberries contain folacin. Magnesium and vitamin $B_6$ are found in bananas.

Fruit may be used fresh, dried, canned or frozen, cooked or raw, as long as no sugar is added. Read the label on the can or package to be certain no sugar or sorbitol has been added.

**This list shows the kinds and amounts of fruits to use for one fruit exchange:**

| | *Amount to use* | | *Amount to use* |
|---|---|---|---|
| **Apple** | 1 small | **Mango** | ½ small |
| **Apple juice** | ⅓ cup | **Melon** | |
| **Applesauce** | | Cantaloupe | ¼ small |
| (unsweetened) | ½ cup | Honeydew | ⅛ medium |
| **Apricots, fresh** | 2 medium | Watermelon | 1 cup |
| **Apricots, dried** | 4 halves | **Nectarine** | 1 small |
| **Banana** | ½ small | **Orange** | 1 small |
| **Berries** | | **Orange juice** | ½ cup |
| Blackberries | ½ cup | **Papaya** | ¾ cup |
| Blueberries | ½ cup | **Peach** | 1 medium |
| Raspberries | ⅔ cup | **Pear** | 1 small |
| Strawberries | ¾ cup | **Persimmon, native** | 1 medium |
| **Cherries** | 10 large | **Pineapple** | ½ cup |
| **Cider** | ⅓ cup | **Pineapple juice** | ⅓ cup |
| **Dates** | 2 | **Plums** | 2 medium |
| **Figs, dried** | 1 | **Prunes** | 2 medium |
| **Figs, fresh** | 1 | **Prune juice** | ¼ cup |
| **Grapefruit** | ½ | **Raisins** | 2 tbsp |
| **Grapefruit juice** | ½ cup | **Tangerine** | 1 medium |
| **Grapes** | 12 | | |
| **Grape juice** | ¼ cup | | |

For variety serve fruit as a salad or in combination with other foods for dessert.

Cranberries may be used as desired if no sugar is added.

---

**List 4—Bread, Cereal, and Starchy Vegetables Exchange**

One Exchange contains 15 grams of carbohydrate, 2 grams of protein and 70 kilocalories

---

Whole grain or enriched breads and cereals are good sources of iron and some of the B vitamins, as are dried beans and peas and the vegetables on this list. Magnesium is found in dried cooked beans and whole grain cereals. Dried beans, peas, and lentils are sources of zinc. Dried peas and beans, and whole grain breads and cereals are excellent sources of fiber.

---

**This list shows the many kinds and amounts of breads, cereals, and starchy vegetables to use for one Bread Exchange:**

| | *Amount to use* | | *Amount to use* |
|---|---|---|---|
| *BREAD* | | *CEREAL* | |
| **White (including French** | | **Bran flakes** | ½ cup |
| **and Italian)** | 1 slice | **Other ready to eat** | |
| **Whole wheat** | 1 slice | **unsweetened cereal** | ¾ cup |
| **Rye or pumpernickel** | 1 slice | **Puff cereal, unfrosted** | 1 cup |
| **Raisin** | 1 slice | **Cereal, cooked** | ½ cup |
| **Bagel, small** | ½ | **Grits, cooked** | ½ cup |
| **English muffin, small** | ½ | **Rice or barley, cooked** | ½ cup |
| **Plain roll, bread** | 1 | **Pastas, cooked** | |
| **Frankfurt roll** | ½ | **spaghetti, noodles** | ½ cup |
| **Hamburger bun** | ½ | **macaroni** | ½ cup |
| **Dry bread crumbs** | 3 tbsp | **Cornmeal, dry** | 2 tbsp |
| | | **Flour** | 2½ tbsp |
| **Pancake, 5″** | 1 | **Wheat germ** | ¼ cup |
| **Waffle, 5″** | 1 | | |
| **Tortilla, 6″** | 1 | | |

| | Amount to use | | | Amount to use |
|---|---|---|---|---|
| *CRACKERS* | | | *MISCELLANEOUS* | |
| **Arrowroot** | 3 | | Biscuit, 2″ dia. | 1 |
| **Graham 2½″** | 2 | | (Omit 1 Fat Exchange) | |
| **Matzoth 4″ × 6″** | ½ | | Corn muffin 2″ dia. | 1 |
| **Oyster** | 20 | | (Omit 1 Fat Exchange) | |
| **Pretzels 3⅛″ long** | 25 | | Crackers, round butter type | 5 |
| **⅛″ dia.** | | | (Omit 1 Fat Exchange) | |
| | | | Muffin, plain small | 1 |
| *DRIED BEANS, PEAS, AND* | | | (Omit 1 Fat Exchange) | |
| *LENTILS* | | | Popcorn, popped | 3 cups |
| **Beans, peas, lentils,** | | | Potatoes, French fried, length | 8 |
| **dried and cooked** | ½ cup | | 2 to 3½″ (Omit 1 Fat | |
| **Baked beans, no pork** | ¼ cup | | Exchange) | |
| *STARCHY VEGETABLES* | | | Potato or corn chips | 15 |
| **Corn** | ⅓ cup | | (Omit 2 Fat Exchanges) | |
| **Corn on cob** | 1 small | | | |
| **Lima beans** | ½ cup | | | |
| **Parsnips** | ⅔ cup | | | |
| **Peas, green—canned or** | | | | |
| **frozen** | ½ cup | | | |
| **Potato, white** | 1 small | | | |
| **Potato, mashed** | ½ cup | | | |
| **Pumpkin** | ¾ cup | | *CRACKERS* | |
| **Winter squash, acorn or** | | | **Rye wafers 2″ × 3½″** | 3 |
| **butternut** | ½ cup | | **Saltines** | 6 |
| **Yam, or sweet potato** | ¼ cup | | **Soda 2½″ sq.** | 4 |

**List 5—Lean Meat, Protein Rich Exchanges**

One Exchange of meat (1 oz) contains 7 grams of protein, 3 grams of fat, and 55 kilocalories

Meat, poultry, fish, cheese and eggs are important sources of protein, iron, vitamin $B_{12}$, and other B-complex vitamins. Liver and eggs also contain Vitamin A. Oysters and peanut butter contain magnesium. Liver is a good source of iron and both liver and peanut butter contain folacin. Zinc is found in lean beef, cheddar type cheese, crab, liver, peanut butter, oysters, and the dark meat of turkey.

Cholesterol is of animal origin; therefore, peanut butter and dried peas and beans contain no cholesterol.

To plan a diet low in saturated fat and cholesterol, choose only those exchanges in **bold type.**

You may use the meat, fish, etc. that is prepared for the family when no fat or flour have been added. If meat is fried, use the fat included in the meal plan. Meat juices with the fat removed may be used with your meat or vegetables for added flavor. Be certain to trim off *all* visible fat and measure meat after it has been cooked. A 3-oz serving of cooked meat is about equal to 4 oz of raw meat.

This list shows the kinds and amounts of meat and protein rich foods to use for one Low Fat Meat Exchange:

| | | |
|---|---|---|
| **Beef:** | Baby beef; chipped beef; chuck; flank steak; tenderloin; plate ribs: plate skirt steak: round (bottom, top); all cuts rump; spare ribs; tripe | **1 oz** |
| **Lamb:** | Leg; rib; sirloin; loin (roast and chops); shank; shoulder | **1 oz** |
| **Pork:** | Leg (whole rump, center shank); ham, smoked (center slices) | **1 oz** |
| **Veal:** | Leg; loin; rib; shank; shoulder; cutlets | **1 oz** |
| **Poultry:** | Meat without skin of chicken, turkey, cornish hen, guinea hen, pheasant | **1 oz** |
| **Fish:** | Any fresh or frozen; | **1 oz** |
| | canned salmon, tuna, mackerel, crab, and lobster; | **¼ cup** |
| | clams, oysters, scallops, shrimp; | **5 or 1 oz** |
| | sardines, drained | **3** |

| | |
|---|---|
| **Cheeses containing less than 5% butterfat** | **1 oz** |
| **Cottage cheese, dry and 2% butterfat** | **¼ cup** |
| **Dried peas and beans (Omit 1 Bread Exchange)** | **½ cup** |

---

Medium Fat Meat and Protein Rich Exchanges contain 7 grams of protein, 5 grams of fat, and 75 kilocalories (1 oz)

---

This list shows the kinds and amounts of meat and protein rich foods to use for one Medium Fat Meat Exchange:

| | | |
|---|---|---|
| Beef: | Ground, 15% fat; corned beef, canned; rib eye; round, ground (commercial) | 1 oz |
| Pork: | Loin (all cuts); tenderloin; shoulder arm, picnic; shoulder blade (Boston butt); Canadian bacon, boiled ham; loin, shoulder, picnic ham | 1 oz |

| | |
|---|---|
| Liver, heart, kidney and sweetbreads (these are high in cholesterol). | 1 oz |
| Cottage cheese, creamed | ¼ cup |
| Cheese, mozzarella, ricotta, farmer's cheese, Neufchâtel | 1 oz |
| Cheese, Parmesan | 3 tbsp |
| Egg (high in cholesterol). | 1 |
| Peanut butter (Omit 2 Fat Exchanges) | 2 tbsp |

---

High Fat Meat and Protein Rich Exchanges contain 7 grams of protein, 8 grams of Fat, and 100 kilocalories (1 oz)

---

This list shows the kinds and amounts of meat and protein rich foods to use for one High Fat Meat Exchange:

| | | |
|---|---|---|
| Beef: | Brisket; corned beef (brisket); ground beef, more than 20% fat; hamburger (commercial); chuck, ground (commercial); roasts, rib; steaks, club and rib | 1 oz |
| Lamb: | Breast | 1 oz |
| Pork: | Spare ribs; loin (back ribs); pork, ground; country style ham; deviled ham; spare ribs | 1 oz |
| Veal: | Breast | 1 oz |
| Poultry: | Capon, duck (domestic); goose | 1 oz |

| | |
|---|---|
| Cheese, cheddar type | 1 oz |
| Cold cuts | 4½" × ⅛" slice |
| Frankfurter | 1 |

**List 6—Fat Exchanges**   One Exchange of fat contains 5 grams of fat and 45 kilocalories.

Since all fats are high in kilocalories, foods on this list should be measured carefully to control weight. Margarine, butter, cream and cream cheese contain vitamin A. Use the fats on this list in the amounts on the meal plan.

To plan a diet low in saturated fat select only those exchanges which appear in **bold type** and are polyunsaturated.

This list shows the kinds and amounts of fat containing foods to use for one Fat Exchange:

|  | *Amount to use* |
|---|---|
| **Margarine,** Soft, tub or stick* | 1 tsp |
| **Avocado** (4″ in diameter)† | ⅛ |
| **Oil, corn, cottonseed, safflower, soy, sunflower** | 1 tsp |
| **Oil, olive**† | 1 tsp |
| **Oil, peanut**† | 1 tsp |
| **Walnuts** | 6 small |
| **Nuts, other**† | 6 small |
| **Olives**† | 5 small |
| Margarine, regular stick | 1 tsp |
| Butter | 1 tsp |
| Bacon fat | 1 tsp |
| Bacon, crisp | 1 strip |
| Cream, light | 2 tbsp |
| Cream, sour | 2 tbsp |
| Cream, heavy | 1 tbsp |
| Cream cheese | 1 tbsp |
| French dressing‡ | 1 tbsp |
| Italian dressing‡ | 1 tbsp |
| Lard | 1 tsp |
| Mayonnaise† | 1 tsp |
| Salad dressing, mayonnaise type‡ | 2 tsp |
| Salt pork | ¾″ cube |

*Source*:   Reprinted from Exchange Lists for Meal Planning [2].
* Made with corn, cottonseed, safflower, soy or sunflower oil only.
† Fat content is primarily monounsaturated.
‡ If made with corn, cottonseed, safflower, or soy oil, can be used on fat modified diet.

**Sample Menu for 1,800 Kcal Diet (Approximately 90 g protein, 60 g fat, 225 g carbohydrate)**

A.M.

12 oz orange juice
½ cup farina with 2 tsp corn oil margarine
1 soft cooked egg
1 slice toast with 1 tsp corn oil margarine
½ cup nonfat milk
Coffee or tea

NOON

⅓ cup unsweetened pineapple juice
Turkey sandwich: 2 slices whole wheat bread, 3 oz sliced turkey, 2 tsp mayonnaise,
    and sliced tomato and lettuce
½ cup green beans
1 banana, small
½ cup nonfat milk
Coffee or tea

P.M.

3 oz round steak
½ cup mashed potato
2 slices bread with 1 tsp corn oil margarine
½ cup broccoli with lemon
¾ cup fresh strawberries
½ cup nonfat milk
Coffee or tea

BETWEEN MEALS

½ cup nonfat milk
6 saltines
1 oz Neufchâtel cheese

References

1. West, K. M.: Diet therapy of diabetes: an analysis of failure. Ann. Intern. Med. 79: 425, 1973.
2. Committees of the American Diabetes Association, Inc., and the American Dietetic Association: Exchange Lists for Meal Planning. Chicago: The American Dietetic Association and the American Diabetes Association, in cooperation with the National Institute of Arthritis, Metabolism and Digestive Diseases and the National Heart, Blood and Lung Institute, Public Health Service, U.S. Department of Health, Education and Welfare, 1976.
3. Committee of Food and Nutrition, American Diabetes Association: Principles of nutrition and dietary recommendations for patients with diabetes mellitus. Diabetes 20: 633, 1971.
4. Weinsier, R. L.; Seeman, A.; Herrera, M. G.; Assal, J. P.; Soeldner, J. S.; and Gleason, R. E.: High and low carbohydrate diets in diabetes mellitus. Ann. Intern. Med. 80: 322, 1974.
5. Brunzell, J. D.; Lerner, R. L.; Porte, D.; and Bierman, E. L.: Effect of a fat free, high carbohydrate diet on diabetic subjects with fasting hyperglycemia. Diabetes 23: 138, 1974.
6. Arky, R. A.: Diet and diabetus mellitus. Postgrad. Med. 63: 72, June 1978.
7. Anderson, J. W.: Effect of carbohydrate restriction and high carbohydrate diets on men with chemical diabetes. Am. J. Clin. Nutr. 30: 402, 1977.
8. Crapo, P. A.; Reaven, G.; and Olefsky, J.: Plasma glucose and insulin responses to orally administered simple and complex carbohydrates. Diabetes 25: 741, 1976.
9. Anderson, J. W., and Ward, K.: Long term effects of high carbohydrate, high fiber diets on glucose and lipid metabolism. A preliminary report on patients with diabetes. Diabetes Care 1: 77, March 1978.
10. Davidson, J. K.: Controlling diabetes mellitus with diet therapy. Postgrad. Med. 59: 114, 1976.
11. Bacon, G. E., and Parkhurst, R. D.: Med. Clin. N. Am. 53: 1367, 1969.

12. Coustan, D. R.: Clinical approaches to diabetes in pregnancy. Cont. Obstet. Gynecol. 7: 27, 1976.
13. The American Diabetes Association and the American Dietetic Association: A Guide for Professionals: The Effective Application of "Exchange Lists for Meal Planning," 1977.
14. Huckaday, T. D. R.: Diabetes Mellitus. Practitioner 213: 5, 1974.
15. Petrie, J. C.; Stowers, J. M.; and Wood, R. A.: Diabetes mellitus—obesity and dietary management. Br. Med. J. 2: 706, 1972.
16. Saperstein, M. D.: The glucose tolerance test: a pitfall in the diagnosis of diabetes mellitus. Adv. Intern. Med. 20: 297, 1975.
17. Gordon, E. S.: Diabetes mellitus—new developments. Postgrad. Med. 55: 145, Mar. 1974.
18. Alford, F. P.; Bloom, S. R.; Nabarro, J. D. N.; Hall, P.; Besser, G. M.; Coy, D. H.; Kastin, A. J.; and Schally, A. V.: Glucagon control of fasting glucose in man. Lancet 2: 974, 1974.
19. Gerich, J. E.; Lorenzi, M.; Schweider, V.; Karam, J. H.; Rivier, J.; Guillemin, R.; and Forsham, P. H.: Effects of somatostatin on plasma glucose and glucagon levels in diabetes mellitus. N. Engl. J. Med. 291: 544, 1974.
20. Unger, R. H., and Orci, L.: The essential role of glucagon in the pathogenesis of diabetes mellitus. Lancet 1: 14, 1975.
21. Felig, P.; Wahren, J.; Sherwin, R.; and Hendler, R.: Insulin, glucagon, and somatostatin in normal physiology and diabetes mellitus. Diabetes 25: 1091, 1976.
22. Sherwin, R., and Felig, P.: Pathophysiology of diabetes mellitus. Med. Clin. N. Am. 62: 695, 1978.
23. Poffenbarger, P. L., and White, F. A.: Guidelines for use of oral hypoglycemic drug therapy: the balance of risks vs. benefits. Conn. Med. 39: 137, 1975.
24. Bruck, E., and MacGillivray, M. H.: Interaction of endogenous growth hormone, cortisol, and catecholamines with blood glucose in children with brittle diabetes mellitus. Pediatr. Res. 9: 535, 1975.
25. Coelingh Bennink, H. J. T., and Schreurs, W. H. P.: Improvement of oral glucose tolerance in gestational diabetes by pyridoxine. Br. Med. J. 3: 13, 1975.
26. Henquin, J. C., and Lambert, A. E.: Catonic environment and dynamics of insulin secretion. II. Effect of a high concentration of potassium. Diabetes 23: 933, 1974.
27. Tandon, R. K.; Srivastava, L. M.; and Pandey, S. C.: Increased disaccharidase activity in human diabetics. Am. J. Clin. Nutr. 28: 621, 1975.
28. Oakley, W. G.; Pyke, D. A.; and Taylor, K. W.: Diabetes and Its Management. Oxford: Blackwell, 1973.
29. Bates, G. W.: Management of gestational diabetes. Postgrad. Med. 55: 55, June 1974.
30. Assal, J.; Aoki, T. T.; Manzano, F. M.; and Kozak, G. P.: Metabolic effects of sodium bicarbonate in management of diabetic ketoacidosis. Diabetes 23: 405, 1974.
31. Scoville, A. B.: Oral therapy in diabetes mellitus. South. Med. J. 67: 635, 1974.
32. Guthrie, R. A.; Guthrie, D. W.; Baker, H. W.; and Jackson, R. L.: Criteria for the selection of patients for treatment with tolbutamide. Metabolism 22: 387, 1973.
33. Emerson, K.; Saxena, B. N.; Varma, S. K.; and Poindexter, E. L.: Caloric cost and sources of energy in diabetic pregnancy. Obstet. Gynecol. 43: 354, 1974.
34. Fulop, M.; Tannenbaum, H.; and Dreyer, N.: Ketotic hyperosmolar coma. Lancet 1: 635, 1973.
35. Albrink, M. J.: Dietary and drug treatment of hyperlipidemia in diabetes. Diabetes 23: 913, 1974.
36. Levine, R., and Pfeiffer, E. F., eds.: Lipid Metabolism Obesity and Diabetes Mellitus, Impact upon Atherosclerosis. Stuttgart: Georg Thieme, 1974.
37. Stimmler, L.: Diabetes in childhood. Guy's Hosp. Rep. 122: 17, 1973.
38. Felig, P.: Diabetic ketoacidosis. N. Engl. J. Med. 290: 1360, 1974.
39. Lazarus, N. R., and Davis, B.: Model for extrusion of insulin B granules. Lancet 1: 143, 1975.
40. Kissebah, A. H.; Hope-Gill, H.; Vydelingum, N.; Tulloch, B. R.; Clarke, P. V.; and Fraser, T. R.: Mode of insulin action. Lancet 1: 144, 1975.
41. Cox, B. D.; Whichelow, M. J.; Butterfield, W. J. H.; and Nicholas, P.: Peripheral vitamin C metabolism in diabetics and non-diabetics: effect of intra-arterial insulin. Clin. Sci. Mol. Med. 47: 63, 1974.

42. MacCuish, A. C.; Irvine, W. J.; Barnes, E. W.; and Duncan, L. J. P.: Antibodies to pancreatic islet cells in insulin dependent diabetics with coexistent autoimmune disease. Lancet 2: 1529, 1974.

43. Vinik, A. I.; Kalk, W. J.; and Jackson, W. P. U.: A unifying hypothesis for heriditary acquired diabetes. Lancet 1: 485, 1974.

44. Knatterrud, G. I.; Klimt, C. R.; Osborne, R. K.; Meinert, C. I.; Martin, D. B.; and Hawkins, B. S.: A study of the effects of hypoglycemic agents on vascular complications in patients with adult-onset diabetes. V. Evaluation of phenformin therapy. Diabetes 24: 65, 1975.

45. Albisser, A. M.; Leibel, B. S.; Ewart, T. G.; Davidovac, Z.; Botz, C. K.; Zingg, W.; Schipper, H.; and Gander, R.: Clinical control of diabetes by the artificial pancreas. Diabetes 23: 397, 1974.

46. Doar, J. W. H.; Wilde, C. E.; Thompson, M. E.; and Sewell, P. F. J.: Influence of treatment with diet alone on oral glucose-tolerance test and plasma sugar and insulin levels in patients with maturity-onset diabetes mellitus. Lancet 1: 1263, 1975.

47. Burman, K. D.: What's new for diabetes? Med. Times 103: 123, July 1975.

48. Bray, G. A.; Rimoin, D. L.; Sperling, M. A.; Fiser, R. H.; Swerdloff, R. S.; Fisher, D. A.; and Odell, W. D.: The obese diabetic. Calif. Med. 119: 14, Oct. 1973.

49. University Group Diabetes Study Program: A study of the effects of hypoglycemic agents and vascular complications in patients with adult onset diabetes. Diabetes 19: 747, 1970.

50. Matz, R.: The limited usefulness of oral hypoglycemic agents. Med. Counterpoint 5: 26, 1973.

51. Schmitt, B. D.: An argument for the unmeasured diet in juvenile diabetes mellitus. Clin. Pediatr. 14: 68, 1975.

52. Brunzell, J. D.; Lerner, R. L.; and Hazzard, W. R.: Improved glucose tolerance with high carbohydrate diets with high carbohydrate feeding in mild diabetes. N. Engl. J. Med. 284: 521, 1971.

53. Lerner, R. L.; Brunzell, J. D.; and Hazzard, W. R.: Mechanism of improved glucose tolerance on high carbohydrate diets in normal and mild diabetics. Diabetes 20: 342, 1971.

54. Anderson, J. W.: Metabolic abnormalities contributing to diabetic complications. I. Glucose metabolism in insulin-insensitive pathways. Am. J. Clin. Nutr. 28: 273, 1975.

55. Saudek, C. D.; Boulter, P. R.; Knopp, R. H.; and Arky, R. A.: Sodium retention accompanying insulin treatment of diabetes mellitus. Diabetes 23: 240, 1974.

56. Ball, S.; Woods, H. F.; and Alberti, M. M.: Lacticacidosis, ketoacidosis, and hyperalaninaemia in a phenformin treated diabetic patient. Br. Med. J. 4: 699, 1974.

57. Albisser, A. M.; Leibel, B. S.; Ewart, T. G.; Davidovac, Z.; Botz, C. K.; and Zingg, W.: An artificial endocrine pancreas. Diabetes 23: 389, 1974.

58. Walsh, C. H.; Solder, N. G.; James, H.; Fitzgerald, M. G.; and Malins, J. M.: Studies on whole-body potassium in non-ketoacidotic diabetes before and after treatment. Br. Med. J. 4: 738, 1974.

59. Taft, P.: Diet in management of diabetes. Why restrict carbohydrate? Med. J. Aust. 1: 838, 1976.

60. Colwell, J. A.: Use of oral agents in treating diabetes mellitus. Postgrad. Med. 59: 139, Jan. 1976.

61. Federal Register 42 (73): 1996–2009, Apr. 15, 1977.

62. Maruhama, X.; Abe, R.; Orvenchi, F.; and Omneda, A.: Dietary intake and hyperlipidemia in controlled diabetic outpatients. Diabetes 26: 94, 1970.

63. Kaufmann, R. L.; Assal, J. P.; Soeldner, J. S.; Wilmshurst, E. G.; Lemaire, J. R.; Gleason, R. E.; and White, P.: Plasma lipid levels in diabetic children. Diabetes 24: 672, 1975.

64. Peterson, C. M.; Koenig, R. J.; and Jones, R. L.: Correlation of serum triglyceride levels and hemoglobin $A_{1C}$ concentration in diabetes mellitus. Diabetes 26: 507, 1977.

65. Drash, A. L.: Managing the child with diabetes mellitus. Postgrad. Med. 63: 85, 1978.

66. Jenkins, D. J. A.; Leeds, A. R.; Gassull, M. A.; Cochet, B.; and Alberti, G. M. M.: Decrease in postprandial insulin and glucose concentrations by guar and pectin. Ann. Intern. Med. 86: 20, 1977.

67. Boshell, B. R., and Gomez, P.: Diabetes mellitus. Conn, H. F., and Conn, R. B., eds. Current Diagnosis. Philadelphia: W. B. Saunders, 1974.
68. Felig, Phillip, M.D., Yale School of Medicine: Personal communication.
69. American Diabetes Association: Blood glucose in diabetes. Diabetes 25: 237, 1976.
70. Owen, O. E.; Boden, G.; and Shuman, C. R.: Managing insulin dependent diabetic patients. Postgrad. Med. 59: 127, Jan. 1976.
71. Bosso, J. A., and Pearson, R. E.: Sugar content of selected liquid medicinals. Diabetes 22: 776, 1973.
72. Bruhn, J. G.: Psychosocial influences in diabetes mellitus. Postgrad. Med. 56: 113, Aug. 1974.
73. Dwyer, L. S., and Fralin, F. G.: Simplified meal planning for hard to teach patients. Am. J. Nurs. 74: 664, 1974.
74. Weinsier, R. L.; Seeman, A.; Guillermo Herrera, M.; Simmons, J. J.; and Collins, M. E.: Diet therapy of diabetes—description of successful methodologic approach to gaining diet adherence. Diabetes 23: 669, 1974.
75. Davenport, R. R.; Ferguson, D. E.; Fitzpatrick, E. O.; and White, B. W.: Dietitians, nurses teach diabetic patients. Hospitals 48: 81, Dec. 1, 1974.
76. Behrman, D. M.: A Cookbook for Diabetics. New York: American Diabetes Association, 1959.
77. Revele, D. T.: Gourmet Recipes for Diabetics. Springfield: Charles C. Thomas, 1971.
78. Olefsky, J. M., and Crapo, P.: Fructose, xylitol and sorbitol. Diabetes Care 3: 390, 1980.
79. American Diabetes Association: Saccharin. Diabetes Care 2: 380, 1979.
80. Morrison, A. S., and Buring, J. E.: Artificial sweeteners and cancer of the lower urinary tract. New. Engl. J. Med. 302: 537, 1980.
81. Graber, A. L.; Christman, B. G.; Alogna, M. T.; and Davidson, J. K.: Evaluation of diabetes patient-education programs. Diabetes 26: 61, 1977.
82. West, K. M.: Diet and diabetes. Postgrad. Med. 60: 209, 1976.

# Kilocalorie Restricted Diet

*Definition*    A diet limited in total kilocalories to a prescribed level significantly below normal requirements.

*Characteristics of the diet*    Most foods are restricted, and highly concentrated sources of kilocalories, such as pies, pastries, etc., are eliminated. The exchange lists used to calculate diets for individuals with diabetes are used for the low kilocalorie diet as well.

*Purpose of the diet*    (1) Reduction in body weight and fat and (2) weight loss maintenance. Obesity has a genetic component [1], and overfeeding in infancy may lead to excessive secretion of insulin and growth hormone and to increases in fat cell size and number. Many fat babies become fat adults [2]. Weight loss results in a reduction of fat cell size. However, changes in fat cell number that have been attributed to weight loss are not clearly established [3]. Obesity is associated with insulin, cholesterol, and triglyceride levels [4,5]. Many metabolic factors are involved in the control of energy stores [6–10].

*Effects of the diet*    A reduction in caloric intake of 3,500 kcal is required in order for the loss of 1 lb of body weight to occur; for example, if the diet is designed to provide 500 kcal less than the person requires to maintain his present weight, he would have to follow the diet for 7 days in order to lose 1 lb: $3,500 \div 500 = 7$.

In terms of the clinical treatment of obesity, there appears to be no advantage in selecting a high protein diet on the basis of obtaining an increase in the caloric costs of digestion and assimilation or a lower net caloric value for the diet [11–14]. The effectiveness of the protein sparing modified fast has been disputed [14]. Weight reduction in the obese patient with an abnormal glucose tolerance test and elevated serum lipids often brings dramatic improvements [8,9].

*Indications for use*    A kilocalorie restricted diet should be part of an overall program of weight reduction in any person who is overweight as determined by skinfold thickness measurements with calipers and the use of a height-weight table. Exercise, which is of little value when used without a concomitant reduction in energy intake, can make a contribution to the achievement of weight loss when used as an adjunct to dietary control [15,16].

Among other specific indications for weight reduction of overweight persons are the following:

1. *Respiratory difficulties*    Very marked obesity may lead to the Pickwickian syndrome, where, through decreased ventilation, accumulation of carbon dioxide in blood leads to lethargy and somnolence. The removal of obesity is essential to the treatment of this syndrome [8].

2. *Hypertension*    Hypertension in an obese patient is a compelling indication for weight reduction. A weight loss of 15 lb may result in a decrease in diastolic pressure of 15 mm mercury. The favorable effects of weight reduction on survival of post coronary patients have been also documented [8].

3. *Endocrine and metabolic disturbances*    Hirsutism and menstrual irregularities among obese women can often be mitigated by weight loss [8]. The improvement in glucose tolerance that accompanies weight loss in the obese person with maturity-onset diabetes has been discussed on pp. F11–F29.

4. *Other conditions*    Certain bone and joint diseases, such as rupture of intravertebral disks, osteoarthritis, and intermittent claudication, are benefited by weight reduction [8].

***Possible adverse reactions***    Iron and thiamine intake may be marginal even on a well balanced diet, and many unbalanced fad diets that exclude major groups of foods with essential nutrients or are disproportionate in their nutrient composition can cause untoward reactions [16–18]. For example, diets composed exclusively of protein and animal fat can produce hypercholesterolemia, particularly in patients with overt or subclinical coronary artery disease [19]. Semistarvation programs should be attempted only with close biochemical and clinical monitoring of the patient [20,21]. Little is known about the long-term effects of ketogenic and semistarvation diets.

***Contraindications***    In the obese pregnant woman. Severe caloric restrictions during pregnancy, even of an obese woman, may compromise the well-being of both the developing fetus and the mother, particularly if the caloric level is so low that protein is used for energy rather than growth. Despite the added risk of obesity, weight reduction regimens should not be instituted during pregnancy [22].

***Suggestions for dietitians***    The dietitians' efforts in assisting patients call for a well coordinated program that begins with insight gained from a dietary history and provides the modification needed for weight control and long-term guidance that will lead to new food preferences.

Caloric reduction along with an exercise program remains the mainstay of treatment for obesity. No drugs, including chorionic gonadotropin [23,24], are considered to be of value in treating obesity at the present time. In addition, ileal bypass surgery carries inherent risks and long-term consequences and should be reserved for a carefully selected group of patients with massive, refractory obesity [25–37].

The use of behavior modification therapy techniques have produced encouraging results, but they too are based on a kilocalorie restricted diet [38–41]. Several excellent low kilocalorie recipe books are now available [42–44].

# Kilocalorie Restricted Diet

**1,200 Kcal Diet (approximately 65 g protein, 50 g fat, 130 g carbohydrate)**

| **Sample Meal Plan*** | **Sample Menu** |
|---|---|
| A.M. | A.M. |
| 1 fruit exchange | ½ cup orange juice |
| 1 medium fat meat exchange | 1 soft cooked egg |
| 1 bread exchange | 1 slice toast |
| 1 fat exchange | 1 tsp butter or fortified margarine |
| Coffee or tea | Coffee or tea |
| NOON | NOON |
| 2 lean meat exchanges | 2 oz sliced turkey |
| 1 bread exchange | 1 slice enriched bread |
| 2 fat exchanges | 2 tsp butter or fortified margarine |
| 1 vegetable exchange | ½ cup broccoli |
| 1 fruit exchange | 2 unsweetened whole apricots |
| 1 milk exchange | 1 cup skim milk |
| Coffee or tea | |
| P.M. | P.M. |
| 2 lean meat exchanges | 2 oz round steak |
| 1 bread exchange | 1 small baked potato with skin |
| 2 fat exchanges | 2 tsp butter or fortified margarine |
| 2 vegetable exchanges | ½ cup carrots |
| | ½ cup lettuce and cucumber salad with |
| 1 fat exchange | 1 tbsp Italian dressing |
| 1 fruit exchange | ¼ cantaloupe |
| Coffee or tea | Coffee or tea |
| BETWEEN MEALS | BETWEEN MEALS |
| 1 milk exchange | 1 cup skim milk |
| 1 bread exchange | 2 graham crackers |

* Exchange Lists, pp. F20–F25.

## References

1. Mann, G. V.: The influence of obesity on health. N. Engl. J. Med. 291: 178, 1974.
2. Collins, T. R.: Infantile obesity. Am. Fam. Phys. 11: 162, March 1975.
3. Widdowsen, E.: Full and empty fat cells. Lancet 2: 905, 1973.
4. Olefsky, J.; Crapo, P. A.; Ginsberg, H.; and Reaven, G. M.: Metabolic effects of increased caloric intake in man. Metabolism 24: 495, March 1975.
5. Freeman, J. B.; Meyer, P. D.; Printen, K. J.; Mason, E. E.; and Den-Besten, L.: Analysis of gallbladder bile in morbid obesity. Am. J. Surg. 129: 163, 1975.
6. Bray, G. A., and Campfield, L. A.: Metabolic factors in the control of energy stores. Metabolism 24: 99, 1975.
7. Schultz, R. B.: Metabolic aspects of obesity. Metabolism 22: 359, 1973.
8. Mayer, J.: Obesity. Goodhart, R. S., and Shils, M. E, eds. Modern Nutrition in Health and Disease. 5th ed. Philadelphia: Lea & Febiger, 1973.
9. Robinson, C., and Lawler, M. R.: Normal and Therapeutic Nutrition. 15th ed. New York: Macmillan, 1977.
10. Stricker, E. M.: Hyperphagia. N. Engl. J. Med. 298: 1010, 1978.
11. Bradfield, R. B., and Jourdan, M. H.: Relative importance of specific dynamic action in weight-reduction diets. Lancet 2: 640, 1973.
12. Worthington, B. S., and Taylor, L. E.: Balanced low-calorie vs. high protein-low-carbohydrate reducing diets. J. Am. Diet. Assoc. 64: 52, 1974.
13. Worthington, B. S., and Taylor, L. E.: Balanced low-calorie vs. low-protein-low-carbohydrate reducing diets. J. Am. Diet. Assoc. 64: 52, 1974.
14. Van Itallie, T. B., and Yang, M. U.: Diet and weight loss. N. Engl. J. Med. 298: 1158, 1977.
15. Harger, B. S.; Miller, J. B.; and Thomas, J. C.: The caloric cost of running: its impact on weight reduction. JAMA 228: 482, 1974.
16. Gwinup, G.: Effect of exercise alone on the weight of obese women. Arch. Intern. Med. 135: 676, 1975.

17. Sherman, D. G., and Easton, J. D.: Dieting and peroneal nerve palsy. JAMA 238: 230, 1977.
18. Michiel, R. R.; Snieder, J. S.; Dickstein, R. A.; Hayman, H.; and Eich, R.: Sudden death on a liquid protein diet. N. Engl. J. Med. 298: 1005, 1978.
19. Rickman, F.; Mtchell, N.; Dingman, J.; and Dalen, J. E.: Changes in serum cholesterol during the Stillman Diet. JAMA 228: 54, 1974.
20. Sapir, D. G.; Owen, O. E.; Pozefsky, T.; and Walser, M.: Nitrogen sparing induced by a mixture of essential amino acids given chiefly as their keto-analogues during prolonged starvation in obese subjects. J. Clin. Invest. 54: 974, 1974.
21. Genuth, S. M.; Castro, J. H.; and Vertes, V.: Weight reduction in obesity by outpatient semistarvation. JAMA 230: 987, 1974.
22. Committee on Maternal Nutrition, Food and Nutrition Board, National Research Council: Maternal Nutrition and the Course of Pregnancy. Washington, DC: National Academy of Sciences, 1970.
23. Young, R. L.; Fuchs, R. J.; and Woltjen, M. J.: Chorionic gonadotropin in weight control. JAMA 236: 2495, 1976.
24. Stein, M. R.; Julis, R. E.; Peck, C. C.; Hinshaw, W.; Sawicki, J. E.; and Deller, J. J.: Ineffectiveness of human chorionic gonadotropin in weight reduction: a double blind study. Am. J. Clin. Nutr. 29: 940, 1976.
25. Hirsch, J.: Jejunoileal shunt for obesity. N. Engl. J. Med. 290: 962, 1974.
26. Brewer, C.; White, H.; and Braddeley, M.: Beneficial effects of jejunoileostomy on compulsive eating and associated psychiatric symptoms. Br. Med. J. 3: 314, 1974.
27. Randolph, J. G.; Weintraub, W. H.; and Rigg, A.: Jejunoileal bypass for morbid obesity in adolescents. J. Pediatr. Surg. 9: 341, 1974.
28. Heydman, A. H.: Intestinal bypass for obesity. Am. J. Nurs. 74: 1102, 1974.
29. Bleicher, J. E.; Cegielski, M.; and Saporta, J. A.: Intestinal bypass operation for massive obesity. Postgrad. Med. 55: 65, Apr. 1974.
30. Swenson, S. A., and Oberst, B.: Pre- and postoperative care of the patient with intestinal bypass for obesity. Am. J. Surg. 129: 225, 1975.
31. Buchwald, H.; Moore, R. B.; and Varco, R. L.: Surgical treatment of hyperlipidemia. III. Clinical status of the partial ileal bypass operation. Circulation 49: I-22, 1974.
32. Chandler, J. G.: Surgical treatment of massive obesity. Postgrad. Med. 56: 124, Aug. 1974.
33. Gazet, J. C.; Pilkington, T. R. E.; Kalucy, R. S.; Crisp, A. H.; and Day, S.: Treatment of gross obesity by jejunal bypass. Br. Med. J. 4: 311, 1974.
34. Lockwood, D. H.; Amatruda, J. M.; Moxley, R. T.; Pozefsky, T.; and Boitmott, J. K.: Effect of oral amino acid supplementation on liver disease after jejunoileal bypass for morbid obesity. Am. J. Clin. Nutr. 30: 58, 1977.
35. Barry, R. E.; Barisch, J.; Bray, G. A.; Sperling, M. A.; Morin, R. J.; and Benefield, J.: Intestinal adaptation after jejunoileal bypass in man. Am. J. Clin. Nutr. 30: 32, 1977.
36. Stauffer, J. Q.: Hyperoxaluria and calcium oxalate nephrolithiasis after jejunoileal bypass. Am. J. Clin. Nutr. 30: 64, 1977.
37. Griffin, W. O.; Young, L.; and Stevenson, C. C.: A prospective comparison of gastric and jejunoileal bypass procedures for marked obesity. Ann. Surg. 186: 500, 1977.
38. Brightwell, D. R.: Treating obesity with behavior modification. Postgrad. Med. 55: 52, Apr. 1974.
39. Katz, R. C., and Zlutnick, S.: Behavior Therapy and Health Care: Principles and Applications. New York: Pergamon, 1975.
40. Ferguson, J. M.: Habits, Not Diets. Palo Alto: Buil, 1976.
41. Guggenheim, F. G.: Basic considerations in the treatment of obesity. Med. Clin. N. Am. 61: 781, 1977.
42. Better Homes and Gardens: Eat and Stay Slim. New York: Meredith, 1968.
43. Nidetch, J.: Weight Watchers Program Cookbook. New York: Hearthside, 1972.
44. MacRae, N. M.: How to Have Your Cake and Eat It Too: Anchorage: Alaska Northwest, 1975.

PART G        Modifications in Mineral Content

# Sodium Restricted Diet

***Definition***    A diet in which the sodium content is limited to a prescribed level [1].

***Characteristics of the diet***    Vary with the degree of restriction. Foods containing large amounts of natural sodium or commercially processed foods to which a sodium containing compound has been added are either eliminated or restricted in amount. Fruits are generally used liberally, as they are insignificant sources of sodium. Low sodium foods permitted on the diet have been grouped into lists according to their sodium content by a joint committee of the American Heart Association and the U.S. Public Health Service.

**Table 1. Sodium Expressed in Milligrams, Milliequivalents, or Sodium Chloride**

| Sodium (mg) | Sodium (meq) | Sodium chloride (g) |
|---|---|---|
| 250 | 11 | 0.65 |
| 500 | 22 | 1.30 |
| 1,000 | 44 | 2.50 |
| 1,500 | 65 | 3.75 |
| 2,000 | 87 | 5.00 |
| 2,400–4,500 | 105–197 | 6.10–11.44 |

***Aims of sodium restriction***    To restore normal sodium balance to the body by effecting loss of excess sodium and water from extracellular fluid compartments.

Sodium is the principle cation of extracellular fluid and is involved in the maintenance of normal blood fluid volume [2]. Normally, moderate sodium loads are promptly excreted in the urine [3]. In certain conditions, however, there is a breakdown of the body's normal homeostatic mechanism, resulting in sodium and water retention and necessitating a reduction in dietary sodium intake [3].

***Indications for use***    *In liver disease*    The accumulation of massive quantities of fluid in the peritoneal cavity, ascites with or without edema, is a frequent complication of cirrhosis [4]. Portal hypertension, hypoalbuminemia (a serum albumin level of less than 3.5 g/100 ml), and other factors that tend to reduce plasma colloid osmotic pressure will upset the body's control of sodium and water balance; retention of sodium and water leads to ascites [5]. Restriction of dietary sodium is usually mandatory [5] and has proven to be an effective method of promoting diuresis and preventing reaccumulation of fluid [4,6].

These patients should be categorized according to their abilities to excrete water and sodium; those with a high urinary sodium excretion rate can be treated by low sodium diet alone, while those with a low sodium excretion rate but a high water excretion rate should be put on a low sodium diet, with the addition of distal potassium sparing diuretics such as spironolactone or triamterene [7,8]. Furthermore, hyperaldosteronism with edema may be a complication of cirrhosis, for which the latter diuretics are particularly useful, since they block the sodium retaining effect of aldosterone on the distal tubule and collecting duct of the kidney [9]. Rapid diuresis with more potent agents can have an effect similar to that of a high protein intake—resulting in hepatic encephalopathy [10]. Daily protein intake should not exceed the Recommended Dietary Allowances.

A diet containing as little as 230 mg (10 meq) sodium may be necessary initially [4,11]. Under these conditions, severe sodium restriction enhances water excretion even when serum sodium is moderately low (125—30 meq/litre). As recovery progresses, the diet may be liberalized. Repair of liver tissue mass is associated with an increase in plasma albumin to a normal level, which in turn results in an increase in plasma colloid osmotic pressure. Normalization of plasma colloid osmotic pressure permits a slow steady loss of water and a gradual return to a normal diet [6].

*Sodium as an etiological factor in hypertension*    The role of sodium intake in the genesis of hypertension is controversial. An interesting new theory—the high sodium, low potassium environment theory—suggests that the excessive consumption of dietary sodium, along with a reduction in dietary potassium intake, induces an increase in extracellular fluid volume that causes hypertension in genetically susceptible individuals [12]. As of 1978, except for epidemiological data, circumstantial evidence, and data from certain animal studies [13], there remains no proof that a high sodium diet *alone* will result in hypertension in normal man [14,15].

*Sodium restriction as a treatment for established hypertension*    The fact that excess sodium ingestion may increase the severity of hypertension once it has developed in certain salt sensitive patients is not disputed [15]. In the hypertensive patient, sodium restricted diets have a mechanism of action similar to that of diuretic drugs. Both forms of therapy produce a negative salt and water balance during long-term treatment and prevent sodium retention [16]. Consequently, they both result in volume depletion and short- and long-term hemodynamic adjustments that produce arterial blood pressure reductions [16]. Some forms of hypertension, however, respond to this form of therapy less favorably than others. Primary aldosteronism, hypervolemic essential hypertension, and hypertension associated with chronic renal parenchymal disease are three forms of the disorder that benefit from the induction of a negative salt and water balance [16].

*Severe dietary sodium restrictions vs. mild restrictions*    Advances in drug therapy have reduced the need for extremely low sodium diets [9,17,18]. When renal function is sufficient to permit a diuretic to be effective, severely restricted sodium diets are unnecessary and serve no purpose. Conversely, in the absence of diuretics, sodium restriction has to be as rigid as 200 mg (9 meq)/day in order to have a therapeutic effect in severely affected patients [16]. Furthermore, many low sodium diets are unpalatable, difficult to implement, and associated with a very low rate of patient compliance [19,20]. On the other hand, the use of mild and moderately restricted sodium diets has recently been rediscovered as an adjunct to drug therapy in treating certain forms of hypertension. Reduction of sodium intake to a level of 1,100 mg/day has been shown to enhance the effectiveness of propranolol [21].

Avoidance of sodium excesses or mild sodium restriction has been shown to be helpful against the possibility of overriding the diuretic effect of drug therapy [16]. Because of the side effects of certain diuretics, many treatment centers now advocate mild degrees of sodium restriction in order to reduce drug dosage [19].

In general, it has been suggested that a sodium intake of 85–87 meq or approximately 2,000 mg sodium/day will enhance the effectiveness of diuretic agents in treating certain forms of hypertension [16, 22]. Most physicians now agree that patients with arterial blood pressures consistently above 160/95 mm mercury should be treated. Levels between 140/90 and 160/95 mm mercury constitute a gray zone where the age of the patient, his individual problems, and the judgment of the physician determine the decision [22]. A recent study of individuals not on any drugs with borderline hypertension noted a 7.3 mm mercury decrease in diastolic pressure while they were on a mild degree of sodium restriction. The diet prescribed was a 1,600–2,300 mg sodium diet, but the level of compliance was closer to 3,450 mg sodium/day. The author postulated that the therapeutic effect would have been even more significant with greater dietary compliance and that in persons with a diastolic blood pressure between 90 and 105 mm mercury, sodium restriction should be tried before drugs [20]. With increasing severity of hypertensive disease the patient's ability to excrete water and sodium decreases [23,24], and diet alone is ineffective.

*In congestive heart failure* Sodium retention and edema occur in congestive heart failure as a result of inadequate cardiac output [25], and congestion of fluid in the lungs leads to pulmonary edema. The kidneys are unable to excrete salt and water adequately because of impaired renal hemodynamics and hormonal factors. The deficient cardiac output results in an imbalance in the capillary fluid shift mechanism and production of the hormone aldosterone, which promotes sodium reabsorption. Consequently, excess sodium and water are stored in tissue spaces as edema fluid [25]. Whenever myocardial infarction is complicated by congestive heart failure, sodium intake must be restricted. Fortunately, the availability of potent diuretics such as furosemide and ethacrynic acid has obviated the need for severe dietary restrictions in most instances [26,27]. A diet containing 2,100 mg or approximately 90 meq sodium is probably as restrictive as is necessary for the majority of patients who are ambulatory or who are responding to diuretic treatment [25,28]. On the other hand, sodium intakes of less than 500 mg (22 meq) or even 250 mg (11 meq) daily have been advoated for patients with severe, refractory pulmonary edema, particularly if they are not being treated with the more potent diuretics [25].

*In renal disease* Whenever renal disease is complicated by edema or diastolic blood pressure above 110 mm mercury (moderate hypertension), sodium intake should be restricted to 40–90 meq or 900–2,100 mg daily [29]. Patients whose renal failure is caused by glomerulonephritis are more prone to develop hypertension and edema than others; thus, they are more likely to require sodium restricted diets. Such diets may not be indicated at all in other types of renal disease. The nephrotic syndrome, by definition, is characterized by low levels of plasma albumin that provoke sodium retention and edema in some cases [30]. Some of these patients, however, lose the ability to conserve sodium on low intakes, as well as the capacity to excrete excess sodium while on high intakes [31]; thus, it may be more important to attempt to restore serum proteins by adequate diet than to restrict sodium. Therefore, the sodium component of the diet prescription for patients with renal disease should be formulated only after an evaluation of the 24-hour urinary sodium output, blood pressure, and weight changes [29]. If the patient is gaining weight unaccounted for by his caloric intake, if his urinary sodium output is less than his intake, or if he has hypertension, a sodium restricted diet is indicated.

In a recent study of individuals with essential hypertension and impaired renal function, mild to moderate sodium restriction and the use of furosemide produced better control of arterial pressure without changes in renal functions than did sodium restriction alone [32].

*With adrenocortical therapy*    The adrenocortical hormones of the anterior pituitary gland and the steroids of the adrenal cortex are used to treat a variety of diseases. However, their continued use may result in sodium retention and edema [33, 34]. In order to counteract this effect, mild sodium restrictions may be indicated.

***Possible adverse reactions***    *Sodium depletion*    Abrupt withdrawal of dietary sodium in normal subjects activates homeostatic mechanisms that increase renal sodium conservation. Diets that are very low in sodium must be used with caution, however, as they can result in depletion of body sodium stores, particularly in those patients with chronic renal insufficiency [35]. Some of these patients may lose the ability to reabsorb sodium in a normal fashion; these salt wasters become sodium depleted on a severely restricted sodium diet [33]. The excretion of urinary sodium greater than intake accompanied by weight loss and a decrease in renal function indicates that more sodium is needed [35]. Too little sodium in the diet can produce muscle cramps, convulsions, hypovolemia, hypotension, and further deterioration of renal function in patients with renal disease [31].

Age also modifies factors that determine renal sodium handling, such as the rate of glomerular filtration, renal hemodynamics, and responsiveness to the renin–angiotensin–aldosterone system. A group of normal persons over 60 were recently found to have a more sluggish conservation response to sodium restriction than subjects in their late teens and twenties [36]; thus, elderly patients may be more vulnerable to abrupt dietary sodium withdrawal than younger persons. In addition, in the period immediately following myocardial infarction, severe sodium restriction may precipitate or aggravate shock by complementing the extensive loss of salt occurring as a result of profuse diaphoresis [37].

*Contraindications*    *In uncomplicated renal disease*    Vigorous sodium restriction should never be employed in renal disease in the absence of complications such as hypertension and edema [38]. Patients with tubular involvement, such as pyelonephritis or interstitial nephritis, polycystic renal disease, or bilateral hydronephrosis, will lose more sodium than patients with glomerulonephritis [29,31]. If normotension or hypotension is demonstrated, sodium intake may need to be increased rather than decreased [23]. In addition, one study has suggested that treatment of renal disease with oral calcium carbonate is associated with an increased urinary sodium excretion [39].

*In normal pregnancies*    The practice of routine administration of sodium restricted diets in pregnancy is counterproductive [40]. Sodium conservation is a normal physiological adjustment to increased need occurring during pregnancy [41]. Severe limitations in dietary sodium may compromise the delicate biochemical and physiological adjustments normally associated with increased nutrient requirements that occur. Furthermore, some pregnant women with chronic hypertension may be sodium wasters [42].

*In ileostomized patients*    Both the ileum and the colon play an important role in sodium and water conservation. Chronic dehydration and sodium depletion can occur in patients with ileostomies who are receiving inadequate sodium intakes [43–46]. Results of one study have led the authors to propose that patients with ileorectal anastomoses are less at risk than those with ileostomies [47].

*In myxedema*    Myxedema and severe hypothyroidism may be associated with hyponatremia. In addition, total body depletion of sodium has been reported as a result of diarrhea in myxedema crisis [48]. Severely affected patients exhibit impaired tubular reabsorption of sodium and are consequently less able to conserve sodium on low intakes [49–51]; they should not be subjected to further sodium losses via a sodium restricted diet.

**Suggestions for dietitians**    In addition to the sodium naturally occurring in foods, many sodium containing compounds, such as monosodium glutamate, baking powder, sodium chloride, baking soda, disodium phosphate, sodium propionate, and sodium benzoate, are used in food manufacturing. There are excellent materials available to dietitians that provide detailed descriptions of the uses of sodium containing additives [52], as well as patient education materials [53,54] and cookbooks [55,56]. Furthermore, dietitians should be aware of the sodium content of the water supply in the regions in which they practice. In areas where the sodium content of the water supply is high, locally bottled carbonated beverages, wines, and other alcoholic beverages may contribute appreciably to the sodium content of the diet [57–59]. Drugs and medicinals may also have appreciable amounts of sodium [60]. Depending upon the water content and the level of sodium restriction, drinking water may have to be either restricted or distilled [61].

Particularly on the less severely restricted diets, the meal patterns presented in table 4 are meant to be used only as a guide; several other combinations of food groups are possible within the confines of a nutritionally adequate sodium restricted diet. At the level of 1 g sodium daily and above, the diet can be further modified to suit the individual and his circumstances by using the food groups listed. For example, a patient on a 2 g sodium diet who desires natural cheddar cheese may substitute 2 oz of it for two slices of regular bread. He should then reduce his intake of regular bread from five slices daily to three. The inclusion of the basic food groups in appropriate amounts provides insurance against nutritional deficits; the only other absolute in calculating the diet is that it truly reflect the amount of sodium mandated by the diet prescription. Finally, in light of the evidence implicating potassium deficits and hypertension [62], dietary assessment and counseling strategies should focus on potassium as well as sodium intakes.

**Table 2.  Approximate Sodium Content of Certain Food Groups That May Be Calculated into Sodium Restricted Diets**

| *Foods containing 500 mg Na/serving* | *Foods containing 250 mg Na/serving* | *Foods containing 200 mg Na/serving* | *Foods containing 100 mg Na/serving* | *Foods containing 50 mg Na/serving* |
|---|---|---|---|---|
| scant ¼ tsp salt | 1 oz canned tuna | 1 slice regular bakery bread or roll | ½ cup of the following unsalted vegetables: beet greens, frozen mixed peas and carrots, Swiss chard | ½ cup of the following fresh, frozen, or canned vegetables, canned without salt: |
| ¾ tsp monosodium glutamate | 2 oz canned sardines or salmon | 2 thin slices bacon, crisp and drained | | 1 artichoke, edible base and leaves |
| ½ bouillon cube | ⅔ cup buttermilk | 3 oz canned shrimp cooked in salted water | 1 oz fresh koshered meat | beets carrots celery dandelion greens |
| 1 cup tomato juice | ½ cup canned or regularly seasoned carrots, spinach, beets, celery, kale, or white turnips | ½ cup canned or regularly seasoned vegetables not listed elsewhere | 1 oz frozen fish fillets | kale mustard greens peas, black eyed spinach |
| 1 average serving ½ cup cooked rice, spaghetti, noodles, hominy, etc., seasoned with salt | 5 salted crackers (2 in. square) | 1 days's supply of drinking water if it contains 100 mg Na/qt | | succotash turnip greens turnip, white |
| ½ cup drained sauerkraut | ¾ cup tomato juice | ½ cup frozen peas or lima beans | | 1 day's supply of drinking water if it contains 40 mg Na/qt |
| 1 average frankfurter (1½ oz) | 1 day's supply of drinking water if it contains 120 mg Na/qt | 1 oz natural cheddar cheese | | |
| 1 day's supply of drinking water if it contains 220 mg Na/qt | | 1 tbsp catsup | | |

**Table 3.  Approximate Nutritive Values of Food Lists for Planning Sodium Restricted Diets (500 mg)**

| List | Amount | Energy (kcal) | Protein (g) | Fat (g) | Carbo-hydrate (g) | Sodium (mg) |
|---|---|---|---|---|---|---|
| 1. Milk, whole | 1 cup reg. | 170 | 8 | 10 | 12 | 120 |
|  | 1 cup LS* | 170 | 8 | 10 | 12 | 7 |
| Milk, nonfat | 1 cup reg. | 85 | 8 | 0 | 12 | 120 |
|  | 1 cup LS | 85 | 8 | 0 | 12 | 7 |
| 2. Vegetables List 2 | ½ cup | 25 | 2 | 0 | 5 | 9 |
| Starchy vege-tables | Varies with choice | 70 | 2 | 0 | 15 | 5 |
| 3. Fruits | Varies with choice | 40 | 0 | 0 | 10 | 2 |
| 4. LS breads, cereals | Varies with choice | 70 | 2 | 0 | 15 | 5 |
| 5. Meat, poultry, fish, eggs, or cheese | 1 oz meat or equivalent | 75 | 7 | 5 | 0 | 25 |
| 6. Fats | 1 tsp butter or equivalent | 45 | 0 | 5 | 0 | tr. |
| 7. Free choice | Varies with choice | 75 | See list: depends on selection made. | | | 10 |

*Source*:  Adapted from Your 500 Milligram Sodium Diet [53].
*Note*:  This level of sodium restriction and the food groups listed form the basis for the other levels of sodium restriction as well. By the addition of certain foods to the basic lists, many other modifications are possible. (See tables 2, 4, and 6 and the suggestions for dietitians.)
* LS = low sodium.

## Food Lists for Sodium Restricted Diets

See Exchange Lists for Meal Planning (pp. F20–F25) for food groupings and portion sizes. For each list, note the items listed here that must be avoided.

**Foods allowed**                                        **Foods excluded**

*List 1. Milk*

Skim, whole, evaporated, low sodium          Commercial foods made with milk—chocolate milk, condensed milk, ice cream, malted milk, milk mixes, milk shakes, sherbet (if kilocalories are not restricted, chocolate milk and condensed milk are also permitted)

*List 2. Vegetables*

Fresh, frozen, or dietetic canned with no salt or other sodium compounds (see List 2, Exchange Lists for Meal Planning, p. F21); starchy vegetables (see Bread Lists, Exchange Lists for Meal Planning, pp. F22–F23)          Canned vegetables or juices except low sodium dietetic; artichokes, beet greens, celery, Swiss chard, dandelion greens, kale, mustard greens, sauerkraut, spinach; beets, carrots, frozen peas if processed with salt, white turnips; frozen lima beans if processed with salt, hominy, potato chips

*List 3. Fruits*

Fresh, frozen, canned, or dried (see Exchange Lists for Meal Planning, pp. F21–F22)          Crystallized or glazed fruit, maraschino cherries, dried fruit with sodium sulfite added

| Foods allowed | Foods excluded |
|---|---|

### List 4. Bread

Low sodium breads, cereals, and cereal products: bread and rolls (yeast) made without salt; quick breads made with sodium free baking powder or potassium bicarbonate and without salt, or made from low sodium dietetic mix; cereals, cooked, unsalted; dry cereals; puffed rice, puffed wheat, shredded wheat; barley; cornmeal; cornstarch; low sodium crackers; matzoth, plain, unsalted; yeast waffle

Yeast bread, rolls, or melba toast made with salt or from commercial mixes; quick breads made with baking powder, baking soda, salt, or monosodium glutamate or made from commercial mixes; quick cooking and enriched cereals that contain a sodium compound (read labels); dry cereals except as listed; graham crackers or any other except low sodium dietetic; salted popcorn; self-rising cornmeal; pretzels; waffles containing salt, baking powder, baking soda, or egg white

### List 5. Meat

Meat, poultry, fish, eggs, and low sodium cheese and peanut butter: meat or poultry: fresh, frozen, or canned low sodium; liver (only once in 2 weeks); tongue, fresh; fish or fish fillets, fresh only—bass, bluefish, catfish, cod, eels, flounder, halibut, rockfish, salmon, sole, trout, tuna; salmon, canned low sodium dietetic; tuna, canned low sodium dietetic; cheese, cottage, unsalted; cheese, processed low sodium dietetic; egg (limit 1 per day); peanut butter, low sodium dietetic

Brains or kidneys; canned, salted, or smoked meat: bacon, bologna, chipped or corned beef, frankfurters, ham, kosher meats, luncheon meat, salt pork, sausage, smoked tongue, etc.; frozen fish fillets; canned, salted, or smoked fish—anchovies, caviar, salted and dried cod, herring, canned salmon (except dietetic low sodium): shellfish—clams, crabs, lobsters, oysters, scallops, shrimp, etc.; cheese except low sodium dietetic; egg substitutes, frozen or powdered; peanut butter unless low sodium dietetic

### List 6. Fat

Spreads, oils, cooking fats, unsalted

Salted butter or margarine, bacon and bacon fat, salt pork, olives, commercial French or other dressings except low sodium, commercial mayonnaise, except low sodium, salted nuts

### List 7. Free choice

Bread list (1 unit)
Candy, homemade, salt free, or special low sodium (75 kcal)
Fat list (2 units)
Fruit list (2 units)
Sugar, white or brown (4 tsp)
Syrup, honey, jelly, jam, or marmalade (4 tsp)
Vegetable list, Group C (1 unit)

| Foods allowed | Foods excluded |
|---|---|

*Miscellaneous foods*

Beverages: alcoholic with doctor's permission; cocoa made with milk from diet; coffee, instant, freeze dried, or regular; coffee substitutes; lemonade; Postum; tea

Candy, homemade, salt free, or special low sodium

Gelatin, plain unflavored

Fountain beverages; instant cocoa mixes; prepared beverage mixes, including fruit flavored powders
Commercial candies, cakes, cookies
Commercial sweetened gelatin desserts
Mixes of all types
Pastries

*Leavening agents*

Cream of tartar, sodium free baking potassium bicarbonate, yeast; rennet dessert powder (not tablets)

Regular baking powder, baking soda (sodium bicarbonate); rennet tablets; pudding mixes; molasses

*Flavoring aids*

Allspice; almond extract; anise seed; basil; bay leaf; bouillon cube (low sodium); caraway seed; cardamom; chives; cinnamon; cloves; cocoa (1–2 tsp); cumin; curry; dill; fennel; garlic; ginger; horseradish (prepared without salt); juniper; lemon juice or extract; mace; maple extract; marjoram; mint; mustard, dry; nutmeg; onion, fresh, juice or slices; orange extract; oregano; paprika; parsley; pepper; peppermint extract; poppy seed; poultry seasoning; purslane; rosemary; saffron; sage; salt substitute (with doctor's approval); savory; sesame seeds; sorrel; sugar; tarragon; thyme; turmeric; vanilla extract; vinegar; walnut extract; wine, if allowed by physician

Barbecue sauce; bouillon cube, regular; catsup; celery salt, seed, leaves; chili sauce; cyclamates; garlic salt; horseradish, prepared with salt; meat extracts, sauces, tenderizers; monosodium glutamate; mustard, prepared; olives; onion salt; pickles; relishes; Saccharin; salt; soy sauce; sugar substitutes containing sodium; Worcestershire sauce

**Table 4. Sample Meal Patterns for Various Levels of Sodium Restriction**

| Food group | Serving unit | Na (mg per unit) | 250 mg Na diet No. of serv. | 250 mg Na diet Total mg Na | 500 mg Na diet No. of serv. | 500 mg Na diet Total mg Na | 1,000 mg Na diet No. of serv. | 1,000 mg Na diet Total mg Na | 1,500 mg Na diet No. of serv. | 1,500 mg Na diet Total mg Na | 2,000 mg Na diet No. of serv. | 2,000 mg Na diet Total mg Na |
|---|---|---|---|---|---|---|---|---|---|---|---|---|
| Milk, fresh | 1 cup | 120 | 0 | 0 | 2 | 240 | 2 | 240 | 2 | 240 | 2 | 240 |
| Low sodium milk* [61] | 1 cup | 7 | 2 | 14 | 0 | 0 | 0 | 0 | 0 | 0 | 0 | 0 |
| Meat, fish, poultry, cheese, unsalted | 1 oz | 25 | 4 | 100 | 4 | 100 | 4 | 100 | 5 | 125 | 6 | 150 |
| Egg | 1 egg | 60 | 1 | 60 | 1 | 60 | 1 | 60 | 1 | 60 | 1 | 60 |
| Salted bread or ready to eat cereals not listed elsewhere | 1 slice bread or ¾ oz cereal | 200 | 0 | 0 | 0 | 0 | 2 | 400 | 4 | 800 | 5 | 1,000 |
| Low sodium breads, cereals, or cereal products | varies | 5 | 7 | 35 | 7 | 35 | 7 | 35 | 3 | 15 | 4 or more | 20 |
| Group A veg.† | ½ cup | 9 | ½ cup | 9 | ½ cup | 9 | ½ cup | 9 | ½ cup | 9 | not | 9 |
| Group B veg.† | ½ cup | 9 | ½ cup | 9 | ½ cup | 9 | ½ cup | 9 | ½ cup | 9 | re- | 9 |
| Group C veg.† | ½ cup | 5 | ½ cup | 5 | ½ cup | 5 | ½ cup | 5 | ½ cup | 5 | stricted | 5 |
| Canned or reg. seasoned vegetables not listed elsewhere. | ½ cup | 200 | 0 | 0 | 0 | 0 | 0 | 0 | 0 | 0 | ½ cup | 200 |
| Fruits | varies | 2 | 4 | 8 | 4 | 8 | 4 | 8 | 4 | 8 | 4 | 8 |
| Unsalted fats | varies | 0 | un-limited | 0 | un-limited | 0 | un-limited | 0 | un-limited | 0 | un-limited | 0 |
| Salted butter or margarine or regular mayonnaise | 1 tsp / 1 tsp / 1½ tsp | 50 | 0 | 0 | 0 | 0 | 2 | 100 | 4 | 200 | 6 | 300 |
| Total Na (mg) | | | | 240 | | 466 | | 966 | | 1,471 | | 2,001 |

\* Low sodium milk made by ion exchange process has an increased potassium content and may be contraindicated in renal disease [61].
† See Exchange Lists for Meal Planning, pp. F20–F25.

**Table 5. Guidelines for a Mildly Restricted Sodium Diet: 2,400–4,500 mg Sodium Diet (105–97 meq)**

1. Estimate the usual daily salt and monosodium glutamate intake of the individual and adjust accordingly.

2. Use only in baking: baking powder, baking soda, cream of tartar.

3. Do not worry about the following:
    Disodium phosphate
    Sodium alginate
    Sodium propionate
    Sodium benzoate
    Sodium sulfite

4. Eliminate especially the following foods unless the diet has been recalculated to permit the substitution of one of the following foods for a certain amount of regular salted bread and butter or table salt (see the suggestions for dietitians):

    Salty or smoked meat such as bacon, bologna, chipped beef or corned beef, frankfurters, ham, meats koshered by salting, luncheon meats, salt pork, sausage, smoked tongue

    Salty or smoked fish, anchovies, caviar, salted cod, herring, sardines, etc.

    Processed cheese or cheese spreads unless low sodium dietetic

    Cheese, such as Roquefort, Camembert, or Gorgonzola

    Regular peanut butter

    Sauerkraut, pickles, or other vegetables prepared in brine or heavily salted

    Breads and rolls with salt toppings

    Regular salted popcorn

    Potato chips

    Corn chips

    Pretzels

    Olives

    Salted nuts

    Party spreads and dips and other heavily salted snack food, such as potato chips and sticks, crackers

    Canned soups, stews, and any kind of commercial bouillon

    Instant cocoa mixes

    Cooking wine

    Pickles and relishes

    Celery salt, garlic salt, and onion salt

    Catsup

    Chili sauce

    Commercial seasonings made of meat and vegetable extracts

    Barbecue sauces and meat sauces

    Meat tenderizers

    Soy sauce

    Worcestershire sauce

*Source*: Adapted from Your Sodium Mild Restricted Diet [53].

**Table 6.  Sample Modifications of One Basic Menu for Varying Degrees of Sodium Restriction**

| *500 mg Na diet** | *1,000 mg Na diet* | *1,500 mg Na diet* | *2,000 mg Na diet* |
|---|---|---|---|
| **A.M.** | | | |
| Baked apple with sugar | Baked apple with sugar | Baked apple with sugar | Baked apple with sugar |
| Soft cooked egg | Soft cooked egg | Soft cooked egg | Soft cooked egg |
| Puffed wheat | Puffed wheat | Puffed wheat | *Cornflakes* |
| 1 slice low sodium toast | 1 slice low sodium toast | *1 slice regular bread* | *1 slice regular bread* |
| 1 tsp unsalted margarine | 1 tsp unsalted margarine | 1 tsp unsalted margarine | *1 tsp regular margarine* |
| 1 cup whole milk | 1 cup whole milk | 1 cup whole milk | 1 cup whole milk |
| Coffee with sugar | Coffee with sugar | Coffee with sugar | Coffee with sugar |
| **Noon** | | | |
| 2 oz broiled fresh flounder | 2 oz broiled fresh flounder | 2 oz broiled fresh flounder | *3 oz fresh flounder* |
| Fresh broccoli unsalted | Fresh broccoli unsalted | Fresh broccoli unsalted | Fresh broccoli unsalted |
| Baked potato | Baked potato | Baked potato | Baked potato |
| 1 slice low sodium bread | 1 slice low sodium bread | *1 slice regular bread* | *1 slice regular bread* |
| 2 tsp unsalted margarine | *2 tsp regular margarine* | *2 tsp regular margarine* | *2 tsp regular margarine* |
| ½ cup whole milk | ½ cup whole milk | ½ cup whole milk | ½ cup whole milk |
| Peaches | Peaches | Peaches | Peaches |
| **P.M.** | | | |
| 2 oz roast beef | 2 oz roast beef | *3 oz roast beef* | *3 oz roast beef* |
| ½ cup fresh green beans | ½ cup fresh green beans | ½ cup fresh green beans | *½ cup regular canned green beans* |
| ½ cup steamed rice | ½ cup steamed rice | ½ cup steamed rice | ½ cup steamed rice |
| 2 low sodium rolls | *2 slices regular bread* | *2 slices regular bread* | *1 slice regular bread* |
| 2 tsp unsalted margarine | 2 tsp unsalted margarine | *2 tsp regular margarine* | *2 tsp regular margarine* |
| 1 tsp currant jelly | 1 tsp currant jelly | 1 tsp currant jelly | 1 tsp currant jelly |
| Banana | Banana | Banana | Banana |
| ½ cup milk | ½ cup milk | ½ cup milk | ½ cup milk |
| Tea with lemon | Tea with lemon | Tea with lemon | Tea with lemon |
| **Between meals** | | | |
| ½ cup orange juice | ½ cup orange juice | ½ cup orange juice | ½ cup orange juice |
| Low sodium muffin | Low sodium muffin | Low sodium muffin | *1 slice regular bread* |
| 1 tsp low sodium margarine | 1 tsp low sodium margarine | 1 tsp low sodium margarine | *1 tsp regular margarine* |

* Diet for 250 mg Na diet is same except for use of low sodium milk rather than fresh whole milk.

References

1. Turner, D.:  Handbook of Diet Therapy. 5th ed. Chicago:  University of Chicago Press, 1970.
2. Newburgh, L. H., and Reimer, A.:  The rationale and administration of low sodium diets.  J. Am. Diet. Assoc. 23: 1047, 1947.
3. Food and Nutrition Board, National Research Council:  Recommended Dietary Allowances. 9th ed. Washington, DC:  National Academy of Sciences, 1980.
4. Davidson, C. S.:  Dietary treatment of hepatic disease.  J. Am. Diet. Assoc. 62: 515, 1973.
5. Summerskill, W. H. J.; Barnardo, D. E.; and Baldus, W. P.:  Disorders of water and electrolyte metabolism in liver disease.  Am. J. Clin. Nutr. 23: 499, 1970.
6. Davidson, C. S.:  Diseases of the liver.  Goodhart, R. S., and Shils, M. E., eds. Modern Nutrition in Health and Disease. 5th ed. Philadelphia:  Lea & Febiger, 1973.
7. Vesin, P.:  Potassium metabolism and diuretics administration in liver cirrhosis.  Postgrad. Med. J. 51: 545, 1975.
8. Arroyo, V., and Rodes, J.:  A rational approach to the treatment of ascites.  Postgrad. Med. J. 51: 558, 1975.
9. Krumlovsky, F. A., and del Greco, F.:  Diuretic agents; mechanisms of action and clinical uses.  Postgrad. Med. 59(4): 105, 1976.
10. Conn, H. O.:  Diuresis of ascites: fraught with or free from hazard.  Gastroenterology 73: 619, 1977.
11. Sherlock, S.:  Diuretics in hepatic disease.  Lant, A. F., and Wilson, G. M., eds.  Modern Diuretic Therapy in the Treatment of Cardiovascular and Renal Disease. Amsterdam:  Excerpta Medica, 1973.

12. McNeely, G. R., and Batterbee, H. D.: High sodium-low potassium environment and hypertension. Am. J. Cardiol. 38: 768, 1976.
13. Freis, E. D.: Salt, volume and the prevention of hypertension. Circulation 53: 589, 1976.
14. Kirkendall, W. M.; Connor, W. E.; Abboud, F.; Rastogi, S. P.; Anderson, T. A.; and Fry, M.: The effect of dietary sodium chloride on blood pressure, body fluids, electrolytes, renal function, and serum lipids of normotensive man. J. Lab. Clin. Med. 87: 418, 1976.
15. Kawasaki, T.; DeLea, C. S.; Bartter, F. C.; and Smith, H.: The effect of high sodium and low sodium intakes on blood pressure and other related variables in human subjects with idiopathic hypertension. Am. J. Med. 64: 193, 1978.
16. Dustan, H. R.; Tarazi, R. C.; and Bravo, E. L.: Diuretic and diet treatment of hypertension. Arch. Intern. Med. 133: 1007, 1974.
17. Gordon, E. S.: Dietary problems in hypertension. Geriatrics 29(5): 139, 1974.
18. Wilson, W. R.: Diuretic drugs in the treatment of hypertension. Lant, A. F., and Wilson, G. M., eds. Modern Diuretic Therapy in the Treatment of Cardiovascular and Renal Disease. Amsterdam: Excerpta Medica, 1973.
19. Buccicone, J., and McAllister, R. G.: Failure of single session dietary counseling to reduce salt intake in hypertensive patients. South Med. J. 70: 1436, 1977.
20. Morgan, T.; Gillies, A.; Morgan, G.; Adam, W.; Wilson, M.; and Carney, S.: Hypertension treated by salt restriction. Lancet 1: 227, 1978.
21. Owens, C. J., and Brackett, N. C.: Role of sodium intake in the antihypertensive effect of propranolol. South. Med. J. 71: 43, 1978.
22. Munro, A. B., and Woods, J. W.: Present day management of hypertension. South. Med. J. 67: 847, 1974.
23. Berglund, G.; Wallentin, I.; Wikstrand, J.; and Wilhelmsen, L.: Sodium excretion and sympathetic activity in relation to severity of hypertensive disease. Lancet 1: 324, 1976.
24. Editorial: Hypertension—the chicken and the egg. Lancet 1: 345, 1976.
25. Kark, R. M., and Oyama, J. H.: Nutrition and cardiovascular renal diseases. Goodhart, R. S., and Shils, M. E., eds. Modern Nutrition in Health and Disease. 5th ed. Philadelphia: Lea & Febiger, 1973.
26. Julian, D. G.: Cardiology. 2d ed. London: Balliere Tindall, 1973.
27. Alstead, S., and Girdwood, R. H.: Textbook of Medical Treatment. 13th ed. Edinburgh: Churchill Livingstone, 1974.
28. Schattenberg, T. T., and Brandenberg, R. O.: Nutrition and cardiovascular disease. Med. Clin. N. Am. 54: 1449, 1970.
29. Anderson, C. F.; Nelson, R. A.; Margie, J. D.; Johnson, W. J.; and Hunt, J. C.: Nutritional therapy for adults with renal disease. JAMA 223: 68, 1973.
30. Robson, J. S.: The nephrotic syndrome. Practitioner 212: 37, 1974.
31. David, D. S.: Dietary treatment of renal failure. Am. Heart J. 86: 1, 1973.
32. Mroczek, W. J.; Moir, D.; Davidov, M. E.; and Finnerty, F. A.: Sodium intake and furosemide administration in hypertensive patients with renal insufficiency. Am. J. Cardiol. 39: 808, 1977.
33. Robinson, C. H., and Lawler, M. R.: Normal and Therapeutic Nutrition. 15th ed. New York: Macmillan, 1977.
34. National Research Council: Sodium Restricted Diets. Publ. 325. Washington, DC: National Academy of Sciences, 1954.
35. Yium, J. J.: Determination of diet orders by analysis of lab values. Tex. Med. 69: 71, July 1973.
36. Epstein, M., and Hollenberg, N. K.: Age as a determinant of renal sodium conservation in normal man. J. Lab. Clin. Med. 87: 411, 1976.
37. Christakis, G., and Winston, M.: Nutritional therapy in acute myocardial infarction. J. Am. Diet. Assoc. 63: 233, 1973.
38. Chan, J. C. M.: Dietary management of renal failure in infants and children. Clin. Pediatr. 12: 707, 1973.
39. Popovtzer, M. M., and Robineete, J. B.: Effect of oral calcium carbonate on urinary excretion of Ca, Na, and Mg in advanced renal disease. Proc. Soc. Exp. Biol. Med. 145: 222, 1974.
40. Lindheimer, M. D., and Katz, A. I.: Sodium and diuretics in pregnancy. Obstet. Gynecol. 44: 434, 1974.
41. Pike, R. L., and Smicklas, H. A.: A reappraisal of sodium restriction during pregnancy. Int. J. Obstet. Gynecol. 10: 1, 1972.
42. Foote, R. G.: The use of liberal salt diet in preeclamptic toxemia and essential hypertension with pregnancy. N. Z. Med. J. 77: 242, 1973.

43. Edmonds, C. J.: Sodium transport by mammalian colon. Lant, A. F., and Wilson, G. M., eds. Modern Diuretic Therapy in the Treatment of Cardiovascular and Renal Disease. Amsterdam: Excerpta Medica, 1973.

44. Kramer, P.: The effect of varying sodium loads on the ileal excreta of human ileostomized subjects. J. Clin. Invest. 45: 1710, 1966.

45. Hill, G. L.; Mair, W. S. J.; and Goligher, J. C.: Cause and management of high volume output salt-depleting ileostomy. Br. J. Surg. 62: 720, 1975.

46. Wright, H. K.: The functional consequences of colectomy. Am. J. Surg. 130: 532, 1975.

47. Hill, G. L.; Watts, J. M.; Iseli, A.; Clarke, A. M.; and Hughes, E. S. R.: Total body water and total exchangeable sodium in patients after ileorectal anastomosis. Br. J. Surg. 61: 189, 1974.

48. Mataverde, A. Q.; Abbasi, A. A.; Hossain, Z.; and Bissell, G. W.: Hydrochlorthiazide-induced water intoxication in myxedema. JAMA 230: 1014, 1974.

49. Jones, E. R.; Cook, W.; and Lizzaralde, G.: Myxedema crisis. South. Med. J. 67: 1481, 1974.

50. Vaamonde, C. A.; Oster, J. R.; Lohavichan, C.; Carroll, K. E.; Sebastianelli, M. J.; and Papper, S.: Renal response to sodium restriction in myxedema. Proc. Soc. Biol. Med. 146: 936, 1974.

51. Vaamonde, C. A.; Sebastianelli, M. J.; Vaamonde, L. S.; Pellegrini, E. L.; Watts, R. S.; Klinger, E. L.; and Papper, S.: Impaired renal tubular reabsorption of sodium in hypothyroid man. J. Lab. Clin. Med. 85: 452, 1975.

52. Food and Nutrition Board, National Research Council: The Use of Chemicals in Food Production, Processing, Storage and Distribution. Washington, DC: National Academy of Sciences, 1973.

53. American Heart Association. Your 500 Milligram Sodium Diet (1968); Your Mild Sodium Restricted Diet (1969).

54. American Heart Association Fold Out Charts: Sodium Restricted Diet, 500 mg. (1965); Sodium Restricted Diet, 1000 mg. (1966); Sodium Restricted Diet, Mild Restriction, (1967).

55. Payne, A. S., and Callahan, D.: The Low Sodium, Fat Controlled Cookbook. 4th ed. Boston: Little, Brown, 1975.

56. Bagg, E.: Cooking without a Grain of Salt. New York: Bantam, 1973.

57. McGarvey, J. F. X.: Sodium content of water softened water. JAMA 227: 1258, 1974.

58. Newborg, B.: Sodium restricted diet. Arch. Intern. Med. 123: 692, 1969.

59. Siegel, N. J., and Myketey, N.: Sodium, potassium and calorie contents of some commercial beverages. Clin. Pediatr. 11: 482, 1972.

60. Diet Committee of the San Francisco Heart Association: Sodium in Medicines. San Francisco: San Francisco Heart Association, 1973.

61. Heap, B.: Low Sodium Milk. J. Am. Diet. Assoc. 53: 43, 1968.

62. Walker, W. G.; Whelton, P. K.; Saito, H.; Russell, R. P.; and Hermann, J.: Relation between blood pressure and renin, renin substrate, angiotensin II, aldosterone and urinary sodium and potassium in 574 ambulatory subjects. Hypertension 1: 287, 1979.

# High Potassium Diet (170 meq or 6,630 mg potassium)

*Definition*    A diet that provides a minimum of 170 meq (6,630 mg) of potassium daily. The normal daily intake varies from 50–150 meq [1] and is usually less than 100 meq.

*Characteristics of the diet*    Increased amounts of fruits and vegetables that are good sources of potassium are included daily, such as prunes, oranges, melons, spinach, collard greens, mushrooms, etc. Potassium intake is also augmented by extra servings of protein and potassium containing foods such as meat, fish, and milk. The diet does not necessarily have to be high in kilocalories; however, it is incompatible with a very low kilocalorie, low sodium diet. If kilocalories must be restricted, a high potassium diet may be expensive and lacking in variety.

*Purpose of the diet*    To prevent the depletion of body potassium reserves as a result of therapy with potassium wasting diuretics. Dietary measures alone are generally unsuccessful in reversing a preexisting potassium deficit once it has occurred [2–4]. However, prophylactic use of a high potassium diet at the onset of diuretic therapy may have a sparing effect on body potassium stores [5].

*Effects of potassium depletion*    The incidence and extent of potassium deficits induced by diuretic therapy vary considerably, depending upon the amount and type of drug used, the physiologic status of the patient, and his dietary potassium intake. Sustained and untreated potassium losses will lead to the development of hypochloremic alkalosis and eventually a catabolic state with progressive nitrogen loss [6]. When the serum potassium drops below 3.5 meq/litre, symptoms of lethargy, weakness, muscle hypotonicity, loss of libido, and mental depression may occur. Serum levels of less than 2.7 meq/litre may result in cardiac arrhythmias [2], and paralysis can occur at lower levels.

Potassium plays a role in insulin secretion; its depletion may play a contributing role in impaired insulin release. In addition, in certain conditions potassium deficiency has been implicated in abnormal glucose tolerance test results. Children suffering from protein kilocalorie malnutrition may be particularly susceptible to hypokalemia [7]. Patients stricken with acute myocardial infarction who are hypokalemic may also be prone to the development of certain ectopic heart rhythms [8]. Potassium deficits have been implicated in the pathogenesis of essential hypertension [9].

*Indications for use*    Concomitantly with the administration of potassium wasting diuretics, such as the thiazides, furosemide, and ethacrynic acid. Controversy exists over the necessity and efficiency of routine administration of potassium supplements to all persons taking potassium wasting diuretics [2–6,9–11]. Greater reliance on preventative diet therapy has been advocated in some instances as an alternative to the risks of administering potassium chloride prior to the demonstration of any great total body potassium losses [5,6,9].

*Conditions in which potassium diet therapy may be unsuccessful*
It is generally agreed that under the following conditions oral potassium chloride supplements are indicated rather than a high potassium diet: (1) whenever a combination of drugs that potentiate each other's potassium wasting effect is administered, e.g., digitalis plus a diuretic; (2) whenever a potassium depleting disease is present and a preexisting deficit exists, e.g., cirrhosis of the liver associated with hyponatremia and hypokalemia or secondary aldosteronism [5]; (3) whenever an incompatible dietary restriction must take precedence over the need for a high potassium diet, e.g., a low protein diet or a low kilocalorie diet; (4) in the patient with severe anorexia; (5) in hypokalemia associated with watery diarrhea and non-beta cell tumors of the pancreas [12].

*Possible adverse reactions*     *Hyperkalemia, hyperkalemic acidosis, and cardiac toxicity*     A hyperkalemic response to the diet is very unlikely except in the person who is taking potassium supplements or a potassium sparing diuretic. However, in any clinical state in which there is a tendency toward hyperkalemia, a high potassium diet will aggravate the condition. Symptomatic hyperkalemia occurs when the serum potassium level exceeds 6.5 meq/litre [13]. Lassitude, fatigue, weakness, and devastating effects on the cardiovascular system may occur when serum potassium levels become markedly elevated [13,14].

*Contraindications*     A high potassium diet is contraindicated under the following conditions: (1) whenever the serum potassium level exceeds 5.0 meq/litre; (2) in certain persons with renal failure or adrenal insufficiency [13]; (3) whenever the patient is taking substantial doses of potassium sparing diuretics, such as spironolactone or triamterene (Individuals with diabetes on these drugs are particularly prone to develop hyperkalemia, possibly because of renal insufficiency [3]); (4) whenever the patient is taking potassium supplements [14,15].

*Suggestions for dietitians*     *Avoiding excessive kilocalories in planning the diet*     In planning the diet for the patient who must avoid excessive kilocalories, skim milk and water packed fruits should be used as substitutes for whole milk and sweetened canned fruits. Further reductions in caloric intake may be made by limiting the choices from the miscellaneous list to coffee and tea only.

*Use of salt substitutes*     For those patients whose sodium intake must be restricted, the use of potassium containing salt substitutes deserves special attention. These substances provide significant amounts of potassium. For example, ¼ tsp Morton's Salt Substitute* contains approximately 655 mg potassium. The daily addition to the diet of ¼ tsp of this product would increase the potassium intake to 187 meq, or 7,285 mg. However, if it is not desirable to increase the potassium intake beyond 170 meq daily, milk intake should be limited to 2 cups instead of 3 daily and meat choices reduced from eight to six. Thus, in the latter instance the addition of ¼ tsp salt substitute to the diet would also permit a reduction of sodium and caloric intakes.

*Morton-Norwich Products, Chicago, IL 60606.

*Emphasis on variety in the choice of foods*   In order to limit the total number of food lists used on the diet and thus facilitate its comprehension and use by patients, foods with a wide range of potassium content were sometimes included in the same group (see ranges for each food group). Formulation of a high potassium diet to achieve a narrower range of potassium content would necessitate a greater number of food lists. Variety in food choices should be stressed to minimize the deviations of actual daily potassium intake from calculated intake.

## High Potassium Diet

### Daily Food Plan

| Food list | Potassium per equivalent (mg) | No. of equivalents | Total potassium (mg) |
|---|---|---|---|
| Milk list | 355 | 3 cups | 1,065 |
| Meat and meat substitute lists 1 and 2 | 130 | 8 | 1,040 |
| Fruit list 1 | 115 | As desired | — |
| Fruit list 2 | 195 | 2 | 390 |
| Fruit list 3 | 380 | 4 | 1,520 |
| Vegetable list 1 | 110 | As desired | — |
| Vegetable list 2 | 230 | 2 | 460 |
| Vegetable list 3 | 360 | 3 | 1,080 |
| Bread and bread substitutes list 1 | 45 | 4 | 180 |
| Bread and bread substitutes list 2 | 230 | 2 | 460 |
| Miscellaneous list | 135 | 3 | 405 |
| Fat list | 10 | 3 or more | 30 |
| Total potassium (mg) | | | 6,630 |

*Milk list*

Potassium content per cup = 350–55 mg

   Milk (skim or whole), buttermilk, or yogurt

*Meat and meat substitute list 1*

Potassium content per equivalent = 100–80 mg.   Average = 130 mg.
Unless otherwise stated, 1 choice equals 1 oz.

| | |
|---|---|
| Beef | Bologna, 2⅓ in. slices |
| Chicken, light meat | Chicken, dark meat, 1½ oz |
| Cod | Clams, ½ cup |
| Flounder | Frankfurter, 1 |
| Goose | Lamb, 1½ oz |
| Haddock | Oysters, 5–8 medium |
| Halibut | Peanut butter, 1 tbsp |
| Liver, calves | Scallops, 1 piece, 12 per lb |
| Pork | Shrimp, ¼ cup |
| Salmon, regular or unsalted | Tuna, 1½ oz, regular or unsalted |
| Sole | |
| Turkey | |
| Veal | |

*Meat and meat substitute list 2*

Potassium content per equivalent = 25–60 mg.   Average = 35 mg.
Unless otherwise stated, 1 choice equals 1 oz.

   Cheese, American processed
   Cheese, cheddar
   Cheese, cottage
   Cheese, Swiss
   Egg, 1 whole, medium
   Lobster

*Fruit list 1*

Potassium content per equivalent equals 80–145 mg.   Average equals 115 mg.

Apple, 1 small, 2 in. diameter
Apple juice, ½ cup
Applesauce, sweetened or unsweetened, canned, ¾ cup
Blackberries, fresh or frozen, ½ cup
Blueberries, fresh or frozen, ½ cup
Boysenberries, frozen, sugar added, ⅔ cup
Cherries, canned in heavy syrup, ½ cup
Cherries, sour, canned in heavy syrup, scant ½ cup
Cherries, sweet, 10 large
Cranberries, raw, 1 cup
Currants, red, ¼ cup
Grapefruit, ½ medium
Grapefruit, canned in syrup or water packed, ½ cup
Grape juice, 4 oz
Grapes, American, 17 medium or ½ cup
Grapes, European, 12 medium or ½ cup
Grapes, Thompson Seedless, ½ cup
Pear Nectar, 8 oz
Pears, canned in syrup, 3 halves
Pears, water packed, 3 halves
Pineapple, canned, water packed or sweetened, 1 large slice
Pineapple, raw, 1 slice, 3½ in. diameter
Tangerine, 1 large or 2 small

*Fruit list 2*

Potassium content per equivalent equals 160–260 mg.   Average equals 195 mg.

Apricot juice, ⅔ cup
Fruit cocktail, water packed or in syrup, ½ cup
Grapefruit juice, 4 oz
Kumquats, 4 medium
Mango, ½ medium
Orange juice, ½ cup
Papaya, ⅓ medium
Peaches, canned, sweetened or unsweetened, ¾ cup
Peach, raw, 1 medium
Pear, raw, 1 medium
Persimmon, Japanese, 1 medium
Pineapple juice, 4 oz
Plum, damson, 1 large
Plums, canned in heavy syrup, 3 medium
Plums, prune type, 3 medium
Pomegranate, 1 medium
Raspberries, black, raw, ⅔ cup
Raspberries, red, raw, ¾ cup
Raspberries, red, frozen, ¾ cup
Rhubarb, frozen, sugar added, ⅜ cup
Strawberries, 10 large
Tangerine juice, 4 oz
Watermelon, 1 cup

*Fruit list 3*

Potassium content per equivalent equals 300–490 mg.   Average equals 380 mg.

Apricots, canned, 3 medium halves
Apricots, dried, sulfured, 8 halves
Avocado, ⅓ whole
Banana, 1 small
Cantaloupe, ¾ cup
Dates, 5 medium
Figs, dried, 3 medium
Honeydew melon, 1 piece 2 in. wide, 6½ in. diameter
Orange, 1 medium or ¾ cup canned
Peaches, dried, cooked, sugar added, ½ cup
Prune juice, 5 oz
Prunes, not cooked, 5 large
Raisins, ⅓ cup

*Vegetable list 1*

Potassium content per equivalent equals 80–140 mg.　Average equals 110 mg.

Beans, snap green, 1-in. pieces, cooked, canned, drained solids, ½ cup
Beans, waxed, canned, drained solids, ½ cup
Beets, canned, drained solids, ½ cup
Cabbage, cooked or shredded raw, ½ cup
Carrots, canned, drained solids, ⅔ cup
Celery, raw inner stalks, 2 small
Celery, cooked, ⅖ cup
Corn, canned, drained solids, ½ cup
Cress, water, 10–16 sprigs
Cucumber, ½ medium
Onion, cooked, ½ cup
Onions, scallions, two 5-in. long, ½ in. diameter
Radishes, 3 small
Squash, summer, raw; cooked, drained, ½ cup


*Vegetable list 2*

Potassium content per equivalent equals 185–270 mg.　Average equals 230 mg.

Asparagus, canned, 6 medium spears
Asparagus, cooked, 6 medium spears
Asparagus, frozen, cooked, ⅔ cup
Beans, dry, white, canned with pork and tomato, ½ cup
Beans, dry, red kidney, canned, drained solids, ⅖ cup
Beans, lima, canned, drained solids, ½ cup
Broccoli, cooked, 1 large stalk
Broccoli, frozen, ⅔ cup
Brussels sprouts, cooked, ½ cup
Carrots, raw, shredded, or grated, ⅔ cup
Carrots, cooked, ⅔ cup
Cauliflower, ⅞ cup
Collards, cooked, leaves and stems, ½ cup
Corn on the cob, cooked, 1 ear 4 in. long
Eggplant, ¾ cup
Kale, cooked, ¾ cup
Kohlrabi, cooked, drained, ⅔ cup
Lentils, dry, cooked, drained, ½ cup
Lettuce, 4 large leaves
Mushrooms, canned, solids and liquid, ½ cup
Mustard greens, cooked, ½ cup
Okra, cooked, 8–9 pods
Peas, cooked, ⅔ cup
Pepper, green, empty shell, raw, 1 large
Pumpkin, canned, ⅖ cup
Squash, winter, frozen, cooked, ½ cup
Sweet potatoes, candied, 2 halves
Tomatoes, canned, ½ cup
Turnip greens, solids and liquid, ½ cup
Vegetable juice cocktail, 4 oz


*Vegetable list 3*

Potassium content per equivalent equals 300–500 mg.　Average equals 360 mg.

Artichoke, French, cooked, edible portion, base and soft ends of leaves of 1 artichoke
Bamboo shoots, ½ cup
Beans, white, cooked, ½ cup
Beans, canned without pork, ½ cup
Beans, dry, red kidney, ⅖ cup
Beans, lima, cooked, ½ cup
Beans, baby lima, frozen, cooked, ½ cup
Beans, Fordhook, baby lima, cooked, ⅝ cup
Beet greens, cooked, ½ cup
Chard, cooked, ⅗ cup

Chick peas, dry, uncooked, ¼ cup
Cowpeas, canned, solids and liquids, ½ cup
Cowpeas, cooked, ¼ cup
Escarole, 4 large leaves
Leeks, 3–4
Mushrooms, cooked, 4 large
Parsnips, cooked, ½ cup
Potato, baked, one 2¼ in. diameter
Potato, boiled in skin, 1 medium
Spinach, chopped, frozen, cooked, ½ cup
Spinach, leaf, frozen, cooked, ½ cup
Squash, winter, baked, ½ cup
Sweet potato, baked in skin, 1 small
Tomato, raw, 1 medium
Tomato juice, 5 oz

*Bread and bread substitutes list 1*

Potassium content per equivalent equals 20–65 mg.   Average equals 45 mg.

Biscuit, baking powder, one 2 in. diameter
Bread, Italian, 1 slice
Bread, rye, 1 slice
Bread, white, 1 slice
Bread, whole wheat, 1 slice
Cornflakes, 1 cup
Frosted Mini-Wheats, 4 biscuits
Graham crackers, 2
Macaroni, cooked, ½ cup
Muffin, 1
Noodles, cooked, ½ cup
Oatmeal, cooked, ½ cup
Rice, cooked, ½ cup
Roll, hard or panroll, 1

*Bread and bread substitutes list 2*

Potassium content per equivalent equals 185–260 mg.   Average equals 230 mg.

All-Bran, ½ cup
Boston brown bread, 2 slices
Bran Buds, ⅓ cup
Bran Flakes, 40%, 1 cup
Bread, pumpernickel, 1½ slices
Raisin Bran, ¾ cup

*Miscellaneous list*

Potassium content per equivalent equals 105–200 mg.   Average equals 135 mg.

Almonds, dried, unblanched, 12–15 nuts
Brazil nuts, 5 medium
Cashew nuts, 12–16 nuts
Chestnuts, 4 large
Coconut, shredded, 2 tbsp
Coffee, 10 oz
Filberts, hazelnuts, 20–24
Fruit cake, dark, enriched, 1 piece 3 in. x 3 in. x ½ in.
Litchi nuts, dried, 6 nuts
Molasses, blackstrap, ¾ tsp
Molasses, medium extraction, 2 tsp
Peanuts, roasted with skin, 1 tbsp
Pecans, 24 halves or 4 tbsp
Tea, 14 oz
Walnuts, English, 16–30 halves

*Fat list—as desired*

Potassium content per equivalent equals 0–20 mg.   Average equals 10 mg.
Unless otherwise stated, 1 choice equals 1 tsp.

Bacon, fried crisp, 1 strip
Butter

Cream cheese, 1 oz or 2 tbsp
Cream, light or heavy, 1 tbsp
French dressing
Half and half, 1 tbsp
Italian dressing
Low kilocalorie dressing
Margarine
Mayonnaise
Oils
Olives, black, ripe, 2 large
Olives, green, 2 medium
Thousand Island dressing

*As desired*

Lemons
Salt
Sugar
Vinegar
Any food not specifically omitted

References

1. Food and Nutrition Board Research Council: Recommended Dietary Allowances. 9th ed. Washington, DC: National Academy of Sciences, 1980.
2. Schwartz, A. B.: Diuretic-induced hypokalemia. Am. Fam. Phys. 11: 101, Jan. 1975.
3. Kosman, M. E.: Management of potassium problems during long-term diuretic therapy. JAMA 230: 743, 1974.
4. Schwartz, A. B.: Dosage of potassium chloride elixir to correct thiazide-induced hypokalemia. JAMA 230: 702, 1974.
5. Gray, F. D.: Counterpoint: the management of uncomplicated K$^+$ wasting. Med. Counterpoint 4: 27, 1972.
6. Walker, W. G.; Sapir, D. G.; Turin, M.; and Cheng, J. T.: Potassium homeostasis and diuretic therapy. Lant, A. F., and Wilson, G. M., eds. Modern Diuretic Therapy in the Treatment of Cardiovascular and Renal Disease. Amsterdam: Excerpta Medica, 1973.
7. Mann, M. D.; Becker, D. J.; Pimstone, B. L.; and Hansen, J.: Potassium supplementation, serum immunoreactive insulin concentrations and glucose tolerance in protein-energy malnutrition. Br. J. Nutr. 33: 55, 1975.
8. Dyckner, T.; Helmers, C.; Lundman, T.; and Wester, P. O.: Initial serum potassium level in relation to early complications and prognosis in patients with acute myocardial infarction. Acta Med. Scand. 197: 207, 1975.
9. Walker, W. G.; Whelton, P. K.; Saito, H.; Russell, R. P.; and Hermann, J.: Relation between renin, renin substrate, angiotensin II, aldosterone, and urinary sodium and potassium in 574 ambulatory patients. Hypertension 1: 287, 1979.
10. Dargie, H. J.; Boddy, K.; Kennedy, A. C.; King, P. C.; Read, P. R.; and Ward, D. M.: Total body potassium in long-term furosemide therapy: is potassium supplementation necessary? Br. Med. J. 4: 316, 1974.
11. Wilkinson, P. R.; Hesp, R.; Issler, H.; and Raftery, E. B.: Total body and serum potassium during prolonged thiazide therapy for essential hypertension. Lancet 1: 759, 1975.
12. Semb, L. S.: Watery diarrhea, hypokalemia, and achlorhydria associated with non-beta cell tumor of the pancreas. Nyhus, L. M., ed. Surgery Annual: 1976. New York: Appleton-Century-Crofts, 1976.
13. Newmark, S. R., and Dluhy, R. G.: Hyperkalemia and hypokalemia. JAMA 231: 631, 1975.
14. Kalbian, V. V.: Iatrogenic hyperkalemic paralysis with electrocardiographic changes. South. Med. J. 67: 342, 1975.
15. Lawson, D. H.: Adverse reactions to potassium chloride. Q. J. Med. 43: 433, 1974.

# PART H    Miscellaneous

# Interactions between Diet and Drugs

When drugs and nutrients are taken concurrently, the biological availability of either or each one may be affected by the other. These effects may become clinically significant in patients with poor nutritional status and in patients taking the interacting drugs for chronic or prolonged indications.

Drugs affect the bioavailability of nutrients by both indirect and direct means. Indirect ways in which drugs decrease the absorption of nutrients include induction of nausea, vomiting, diarrhea, and anorexia.

Gastrointestinal upset caused by drugs is usually secondary either to direct chemical insult to the gastrointestinal mucosa or to drug induced changes in the gut flora. The former effect can often be minimized by administration of the drug in smaller, more frequent doses and by the patient's drinking a full glass of water with oral solid drugs to aid dissolution. When not specifically contraindicated by the pharmaceutic or pharmacological characteristics of the drug, a medication that causes troublesome gastrointestinal upset may be taken with a small quantity of food or milk. Some drugs that have a high potential for gastrointestinal upset should routinely be taken with meals (see "Timing of Oral Medication Devices," in this article).

Oral antiinfective agents are seldom completely absorbed. Any quantity of drug that does not enter the blood stream dumps into the colon. Thus, the colonic flora that are susceptible to the drug are decreased and the resulting overgrowth of nonsusceptible organisms frequently results in diarrhea. These effects can usually be lessened by lowering the dose of the drug or by the use of better absorbed and/or narrower spectrum antiinfectives.

Drug induced anorexia is often dose related or due to pharmacologically predictable side effects. When drug induced anorexia becomes clinically significant, discussion of alternative drugs or dosage adjustments should be initiated between the prescribing pharmacist and dietitian.

## Interference with Absorption

Drugs may directly interfere with the biological availability of nutrients by decreasing gastrointestinal absorption. All laxatives may decrease absorption of nutrients by lessening gastrointestinal transit time [1]. The most troublesome type of laxative in this regard is the peristaltic stimulant. These include, among others:

| | |
|---|---|
| Bisacodyl | (Dulcolax) |
| Senna | (Senokot) |
| Phenolphthalein | (in Exlax) |

Arthur G. Lipman, who prepared this article, is Associate Professor of Clinical Pharmacology and Chairman of the Department of Pharmacy Practice, College of Pharmacy, The University of Utah, Salt Lake City, UT; he was formerly Drug Information Director, Yale-New Haven Hospital, New Haven, CT.

Laxative overuse is extremely common in contemporary American society. Chronic laxative abusers whose nutritional status is compromised by laxative use may require retraining in normal bowel habits and agressive dietary therapy.

Intestinal lubricants taken orally as laxatives impede absorption of the fat soluble vitamins (A, D, E, K) [2]. Such laxatives include:

Mineral oil
Haleys MO

Saline cathartics are hypertonic solutions that draw extralumenal water into the gut. These drugs are not as apt to cause malabsorption of nutrients as the peristaltic lubricants, but chronic abuse can decrease nutrient availability. These drugs include:

Milk of magnesia
Citrate of Magnesia
Epsom salts

The vegetable bulk producers (psyllium—Metamucil) are the laxatives least apt to cause malabsorption of nutrients.

## Alteration of Gastrointestinal pH

Most drugs are weak acids or bases that do not significantly alter physiological pH. However, some drugs can induce metabolic pH changes secondary to direct effects on gastrointestinal pH or by induction of urinary alkalosis or acidosis [1]. Drugs frequently implicated in such changes are:

Ascorbic acid   (vitamin C in high doses decreases pH)
Diuretics   (cause urinary pH changes due to electrolyte wasting)
Antacids   (raise gastrointestinal pH)
Glaucoma drugs   (cause urinary pH changes due to electrolyte wasting)

## Drugs Affecting the Autonomic and Central Nervous Systems

Significant changes in gastrointestinal motility (and secretions with anticholinergic agents) often accompany drugs that affect the autonomic [3] and central nervous systems. These are effects which:

Block the parasympathetic branch of the autonomic nervous system (anticholinergic drugs, i.e., atropine)
Stimulate the sympathetic branch of the autonomic nervous system (adrenergic drugs, i.e., epinephrine)
Depress the central nervous system (i.e., barbiturates, opiates)

These effects are dose related and thus can frequently be managed with dosage adjustments.

Cerebral stimulants (i.e., amphetamines) and chemically related drugs (i.e., ephedrine) frequently induce anorexia. Alternative drug therapy may be indicated when such anorexia becomes clinically significant.

Cytotoxic Drugs    Cytotoxic drugs used to treat neoplastic disease, severe psoriasis, autoimmune disorders, and gout may cause significant morphological changes in the gut mucosa. Villous atrophy, arrest of mitosis, inhibitance of mucosal enzyme production, and impaired transport systems are generally unavoidable side effects [4–7]. In such diseases the potential benefit of the drugs is generally greater than the potential risk of malnutrition. To minimize this risk, dietary therapy is often necessary.

Tetracycline Interactions    The tetracyclines are a commonly used class of antibiotics. Tetracyclines have been shown experimentally to stimulate pancreatic lipase in low doses. High doses of the drugs appear to inhibit proteolytic systems.

All tetracyclines chelate di- and trivalent cations. Thus antacids containing $Mg^{++}$, $Al^{+++}$, $Ca^{++}$, or iron salts $Fe^{++}$ will prevent oral tetracycline from being absorbed, since the chelate is not biologically available. Dairy foods have the same effect because of the presence of calcium [8,9]. This interaction can be obviated by the patient not taking any di- or trivalent cation containing food or drug within 2 hours of each dose of tetracycline.

Miscellaneous Interactions    Other interactions have been demonstrated to be potentially significant. Inactivation of mucosal enzymes, decreased intralumenal lipolysis, and precipitation of bile salts may follow oral aminoglycoside antibiotic (neomycin, kanamycin) therapy.

Hypocholesterolemic agents, notably cholestyramine resin (Questran, Cuemid), may lead to malabsorption of long chain triglycerides and fat soluble vitamins. The addition of medium chain triglycerides (MCT oil) to the diets of patients receiving these drugs may help to alleviate this problem.

Hydantoin anticonvulsants (phenytoin—Dilantin, ethotoin—Peganone, mephenytoin—Mesantoin) appear to decrease folic acid absorption. The lowered folate levels are significant but reversible upon discontinuation of the drugs.

Phenothiazine tranquilizers (chlorpromazine—Thorazine, etc.) appear to decrease gastrointestinal absorption of both vitamin $B_{12}$ and xylose.

Effects of Nutrients on Biological Availability of Drugs    Nutrients may decrease the biological availability of drugs taken concurrently by both indirect and direct means. The major indirect mechanism is the lowering of gastric pH in response to the presence of foods in the stomach. Many drugs are acid labile to some degree. The physical presence of food in the stomach and proximal intestine will often delay the absorption of drugs from the gut, but will not necessarily decrease the total amount of drug absorbed. Thus, drugs for which rapid high serum level peaks are desired (antiinfectives for acute infections) are best taken on an empty stomach. Drugs from which a rapid effect is desired (analgesics, hypnotics) should also be taken on an empty stomach for this reason. Drugs for which the mean serum level is more important than a rapid peak may usually be taken with food without significant loss of activity. This latter group includes antiinfectives for many chronic processes (tuberculosis, fungal infections) and many drugs for chronic diseases (anticonvulsants, antidiabetic agents, etc.) [10–13]. Food in the gastrointestinal tract may also affect drug absorption because of food induced changes in gastrointestinal secretions and motility.

Most drugs are hydrophilic. Thus, fatty meals tend to delay absorption. A notable exception to this is griseofulvin, an oral agent used to treat deep fungal infections of the skin and nails. This drug is highly lipophilic and is absorbed better when taken with a fatty meal than when taken on an empty stomach [14].

Drugs are commonly absorbed by nonionic diffusion. Thus, significant gastrointestinal pH changes induced by foods may impede drug absorption. Changes in urinary pH due to diet may also significantly affect the renal tubular reabsorption of drugs that undergo glomerular filtration [15].

## Interactions between Food and Monoamine Oxidase Inhibitors

Monoamine oxidase (MAO) is one of the two major enzymes responsible for the re-uptake and destruction of released catecholamines *in vivo*. Tyramine and related biologically active amines in food act similarly to catecholamines in the absence of MAO. Thus severe, life threatening hypertension may occur in patients taking MAO inhibiting drugs who eat tyramine containing foods [16–18].*

DOCUMENTED INTERACTIONS

*Meats and fish*

Chicken liver
Pickled herring

*Vegetables and fruits*

Broad beans (fava beans, pasta fasula)
Canned figs*
Bananas
Avocados*

*Dairy products*

Cheese—especially sharp or aged cheeses (cream cheese and cottage cheese are allowed)

*Beverages*

Beer
Chianti wine
Sherry
Other wines in large quantities

*Miscellaneous*

Active yeast preparations (bread is allowed)
Soy sauce

POSSIBLE INTERACTIONS

Cola beverages
Chocolate

* See tyramine restricted diet on pp. C49–C53.

Coffee
Raisins
Soured cream

Timing of Oral
Medication Doses

Proper timing of oral dosage form administration may prevent many potential drug–diet interactions. The following table lists such considerations.

I. Drugs to be taken on an empty stomach (1 hour before or 2 hours after meals)
    Oral antibiotics*
     (sulfonamides may be taken with food)
    Penicillamine (Cuprimine)
    Prophylactic coronary vasodilators
      Pentaerythritol tetranitrate (Peritrate)
      Erythrityl tetranitrate (Cardilate)

* Some antibiotics are more acid stable than others, but all antibiotics provide optimum serum levels when taken on an empty stomach ("The Effects of Food on the Absorption of Antibiotics," p. H9).

> Note: If gastrointestinal upset precludes the patient's taking the drug on an empty stomach, he should take it with a small amount of food or milk (no milk with tetracyclines).

II. Drugs to be taken ½ hr before meals
    Anticholinergics prescribed for gastrointestinal disorders (to decrease gastrointestinal motility)
      Belladonne alkaloids (including atropine)
      Propantheline bromide (probanthine)
      Donnatal
      Etc.

    Anorexiants (to decrease appetite)
      Phenmetrazine (Preludin)
      Diethylpropion (Tenuate, Tepanil)
      Chlorphentermine (Pre-Sade)
      Etc.

III. Drugs to be taken with meals (to lessen gastrointestinal upset)
    Iron preparations
      Ferrous sulfate (Feosol, Fer In Sol, etc.)
      Ferrous gluconate (Fergon)
      Etc.

*Theophylline and its salts*
    Aminophyllin
    Oxtriphylline (Choledyl)
    Etc.

*Corticosteroids*
    Prednisone
    Hydrocortisone
    Etc.

*Tuberculosis drugs*
    Aminosalicylic acid   (PAS)
    Ethambutol          (Myambutol)
    Isoniazid           (INH)
    Rifampin            (Rifadin, Rimactane)

*Antiinflammatory agents*
    Ibuprofen           (Motrin)
    Indomethacin        (Indocin)
    Oxyphenbutazone     (Tandearil, Oxalid)
    Phenylbutazone      (Burazolidin, Azolid)

*Urinary antiinfectives*
    Nalidixic acid      (NegGram)
    Oxilinic acid       (Utibid)
    Nitrofurantoin      (Furadantin, Macrodantin)

*Miscellaneous agents*
    Rauwolfia serpentina (Raudixin)
    Reserpine
    Potassium supplements

IV.   Drugs to be taken 30–45 minutes after meals
            Antacids

V.   Avoid alcoholic beverages when taking
        Antihistamines
        Sedatives or hypnotics
        Anticonvulsants
        Narcotic analgesics
        Tranquilizers
        Oral antidiabetic agents
        Sulfonamide
        Metronidazole (Flagyl)
        Disulfiram (Antabuse—except under physician's direct observation)

VI.   Drugs to be taken with a full glass of water—with or without meals
        Sulfonamides (Gantrisin, etc.), to prevent crystalluria
        Salicylates (aspirin, etc.), to aid dissolution
        Laxatives, to help soften the stool

Urinary pH and Kidney Tubular Reabsorption    The pH of glomerular filtrate significantly affects the amounts of ionizable drug that might be reabsorbed into the bloodstream and that might be excreted in the urine. Most drugs are ionizable. The un-ionized form is relatively lipophillic and therefore is more apt to be reabsorbed across the lipoid tubule membrane than the relatively hydrophillic ionized form. Alterations in the pH of the glomerular filtrate can be induced by food and electrolyte ingestion. A drug with a $pK_a$ of 6.5 (e.g., phenobarbital) is 50% ionized at pH 6.5. At pH 7.5, the drug is 90% ionized. Thus a 1 unit pH shift results in 40%

more of the drug being in the form that is preferentially excreted. Duration of effect and biological activity of the drug are significantly affected.

Tables of potentially acid or acid ash and potentially basic or alkaline ash foods are available in many diet manuals and should be consulted if a diet induced shift in urinary pH is a concern.

Vitamin Interactions

Most Americans who eat a normal diet do not require vitamin supplementation. Many Americans take vitamins needlessly. However, vitamin supplements are often clinically indicated, and a real potential for interference with vitamins by other drugs, or vice versa, exists.

Levodopa is the pharmacological mainstay of the management of Parkinson's Disease. Exogenous pyridoxine (vitamin $B_6$) has been shown to decrease the effect of Levodopa significantly [19]. Elimination of the vitamin from the diet is also contraindicated, since small levels of the vitamin appear to be necessary for normal drug metabolism [20]. Patients on Levodopa should not take $B_6$ containing vitamin dosage forms. A commercially available vitamin B complex plus vitamin C without pyridoxine (Larobec) tablet is available for patients requiring Levodopa and vitamin supplementation.

Excessive use of mineral oil or other undigestible fat may induce hypovitaminosis A, D, E, or K (the fat soluble vitamins) as discussed previously under "Interference with Absorption."

Hydantoin anticonvulsants (phenytoin—Dilantin, ethotoin—Peganone, mephenytoin—Mesantoin) appear to decrease folic acid absorption. The lowered folate levels are significant but reversible upon discontinuation of the drugs [21].

Phenothiazine tranquilizers (chlorpromazine—Thorazine, etc.) appear to decrease gastrointestinal absorption of both vitamin $B_{12}$ and xylose.

Leafy vegetables such as spinach and kale are high in vitamin K [22]. This vitamin is an antagonist to oral anticoagulant drugs. Thus, patients who are stabilized on oral anticoagulants should avoid excessive consumption of these and other foods containing significant amounts of vitamin K.

The Effects of Food on the Absorption of Antibiotics

In general food tends to reduce the efficiency of absorption of orally administered antibiotics. Antibiotics which are not acid stable will show decreased absorption in the presence of food because of the decrease in gastric pH (increased acidity) associated with food. For those antibiotics which are acid stable food will quite often delay the time required to reach peak serum concentrations relative to the fasting state. Food may also decrease the peak serum concentrations. Optimal absorption of antibiotics can usually be achieved by administration of the antibiotics 1–2 hr before or 2 hr after food. The following table is a summary of some of the available information concerning the effects of food on antibiotic absorption.

| Antibiotic | | Effect of food on percent Absorption | Comments | Ref. |
|---|---|---|---|---|
| Generic name | Brand name | | | |
| Amoxicillin | Larocin Amoxil | None | | 23 |
| Ampicillin | Various | Decrease | Peak levels in one study decreased by about 40% (from 5 µg/ml to 3 µg/ml) when given with food | 24 |
| Cephalexin | Keflex | 82%—fasting 73%—with food | Other authors reported 95% absorption when given with food or fasting | 25,26 |
| Cephradine | Anspor Velosef | None | Absorption slightly more rapid when patient was fasting. However, the peak serum concentration and total amount of drug absorbed was not affected by food. | 27 |
| Clindamycin | Cleocin | None | Peak serum levels may be delayed if given with food, but total amount absorbed unchanged | 28 |
| Demethy-chlortetra-cycline | Declomycin | Non-dairy food produced about a 50% decrease in absorption | Milk decreased absorption by about 70% | 29 |
| Doxycyline | Vibramycin Doxy-11 | None; non-dairy food did not affect absorption | Milk or other products containing calcium, zinc, iron or other divalent or trivalent cations may decrease absorption | 29 |
| Erythromycin estolate | Illosone | None | Absorption with food comparable to that achieved while fasting | 30 |
| Erythromycin base (enteric coated) | E-Mycin Erythrocin | Decrease | Peak serum concentrations when 500 mg given 2 hr before a meal about 2.3 µg, 1 hr before a meal about 1.00 µg/ml, immediately after a meal 1.7 µg/ml, 1 hr after a meal 1.71 µg/ml | 31 |
| Erythromycin propionate | | Decrease | Marked decrease in absorption when given with food | 32 |
| Erythromycin sterate | Bristamycin Ethril SK-Erythromycin | Decrease | Marked decrease in absorption when given with food | 32,33 |
| Hetacillin | Versapen | Decrease | Peak blood level decreased by 50% when taken with food | 24 |
| Lincomycin | Lincocin | Decrease | Give the drug at least 2 hr before or after meals | 34,35 |
| Minocycline | Minocin | None | Claim by Lederle (Minocin) and Parke-Davis (Vectrin) "food did not effect the absorption." No published clinical data available. | 36,37 |

| Antibiotic | | Effect of food on percent Absorption | Comments | Ref. |
|---|---|---|---|---|
| Generic name | Brand name | | | |
| Oxytetra-cycline | Terramycin | None | No difference in serum levels 3 hr after an oral dose with or without food | 38 |
| Penicillin G | Various | Decrease | Only about 35% absorption under optimal conditions. Gastric pH of 2.0 rapidly destroys drug. If used it should be given no later than ½ hr before a meal and no earlier than 2–3 hr after a meal. | 38,39 |
| Rifampin | Rifadin Rimactane | Decrease | Absorption was delayed by food and total amount and peak serum concentrations were decreased. However, the authors felt that food did not significantly decrease the time for which the serum rifampin levels remained above the MIC and therefore, it is not necessary to insist that rifampin be taken in the fasting state. | 31,32 |
| Triacetyl-oleandomycin | TAO Cyclamycin | None | Delay in peak serum concentration when given with food. However, total amount absorbed appeared comparable to fasting state. | 10 |

*Source*: Reprinted with permission from Drug and therapeutic information bulletin [40].

## Managing Drug–Diet Interactions

A few drug–diet interactions are highly significant and must be avoided in all patients, i.e., MAO inhibitors and tyramine containing foods, tetracyclines and milk. Most drug–diet interactions that have been reported may occur, but will not necessarily occur, in any one patient.

Many other drug–food interactions have been suggested, but few have been documented to be clinically significant through controlled studies.

Patients with malnutrition or marginal nutritional status and patients with impaired metabolic or excretory functions are at greatest risk of experiencing significant drug–food interactions. An index of suspicion of such interactions should be maintained for these patients. An awareness of possible drug–food interactions is also important in the proper management of patients taking oral drugs that provide only marginal levels. *In vivo* interference with the absorption, distribution, or metabolism of such drugs by diet may lead to drug treatment failures.

Drugs may also affect patients' nutritional status by disturbing electrolyte balance (e.g., diuretics), taste and odor of foods, or appetite. Drug induced nausea and vomiting or diarrhea may obviate a well planned diet regimen.

Foods may contain pharmacologically active substances and the effects may be significant when the foods are taken by highly sensitive individuals or in excessive quantities. Examples of these effects are seen with coffee or cola (containing caffeine) and tea (containing theophylline).

It is, therefore, appropriate that radical changes in drug therapy or diet not be undertaken to avoid most potential interactions, but rather that a suspicion of drug–diet interactions be maintained. When patients respond to their drugs or diet in unexpected ways, potential drug–diet interactions should be considered and drugs or diet altered appropriately at that time.

References

1. Krondl, A.: Present understanding of the interaction of drugs and food during absorption. Can. Med. Assoc. J. 103: 360, 1970.
2. Christakis, G., and Miridjamian, A.: Diet, drugs, and their interrelationships. J. Am. Diet. Assoc. 52: 2, 1968.
3. Fordtsan, J. S., and Locklear, T. W.: Ionic constituents and osmolality of gastric and small intestinal fluids after eating. Am. J. Dig. Dis. 11: 503, 1966.
4. Waxman, S. D.; Goldberg, L. S.; and Fudenberg, H. N.: Clinical, serologic and leucocyte function studies on patients with idiopathic "acquired" agammaglobulinemia and their families. Am. J. Med. 48: 600, 1970.
5. Trier, J. S.: Morpholocic alterations induced by methotrexate in the mucosa of human proximal intestine. Gastroenterology 43: 407, 1962.
6. Race, T. R.; Paes, I. C.; and Faloon, W. W.: Intestinal malabsorption induced by oral colchicine. Am. J. Med. Sci. 259: 32, 1970.
7. Webb, D. I.; Chodos, R. B.; Mahar, C. Q.; and Faloon, W. W.: Mechanism of vitamin $B_{12}$ malabsorption in patients receiving colchicine. N. Engl. J. Med. 279: 845, 1968.
8. Seneca, H.: Biological Basis of Chemotherapy of Infections and Infestations. Philadelphia: F. D. Davis, 1971.
9. Neuvonen, P. J.; Gothoni, G.; Hackman, R.; and Bjorksten, K.: Interference of iron with the absorption of tetracyclines in man. Br. Med. J. 4: 532, 1970.
10. Hirsch, H. H., and Finland, M.: Effect of food on the absorption of erythromycin propionate and erythromyxin stearate and triacetyloleandomycin. Am. J. Med. Sci. 237: 693, 1959.
11. Klein, J. O., and Finland, M.: Ampicillin activity in vitro and absorption and excretion in normal young men. Am. J. Med. Sci. 245: 544, 1963.
12. Klein, J. O., and Finland, M.: Nafcillin antibacterial action in vitro and absorption and excretion in normal young men. Am. J. Med. Sci. 246: 10, 1963.
13. Macdonald, V. A.; Place, V. A.; Falk, H.; and Darken, M. A.: Effect of food on absorption of sulfonamides in man. Chemotherapia 12: 282, 1967.
14. Crounse, R. G.: Effective use of griseofulvin. Arch. Dermatol. 87: 176, 1963.
15. Zinn, M.: Quinidine intoxication from alkali ingestion. Tex. Med. 66(12): 64, 1970.
16. Horowitz, D.; Lovenberg, W.; Engelman, K.; and Sjoerdsma, K.: Monoamine oxidase inhibitors, tyramine and cheese. JAMA 188(13): 1109, 1964.
17. Blackwell, B., and Mabbitt, L. A.: Tyramine in cheese related to hypertensive crises after monoamine-oxidase inhibition. Lancet 1: 938, 1965.
18. Sjoquist, F.: Psychotic drugs. Interaction between monoamine oxidase (MAO) inhibitors and other substances. Proc. R. Soc. Med. 58: 967, 1965.
19. Mars, H.: Levodopa, carbidopa, and pyridoxine in Parkinson disease. Arch. Neurol. 30(6): 444, 1974.
20. Van Woert, M. H.: Low pyridoxine diet in Parkinsonism. JAMA 219, 1211, 1972.
21. Jensen, O., and Olesen, O. V.: Subnormal serum folate due to anticonvulsive therapy. Arch. Neurol. 22: 181, 1970.
22. Medical News. Anticoagulant therapy—a clinical dilemma. JAMA 187, 27, 1964.
23. Wagner, J. G.: Can. J. Pharm. Sci. 1: 55, 1966.

24. McGehee, R. F., Jr.; Smith, C. B.; Wilcox, C.; and Finland, M.: Comparative studies of antibacterial activity in vitro and absorption and excretion of lincomycin and clinimycin. Am. J. Med. Sci. 256: 279, 1968.
25. Wagner, J. G.; Novak, E.; Patel, N. C.; Chidester, C. G.; and Lummis, W. L.: Absorption, excretion and half-life of clinimycin in normal male adults. Am. J. Med. Sci. 256: 25, 1968.
26. Rosenblatt, J. E.; Barritt, J. E.; Brodie, J. L.; and Kirby, W. M. M.: Comparison of in vitro activity and clinical pharmacology of doxycycline with other tetracyclines. Antimicrob. Agents Chemother., 1966: 134.
27. Minocin clinical brochure, Lederle Laboratories, 1971: 14.
28. Vectrin formulary monograph, Parke-Davis, 1974: 4.
29. Gower, P. E., and Dash, C. H.: Cephalexin: human studies of absorption and excretion of a new cephalosporin antibiotic. Br. J. Pharmacol. 37: 738, 1969.
30. Griffith, R. S., and Black, H. R.: Cephalexin: a new antibiotic. Clin. Med. 75(11): 14, 1968.
31. Dans, P. E.; McGehee, R. F., Jr.; Wilcox, C.; and Finland, M.: Ramfin: antibacterial activity in vitro and absorption and excretion in normal young men. Am. J. Med. Sci. 259: 120, 1970.
32. Siegler, D. I.; Bryant, M.; Burley, D. M.; Citron, K. M.; and Standen, S. M.: Effect of meals on rifampicin absorption. Lancet 2: 197, 1974.
33. Sutherland, R., and Robinson, O. P. W.: Laboratory and pharmacological studies in man with hetacillin and ampicillin. Br. Med. J. 2: 804, 1967.
34. Neu, H. C., and Winshelleb, E. B.: Pharmacological studies of 6 (D(-) α Amino-p-Hydroxyphenylacetamido) penicillanic acid in humans. Antimicrob. Agents Chemother., 1970: 423.
35. Michel, J. C.; Sayer, R. J.; and Kirby, M. M.: Effect of food and antacids on blood levels of aureomycin and terramycin. J. Lab. Clin. Med. 36: 632, 1950.
36. Hirsch, H. A.; Pryles, C. V.; and Finland, M.: Effect of food on absorption of a new form of erythromycin propionate. Am. J. Med. Sci. 239: 198, 1960.
37. Upjohn study (Protocol N. 058) per letter by Alan B. Varley, M.D., Medical Director, The Upjohn Co., 1970.
38. McDermott, W.; Bunn, P. A.; Benoit, M.; DuBois, R.; and Reynolds, M. E.: The absorption, excretion and destruction of orally administered penicillin. J. Clin. Invest. 25: 190, 1946.
39. Goodman, L. S., and Gilman, A.: The Pharmacological Basis of Therapeutics. New York: Macmillan, 1970: 1212.
40. PRN: Drug and therapeutic information bulletin. Memorial Medical Center, Long Beach, CA, December 1974.

**Additional References**   Griffith, R. S., and Black, H. R.: Comparison of the blood levels obtained after single and multiple doses of erythromycin estolate and erythromycin stearate. Am. J. Med. Sci. 247: 69, 1964.

Harvengt, C.; DeSchepper, P.; Lahy, F.; and Hansen, J.: Cephradine absorption and excretion in fasting and non-fasting volunteers. J. Clin. Pharmacol. 13: 36, 1973.

Pierpaoli, P. G.: Drug therapy and diet. Drug Intelligence Clin. Pharmacy 6: 89, 1972.

Symposium on drug-nutrient relationships. Am. J. Clin. Nutr. 26: 103, 1973.

# Test Diets

Diet and Vanillylmandelic
Acid Excretion

Measurement of urinary 4-hydroxy-3 methoxymandelic acid (VMA) is a diagnostic test widely used in the assessment of pheochromocytoma [1,2]. Until recently, patients were advised to abstain from certain foods during the period just prior to and during their urine collections. Coffee, tea, chocolate, nuts, bananas, citrus fruits, raisins, and vanilla were often eliminated from the diets of tested patients in order to prevent any interference with the test or misinterpretation of results [1,3]. The older and less specific tests that, in addition to VMA or total catecholamines, also measured phenolic acids of dietary origin are now being replaced by more specific fluorescence assays [4]. The use of a method of analysis that converts VMA to vanillin or one that relies on the measurement of metanephrines rather than VMA obviates the need for any dietary restrictions at all [1,3,5,6]. Patients whose urines are analyzed by the latter methods may be maintained on normal diets prior to and during the period of their urine collections without fear of compromising the validity of the test.

References

1. Rayfield, E. J.; Cain, J. P.; Casey, M. P.; Williams, G. H.; and Sullivan, J. M.: Influence of diet on urinary VMA excretion. JAMA 221: 704, 1972.
2. Remine, W. H.; Chong, G. C.; Van Heerden, J. A.; Sheps, S. G.; and Harrison, E. G.: Current management of pheochromocytoma. Ann. Surg. 179: 740, 1974.
3. Page, L. B., and Copeland, R. B.: Pheochromocytoma. Disease a Month 1: 1, 1968.
4. Sjoerdsma, A.; Engelman, K.; Waldmann, T. A.; Cooperman, L. H.; and Hammond, W. G.: Pheochromocytoma: current concepts of diagnosis and treatment. Ann. Intern. Med. 65: 1305, 1966.
5. Pisano, J. J.; Crout, J. R.; and Abraham, D.: Determination of 3-methoxy-4-hydroxymandelic acid in urine. Clin. Chim. Acta. 7: 285, 1962.
6. Amery, A., and Conway, J.: A critical review of diagnostic tests for pheochromocytoma. Am. Heart J. 73: 129, 1967.

Test for Fat Malabsorption:
100 g Fat Diet

The fecal excretion of more than 5–7 g fat/24 hr over a 3-day period in patients ingesting 100 g of dietary fat daily is generally considered to be evidence of fat malabsorption [1–3]. A marker should be ingested by the patient at the beginning and end of the stool collection. Otherwise, stool collections should be begun only after the patient has been on the diet for 3 days [1]. The actual fat intake must be estimated [1], as knowledge of the fat consumed is imperative in determining fat malabsorption. In chronic pancreatic disease, more than 10 g fat are excreted per 24 hr [4], and 10–40 g/day are excreted in patients with celiac disease [5]. Other less definitive indices of fat malabsorption include a positive Sudan stain of stool for fat as well as a serum carotene level of less than 60 $\mu$g/100 ml [1,2].

**100 G Fat Diet** *Include at Least the Following Foods or Their Nutritive Equivalents Daily for 3 Days:*

| Food | Fat (g) |
|---|---|
| 2 cups whole milk | 20 |
| 8 oz lean meat | 24 |
| 1 egg | 5 |
| 4 or more servings fruits and vege-tables | 0 |
| 4 or more servings whole grain breads or enriched bread and cereals | 0 |
| 10 fat choices, such as 10 tsp butter, margarine, oils, etc. | 50 |
| Total | 99 |

**Sample Menu**

A.M.

½ cup orange juice
½ cup farina with 2 tsp butter or fortified margarine
1 soft cooked egg
1 slice toast with 1 tsp butter or fortified margarine
Coffee or tea
1 cup whole milk

Noon

4 oz sliced turkey on 2 slices whole wheat bread with 1 tsp butter or margarine
½ cup spinach with 1 tsp butter or fortified margarine
Lettuce and tomato salad with 2 tsp mayonnaise
½ cup fruit cocktail
½ cup whole milk

P.M.

4 oz lean roast beef
½ cup mashed potato with 1 tsp butter or fortified margarine
½ cup carrots with 1 tsp butter or fortified margarine
1 raw apple
1 slice white bread with 1 tsp butter or fortified margarine
Coffee or tea
½ cup whole milk

References

1. Wright, H. K., and Tilson, M. D.: Postoperative Disorders of the Gastrointestinal Tract. New York: Grune & Stratton, 1973.
2. Westergaard, H., and Dietschy, J. M.: Normal mechanisms of fat absorption and derangements induced by various gastrointestinal diseases. Med. Clin. N. Am. 58: 1513, 1974.
3. Ravel, R.: Clinical Laboratory Medicine. 2d ed. Chicago: Year Book Medical Publishers, 1974.
4. Wallach, J.: Interpretation of Diagnostic Tests. 2d ed. Boston: Little, Brown, 1974.
5. Conn, H. G., and Conn, R. B.: Current Diagnosis. Philadelphia: W. B. Saunders, 1974.

Status of Fat Free Test Diet

Preparation for gallbladder X-ray has often included a preparatory fat free test meal, on the premise of its necessity for adequate visualization of gall stones. New studies, however, indicate that dietary preparation prior to cholecystographic examination is not necessary [1]. Two groups of patients undergoing the X-ray procedure, one of which had received the dietary preparation, one of which, had not were compared. Results were similar, with those persons who had not been on the diet receiving a slightly higher percentage of adequate visualizations [1].

References

1. Mauthe, H.: The low fat meal in gallbladder examinations. Radiology 112: 5, 1974.

Dietary Preparation for the Glucose Tolerance Test

The need for a high carbohydrate diet prior to the glucose tolerance test has been exaggerated. An early report that patient preparation with a 300 g carbohydrate diet is necessary for valid glucose tolerance test results [1] has been contraindicated by later publications [2–8]. As long as the patient is on an adequate diet [2] that contains at least 150 g carbohydrate daily, patient adherence to a 300 g test diet for 3 days prior to the test is unnecessary [2–8], except in the individual who has been on an inadequate, hypocaloric diet [8].

References

1. Conn, J. W.: Interpretation of the glucose tolerance test. The necessity of a standard and preparatory diet. Am. J. Med. Sci. 199: 555, 1946.
2. Nievadlik, D. C.: The glucose tolerance test. An evaluation. Postgrad. Med. 55: 73, June 1974.
3. Siperstein, M. D.: The glucose tolerance test: a pitfall in the diagnosis of diabetes mellitus. Adv. Intern. Med. 20: 297, 1975.
4. Hecht, A.; Weisenfield, S.; and Goldner, M. G.: Factors affecting oral glucose tolerance: experience with chronically ill patients. Metabolism 10: 712, 1961.
5. Wilkerson, H. L. C.; Hyman, H.; Kaufman, M.; McCuestion, A. C.; and Frances, J. O. S.: Diagnostic evaluation of oral glucose tolerance tests in non-diabetic subjects after various levels of carbohydrate intake. N. Engl. J. Med. 262: 1047, 1960.
6. Unger, R. H.: The standard two hour glucose tolerance test in the diagnosis of diabetes mellitus in subjects without fasting hyperglycemia. Ann. Intern. Med. 47: 1138, 1957.
7. Klint, C. R.; Prout, T. E.; Bradley, R. F.; Dalger, H.; Fisher, C.; Gastineau, C. F.; Marks, H.; Meinert, C. L.; and Schumacher, O. P.: Standardization of the oral glucose tolerance test. Diabetes 18: 299, 1969.
8. Conn, H. F., and Conn, R. B.: Current Diagnosis. Philadelphia: W. B. Saunders, 1974.

5-Hydroxyindoleacetic Acid and Serotonin Restricted Diet

The diet is used in conjunction with urinalysis for 5-hydroxyindoleacetic acid (5-HIAA). Some, but not all, patients having malignant carcinoid tumors excrete elevated levels of 5-hydroxyindoleacetic acid as a result of increased serotonin synthesis by the tumor [1]. The diet eliminates foods containing 5-HIAA and its precursor serotonin, a by-product of tryptophan metabolism in the body; ingestion of these foods results in elevated levels of 5-HIAA in the urine and may lead to false positive results in the diagnostic test for the carcinoid syndrome [2,3]. Consequently, the following foods should be excluded for at least 24 hours prior to the test: bananas, plantains, tomato, red plums, red blue plums, avocados, pineapples, pineapple juice, walnuts, and passion fruit [3,4].

References
1. Dickie, R. S.: Diet in Health and Disease—Rationale and Practice. Springfield: Charles C. Thomas, 1974.
2. Bruce, D. W.: Carcinoid tumours and pineapples. J. Pharm. Pharmacol. 13: 256, 1961.
3. Lovenberg, W.: Some vasoactive and psychoactive substances in foods: amines, stimulants, depressants and hallucinogens. National Research Council: Toxicants Occurring Naturally in Foods. Washington, DC: National Academy of Sciences, 1973.
4. Oats, J. A.: The carcinoid syndrome. Thorn, G. W.; Adams, R. D.; Braunwald, E.; Iselbacher, K. J.; and Peterdorf, R. G. Harrison's Principles of Internal Medicine. 8th ed. New York: McGraw-Hill, 1977.

## Use of High-Normal Calcium Intake in Screening for Hypercalciuria

The use of a low calcium diet has no place among the diagnostic tools for hypercalciuria. When screening for hypercalciuria, the only rational dietary preparation is that of a high-normal calcium intake. A potentially hypercalciuric patient must be screened under circumstances that allow him to express his abnormality. Studies have shown this to be true [1]. At low calcium intakes little differences were found in the urinary calcium excretion of stone forming and non–stone forming patients. However, as the calcium intake was increased, the urinary calcium levels rose more steeply in the stone formers than in the non–stone formers [1]. Thus, hypercalciuria was detectable only at moderately high calcium intakes [1].

A logical approach is to define hypercalciuria on a 1,000 mg calcium diet. Food sources contribute 400 mg calcium daily, and the remaining 600 mg is derived from the oral administration of calcium gluconate [2]. Such an approach increases the likelihood that the actual intake will be as close to 1,000 mg calcium as is possible.

Adapted from Nutrition Care Manual, Yale-New Haven Medical Center, New Haven—Hospital of St. Raphael, New Haven—West Haven VA Medical Center, West Haven—The Waterbury Hospital, Waterbury, 1980.

References
1. Peacock, M.; Hodgkinson, A.; and Nordin, B. D. C.: Importance of dietary calcium in the definition of hypercalciuria. Br. Med. J. 3: 469, 1967.
2. Broadus, A. E.; Dominguez, M.; and Bartter, E. F. C.: Pathiophysiologic studies in idiopathic hypercalciuria: use of an oral calcium tolerance test to characterize distinctive hypercalciuric subgroups. J. Clin. Endochrinol. Metab. 47: 751, 1978.

Status of Calcium Restricted and Phosphate Restricted Diets

## STATUS OF SEVERELY RESTRICTED CALCIUM DIETS IN TREATING CALCIUM OXALATE RENAL STONES

There is no clear-cut evidence indicating the effectiveness of a severely restricted calcium diet in hypercalciuria. A reduction in calcium intake increases the absorption of dietary oxalate so that the degree of saturation of the urine with respect to calcium oxalate remains unchanged [1].

Studies have shown that a reduction of dietary calcium to approximately 600 mg in 24 hours, especially if prior intake has been excessive, reduces or eliminates hypercalciuria. When combined with increased fluid intake, this program can prevent stone formation in many patients with idiopathic hypercalciuria [2].

## STATUS OF CALCIUM RESTRICTED DIETS IN TREATING HYPERCALCEMIA OF CANCER

Calcium restricted diets are also not indicated in most cases of hypercalcemia, including those associated with certain forms of cancer. Only in situations where increased intestinal absorption of calcium is important in the pathogenesis of hypercalcemia can it be expected that dietary limitations of calcium will be of value. Sarcoidosis and vitamin D intoxication belong in this category [3]. In the great majority of situations where the increased calcium is mostly derived from the skeleton, dietary restriction can be of only marginal value [3]. The diet may be counterproductive if it is so restrictive that it fails to meet the increased nutritional needs of the cachectic cancer patient, who needs more nutrition, not less. Furthermore, a diet limited in calcium is often limited in phosphate, a limitation that leads to augmentation of serum calcium. Finally, the absorption of calcium is already greatly reduced in hypercalcemic states by the adaptive mechanism that maintains a reciprocal relationship between the calcium absorption and serum concentration [3].

## STATUS OF PHOSPHATE RESTRICTED DIETS IN TREATING RENAL LITHIASIS

There is no indication for a low phosphorus diet as part of the treatment for renal lithiasis.

In the past, a combination of a low phosphate diet and phosphate binders has been used in the management of magnesium ammonium phosphate stone formations associated with infection [2]. More recently, it has been shown that such a program may actually increase stone formation in patients who have idiopathic renal lithiasis without infection. With decreased phosphate intake there is a reduction in the urinary excretion of pyrophosphate, an inhibitor of calcium crystal growth and aggregation. In addition, on a low phosphate intake, the serum phosphorus may decrease, thereby stimulating production of 1,25-dihydroxy-vitamin D, leading to mild hypercalcemia and hypercalciuria [2].

References

1. Broadus, A., M.D., Yale School of Medicine: Personal communication.
2. Smith, L. H.; Van Den Berg, C. T.; and Wilson, D. M.: Current concepts in nutrition: Nutrition and urolithiasis. N. Engl. J. Med. 298: 87, 1978.
3. Schneider, A. B., and Sherwood, L. M.: Calcium homeostasis and the pathogenesis and management of hypercalcemic disorders. Metabolism 23: 975, 1974.

Food Additive References

Bayne, H. G., and Michener, H. D.: Growth of staphylococcus and salmonella on frankfurters with and without sodium nitrite. Appl. Microbiol. 30: 844, 1975.

Committee on Food Protection, Food and Nutrition Board, National Research Council: Toxicants Occurring Naturally in Foods. Washington, DC: National Academy of Sciences, 1973.

Committee on Food Protection, Food and Nutrition Board, National Research Council: The Use of Chemicals in Food Production, Processing, Storage and Distribution. Washington, DC: National Academy of Sciences, 1973.

Conners, C. K.; Goyette, C. H.; Southwick, D. A.; Lees, J. M.; and Andrulonis, P. A.: Food additives and hyperkinesis: a controlled double blind experiment. Pediatrics 58: 154, 1976.*

Corwin, E., and Pines, W. L.: Why FDA banned Red N. 2. FDA Consumer 10: 18, 1976.

Echols, B., and Arena, J. M.: Food additives and pesticides in foods. Ped. Clin. N. Am. 24: 175, 1977.

Editorial: Nitrate and human cancer. Lancet 2: 281, 1977.

Feingold, B.: Hyperkinesis and learning disabilities linked to artificial food flavors and colors. Am. J. Nurs. 75: 797, 1975.

Food additives and hyperactivity. Clin. Pediatr. 14: 957, 1975.

Jukes, T. H.: Food additives. N. Engl. J. Med. 297: 427, 1977.

National Academy of Sciences: Sweeteners. Issues and Uncertainties. Washington, DC: National Academy of Sciences, 1975.

National Advisory Committee on Hyperkinesis and Food Additives: Report to the Nutrition Foundation, June 1, 1975.

Noid, H. E.; Schulze, W.; and Windelmann, R. K.: Diet plan for patients with salicylate-induced urticaria. Arch. Dermotol. 109: 867, 1974.

Pines, W. L.: The cyclamate story. FDA Consumer 8: 19, 1974–75.

Reif-Lehrer, L.: Possible significance of adverse reactions to glutamate in humans. Fed. Proc. 35: 2205, 1976.

Shurbik, P.: Potential carcinogenicity of food additives and contaminants. Cancer Res. 35: 3475, 1975.

Spencer, M.: Food additives. Postgrad. Med. J. 50: 620, 1974.

* At the time of this writing, this is the only controlled, double blind study that has been published on the relationship of food additives and hyperkinesis in children. The authors concluded that it is possible that a diet free of food additives may reduce hyperkinetic symptoms in children, but admitted that their results should be interpreted with caution because of several features inherent in the study that need further evaluation. These include objective measures of change, manipulation of the independent variable, and reducing the independent variable to more specific components.

Food Allergy References

Ament, M. E., and Rubin, C. E.: Soy protein, another cause of flat intestinal lesion. Gastroenterology 62: 227, 1974.

Dolowitz, D. A.: Theories of allergy brought up to date: allergy as a biologic process. Ann. Allergy 32: 183, 1974.

Fontana, V. J., and Strauss, M. B.: Allergy and diet. Goodhart, R. S., and Shils, M. E., eds. Modern Nutrition in Health and Disease. 5th ed. Philadelphia: Lea & Febiger, 1973.

Fulton, L., and Davis, C.: Baking for People with Food Allergies, U. S. Department of Agriculture Home and Garden Bulletin, No. 147, rev. Washington, DC: U. S. Government Printing Office, 1975.

Klish, W.; Potts, E.; Ferry, G. D.; and Nichols, B. L.: Modular formula: an approach to management of infants with specific or complex food intolerances. J. Pediatr. 88: 948, 1976.

Lebenthal, E.: Cow's milk protein allergy. Ped. Clin. N. Am. 22: 827, 1975.

Randolph, T. G.: Dynamics, diagnosis, and treatment of food allergy. Otolaryngol. Clin. N. Am. 7: 617, 1974.

Rowe, A. H.: Food Allergy. Its Manifestations and Control and the Elimination Diets. A Compendium. Springfield: Charles C. Thomas, 1972.

Shiner, M.; Brook, C. G. D.; Ballard, J.; and Herman, S.: Intestinal biopsy in the diagnosis of cow's milk protein intolerance without acute symptoms. Lancet 2: 1060, 1975.

Speer, F.: The allergic child. Am. Fam. Phys. 11: 88, 1975.

Speer, F.: Multiple food allergy. Ann. Allergy 32: 71, 1975.

**Burn References**

Curreri, P. W.: Dietary requirements of patients with major burns. J. Am. Diet. Assoc. 65: 415, 1974.

Curreri, P. W.: Metabolic and nutritional aspects of thermal injury. Burns 2: 16, 1975.

Davies, J. W. L.: The fluid therapy given to 1027 patients during the first 48 hours after burning. II. The input of sodium and water and the tonicity of the therapy. Burns 1: 331, 1975.

Larkin. J. M., and Moylan, J. A.: Complete enteral support of thermally injured patients. Am. J. Surg. 131: 722, 1976.

Lennard, E. S.; Alexander, J. W.; Craycraft, T. K.; and MacMillan, B. S.: Association in burn patients of improved antibacterial defense with nutritional support by the oral route. Burns 1: 98, 1975.

McDougal, W. S.; Wilmore, D. W.; and Pruitt, B. A.: Effect of intravenous near isomatic nutrient infusions on nitrogen balance in critically ill injured patients. Surg. Gynecol. Obstet. 145: 408, 1977.

Masterton, J. P.: Nutritional requirements and parenteral nutrition. Burns 1: 245, 1975.

Monies-Chass, I.: Early management of severe burns. Burns 1: 309, 1975.

Rosenthal, A.; Czaja, A. J.; and Pruitt, B. A.: Gastrin levels and gastric acidity in the pathogenesis of acute gastroduodenal disease after burns. Surg. Gynecol. Obstet. 144: 232, 1977.

Sutherland, A. B.: Nitrogen balance and nutritional requirement in the burned patient: a reappraisal. Burns 2: 238, 1976.

Watson, L. C., and Abston, S.: Prevention of upper gastrointestinal hemorrhage in 582 burned children. Am. J. Surg. 132: 790, 1976.

Wilmore, D. W.: Alimentation in injured and septic patients. Heart and Lung 5: 791, 1976.

Wilmore, D. W.: Nutrition and metabolism following thermal injury. Clin. Plast. Surg. 1: 603, 1974.

Wilmore, D. W., and Pruitt, B. A.: Parenteral nutrition in burn patients. Fischer, J. E., ed. Total Parenteral Nutrition. Boston: Little, Brown, 1976.

# Obsolete Diets

*Alvarez Diet*    A "smooth" diet that provided 6 oz of a milk and egg mixture every 2 hours as a means of treating peptic ulcers. Among other foods eventually included were orange juice; coffee and tea; cocoa or chocolate; white bread or toast; cream soups; farina; Cream of Wheat; strained rolled oats; rice; potatoes; pureed beans, peas, or lentils; small portions of meat, fish, and chicken; plain puddings; custards, ice cream; cake and gelatin; ripe banana; and stewed fruits [1].

*Andresen Diet*    A diet prescribed for bleeding peptic ulcers that initially included a 6 oz mixture of milk, cream, gelatin, and dextrose given every 2 hours. After 5 or 6 days, it was liberalized to include eggs, cereal, custard, ice cream, and eventually other foods as well [1].

*Borst Diet*    A diet low in protein advocated for the treatment of acute renal failure or uremia. Equal amounts of sugar and butter were mixed and rolled into butterballs that were often served in the form of "butter soup" [1].

*Caesar's Diet*    A milk and barley water based diet formerly used to treat gout [1].

*Cantani's Diet*    A meat based diet used to treat diabetes [1].

*Coleman–Shaffer Diet*    Eggs, cream, cocoa, milk, sugar, bread, and butter given in small, frequent feedings to patients with typhoid fever [1].

*Gerson–Hermannsdorfer diet*    Initially prescribed as a cure for tuberculosis, and later used as a cure for cancer [1,2]. Essentially all foods, except fresh fruits, vegetables, and oatmeal, were restricted. After the first 6 weeks, proteins from milk products were added, along with vitamins A and D. A dangerous, inadequate diet condemned by the American Cancer Society in 1972 [2].

*Grape diet*    A four-stage diet that provided feedings of grapes alone every 2 hours with the later addition of other fresh fruits and vegetables. The diet was promulgated as a cure for cancer and was condemned by the American Cancer Society. Grape juice was also used in douches, enemas, etc., as part of the treatment [3].

*Guelpa diet*    An earlier dietary treatment for diabetes that was preceded by a 3 day fast followed by milk, then vegetables, and finally gradual return to a completely normal diet [1].

*Hare's diet*    A diet used in the treatment of migraine, "bilious attacks," and asthma. The rationale for the diet was based on the reduction of so-called carbonaceous foods ingested in order to prevent the occurrence of a state of "hyperpyraemia," which was thought to be the cause of symptoms [4].

*Diet for hypoacidity*    A diet that proposed to treat gastric hypoacidity by the elimination of all highly seasoned foods, mustard, pepper, cakes, candy, pastry, and nuts, as well as certain "bulky" vegetables and "the cellulose of fruits" [5].

**Jarotsky diet**    An egg white and olive oil based diet formerly prescribed for patients with peptic ulcers [1].

**Karell diet**    Milk and milk only given in the amount of 200 ml four times daily in the initial stages of congestive heart failure and myocardial infarction. The milk was increased to 1,000 ml, and other foods such as eggs, toast, cereal gruel, gelatin, custard, and fruit and vegetable purees were gradually added after 3 or 4 days [1].

**Kempner rice–fruit diet**    An earlier version of a very rigid sodium, fat, cholesterol, and protein restricted diet prescribed in the treatment of hypertension and renal disease. It included very simply prepared rice as well as sugar and liberal amounts of fruit. Fluids were restricted to less than 1,000 ml/day [1].

**Lenhartz diet**    A diet prescribed for the treatment of bleeding peptic ulcers. It consisted mainly of eggs beaten with sugar and then iced, plus milk and occasionally wine, in increasing amounts until 6–8 eggs and 2 pints of milk were consumed daily [4].

**Meulengracht diet**    Essentially a pureed diet that included milk, eggs, pureed fruits and vegetables, custard, ice cream, gelatin, plain pudding, crackers, bread, and butter. Later stages of the diet permitted the inclusion of minced meats and broiled, baked, or creamed fish. Foods such as pastries, spices, nuts, alcoholic beverages, carbonated beverages, coffee, tea, and cocoa were excluded [1].

**Newburgh diet**    A high fat diet formerly prescribed for patients with diabetes [1].

**Oatmeal cure**    A diet that provided about 3,000 kilocalories/day mainly in the form of oatmeal, egg white, and butter and prescribed for the control of diabetes [6].

**Salisbury diet**    A diet recommended in the treatment of chronic gout, psoriasis, and dyspepsia. It consisted of only lean meat and hot water [4].

**Schemm diet**    An acid ash, sodium restricted diet used to treat edema due to heart and renal diseases. The stated aim of the diet was acidification of the urine in order to promote sodium and water losses via the kidneys. Such losses are best achieved by diuretic therapy in combination with a mildly restricted sodium diet [1].

**Schrath's cure**    A diet formerly prescribed in Europe for dilation of the stomach, chronic peritonitis, and other conditions. The amount of food ingested was gradually reduced until nothing was permitted except dried bread, boiled vegetables, and small amounts of hot wine [6].

**Sippy diet**    A high cholesterol, high fat diet formerly prescribed for patients with ulcers, which included hourly feedings of milk and cream in the early stage and, in addition, eggs, strained cereal, custard, and pureed foods in later stages [1].

**Tuffnell's diet**    A diet used in the treatment of aneurysm, prescribed with the tenuous objectives of diminishing the force of the heart and increasing the coagulability of the blood. The chief characteristic of the diet is "its dryness." It included 4 oz bread and butter; 2–3 oz meat, 4 oz milk, and 3–4 oz claret daily. Water and other liquids were restricted [4].

*Yolk cure*    A diet recommended by Stern for the control of diabetes; it provided 10–40 egg yolks daily, along with some green vegetables [6].

*Zomatherapy*    By the term zomatherapy is meant treatment by raw meat or meat juice. It was suggested that raw meat juice contained a specific "tonic" and stimulant or some antitoxic substance that benefited persons with tuberculosis, anemia, and neurasthenia [4].

An excellent and inexpensive critique of several currently promulgated fad diets has been published [7].

References    1. Lagua, R. T.; Claudio, V. S.; and Thiele, V. F.:   Nutrition and Diet Therapy Reference Dictionary. St. Louis:   C. V. Mosby, 1974.
2. American Cancer Society:   Unproven methods of cancer treatment.   Gersan method of treatment for cancer. CA:   Cancer J. Clinicians 23: 314, 1973.
3. American Cancer Society:   The grape diet. CA:   Cancer J. Clinicians 24: 144, 1974.
4. Hutchinson, R.:   Food and the Principles of Dietetics. 3d ed. New York:   William Wood, 1911.
5. Pope, A. E., and Geraghty, E. M.:   Essentials of Dietetics in Health and Disease. 3d ed. New York:   G. P. Putnam's Sons, 1931.
6. Watson, C.:   Food and Feeding in Health and Disease. 2d ed. London:   Oliver & Boyd, 1915.,
7. Los Angeles District, California Dietetic Association:   A Dozen Diets for Better or Worse. Los Angeles:   California Dietetic Association, 1973.

# PART I    Appendix

# Recommended Daily Dietary Allowances, Revised 1980[a]

## FOOD AND NUTRITION BOARD, NATIONAL ACADEMY OF SCIENCES—NATIONAL RESEARCH COUNCIL

Designed for the maintenance of good nutrition of practically all healthy people in the U.S.A.

| | Age (yr) | Weight (kg) | Weight (lb) | Height (cm) | Height (in.) | Protein (g) | Fat soluble vitamins: Vitamin A (µg R.E.)[b] | Vitamin D (µg)[c] | Vitamin E (mg α T.E.)[d] | Water soluble vitamins: Vitamin C (mg) | Thiamin (mg) | Riboflavin (mg) | Niacin (mg N.E.)[e] | Vitamin B6 (mg) | Folacin[f] (µg) | Vitamin B12 (µg) | Minerals: Calcium (mg) | Phosphorus (mg) | Magnesium (mg) | Iron (mg) | Zinc (mg) | Iodine (µg) |
|---|---|---|---|---|---|---|---|---|---|---|---|---|---|---|---|---|---|---|---|---|---|---|
| Infants | 0.0–0.5 | 6 | 13 | 60 | 24 | kg × 2.2 | 420 | 10 | 3 | 35 | 0.3 | 0.4 | 6 | 0.3 | 30 | 0.5g | 360 | 240 | 50 | 10 | 3 | 40 |
| | 0.5–1.0 | 9 | 20 | 71 | 28 | kg × 2.0 | 400 | 10 | 4 | 35 | 0.5 | 0.6 | 8 | 0.6 | 45 | 1.5 | 540 | 360 | 70 | 15 | 5 | 50 |
| Children | 1–3 | 13 | 29 | 90 | 35 | 23 | 400 | 10 | 5 | 45 | 0.7 | 0.8 | 9 | 0.9 | 100 | 2.0 | 800 | 800 | 150 | 15 | 10 | 70 |
| | 4–6 | 20 | 44 | 112 | 44 | 30 | 500 | 10 | 6 | 45 | 0.9 | 1.0 | 11 | 1.3 | 200 | 2.5 | 800 | 800 | 200 | 10 | 10 | 90 |
| | 7–10 | 28 | 62 | 132 | 52 | 34 | 700 | 10 | 7 | 45 | 1.2 | 1.4 | 16 | 1.6 | 300 | 3.0 | 800 | 800 | 250 | 10 | 10 | 120 |
| Males | 11–14 | 45 | 99 | 157 | 62 | 45 | 1000 | 10 | 8 | 50 | 1.4 | 1.6 | 18 | 1.8 | 400 | 3.0 | 1200 | 1200 | 350 | 18 | 15 | 150 |
| | 15–18 | 66 | 145 | 176 | 69 | 56 | 1000 | 10 | 10 | 60 | 1.4 | 1.7 | 18 | 2.0 | 400 | 3.0 | 1200 | 1200 | 400 | 18 | 15 | 150 |
| | 19–22 | 70 | 154 | 177 | 70 | 56 | 1000 | 7.5 | 10 | 60 | 1.5 | 1.7 | 19 | 2.2 | 400 | 3.0 | 800 | 800 | 350 | 10 | 15 | 150 |
| | 23–50 | 70 | 154 | 178 | 70 | 56 | 1000 | 5 | 10 | 60 | 1.4 | 1.6 | 18 | 2.2 | 400 | 3.0 | 800 | 800 | 350 | 10 | 15 | 150 |
| | 51+ | 70 | 154 | 178 | 70 | 56 | 1000 | 5 | 10 | 60 | 1.2 | 1.4 | 16 | 2.2 | 400 | 3.0 | 800 | 800 | 350 | 10 | 15 | 150 |
| Females | 11–14 | 46 | 101 | 157 | 62 | 46 | 800 | 10 | 8 | 50 | 1.1 | 1.3 | 15 | 1.8 | 400 | 3.0 | 1200 | 1200 | 300 | 18 | 15 | 150 |
| | 15–18 | 55 | 120 | 163 | 64 | 46 | 800 | 10 | 8 | 60 | 1.1 | 1.3 | 14 | 2.0 | 400 | 3.0 | 1200 | 1200 | 300 | 18 | 15 | 150 |
| | 19–22 | 55 | 120 | 163 | 64 | 44 | 800 | 7.5 | 8 | 60 | 1.1 | 1.3 | 14 | 2.0 | 400 | 3.0 | 800 | 800 | 300 | 18 | 15 | 150 |
| | 23–50 | 55 | 120 | 163 | 64 | 44 | 800 | 5 | 8 | 60 | 1.0 | 1.2 | 13 | 2.0 | 400 | 3.0 | 800 | 800 | 300 | 18 | 15 | 150 |
| | 51+ | 55 | 120 | 163 | 64 | 44 | 800 | 5 | 8 | 60 | 1.0 | 1.2 | 13 | 2.0 | 400 | 3.0 | 800 | 800 | 300 | 10 | 15 | 150 |
| Pregnant | | | | | | +30 | +200 | +5 | +2 | +20 | +0.4 | +0.3 | +2 | +0.6 | +400 | +1.0 | +400 | +400 | +150 | h | +5 | +25 |
| Lactating | | | | | | +20 | +400 | +5 | +3 | +40 | +0.5 | +0.5 | +5 | +0.5 | +100 | +1.0 | +400 | +400 | +150 | h | +10 | +50 |

[a] The allowances are intended to provide for individual variations among most normal persons as they live in the United States under usual environmental stresses. Diets should be based on a variety of common foods in order to provide other nutrients for which human requirements have been less well defined. See table Mean Heights and Weights and Recommended Energy Intake (p. 14) for suggested average energy intakes.

[b] Retinol equivalents. 1 retinol equivalent = 1 µg retinol or 6 µg carotene.

[c] As cholecalciferol. 10 µg cholecalciferol = 400 IU vitamin D.

[d] α-tocopherol equivalents. 1 mg d-α-tocopherol = 1 α T.E.

[e] 1 NE (niacin equivalent) is equal to 1 mg of niacin or 60 mg of dietary tryptophan.

[f] The folacin allowances refer to dietary sources as determined by *Lactobacillus casei* assay after treatment with enzymes ("conjugases") to make polyglutamyl forms of the vitamin available to the test organism.

[g] The RDA for vitamin B₁₂ in infants is based on average concentration of the vitamin in human milk. The allowances after weaning are based on energy intake (as recommended by the American Academy of Pediatrics) and consideration of other factors such as intestinal absorption.

[h] The increased requirement during pregnancy cannot be met by the iron content of habitual American diets or by the existing iron stores of many women; therefore the use of 30–60 mg of supplemental iron is recommended. Iron needs during lactation are not substantially different from those of non-pregnant women, but continued supplementation of the mother for 2–3 months after parturition is advisable in order to replenish stores depleted by pregnancy.

## MEAN HEIGHTS AND WEIGHTS AND RECOMMENDED ENERGY INTAKE

| Category | Age (yr) | Weight (kg) | Weight (lb) | Height (cm) | Height (in.) | Energy needs (with range) (kcal) | Energy needs (with range) (MJ) |
|---|---|---|---|---|---|---|---|
| Infants | 0.0 –0.5 | 6 | 13 | 60 | 24 | kg × 115 (95–145) | kg × 0.48 |
| | 0.05–1.0 | 9 | 20 | 71 | 28 | kg × 105 (80–135) | kg × 0.44 |
| Children | 1–3 | 13 | 29 | 90 | 35 | 1300 (900–1800) | 5.5 |
| | 4–6 | 20 | 44 | 112 | 44 | 1700 (1300–2300) | 7.1 |
| | 7–10 | 28 | 62 | 132 | 52 | 2400 (1650–3300) | 10.1 |
| Males | 11–14 | 45 | 99 | 157 | 62 | 2700 (2000–3700) | 11.3 |
| | 15–18 | 66 | 145 | 176 | 69 | 2800 (2100–3900) | 11.8 |
| | 19–22 | 70 | 154 | 177 | 70 | 2900 (2500–3300) | 12.2 |
| | 23–50 | 70 | 154 | 178 | 70 | 2700 (2300–3100) | 11.3 |
| | 51–75 | 70 | 154 | 178 | 70 | 2400 (2000–2800) | 10.1 |
| | 76+ | 70 | 154 | 178 | 70 | 2050 (1650–2450) | 8.6 |
| Females | 11–14 | 46 | 101 | 157 | 62 | 2200 (1500–3000) | 9.2 |
| | 15–18 | 55 | 120 | 163 | 64 | 2100 (1200–3000) | 8.8 |
| | 19–22 | 55 | 120 | 163 | 64 | 2100 (1700–2500) | 8.8 |
| | 23–50 | 55 | 120 | 163 | 64 | 2000 (1600–2400) | 8.4 |
| | 51–75 | 55 | 120 | 163 | 64 | 1800 (1400–2200) | 7.6 |
| | 76+ | 55 | 120 | 163 | 64 | 1600 (1200–2000) | 6.7 |
| Pregnancy | | | | | | +300 | |
| Lactation | | | | | | +500 | |

(The data in this table have been assembled from the observed median heights and weights of children shown on p. I3, together with desirable weights for adults given here for the mean heights of men (70 inches) and women (64 inches) between the ages of 18 and 34 years as surveyed in the U.S. population (HEW/NCHS data).)

The energy allowances for the young adults are for men and women doing light work. The allowances for the two older age groups represent mean energy needs over these age spans, allowing for a 2% decrease in basal (resting) metabolic rate per decade and a reduction in activity of 200 kcal/day for men and women between 51 and 75 years, 500 kcal for men over 75 years and 400 kcal for women over 75. The customary range of daily energy output is shown for adults in parentheses, and is based on a variation in energy needs of ±400 kcal at any one age, emphasizing the wide range of energy intakes appropriate for any group of people.

Energy allowances for children through age 18 are based on median energy intakes of children of these ages followed in longitudinal growth studies. The values in parentheses are 10th and 90th percentiles of energy intake, to indicate the range of energy consumption among children of these ages.

*Source:* Recommended Dietary Allowances, Revised 1980. Food and Nutrition Board National Academy of Sciences—National Research Council, Washington, D.C.

## ESTIMATED SAFE AND ADEQUATE DAILY DIETARY INTAKES OF ADDITIONAL SELECTED VITAMINS AND MINERALS [a]

| | Age (yr) | Vitamins | | | Trace elements [b] | | | | | | Electrolytes | | |
|---|---|---|---|---|---|---|---|---|---|---|---|---|---|
| | | Vitamin K (µg) | Biotin (µg) | Pantothenic acid (mg) | Copper (mg) | Manganese (mg) | Fluoride (mg) | Chromium (mg) | Selenium (mg) | Molybdenum (mg) | Sodium (mg) | Potassium (mg) | Chloride (mg) |
| Infants | 0–0.5 | 12 | 35 | 2 | 0.5–0.7 | 0.5–0.7 | 0.1–0.5 | 0.01–0.04 | 0.01–0.04 | 0.03–0.06 | 115–350 | 350–925 | 275–700 |
| | 0.5–1 | 10–20 | 50 | 3 | 0.7–1.0 | 0.7–1.0 | 0.2–1.0 | 0.02–0.06 | 0.02–0.06 | 0.04–0.08 | 250–750 | 425–1275 | 400–1200 |
| Children | 1–3 | 15–30 | 65 | 3 | 1.0–1.5 | 1.0–1.5 | 0.5–1.5 | 0.02–0.08 | 0.02–0.08 | 0.05–0.10 | 325–975 | 550–1650 | 500–1500 |
| and | 4–6 | 20–40 | 85 | 3–4 | 1.5–2.0 | 1.5–2.0 | 1.0–2.5 | 0.03–0.12 | 0.03–0.12 | 0.06–0.15 | 450–1350 | 775–2325 | 700–2100 |
| adolescents | 7–10 | 30–60 | 120 | 4–5 | 2.0–2.5 | 2.0–3.0 | 1.5–2.5 | 0.05–0.20 | 0.05–0.20 | 0.1–0.30 | 600–1800 | 1000–3000 | 925–2775 |
| | 11+ | 50–100 | 100–200 | 4–7 | 2.0–3.0 | 2.5–5.0 | 1.5–2.5 | 0.05–0.20 | 0.05–0.20 | 0.15–0.50 | 900–2700 | 1525–4575 | 1400–4200 |
| Adults | | 70–140 | 100–200 | 4–7 | 2.0–3.0 | 2.5–5.0 | 1.5–4.0 | 0.05–0.20 | 0.05–0.20 | 0.15–0.50 | 1100–3300 | 1875–5625 | 1700–5100 |

*Source:* Recommended Dietary Allowances, Revised 1980. Food and Nutrition Board National Academy of Sciences—National Research Council, Washington, D.C.
[a] Because there is less information on which to base allowances, these figures are not given in the main table of the RDA and are provided here in the form of ranges of recommended intakes.
[b] Since the toxic levels for many trace elements may be only several times usual intakes, the upper levels for the trace elements given in this table should not be habitually exceeded.

# Abbreviations: Official and Unofficial

| | | | |
|---|---|---|---|
| a | before | f.b. | fingers' breadths |
| a.c. | before meals | F.B.S. | fasting blood sugar |
| A.F. | auricular fibrillation | F.H. | family history |
| A/G | albumin/globulin ratio | F.T.B.S. | finger tip blood sugar |
| A.I.D. | acute infectious disease | G.A. | general appearance |
| | | G.B. | gall bladder |
| A.R.F. | acute rheumatic fever | G.C. | gonococcus |
| A.S. | left ear | gt. | a drop |
| A.S.H.D. | arteriosclerotic heart disease | G.I. | gastrointestinal |
| | | G.U. | genitourinary |
| a-v | auricula-ventricular | Gyn. | gynecology |
| A.V. | arterio-venous | H.A. | headache |
| a & w | alive and well | Hb. or Hgb. | hemoglobin |
| b.i.d. or b.d. | twice daily | H.C. | high calorie |
| b.m. | bowel movement | Hct | hematocrit |
| B.M.R. | basal metabolic rate | H.C.V.D. | hypertensive cardio-vascular disease |
| B.P. | blood pressure | | |
| B.P.H. | benign prostatic hypertrophy | H.E.E.N.T. | head, eye, ear, nose, and throat |
| B.S. | bowel sounds | h.s. | at bedtime |
| B.T. | bedtime | Hx | history |
| B.U.N. | blood urea nitrogen | I.M. | intramuscular |
| c | with | Imp: | impression |
| ca. | approximately | I & O | intake and output |
| Ca | calcium | I.P. | intraperitoneal |
| CA | cancer | I.V. | intravenous |
| C.B.C. | complete blood count | i.c. | in the place cited |
| C.C. | chief complaint | L.E. | lupus erythemstosis |
| C.H.F. | congestive heart failure | L.M.D. | local doctor |
| | | L.P. | lumbar puncture |
| C.I. | color index | L.U.Q. | left upper quadrant |
| c.m. | costal margin | L.V. | left ventricle |
| C.N.S. | central nervous system | L.V.H. | left ventricular hypertrophy |
| CSF | cerebrospinal fluid | L & W | living and well |
| C.T. | clotting time | M. | muscles |
| c.v. | cardiovascular | M.H. | menstrual history |
| C.V.A. | cardiovascular accident | M.S. | multiple sclerosis or morphine sulfate |
| C.V.R. | cardiovascular-renal | | |
| Cx | cervix | N.P.N. | nonprotein nitrogen |
| D/C | discontinue | NR | not remarkable |
| D.&C. | dilatation and curettage | N. & V. | nausea and vomiting |
| d.l. | danger list | O.B. | obstetrics |
| d.p. | diastolic pressure | ob | in front of |
| D.O.B. | Doctor's Order Book | O.D. | right eye |
| Dx | diagnosis | o & o | off and on |
| D/W | dextrose and water | O.S. | left eye |
| E.E.G. | electro-encephalogram | P. | pulse |
| | | P.A. | pernicious anemia |
| E.K.G. or E.C.G. | electrocardiogram | P.&A. | percussion and auscultation |
| | | para | pregnancies |
| E.N.T. | ear, nose and throat | P.B.I. | protein-bound iodine |
| E.S.R. | erythrocyte sedimentation rate | p.c. | after eating |
| | | P.C. | present complaint |
| Ext. | extremities | PH | past history |

| | | | |
|---|---|---|---|
| P.I. | present illness | S.R. | systems review |
| P.M.H. | past medical history | stat | at once |
| P.N.D. | paroxysmal noctur-<br>nal dyspnea | S.W.C. | senior ward clerk |
| | | Sx | symptom |
| p.o. | postoperative or<br>by mouth | T | temperature |
| p.p. | pulse pressure | T.&A. | tonsillectomy and<br>adenoidectomy |
| p.r. | pulse rate or<br>by rectum | T.A.H. | total abdominal<br>hysterectomy |
| p.r.n. | whenever necessary | T.B. | tuberculosis |
| P.T.A. | prior to admission | tbc | tubercle bacillus |
| PZI | protein zinc insulin | t.i.d. | thrice daily |
| q. | every | T.P. | total protein |
| q.d. | every day | T.P.R. | temperature, pulse,<br>respiration |
| q.h. | every hour | | |
| q.i.d. | four times daily | T.U.R. | trans-urethral<br>resection |
| q.o.d. | every other day | | |
| r.b.c. | red blood cells | U.A. | urine analysis |
| R.B.C. | red blood count | U.C.D.<br>or O.C.H.D. | usual childhood<br>diseases |
| R.F. | rheumatic fever | U.R.I. | upper respiratory<br>infection |
| R.H.D. | rheumatic heart<br>disease | | |
| R.O. | rule out | U.R.Q. | upper right quadrant |
| R.O.S. | review of systems | U-V | ultraviolet |
| R.Q. | respiratory quotient | V.D. | venereal disease |
| R.U.Q. | right upper quadrant | v.p. | venous pressure |
| R.V. | right ventricle | w.b.c. | white blood cells |
| R.V.H. | right ventricular<br>hypertrophy | W.B.C. | white blood count |
| | | W.D. | well developed |
| Rx | prescription,<br>treatment | W.N. | well nourished |

Prefixes

| | |
|---|---|
| gastr- | pertaining to stomach |
| chole- | pertaining to gallbladder |
| hyper- | above normal |
| hypo- | below normal |

| | | |
|---|---|---|
| s | without | |
| S.B.E. | subacute bacterial<br>endocarditis | |
| S.D.A. | specific dynamic<br>action | |
| S.H. | social history | |
| S.O.B. | shortness of breath | |
| S.O.B.O.E. | shortness of breath<br>on exertion | |
| s.p. | systolic pressure | |

Suffixes

| | |
|---|---|
| -oma | pertaining to tumor |
| -ectomy | removal of |
| -itis | inflammation of |
| -scopy | examination of |

# Medical Combining Forms

| Form | Pertaining to | Example | Definition |
|------|---------------|---------|------------|
| Aden- | A gland | Adenitis—Inflammation of a gland. |
| Cardi- | The heart | Cardialgia—Pain in the region of the heart. |
| Chole- | Bile | Cholecyst—Gallbladder—Pear-shaped reservoir for the bile on the under surface of the liver. |
| Crani- | The skull | Craniotomy—Cutting up of fetal head to effect delivery. |
| Cyst- | Any fluid containing sac | Cystitis—Inflammation of bladder. |
| Derm- or Dermati- | The skin | Dermatitis—Inflammation of skin. |
| Gastri- | Stomach | Gastrectomy—Excision of part of stomach. |
| Gynec- | Women | Gynecology—Sum of knowledge of women's diseases. |
| Hem- or Hemat- | Blood | Hematology—Sum of what is known regarding the blood. |
| Hyster- | Uterus | Hysterectomy—Excising the uterus— performed either through the abdominal wall or through the vagina. |
| Leuk- or Leuc- | Anything white | Leukocyte—Any colorless, ameboid cell. Mass white blood corpuscle, lymph corpuscle, or wandering connective tissue cell. |
| My- | Muscle | Myoma—Any tumor formed of muscular tissue. |
| Neph- | Kidney | Nephrectomy—Removal of the kidney. |
| Oophor- | Ovary | Oophorectomy—Surgical removal of an ovary. |
| Ophthalm- | Eye | Ophthalmomometer—Instrument for measuring refractive powers of the eye. |
| Oss- | Bone | Osseous—Composed of bone, boney. |
| Oste- | Bone | Osteitis—Inflammation of bone. |
| Ot- | The ear | Otoscope—Instrument for inspecting or for auscultating (listening to) the ear. |
| Ovar- | Ovary | Ovarian—Pertaining to an ovary (female gland in which ova are formed). |
| Path- | Disease | Pathology—Sum of what is known regarding disease. |
| Ped- (Greek) | Children | Pediatrician—Specialist in children's diseases. |
| Ped- (Latin) | Feet | Pedography—Imprint of weight-bearing surface of the foot. |
| Pneum- or Pneumon- | Lung | Pneumococcus—Organism causing lobar pneumonia. |
| Py- | Pus | Pyuria—Passage of urine containing pus. |

| Form | Pertaining to | Example | Definition |
|---|---|---|---|
| Salping- | Tube | Salpingitis—Inflammation of fallopian tube. |
| Septic- | Poison | Septicemia—Morbid condition due to presence of pathogenic bacteria and associated poisons in the blood. |
| Tox- or Toxic- | Poison | Toxemia—Blood poisoning—poisoning by toxins. |
| Trache- | Trachea or neck | Tracheitis—Inflammation of trachea. |

*Prefixes*

| | | | |
|---|---|---|---|
| Brady- | Slow | Bradycardia—Abnormal slowness of pulse. |
| Dys- | Pain or difficulty | Dyspnea—Labored or difficult breathing. |
| Hyper- | Above, excess of | Hyperemia—Excess of blood in any part of body. |
| Hypo- | Under. deficiency of | Hypodermic—Applied under the skin. |
| Tachy- | Fast | Tachycardia—Excessive rapidity of heart's action. |

*Suffixes*

| | | | |
|---|---|---|---|
| -algia | Pain | Cardialgia—Pain in region of the heart or of cardia. |
| -asis or -osis | Being affected with | Leukocytosis—Increase in number of blood leukocytes. |
| -clysis | Injection | Hypedermoclysis—Injection under the skin of fluids. |
| -cyte | Cell | Leukocyte—Colorless, ameboid cell mass. |
| -ectomy | Excision | Adenoidectomy—Excision of adenoid growths. |
| -emia | Blood | Glycemia—Presence of glucose or sugar in blood. |
| -esthesia | Sensation | Anesthesia—Loss of feeling or sensation. |
| -genic | Producing | Pyogenic—Producing a formation of, conversion into, discharge of pus. |
| -itis | Inflammation | Tonsillitis—Inflammation of a tonsil. |
| -logy | Science of | Pathology—Sum of what is known regarding disease. |
| -oma | Tumor | Myoma—Any tumor formed of muscular tissue. |
| -otomy | Cutting into | Laparotomy—Surgical incision through abdominal wall. |
| -penia | Lack of | Leukopenia—Deficiency in number of leukocytes. |
| -ostomy | Creation of an opening | Gastrostomy—Creation of artificial gastric fistula. |
| -phobia | Fear | Hydrophobia—Acute infectious disease communicated to man by bite of infected dog. |

| Form | Pertaining to | Example | Definition |
|------|---------------|---------|------------|
| -pnea | Air or breathing | Dyspnea—Labored or difficult breathing. | |
| -rrhaphy | Suture of | herniorrhaphy—Repaired hernia. | |
| -uria | Urine | Polyuria—Excess amount of urine. | |

*Source*:   Reprinted from Diet Manual, Commonwealth of Pennsylvania, Rev. 1976.

# Guidelines for Recording Nutritional Information in Medical Records

AMERICAN HOSPITAL ASSOCIATION

As the complexity of medical care continues to increase, the integration of care provided to the individual patient by each professional discipline is facilitated through regular and systematic recording in the patient's record of actual care given. Such documentation must include pertinent findings and actions taken, patient's progress and response to therapy, and concluding instructions to the patient and/or family on physical activity, medication, diet, and follow-up care. The patient's medical record is an information-sharing tool that promotes and assists in coordinating the activities of all health team members contributing to the patient's care. It should reflect the health team's ultimate goal of high-quality care and optimal cost effectiveness.

The dietitian, like other members of the health team, cooperates in carrying out the written orders of the responsible physician. By promptly recording in the patient's medical record pertinent, meaningful observations and information on food habits, food acceptance, and dietary treatment, the dietetic staff uses the only reliable means of documenting regular communication with the physician and other professionals participating in the patient's total care.

Although verbal communication is informative, it is sporadic and does not replace the need for documentation that will reach all members of the health team involved in the patient's care. Documented communication is necessary for patients receiving short-term care and of prime importance for those patients requiring prolonged care if a unified appraisal of existing problems is to be made and plans for coordinating management are to be carried out. Traditionally, the medical record is structured according to source of information, with entries in chronological sequence for a close overview of patient care activities by the physician. However, a number of other methods for organization of clinical information in the medical record are in use, including the problem-oriented medical record (POMR). The POMR is an integrated recording system focusing on

Reprinted with permission of the American Hospital Association, 840 North Lake Shore Drive, Chicago, IL 60611. Copyright 1976.
These guidelines are a revision of *Guidelines for Therapeutic Dietitians on Recording in Patient's Medical Records*, published in 1966 as S31 in the American Hospital Association S series leaflets. The guidelines originated in the Joint Committee of the American Hospital Association and the American Dietetic Association and had been approved by both associations as suggested methods for documenting nutritional care information in patients' medical records. The revision includes procedures for ensuring systematic planning for nutritional care and education of patients for whom modified diets have been prescribed and/or for whom continuing care is anticipated. These revised guidelines were approved by the Joint Committee of the American Hospital Association and the American Dietetic Association on April 27, 1976, and by the AHA General Council on October 13–14, 1976.

the patient's problems and profile, plans for care and for patient education, assessment of progress, and results. Regardless of the methodology used, the essentials of recordings are timely, well-organized, definitive entries amenable to peer review in the evaluation of patient care.

The Professional Standards Review Organizations (PSROs), created under P.L. 92-603 in 1972, are required to involve nonphysician health care practitioners in the review of care provided by their peers to recipients of Medicare, Medicaid, maternal, and child health–crippled children programs. This involvement includes development of standards and criteria for use by their peers in reviewing the quality of services delivered by practitioners of their own discipline. Physicians participate in the review of decisions on the medical appropriateness of care ordered by a physician, but delivered by other health practitioners. Thus, qualified dietitians* are reviewers of care provided by other qualified dietitians and their authorized alternates in a continuing study of high-quality patient care.

Criteria developed for an organized and objective assessment of nutritional care given to patients requiring diet modifications will be compared with the documented description in patients' medical records of actual nutritional care provided, such as:

- Type of diet and number of kilocalories, if indicated

- Tolerance to diet, for example, complications and substitutes

- Communications between dietitian and physician and/or nursing service personnel regarding diet

- Diet instructions to patient, family, and/or program personnel inside and outside the institution

- Recommendations, if indicated

- Actual follow-up

Where and How to Record  Regardless of the format used, entries in the patient's medical record should contain sufficient information to support the dietary assessment, to justify the dietetic care, and to document the results accurately. Peer review is facilitated by the centralization of information in the patient's record. The progress note section of the medical record is recommended as the most suitable location for recording dietetic care information and nutritional care plans.

Brevity without sacrifice of essential facts is the essence of effective recording. Dietary progress notes and summaries should be as brief as is consistent with good communication, should avoid professional jargon, and should have meaning for all responsible members of the health care team contributing to the patient's care. When professional opinion is expressed, it should be phrased to indicate clearly that it is the view of the person recording.

* The term *qualified dietitian* means one who is eligible for registration by the Commission on Dietetic Registration *or* has a baccalaureate with major studies in food and nutrition or dietetics.

Remarks that are critical of treatment carried out by others, that indicate bias against the patient, or that are unprofessional should never appear in the medical record.

A "Department of Dietetics" stamp will readily identify the dietetic staff entries on progress notes forms. Patients on normal or near-normal diets occasionally present problems requiring dietetic entries. Such entries should be flagged to apprise the physician of nutrition information or problems.

**Who Is to Record** Entries in patient medical records may be made only by individuals so authorized by the institution's policies, which are usually developed in cooperation with the medical staff. When the services of a qualified dietitian are not available on a regular full-time basis, dietetic technicians or dietetic assistants may be designated as authorized alternates to record current, pertinent nutritional care information commensurate with the responsibility delegated to their position within the institution. All entries should be dated and signed with the name and title of the person making the entry.

**What to Record** The qualified dietitian or authorized alternate is responsible for recording the following subject items for patients on modified diets:

1. Confirmation of diet order
   a. Within 24 hours of admission, a notation that the prescribed modified diet order is being fulfilled (except for those patients not being fed orally).
   b. All subsequent orders by the physician for a modified diet.
2. Summary of dietary history
   a. Evaluation of the patient's diet pattern, nutrient deficit, lifestyle, food allergies, and socioeconomic resources essential for nutritional care planning.
   b. Assessment of the patient's awareness of the relationship of diet to disease, which has a direct bearing on plans for individual nutritional care.
3. Nutritional care therapy
   a. Type of diet and, if indicated, the number of kilocalories or other nutrients, such as sodium, cholesterol, or saturated fat.
   b. Daily record of patient's nutrient intake during a period of quantitative or qualitative control of food and fluid intake, medication, or other pertinent therapy.
   c. Report of the patient's tolerance to the prescribed diet modification, including the effect of the patient's appetite and food habits on food intake and any substitutes made:
   d. Notations of any changes in diet orders and diet instruction plans.
   e. Brief written communications between dietetic staff and physician and/or nursing service personnel pertinent to patient's nutritional care.
   f. Request, if indicated, for referral of patient to appropriate community agency for assistance in following diet at home.

4. Nutritional care discharge plan
   a. Description of diet instructions given to patient and/or family. If preprinted instructions are given to patient or family, a copy should be placed either in the patient's medical record or on file in the medical record department's reference file.
   b. Description or copy of diet pattern forwarded to referral agency or nursing home facility for subsequent patient care.
   c. Plan for patient's continued nutritional care, including any dates for return visits. If nutritional care follow-up reverts to the physician's office practice, this should be noted in the patient's record.
5. Dietetic consultation
   a. The physician's written request for dietetic consultation should be acknowledged.
   b. Consultation reports containing a written opinion by the dietitian that reflects an assessment of the patient's dietary history, examination of the patient's medical record for any previous dietetic care, and any recommendations for normal or modified diet. Subsequent counseling of the patient or family should be recorded in the patient's medical record.

Methods of Recording    The method selected for recording dietary data in the patient's medical record should be compatible with the institution's method for arranging clinical data. If the POMR is used, the procedure described in the appendix is suggested.

References    Chappelle, M. L., and Scholl, R.:   Adapting the problem oriented medical record to the psychiatric hospital.   J. Am. Diet. Assoc. 63: 643, December 1973.

Easton, E.:   Problem Oriented Medical Records Concepts. New York:   Appleton-Century-Crofts, 1974.

Feinstein, A. R.:   The problems of the problem-oriented medical records.   Ann. Intern. Med. 78: 751, May 1973.

Joint Commission on Accreditation of Hospitals:   Accreditation Manual for Hospitals, 1970, updated 1973. Chicago:   JCAH, 1973.

American Dietetic Association:   Professional Standards Review Procedure Manual. Chicago:   ADA, 1976.

Voytovich, A. E.:   Dietitian/nutritionist and the problem-oriented medical record, a physician's viewpoint.   J. Am. Diet. Assoc. 63: 641, December 1973.

Walters, F. M., and DeMarco, M.:   Dietitian/nutritionist and the problem-oriented medical record:   the role of the dietitian.   J. Am. Diet. Assoc. 63: 641, December 1973.

Weed, L. L.:   Quality control and the medical record.   Arch. Intern. Med. 127: 101, January 1971.

Appendix    The distinctive feature of the POMR is that of a problem-structured record rather than an arrangement according to sources of data. Data are structured according to a series of problems identified by the various disciplines. The progress notes are maintained in chronological order, but, as pertinent information and observations are cited, the responsible members of the health team enter their data under the title of that problem. The major advantages of a problem-structured record are: (1) the ability to express each problem in its own observational terms, (2) a patient profile that contains descriptions of the patient's life situation, (3) integration of data recorded by diverse disciplines, (4) deliberate attention to plans for education of the patient about his illness and his part in managing it, and (5) ideas for further application or adaptations.

The three specific information areas in the POMR shown here have been selected to provide guidance to the dietetic staff in improving the adequacy and organization of nutritional care information for effective documentation.

### DATA BASE

The data base includes the relevant admission data from the health team members, that is, chief complaint, present illness, physical examination, and laboratory results. Pertinent facts from the assessment of dietary history, home and family resources, and patient's knowledge of and attitude toward food and nutrition should be recorded in the data base.

### PROBLEM LIST

A complete problem list is maintained and is updated as new information accumulates, which will require problems to be added, deleted, or changed. A problem is any condition (health, socioeconomic, or personal) the patient presents that requires the health team to obtain more information, treat, or educate. Coupled with proper team supervision, the documented problems requiring attention are not overlooked in the day-to-day charting of information.

### PROGRESS NOTES

The progress notes are entered by participating team members in chronological sequence. The narrative entries may be structured according to the SOAP format:

S—Subjective data: Patient's expression of well-being, concern, and current status, which would include interim dietary intake and food habits.
O—Objective data: Actual clinical findings of laboratory tests, screening tests, and other parameters being taken into consideration, such as height, weight, and skin folds that have direct bearing on dietetic treatment.
A—Assessment: Dietitian's appraisal based on subjective and objective data. If the subjective and objective data are consistent, the appraisal may be self-evident.
P—Planning: Recommendations and plans, including the dietitian's, for follow-up care. Three categories of recommendations are: obtain more information, treat, and educate.

An example of an education plan for an obese patient is "Explain caloric deficit in relation to weight loss and provide information on caloric content of snack foods. Design meal plan with patient. Have patient plan menus for several days." An example of a treatment plan is "A 1,500–1,800 kilocalorie diet and exercise regimen is suggested for this patient. He should also be followed for eight visits in the obesity clinic."

Progress notes using the SOAP format inform the health team of the dietitian's plans and promote cooperation among team members in the implementation of the plan.

## Normal Hematologic Values

|  |  |
|---|---|
| Acid hemolysis test (Ham) | No hemolysis |
| Alkaline phosphatase leukocyte | Total score 14–100 |
| Bleeding time | |
|   Ivy | Less than 5 min |
|   Duke | 1–5 min |
| Carboxyhemoglobin | Up to 5% of total |
| Cell counts | |
| Erythrocytes: Males | 4.6–6.2 million/mm³ |
|   Females | 4.2–5.4 million/mm³ |
|   Children (varies with age) | 4.5–5.1 million/mm³ |

| Leukocytes | | Percentage | Absolute (per mm³) |
|---|---|---|---|
| Total | | | 5000–10,000 mm³ |
| Differential | | | |
| Myeloblasts | | 0 | 0 |
| Myelocytes / Juvenile neutrophils | | 3– 5 | 150– 400 |
| Segmented neutrophils | | 54–62 | 3000–5800 |
| Lymphocytes | | 25–33 | 1500–3000 |
| Monocytes | | 3– 7 | 285– 500 |
| Eosinophils | | 1– 3 | 50– 250 |
| Basophils | | 0– 0.75 | 15– 50 |

(Infants and children have greater relative numbers of lymphocytes and monocytes)

|  |  |
|---|---|
| Platelets | 150,000–350,000/mm³ |
| Reticulocytes | 25,000– 75,000/mm³; 0.5–1.5% of erythrocytes |
| Clot retraction, qualitative | Begins in 30–60 min; Complete in 24 hr |
| Coagulation time (Lee-White) | 5–15 min (glass tubes); 19–60 min (siliconized tubes) |
| Cold hemolysin test (Donath-Landsteiner) | No hemolysis |
| Corpuscular values of erythrocytes (Values are for adults; in children, values vary with age) | |
|   M.C.H. (mean corpuscular hemoglobin) | 27–31 pg |
|   M.C.V. (mean corpuscular volume) | 80–105 um³ |
|   M.C.H.C. (mean corpuscular hemoglobin concentration) | 32–36% |
| Fibrinogen | 200–400 mg/100 ml |
| Fibrinolysins | 0 |
| Hematocrit | |
|   Males | 40–54 ml/100 ml |
|   Females | 37–47 ml/100 ml |
|   Newborn | 49–54 ml/100 ml |
|   Children (varies with age) | 35–49 ml/100 ml |

|  |  |
|---|---|
| Hemoglobin | |
|   Males | 14.0–18.0 g/100 ml |
|   Females | 12.0–16.0 g/100 ml |
|   Newborn | 16.5–19.5 g/100 ml |
|   Children (varies with age) | 11.2–16.5 g/100 ml |
|   Hemoglobin, fetal | Less than 1% of total |
|   Hemoglobin A | 1.5–3.0% of total |
|   Hemoglobin, plasma | 0–5.0 mg/100 ml |
|   Methemoglobin | 0.03–0.13 g/100 ml |
| Osmotic fragility of erythrocytes | Begins in 0.45–0.39% NaCl; Complete in 0.33–0.30% NaCl |
| Partial thromboplastin time | |
|   Kaolin activated | 60–70 sec |
| Prothrombin consumption | 35–45 sec; Over 80% consumed in 1 hr |
| Prothrombin content | 100% (calculated from prothrombin time) |
| Prothrombin time (one stage) | 12.0–14.0 sec |
| Sedimentation rate | |
|   Wintrobe: Males | 0–5 mm in 1 hr |
|     Females | 0–15 mm in 1 hr |
|   Westergren: Males | 0–15 mm in 1 hr |
|     Females | 0–20 mm in 1 hr |
| (May be slightly higher in children and during pregnancy) | |
| Thromboplastin generation test | Compared to normal control |
| Tourniquet test | Ten or fewer petechiae in a 2.5 cm circle after 5 min with cuff at 100 mm Hg |

| Bone marrow, differential cell count | Range (%) | Average (%) |
|---|---|---|
| Myeloblasts | 0.3 – 5.0 | 2.0 |
| Promyelocytes | 1.0 – 8.0 | 5.0 |
| Myelocytes: Neutrophilic | 5.0 –19.0 | 12.0 |
|   Eosinophilic | 0.5 – 3.0 | 1.5 |
|   Basophilic | 0.0 – 0.5 | 0.3 |
| Metamyelocytes ("juvenile" forms) | 13.0 –32.0 | 22.0 |
| Polymorphonuclear neutrophils | 7.0 –30.0 | 20.0 |
| Polymorphonuclear eosinophils | 0.5 – 4.0 | 2.0 |
| Polymorphonuclear basophils | 0.0 – 0.7 | 0.2 |
| Lymphocytes | 3.0 –17.0 | 10.0 |
| Plasma cells | 0.0 – 2.0 | 0.4 |
| Monocytes | 0.5 – 5.0 | 2.0 |
| Reticulum cells | 0.1 – 2.0 | 0.2 |
| Megakaryocytes | 0.03– 3.0 | 0.4 |
| Pronormoblasts | 1.0 – 8.0 | 4.0 |
| Normoblasts | 7.0 –32.0 | 18.0 |

*Source:* Adapted from Conn, H. F., and Conn, R. B.: Current Diagnosis. Philadelphia: W. B. Saunders, 1974. Prepared by Rex B. Conn, M.D., The Johns Hopkins School of Medicine, Baltimore.

**Normal Blood, Plasma, and Serum Values**

|  |  |
|---|---|
| Acetone, serum | |
|   Qualitative | Negative |
|   Quantitative | 0.3–2.0 mg/100 ml |
| Aldolase, serum | 0.8–3.0 milliunits/ml (IU) (30°) (Sibley-Lehninger) |
| Amino acid nitrogen, serum | 4–6 mg/100 ml |
| Ammonia nitrogen, blood | 75–196 µg/100 ml |
|   plasma | 56–122 µg/100 ml |
| Amylase, serum | 80–160 Somogyi units/100 ml |
| Ascorbic acid | See Vitamin C |
| Base, total, serum | 145–160 meq/litre |
| Bilirubin, serum | |
|   Direct | 0.1–0.4 mg/100 ml |
|   Indirect | 0.2–0.7 mg/100 ml (Total minus direct) |
|   Total | 0.3–1.1 mg/100 ml |
| Calcium, serum | 4.5–5.5 meq/litre (9.0–11.0 mg/100 ml) (Slightly higher in children) (Varies with protein concentration) |
| Calcium, serum, ionized | 2.1–2.6 meq/litre (4.25–5.25 mg/100 ml) |
| Carbon dioxide content, serum | 24–30 meq/litre; Infants: 20–28 meq/litre |
| Carbon dioxide tension (Pco₂), blood | 35–45 mm Hg |
| Carotene, serum | 50–300 µg/100 ml |
| Ceruloplasmin, serum | 23–44 mg/100 ml |
| Chloride, serum | 96–106 meq/litre |
| Cholesterol, serum | |
|   Total | 150–250 mg/100 ml |
|   Esters | 68–76% of total cholesterol |
| Cholinesterase, serum | 0.5–1.3 pH units |
|   RBC | 0.5–1.0 pH units |
| Copper, serum | |
|   Males | 70–140 µg/100 ml |
|   Females | 85–155 µg/100 ml |
| Cortisol, plasma | 6–16 µg/100 ml |
| Creatine, serum | 0.2–0.8 mg/100 ml |
| Creatine phosphokinase, serum | |
|   Male | 0–50 milliunits/ml (IU) (30°) |
|   Female | 0–30 milliunits/ml (IU) (30°) (Oliver-Rosalki) |
| Creatinine, serum | 0.7–1.5 mg/100 ml |
| Cryoglobulins, serum | 0 |
| Fatty acids, total, serum | 190–420 mg/100 ml |
| Fibrinogen, plasma | 200–400 mg/100 ml |
| Folic acid, serum | 7–16 mg/100 ml |

|  |  |
|---|---|
| Nitrogen, nonprotein, serum | 15–35 mg/100 ml |
| Osmolality, serum | 285–295 mOsm/kg serum water |
| Oxygen, blood | |
|   Capacity | 16–24 vol % (varies with Hb) |
|   Content  Arterial | 15–23 vol % |
|          Venous | 10–16 vol % |
|   Saturation  Arterial | 94–100% of capacity |
|           Venous | 60–85% of capacity |
|   Tension, Po₂ Arterial | 75–100 mm Hg |
| pH, arterial, blood | 7.35–7.45 |
| Phenylalanine, serum | Less than 3 mg/100 ml |
| Phosphatase, acid, serum | 1.0–5.0 units (King-Armstrong) |
| | 0.5–2.0 units (Bodansky) |
| | 0.5–2.0 units (Gutman) |
| | 0.0–1.1 units (Shinowara) |
| | 0.1–0.63 unit (Bessey-Lowry) |
| Phosphatase, alkaline, serum | 5.0–13.0 units (King-Armstrong) |
| | 2.0–4.5 units (Bodansky) |
| | 3.0–10.0 units (Gutman) |
| | 2.2–8.6 units (Shinowara) |
| | 0.8–2.3 units (Bessey-Lowry) |
| | 3.0–10.0 milliunits/ml (IU) |
| | (Values are higher in children) |
| Phosphate, inorganic, serum | 3.0–4.5 mg/100 ml (Children: 4.0–7.0 mg/100 ml) |
| Phospholipids, serum | 6–12 mg/100 ml as lipid phosphorus |
| Potassium, serum | 3.5–5.0 meq/litre |
| Proteins, serum | |
|   Total | 6.0–8.0 g/100 ml |
|     Albumin | 3.5–5.5 g/100 ml |
|     Globulin | 2.5–3.5 g/100 ml |
|   Electrophoresis | |
|     Albumin | 3.5–5.5 g/100 ml; 52–68% of total |
|     Globulin | |
|       Alpha₁ | 0.2–0.4 g/100 ml; 2–5% of total |
|       Alpha₂ | 0.5–0.9 g/100 ml; 7–14% of total |
|       Beta | 0.6–1.1 g/100 ml; 9–15% of total |
|       Gamma | 0.7–1.7 g/100 ml; 11–21% of total |
| Pyruvic acid, plasma | 1.0–2.0 mg/100 ml |

Glucose (fasting)  
  blood, true — 60–100 mg/100 ml  
    Folin — 80–120 mg/100 ml  
  plasma or serum, true — 70–115 mg/100 ml  
Haptoglobin, serum — 40–170 mg/100 ml  
Hydroxybutyric dehydrogenase, serum — 0–180 milliunits/ml (IU) (30°) (Rosalki-Wilkinson); 114–290 units/ml (Wroblewski)  
17-Hydroxycorticosteroids, plasma — 8–18 μg/100 ml  
Icterus index, serum — 4–7  
Immunoglobulins, serum  
  IgG — 800–1500 mg/100 ml  
  IgA — 50–200 mg/100 ml  
  IgM — 40–120 mg/100 ml  
Iodine, butanol extractable, serum — 3.2–6.4 μg/100 ml  
Iodine, protein bound, serum — 3.5–8.0 μg/100 ml (May be slightly higher in infants)  
Iron, serum — 75–175 μg/100 ml  
Iron binding capacity, total, serum — 250–410 μg/100 ml  
  % saturation — 20–55%  
17-Ketosteroids, plasma — 25–125 μg/100 ml  
Lactic acid, blood — 6–16 mg/100 ml  
Lactic dehydrogenase, serum — 0–300 milliunits/ml (IU) (30°) (Wroblewski modified); 150–450 units/ml (Wroblewski); 80–120 units/ml (Wacker)  
Lipase, serum — 0–1.5 units (Cherry-Crandall)  
Lipids, total, serum — 450–850 mg/100 ml  
Magnesium, serum — 1.5–2.5 meq/litre (1.8–3.0 mg/100 ml)

Serotonin, platelet suspension serum — 0.1–0.3 μg/ml blood; 0.10–0.32 μg/ml  
Sodium, serum — 136–145 meq/litre  
Sulfates, inorganic, serum — 0.8–1.2 mg/100 ml (as S)  
Thyroxine, free, serum — 1.0–2.1 ng/100 ml  
Thyroxine, serum — 4.4–9.9 μg/100 ml  
Thyroxine, binding globulin (TBG), serum — 10–26 μg/100 ml  
Thyroxine iodine ($T_1$), serum — 2.9–6.4 μg/100 ml  
Transaminase, serum  
SGOT — 0–19 milliunits/ml (IU) (30°) (Karmen modified); 15–40 units/ml (Karmen); 18–40 units/ml (Reitman-Frankel)  
SGPT — 0–17 milliunits/ml (IU) (30°) (Karmen modified); 6–35 units/ml (Karmen); 5–35 units/ml (Reitman-Frankel)  

Triglycerides, serum — 0–150 mg/100 ml  
Urea, blood — 21–43 mg/100 ml  
  plasma or serum — 24–49 mg/100 ml  
Urea nitrogen, blood (BUN) — 10–20 mg/100 ml  
  plasma or serum — 11–23 mg/100 ml  
Uric acid, serum  
  Male — 2.5–8.0 mg/100 ml  
  Female — 1.5–6.0 mg/100 ml  
Vitamin A, serum — 20–80 μg/100 ml  
Vitamin $B_{12}$, serum — 200–800 pg/ml  
Vitamin C, blood — 0.4–1.5 mg/100 ml  

Calcium  
  Low Ca diet (Bauer-Aub) — Less than 150 mg/24 hr  
  Usual diet — Less than 250 mg/24 hr  
Catecholamines  
  Epinephrine — Less than 10 μg/24 hr  
  Norepinephrine — Less than 100 μg/24 hr  
Chloride — 110–250 meq/24 hr (Varies with intake)  
Chorionic gonadotrophin — 0  
Copper — 0–30 μg/24 hr  
Creatine  
  Male — 0–40 mg/24 hr  
  Female — 0–100 mg/24 hr (Higher in children and during pregnancy)

*Note:* For some procedures the normal values may vary depending upon the methods used.

**Normal Urine Values**

Acetone and acetoacetate — 0  
Addis count  
  Erythrocytes — 0–130,000/24 hr  
  Leukocytes — 0–650,000/24 hr  
  Casts thyaline — 0–2000/24 hr  
Alcapton bodies — Negative  
Aldosterone — 3–20 μg/24 hr  
Amino acid nitrogen — 50–200 mg/24 hr (Not over 1.5% of total nitrogen)  
Ammonia nitrogen — 20–70 meq/24 hr  
Amylase — 35–260 Somogyi units/hr  
Bence Jones protein — Negative  
Bilirubin (bile) — Negative

Creatinine — 15–25 mg/kg of body weight/24 hr
Cystine or cysteine, qualitative — Negative
Delta aminolevulinic acid — 1.3–7.0 mg/24 hr

Estrogens

|  | Male | Female |
|---|---|---|
| Estrone | 3–8 | 4–31 |
| Estradiol | 0–6 | 0–14 |
| Estriol | 1–11 | 0–72 |
| Total | 4–25 | 5–100 |

(Units above are μg/24 hr)
(Markedly increased during pregnancy)

Glucose (reducing substances) — Less than 250 mg/24 hr
Gonadotrophins, pituitary — 5–10 rat units/24 hr
10–50 mouse units/24 hr
(Increased after menopause)

Hemoglobin and myoglobin — Negative
Homogentisic acid, qualitative — Negative

17-Hydroxycorticosteroids
Male — 3–9 mg/24 hr
Female — 2–8 mg/24 hr
(Varies with method used)

5-Hydroxyindole-acetic acid (5-HIAA)
Qualitative — Negative
Quantitative — Less than 16 mg/24 hr

17-Ketosteroids
Male — 6–18 mg/24 hr
Female — 4–13 mg/24 hr
Osmolality — 38–1400 mOsm/kg water
pH — 4.6–8.0, average 6.0
(Depends on diet)

Phenylpyruvic acid, qualitative — Negative

Phosphorus — 0.9–1.3 g/24 hr (Varies with intake)

Porphobilinogen
Qualitative — Negative
Quantitative — 0–0.2 mg/100 ml, Less than 2.0 mg/24 hr

Porphyrins
Coproporphyrin — 50–250 μg/24 hr
Uroporphyrin — 10–30 μg/24 hr

Potassium — 25–100 meq/24 hr (Varies with intake)

Pregnanetriol — Less than 2.5 mg/24 hr in adults

Protein
Qualitative — 0
Quantitative — 10–150 mg/24 hr

Sodium — 130–260 meq/24 hr (Varies with intake)

Solids, total — 30–70 g/litre, average 50 g/litre
(To estimate total solids per litre, multiply last two figures of specific gravity by 2.66, Long's coefficient)

Specific gravity — 1.003–1.030
Sugar — 0
Titratable acidity — 20–40 meq/24 hr
Urobilinogen — Up to 1.0 Ehrlich unit/2 hr (1–3 P.M.), 0–4.0 mg/24 hr

Vanillylmandelic acid (VMA) — 1–8 mg/24 hr

## Normal Values for Semen

Volume — 2–5 ml, usually 3–4 ml
Liquefaction — complete in 15 min
pH — 7.2–8.0; average 7.8
Leukocytes — Occasional or absent
Count — 60–150 million/ml, Below 60 million/ml is abnormal
Motility — 80% or more motile
Morphology — 80–90% normal forms

## Normal Values for Gastric Analysis

Basal gastric secretion (1 hr)

|  | Concentration Mean ± 1 S.D. | Output Mean ± 1 S.D. |
|---|---|---|
| Male | 25.8 ± 1.8 meq/litre | 2.57 ± 0.16 meq/hr |
| Female | 20.3 ± 3.0 meq/litre | 1.61 ± 0.18 meq/hr |

Diagnex blue (Squibb):
Anacidity — 0–0.3 mg in 2 hr
Doubtful — 0.3–0.6 mg in 2 hr
Normal — Greater than 0.6 mg in 2 hr

After histamine stimulation
  Normal          Mean output = 11.8 meq/hr
  Duodenal ulcer  Mean output = 15.2 meq/hr
After maximal histamine stimulation
  Normal          Mean output  22.6 meq/hr
  Duodenal ulcer  Mean output  44.6 meq/hr

| Volume, fasting stomach content | 50–100 ml |
| Emptying time | 3–6 hr |
| Color | Opalescent or colorless |
| Specific gravity | 1.006–1.009 |
| pH (adults) | 0.9–1.5 |

## Normal Values for Cerebrospinal Fluid

| Cells | Fewer than 5/mm$^3$, all mononuclear |
| Chloride | 120–130 meq/litre (20 meq/litre higher than serum) |
| Colloidal gold test | Not more than 1 in any tube |
| Glucose | 50–75 mg/100 ml (20 mg/100 ml less than blood) |
| Pressure | 70–180 mm water |

| Protein, total | 15–45 mg/100 ml |
| Albumin | 52% |
| Alpha$_1$ globulin | 5% |
| Alpha$_2$ globulin | 14% |
| Beta globulin | 10% |
| Gamma globulin | 19% |

## Normal Values for Feces

| Bulk | 100–200 g/24 hr |
| Dry matter | 23–32 g/24 hr |
| Fat, total | Less than 6.0 g/24 hr |

| Nitrogen, total | Less than 2.0 g/24 hr |
| Urobilinogen | 40–280 mg/24 hr |
| Water | Approximately 65% |

## Normal Values for Serologic Procedures

Anti-hyaluronidase  Less than 1:200. Significant if rising titer can be demonstrated at weekly intervals.

| Proteus OX-19 agglutinins | 1:80 | Negative |
| | 1:160 | Doubtful |
| | 1:320 | Positive |

Anti-streptolysin O titer  Normal up to 1:128. Single test usually has little significance. Rise in titer or persistently elevated titer is significant.

| R.A. test (Latex) | 1:40 | Negative |
| | 1:80–1:160 | Doubtful |
| | 1:320 | Positive |

Bacterial agglutinins  Significant only if rise in titer is demonstrated or if antibodies are absent.

Complement fixation tests  Titers of 1:8 or less are usually not significant. Paired sera showing rise in titer of more than two tubes are usually considered significant

| Rose test | 1:10 | Negative |
| | 1:20–1:40 | Doubtful |
| | 1:80 | Positive |

C reactive protein (CRP)  Negative

| Tularemia agglutinins | 1:80 | Negative |
| | 1:160 | Doubtful |
| | 1:320 | Positive |

Heterophile titer

| | Unabsorbed | Absorbed with G.P. | Absorbed with Beef |
| --- | --- | --- | --- |
| Normal | 1:160 | 1:10 | 1:160 |
| Infectious mononucleosis | 1:160 | 1:320 | 1:10 |
| Serum sickness | 1:160 | 1:5 | 1:10 |

## Toxicology

|  |  |
|---|---|
| Arsenic, blood | 3.5–7.2 μg/100 ml |
| Arsenic, urine | Less than 100μg/24 hr |
| Barbiturates, serum | Coma level: phenobarbital approximately 11 mg/100 ml; most other barbiturates 1.5 mg/100 ml |
| Ethanol, blood | Less than 0.005% |
| Marked intoxication | 0.3–0.4% |
| Alcoholic stupor | 0.4–0.5% |
| Coma | Above 0.5% |
| Lead, blood | 0–40 μg/100 ml |
| Lead, urine | Less than 100 μg/24 hr |
| Lithium, serum | 0 |
| | Therapeutic levels 0.5–1.5 meq/litre |
| | Toxic levels above 2 meq/litre |
| Bromides, serum | 0 |
| | Toxic levels above 17 meq/litre |
| Carbon monoxide, blood | Up to 5% saturation |
| | Symptoms occur with 20% saturation |
| Dilantin, blood or serum | Therapeutic levels 1–11 μg/ml |
| Mercury, urine | Less than 10 μg/24 hr |
| Salicylate, plasma | 0 |
| Therapeutic range | 20–25 mg/100 ml |
| Toxic range | Over 30 mg/100 ml |
| Death | 45–75 mg/100 ml |

## Liver Function Tests

|  |  |
|---|---|
| Bromsulphalein (B.S.P.) | Less than 5% remaining in serum 45 min after injection of 5 mg/kg of body weight |
| Cephalin cholesterol flocculation | 0–1 in 24 hr |
| Galactose tolerance | Excretion of not more than 3.0 g galactose in the urine 5 hr after ingestion of 40 g galactose. |
| Glycogen storage | Increase of blood glucose 45 mg/100 ml over fasting level 45 min after subcutaneous injection of 0.01 mg/kg body weight of epinephrine. |
| Hippuric acid | Excretion of 3.0–3.5 g hippuric acid in urine within 4 hr after ingestion of 6.0 g sodium benzoate |
| | *or* |
| | Excretion of 0.7 g hippuric acid in urine within 1 hr after intravenous injection of 1.77 g sodium benzoate |
| Thymol turbidity | 0–5 units |
| Zinc turbidity | 2–12 units |

## Pancreatic (Islet) Function Tests

|  |  |
|---|---|
| Glucose tolerance tests | Patient should be on a diet containing 300 g carbohydrate/day for 3 days prior to test.* |
| Oral | After ingestion of 100 g glucose or 1.75 g glucose/kg of body weight, blood glucose is not more than 160 mg/100 ml after 60 min, 140 mg/100 ml after 90 min, and 120 mg/100 ml after 120 min. Values are for blood; serum measurements are approximately 15% higher. |
| Intravenous | Blood glucose does not exceed 200 mg/100 ml after infusion of 0.5 g glucose/kg of body weight over 30 min. Glucose concentration falls below initial level at 2 hr and returns to preinfusion levels in 3 or 4 hr. Values are for blood; serum measurements are approximately 15% higher. |
| Cortisone–glucose tolerance test | The patient should be on a diet containing 300 g carbohydrate/day for 3 days prior to test. At 8½ and again 2 hr prior to glucose load patient is given cortisone acetate by mouth (50 mg if patient's ideal weight is less than 160 lb, 62.5 mg if ideal weight is greater than 160 lb). An oral dose of glucose, 1.75 g/kg of body weight, is given and blood samples are taken at 0, 30, 60, 90, and 120 min. Test is considered positive if true blood glucose exceeds 160 mg/100 ml at 60 min, 140 mg/100 ml at 90 min, and 120 mg/100 ml at 120 min. Values are for blood; serum measurements are approximately 15% higher. |

* Not necessary in all individuals (see "Dietary Preparation for the Glucose Tolerance Test," p. H17).

# Renal Function Tests

| | | |
|---|---|---|
| Clearance tests (corrected to 1.73 m² body surface area) | | |
| Glomerular filtration rate (G.F.R.) | | |
|   Inulin clearance, | | |
|   Mannitol clearance, or | | |
|   Endogenous creatinine clearance | Males | 110–150 ml/min |
| | Females | 105–132 ml/min |
| Renal plasma flow (R.P.F.) | | |
|   p-Aminohippurate (P.A.H.), or | | |
|   Diodrast | Males | 560–830 ml/min |
| | Females | 490–700 ml/min |
| Filtration fraction (F.F.) | | |
| $FF \quad \dfrac{G.F.R.}{R.P.F.}$ | Males | 17–21% |
| | Females | 17–23% |
| Urea clearance ($C_U$) | Standard | 40–65 ml/min |
| | Maximal | 60–100 ml/min |
| Concentration and dilution | Specific gravity >1.025 on dry day | |
| | Specific gravity <1.003 on water day | |
| Maximal Diodrast excretory capacity $T_{MD}$ | Males | 43–59 mg/min |
| | Females | 33–51 mg/min |
| Maximal glucose reabsorptive capacity $T_{MG}$ | Males | 300–450 mg/min |
| | Females | 250–350 mg/min |
| Maximal PAH excretory capacity $T_{MPAH}$ | 80–90 mg/min | |
| Phenolsulfonphthalein excretion (P.S.P.) | 25% or more in 15 min | |
| | 40% or more in 30 min | |
| | 55% or more in 2 hr | |
| | After injection of 1 ml P.S.P. intravenously | |

# Thyroid Function Tests

| | |
|---|---|
| Protein bound iodine, serum (P.B.I.) | 3.5–8.0 µg/100 ml |
| Butanol extractable iodine, serum (B.E.I.) | 3.2–6.4 µg/100 ml |
| Thyroxine iodine, serum ($T_I$) | 2.9–6.4 µg/100 ml |
| Free thyroxine, serum | 1.4–2.5 ng/100 ml |
| $T_3$ (index of unsaturated T.B.G.) | 10.0–14.6% |
| Thyroxine-binding globulin, serum (T.B.G.) | 10–26 µg $T_4$/100 ml |
| Thyroid-stimulating hormone, serum (T.S.H.) | 0 up to 0.2 milliunit/ml |
| Radioactive iodine ($I^{131}$) uptake (R.A.I.) | 20–50% of administered dose in 24 hr |
| Radioactive iodine ($I^{131}$) excretion | 30–70% of administered dose in 24 hr |
| Radioactive iodine ($I^{131}$), protein bound | Less than 0.3% of administered dose per litre of plasma at 72 hr |
| Basal metabolic rate | Minus 10% to plus 10% of mean standard |

# Gastrointestinal Absorption Tests

| | |
|---|---|
| d-Xylose absorption test | After an 8-hr fast 10 ml/kg of body weight of a 5% solution of d-xylose is given by mouth. Nothing further by mouth is given until the test has been completed. All urine voided during the following 5 hr is pooled, and blood samples are taken at 0, 60, and 120 min. Normally 26% (range 16–33%) of ingested xylose is excreted within 5 hr, and the serum xylose reaches a level between 25 and 40 mg/100 ml after 1 hr and is maintained at this level for another 60 min. |
| Vitamin A absorption test | A fasting blood specimen is obtained and 200,000 units of vitamin A in oil is given by mouth. Serum vitamin A level should rise to twice fasting level in 3 to 5 hr. |

Abbreviations
| | | | | | | |
|---|---|---|---|---|---|---|
| kg | = kilogram | = 1000 g | | ml | = milliliter | = 0.001 litre |
| mg | = milligram | = 0.001 g | | mm | = millimeter | = 0.001 metre |
| μg | = microgram | = 0.000001 g | | μm | = micron | = 0.000001 metre |
| ng | = nanogram | = 0.000000001 g | | meq | = milliequivalent | |
| pg | = picogram | = 0.000000000001 g | | mOsm | = milliosmole | |

References

1. Castleman, B., and McNeely, B. U.: New Engl. J. Med. 283: 1276, 1970.
2. Davidsohn, I., and Henry, J. B.: Clinical Diagnosis by Laboratory Methods. 15th ed. Philadelphia: W. B. Saunders, 1974.
3. Department of Laboratory Medicine, Johns Hopkins Hospital: Clinical Laboratory Handbook, Baltimore, July 1, 1973.
4. Henry, R. J.: Clinical Chemistry—Principles and Techniques. New York: Harper & Row, 1964.
5. Long, C.: Biochemists' Handbook. Princeton: D. Van Nostrand, 1961.
6. Miale, J. B.: Laboratory Medicine—Hematology. 4th ed. St. Louis: C. V. Mosby, 1972.
7. Miller, S. E., and Weller, J. M.: Textbook of Clinical Pathology. 8th ed. Baltimore: Williams & Wilkins, 1971.
8. Stewart, C. P., and Stolman, A.: Toxicology, Mechanisms and Analytic Methods. New York: Academic, 1960.
9. Sunderman, F. W., and Boerner, F.: Normal Values in Clinical Medicine. Philadelphia: W. B. Saunders, 1949.
10. Tietz, N. W.: Fundamentals of Clinical Chemistry. Philadelphia: W. B. Saunders, 1970.
11. Wintrobe, M. M.: Clinical Hematology. 6th ed. Philadelphia: Lea & Febiger, 1967.

# Calculation of Desirable Body Weight

| Build | Women | Men | Children |
|---|---|---|---|
| Medium frame | Allow 100 lb for first 5 ft of height, plus 5 lb for each additional inch | Allow 106 lb for first 5 ft of height, plus 6 lb for each additional inch | Chart growth pattern on Wetzel, Iowa, or Stuart graph, preferably every 3–6 months |
| Small frame | Subtract 10% | Subtract 10% | |
| Large frame | Add 10% | Add 10% | |

*Source*:  Reprinted from Davidson, J. K.:  Postgrad. Med. 59: 114, 1976.

# Height–Weight Tables

**GIRLS: BIRTH TO 36 MONTHS**
**PHYSICAL GROWTH**
**NCHS PERCENTILES***

NAME _____ RECORD # _____

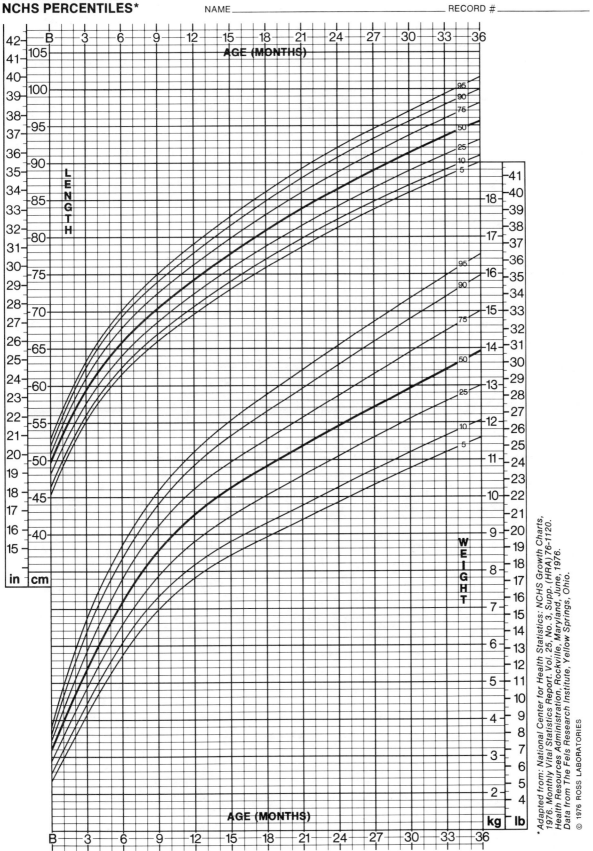

* Adapted from: National Center for Health Statistics: NCHS Growth Charts, 1976. Monthly Vital Statistics Report. Vol. 25, No. 3, Supp. (HRA) 76-1120. Health Resources Administration, Rockville, Maryland, June, 1976. Data from The Fels Research Institute, Yellow Springs, Ohio.

© 1976 ROSS LABORATORIES

# GIRLS: BIRTH TO 36 MONTHS
## PHYSICAL GROWTH
## NCHS PERCENTILES*

NAME _____ RECORD # _____

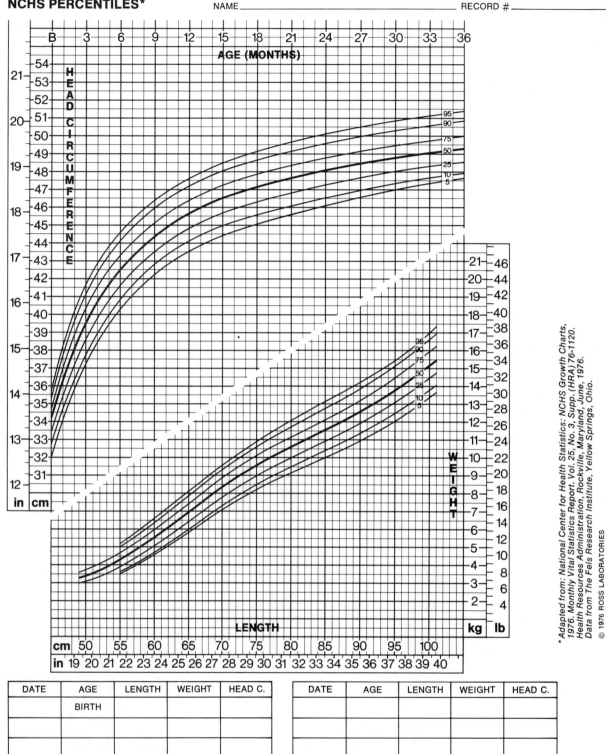

*Adapted from: National Center for Health Statistics: NCHS Growth Charts, 1976. Monthly Vital Statistics Report. Vol. 25, No. 3, Supp. (HRA) 76-1120. Health Resources Administration, Rockville, Maryland, June, 1976. Data from The Fels Research Institute, Yellow Springs, Ohio.

© 1976 ROSS LABORATORIES

| DATE | AGE | LENGTH | WEIGHT | HEAD C. |
|------|------|--------|--------|---------|
|      | BIRTH |        |        |         |
|      |      |        |        |         |
|      |      |        |        |         |
|      |      |        |        |         |
|      |      |        |        |         |

| DATE | AGE | LENGTH | WEIGHT | HEAD C. |
|------|------|--------|--------|---------|
|      |      |        |        |         |
|      |      |        |        |         |
|      |      |        |        |         |
|      |      |        |        |         |
|      |      |        |        |         |

**GIRLS: 2 TO 18 YEARS**
**PHYSICAL GROWTH**
**NCHS PERCENTILES***

NAME _____ RECORD # _____

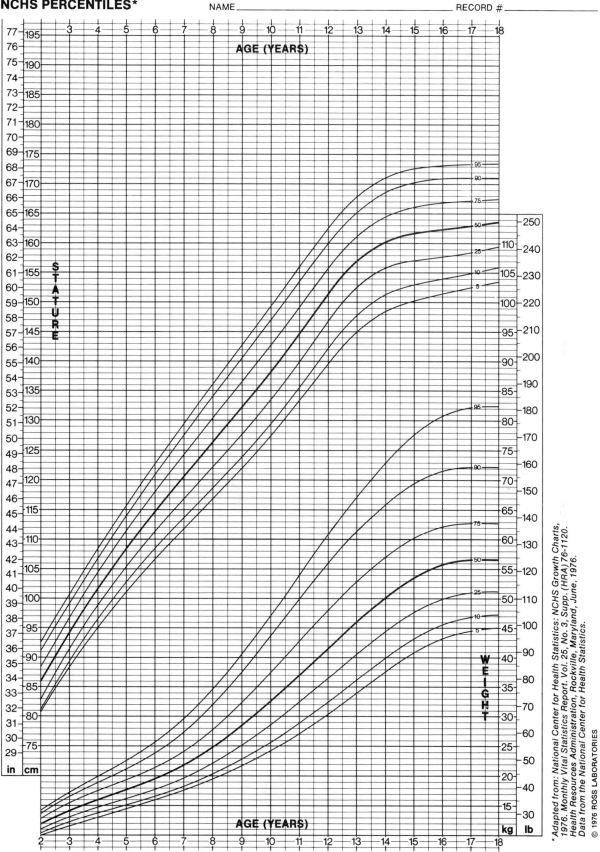

* Adapted from: National Center for Health Statistics: NCHS Growth Charts, 1976. Monthly Vital Statistics Report. Vol. 25, No. 3, Supp. (HRA)76-1120. Health Resources Administration, Rockville, Maryland, June, 1976. Data from the National Center for Health Statistics.

© 1976 ROSS LABORATORIES

# GIRLS: PREPUBESCENT
## PHYSICAL GROWTH
## NCHS PERCENTILES*

NAME _____    RECORD # _____

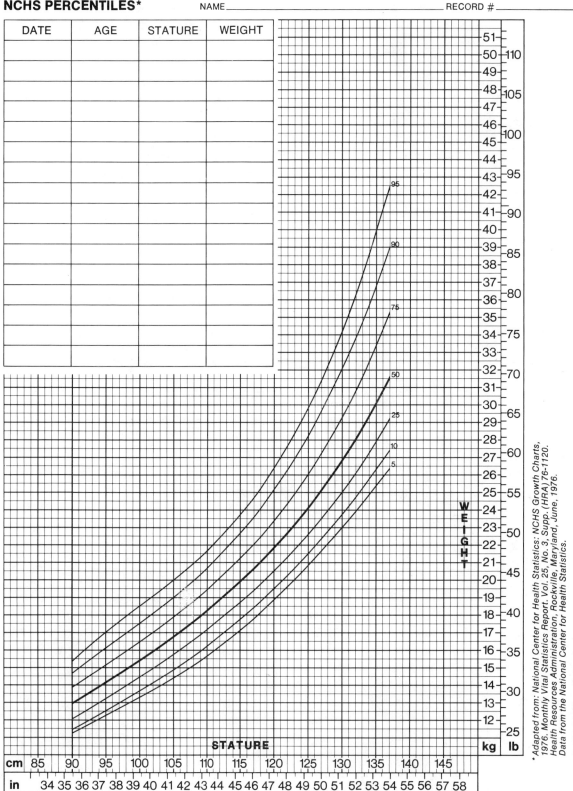

| DATE | AGE | STATURE | WEIGHT |
|------|-----|---------|--------|
|      |     |         |        |
|      |     |         |        |
|      |     |         |        |
|      |     |         |        |
|      |     |         |        |
|      |     |         |        |
|      |     |         |        |
|      |     |         |        |
|      |     |         |        |
|      |     |         |        |
|      |     |         |        |
|      |     |         |        |
|      |     |         |        |

* Adapted from: National Center for Health Statistics: NCHS Growth Charts,
1976. Monthly Vital Statistics Report. Vol. 25, No. 3, Supp. (HRA) 76-1120.
Health Resources Administration, Rockville, Maryland, June, 1976.
Data from the National Center for Health Statistics.

© 1976 ROSS LABORATORIES

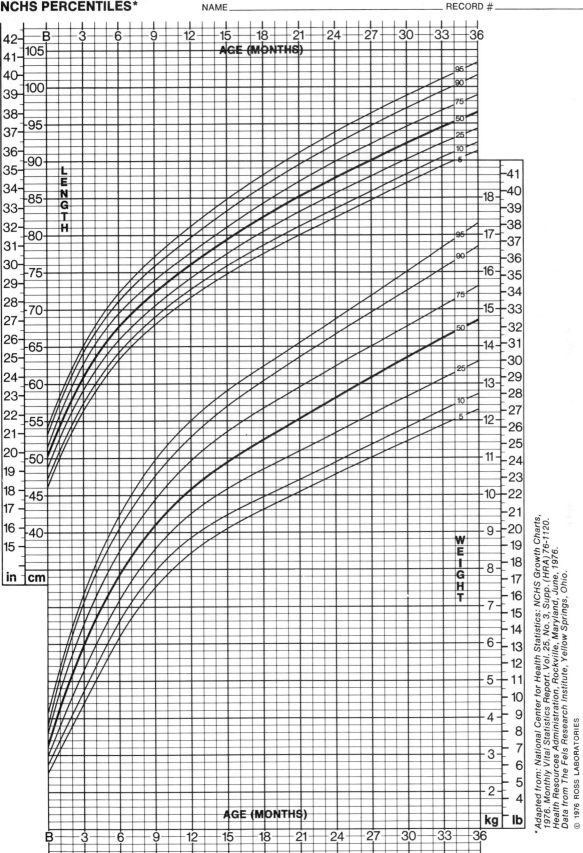

**BOYS: BIRTH TO 36 MONTHS**
**PHYSICAL GROWTH**
**NCHS PERCENTILES***

NAME _____ RECORD # _____

AGE (MONTHS)

LENGTH

AGE (MONTHS)

WEIGHT

* Adapted from: National Center for Health Statistics: NCHS Growth Charts, 1976. Monthly Vital Statistics Report. Vol. 25, No. 3, Supp. (HRA) 76-1120. Health Resources Administration, Rockville, Maryland, June, 1976. Data from The Fels Research Institute, Yellow Springs, Ohio.

© 1976 ROSS LABORATORIES

## BOYS: BIRTH TO 36 MONTHS
## PHYSICAL GROWTH
## NCHS PERCENTILES*

NAME _____     RECORD # _____

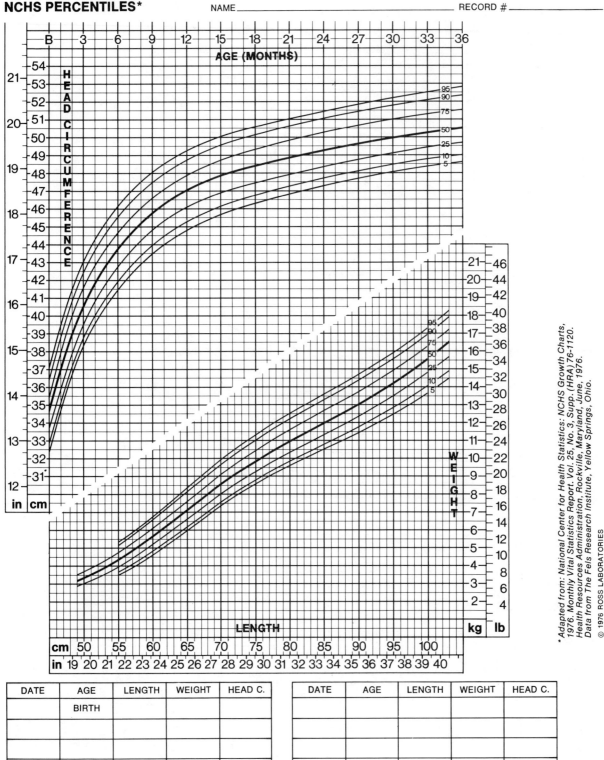

*Adapted from: National Center for Health Statistics: NCHS Growth Charts, 1976. Monthly Vital Statistics Report. Vol. 25, No. 3, Supp. (HRA) 76-1120. Health Resources Administration, Rockville, Maryland, June, 1976. Data from The Fels Research Institute, Yellow Springs, Ohio.

© 1976 ROSS LABORATORIES

| DATE | AGE | LENGTH | WEIGHT | HEAD C. |
|------|-----|--------|--------|---------|
|      | BIRTH |      |        |         |
|      |     |        |        |         |
|      |     |        |        |         |
|      |     |        |        |         |
|      |     |        |        |         |

| DATE | AGE | LENGTH | WEIGHT | HEAD C. |
|------|-----|--------|--------|---------|
|      |     |        |        |         |
|      |     |        |        |         |
|      |     |        |        |         |
|      |     |        |        |         |
|      |     |        |        |         |

**BOYS: 2 TO 18 YEARS**
**PHYSICAL GROWTH**
**NCHS PERCENTILES***

NAME _____ RECORD # _____

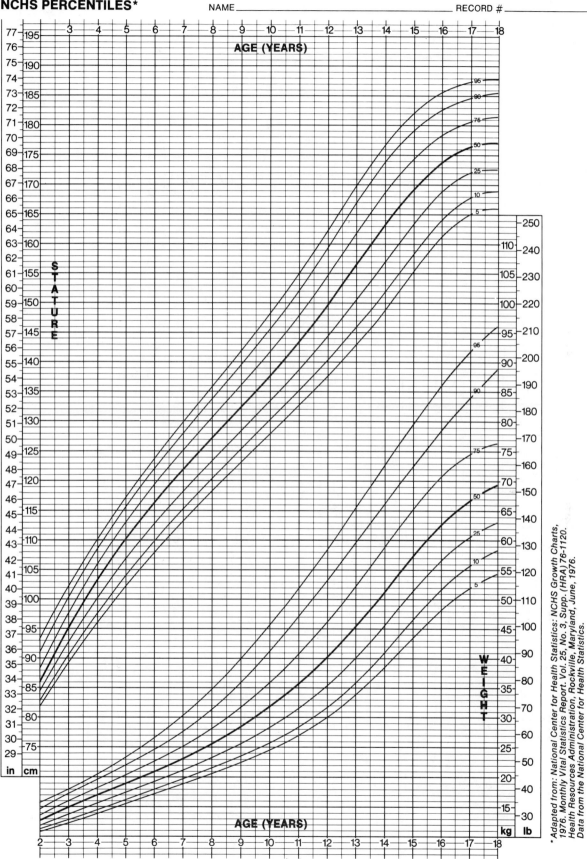

* Adapted from: National Center for Health Statistics: NCHS Growth Charts,
1976. Monthly Vital Statistics Report. Vol. 25, No. 3, Supp. (HRA) 76-1120.
Health Resources Administration, Rockville, Maryland, June, 1976.
Data from the National Center for Health Statistics.

© 1976 ROSS LABORATORIES

**BOYS: PREPUBESCENT**
**PHYSICAL GROWTH**
**NCHS PERCENTILES***

NAME_____ RECORD #_____

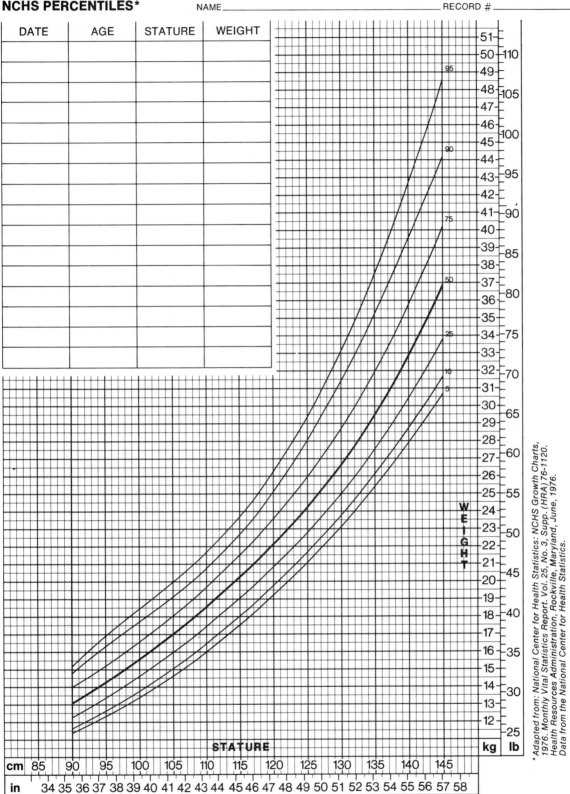

| DATE | AGE | STATURE | WEIGHT |
|------|-----|---------|--------|
|      |     |         |        |
|      |     |         |        |
|      |     |         |        |
|      |     |         |        |
|      |     |         |        |
|      |     |         |        |
|      |     |         |        |
|      |     |         |        |
|      |     |         |        |
|      |     |         |        |
|      |     |         |        |
|      |     |         |        |

* Adapted from: National Center for Health Statistics: NCHS Growth Charts, 1976. Monthly Vital Statistics Report. Vol. 25, No. 3, Supp. (HRA) 76-1120. Health Resources Administration, Rockville, Maryland, June, 1976. Data from the National Center for Health Statistics.

© 1976 ROSS LABORATORIES

# NCHS PERCENTILES*–LENGTH, WEIGHT AND HEAD CIRCUMFERENCE BOYS AND GIRLS: BIRTH TO 36 MONTHS

| AGE months | PERCENTILES, BOYS | | | | | | | MEASUREMENT | PERCENTILES, GIRLS | | | | | | |
|---|---|---|---|---|---|---|---|---|---|---|---|---|---|---|---|
| | 5th | 10th | 25th | 50th | 75th | 90th | 95th | | 5th | 10th | 25th | 50th | 75th | 90th | 95th |
| BIRTH | 46.4 / 18¼ | 47.5 / 18¾ | 49.0 / 19¼ | 50.5 / 20 | 51.8 / 20½ | 53.5 / 21 | 54.4 / 21½ | Length–cm / Length–in | 45.4 / 17¾ | 46.5 / 18¼ | 48.2 / 19 | 49.9 / 19¾ | 51.0 / 20 | 52.0 / 20½ | 52.9 / 20¾ |
| | 2.54 / 5½ | 2.78 / 6¼ | 3.00 / 6½ | 3.27 / 7¼ | 3.64 / 8 | 3.82 / 8½ | 4.15 / 9¼ | Weight–kg / Weight–lb | 2.36 / 5¼ | 2.58 / 5¾ | 2.93 / 6½ | 3.23 / 7 | 3.52 / 7¾ | 3.64 / 8 | 3.81 / 8½ |
| | 32.6 / 12¾ | 33.0 / 13 | 33.9 / 13¼ | 34.8 / 13¾ | 35.6 / 14 | 36.6 / 14½ | 37.2 / 14¾ | Head C–cm / Head C–in | 32.1 / 12¾ | 32.9 / 13 | 33.5 / 13¼ | 34.3 / 13½ | 34.8 / 13¾ | 35.5 / 14 | 35.9 / 14¼ |
| 1 | 50.4 / 19¾ | 51.3 / 20¼ | 53.0 / 20¾ | 54.6 / 21½ | 56.2 / 22¼ | 57.7 / 22¾ | 58.6 / 23 | Length–cm / Length–in | 49.2 / 19¼ | 50.2 / 19¾ | 51.9 / 20½ | 53.5 / 21 | 54.9 / 21½ | 56.1 / 22 | 56.9 / 22½ |
| | 3.16 / 7 | 3.43 / 7½ | 3.82 / 8½ | 4.29 / 9½ | 4.75 / 10½ | 5.14 / 11¼ | 5.38 / 11¾ | Weight–kg / Weight–lb | 2.97 / 6½ | 3.22 / 7 | 3.59 / 8 | 3.98 / 8¾ | 4.36 / 9½ | 4.65 / 10¼ | 4.92 / 10¾ |
| | 34.9 / 13¾ | 35.4 / 14 | 36.2 / 14¼ | 37.2 / 14¾ | 38.1 / 15 | 39.0 / 15¼ | 39.6 / 15½ | Head C–cm / Head C–in | 34.2 / 13½ | 34.8 / 13¾ | 35.6 / 14 | 36.4 / 14¼ | 37.1 / 14½ | 37.8 / 15 | 38.3 / 15 |
| 3 | 56.7 / 22¼ | 57.7 / 22¾ | 59.4 / 23½ | 61.1 / 24 | 63.0 / 24¾ | 64.5 / 25½ | 65.4 / 25¾ | Length–cm / Length–in | 55.4 / 21¾ | 56.2 / 22¼ | 57.8 / 22¾ | 59.5 / 23½ | 61.2 / 24 | 62.7 / 24¾ | 63.4 / 25 |
| | 4.43 / 9¾ | 4.78 / 10½ | 5.32 / 11¾ | 5.98 / 13¼ | 6.56 / 14½ | 7.14 / 15¾ | 7.37 / 16¼ | Weight–kg / Weight–lb | 4.18 / 9¼ | 4.47 / 9¾ | 4.88 / 10¾ | 5.40 / 12 | 5.90 / 13 | 6.39 / 14 | 6.74 / 14¾ |
| | 38.4 / 15 | 38.9 / 15¼ | 39.7 / 15¾ | 40.6 / 16 | 41.7 / 16½ | 42.5 / 16¾ | 43.1 / 17 | Head C–cm / Head C–in | 37.3 / 14¾ | 37.8 / 15 | 38.7 / 15¼ | 39.5 / 15½ | 40.4 / 16 | 41.2 / 16¼ | 41.7 / 16½ |
| 6 | 63.4 / 25 | 64.4 / 25¼ | 66.1 / 26 | 67.8 / 26¾ | 69.7 / 27½ | 71.3 / 28 | 72.3 / 28½ | Length–cm / Length–in | 61.8 / 24¼ | 62.6 / 24¾ | 64.2 / 25¼ | 65.9 / 26 | 67.8 / 26¾ | 69.4 / 27¼ | 70.2 / 27¾ |
| | 6.20 / 13¾ | 6.61 / 14½ | 7.20 / 15¾ | 7.85 / 17¼ | 8.49 / 18¾ | 9.10 / 20 | 9.46 / 20¾ | Weight–kg / Weight–lb | 5.79 / 12¾ | 6.12 / 13½ | 6.60 / 14½ | 7.21 / 16 | 7.83 / 17¼ | 8.38 / 18½ | 8.73 / 19¼ |
| | 41.5 / 16¼ | 42.0 / 16½ | 42.8 / 16¾ | 43.8 / 17¼ | 44.7 / 17½ | 45.6 / 18 | 46.2 / 18¼ | Head C–cm / Head C–in | 40.3 / 15¾ | 40.9 / 16 | 41.6 / 16½ | 42.4 / 16¾ | 43.3 / 17 | 44.1 / 17¼ | 44.6 / 17½ |
| 9 | 68.0 / 26¾ | 69.1 / 27¼ | 70.6 / 27¾ | 72.3 / 28½ | 74.0 / 29¼ | 75.9 / 30 | 77.1 / 30¼ | Length–cm / Length–in | 66.1 / 26 | 67.0 / 26½ | 68.7 / 27 | 70.4 / 27¾ | 72.4 / 28½ | 74.0 / 29¼ | 75.0 / 29½ |
| | 7.52 / 16½ | 7.95 / 17½ | 8.56 / 18¾ | 9.18 / 20¼ | 9.88 / 21¾ | 10.49 / 23¼ | 10.93 / 24 | Weight–kg / Weight–lb | 7.00 / 15½ | 7.34 / 16¼ | 7.89 / 17½ | 8.56 / 18¾ | 9.24 / 20¼ | 9.83 / 21¾ | 10.17 / 22½ |
| | 43.5 / 17¼ | 44.0 / 17¼ | 44.8 / 17¾ | 45.8 / 18 | 46.6 / 18¼ | 47.5 / 18¾ | 48.1 / 19 | Head C–cm / Head C–in | 42.3 / 16¾ | 42.8 / 16¾ | 43.5 / 17¼ | 44.3 / 17½ | 45.1 / 17¾ | 46.0 / 18 | 46.4 / 18¼ |
| 12 | 71.7 / 28¼ | 72.8 / 28¾ | 74.3 / 29¼ | 76.1 / 30 | 77.7 / 30½ | 79.8 / 31½ | 81.2 / 32 | Length–cm / Length–in | 69.8 / 27½ | 70.8 / 27¾ | 72.4 / 28½ | 74.3 / 29¼ | 76.3 / 30 | 78.0 / 30¾ | 79.1 / 31¼ |
| | 8.43 / 18½ | 8.84 / 19½ | 9.49 / 21 | 10.15 / 22½ | 10.91 / 24 | 11.54 / 25½ | 11.99 / 26½ | Weight–kg / Weight–lb | 7.84 / 17¼ | 8.19 / 18 | 8.81 / 19½ | 9.53 / 21 | 10.23 / 22½ | 10.87 / 24 | 11.24 / 24¾ |
| | 44.8 / 17¾ | 45.3 / 17¾ | 46.1 / 18¼ | 47.0 / 18½ | 47.9 / 18¾ | 48.8 / 19¼ | 49.3 / 19½ | Head C–cm / Head C–in | 43.5 / 17¼ | 44.1 / 17¼ | 44.8 / 17¾ | 45.6 / 18 | 46.4 / 18¼ | 47.2 / 18½ | 47.6 / 18¾ |
| 18 | 77.5 / 30½ | 78.7 / 31 | 80.5 / 31¾ | 82.4 / 32½ | 84.3 / 33¼ | 86.6 / 34 | 88.1 / 34¾ | Length–cm / Length–in | 76.0 / 30 | 77.2 / 30½ | 78.8 / 31 | 80.9 / 31¾ | 83.0 / 32¾ | 85.0 / 33½ | 86.1 / 34 |
| | 9.59 / 21¼ | 9.92 / 21¾ | 10.67 / 23½ | 11.47 / 25¼ | 12.31 / 27¼ | 13.05 / 28¾ | 13.44 / 29½ | Weight–kg / Weight–lb | 8.92 / 19¾ | 9.30 / 20½ | 10.04 / 22¼ | 10.82 / 23¾ | 11.55 / 25½ | 12.30 / 27 | 12.76 / 28¼ |
| | 46.3 / 18¼ | 46.7 / 18½ | 47.4 / 18¾ | 48.4 / 19 | 49.3 / 19½ | 50.1 / 19¾ | 50.6 / 20 | Head C–cm / Head C–in | 45.0 / 17¾ | 45.6 / 18 | 46.3 / 18¼ | 47.1 / 18½ | 47.9 / 18¾ | 48.6 / 19¼ | 49.1 / 19¼ |
| 24 | 82.3 / 32½ | 83.5 / 32¾ | 85.6 / 33¾ | 87.6 / 34½ | 89.9 / 35½ | 92.2 / 36¼ | 93.8 / 37 | Length–cm / Length–in | 81.3 / 32 | 82.5 / 32½ | 84.2 / 33¼ | 86.5 / 34 | 88.7 / 35 | 90.8 / 35¾ | 92.0 / 36¼ |
| | 10.54 / 23¼ | 10.85 / 24 | 11.65 / 25¾ | 12.59 / 27¾ | 13.44 / 29¾ | 14.29 / 31½ | 14.70 / 32½ | Weight–kg / Weight–lb | 9.87 / 21¾ | 10.26 / 22½ | 11.10 / 24½ | 11.90 / 26¼ | 12.74 / 28 | 13.57 / 30 | 14.08 / 31 |
| | 47.3 / 18½ | 47.7 / 18¾ | 48.3 / 19 | 49.2 / 19¼ | 50.2 / 19¾ | 51.0 / 20 | 51.4 / 20¼ | Head C–cm / Head C–in | 46.1 / 18¼ | 46.5 / 18¼ | 47.3 / 18½ | 48.1 / 19 | 48.8 / 19¼ | 49.6 / 19½ | 50.1 / 19¾ |
| 30 | 87.0 / 34¼ | 88.2 / 34¾ | 90.1 / 35½ | 92.3 / 36¼ | 94.6 / 37¼ | 97.0 / 38¼ | 98.7 / 38¾ | Length–cm / Length–in | 86.0 / 33¾ | 87.0 / 34¼ | 88.9 / 35 | 91.3 / 36 | 93.7 / 37 | 95.6 / 37¾ | 96.9 / 38¼ |
| | 11.44 / 25¼ | 11.80 / 26 | 12.63 / 27¾ | 13.67 / 30¼ | 14.51 / 32 | 15.47 / 34 | 15.97 / 35¼ | Weight–kg / Weight–lb | 10.78 / 23¾ | 11.21 / 24¾ | 12.11 / 26¾ | 12.93 / 28½ | 13.93 / 30¾ | 14.81 / 32¾ | 15.35 / 33¾ |
| | 48.0 / 19 | 48.4 / 19 | 49.1 / 19¼ | 49.9 / 19¾ | 51.0 / 20 | 51.7 / 20¼ | 52.2 / 20½ | Head C–cm / Head C–in | 47.0 / 18½ | 47.3 / 18½ | 48.0 / 19 | 48.8 / 19¼ | 49.4 / 19½ | 50.3 / 19¾ | 50.8 / 20 |
| 36 | 91.2 / 36 | 92.4 / 36½ | 94.2 / 37 | 96.5 / 38 | 98.9 / 39 | 101.4 / 40 | 103.1 / 40½ | Length–cm / Length–in | 90.0 / 35½ | 91.0 / 35¾ | 93.1 / 36¾ | 95.6 / 37¾ | 98.1 / 38½ | 100.0 / 39¼ | 101.5 / 40 |
| | 12.26 / 27 | 12.69 / 28 | 13.58 / 30 | 14.69 / 32½ | 15.59 / 34¼ | 16.66 / 36¾ | 17.28 / 38 | Weight–kg / Weight–lb | 11.60 / 25½ | 12.07 / 26½ | 12.99 / 28¾ | 13.93 / 30¾ | 15.03 / 33¼ | 15.97 / 35¼ | 16.54 / 36½ |
| | 48.6 / 19¼ | 49.0 / 19¼ | 49.7 / 19½ | 50.5 / 20 | 51.5 / 20¼ | 52.3 / 20½ | 52.8 / 20¾ | Head C–cm / Head C–in | 47.6 / 18¾ | 47.9 / 18¾ | 48.5 / 19 | 49.3 / 19½ | 50.0 / 19¾ | 50.8 / 20 | 51.4 / 20¼ |

*National Center for Health Statistics, Health Resources Administration, DHEW, Hyattsville, Maryland 20782. Data from The Fels Research Institute, Yellow Springs, Ohio; smoothed by least-squares-cubic-spline technique.

Values correspond with NCHS percentile curves displayed in Ross NCHS Percentile Growth Charts. Conversion of metric data to inches and pounds by Ross Laboratories.

© 1977 ROSS LABORATORIES

# NCHS PERCENTILES*–WEIGHT FOR LENGTH
# BOYS AND GIRLS: LESS THAN 4 YEARS

| RECUMBENT LENGTH | WEIGHT PERCENTILES, BOYS—kg and lb | | | | | | | WEIGHT PERCENTILES, GIRLS—kg and lb | | | | | | |
|---|---|---|---|---|---|---|---|---|---|---|---|---|---|---|
| | 5th | 10th | 25th | 50th | 75th | 90th | 95th | 5th | 10th | 25th | 50th | 75th | 90th | 95th |
| **48 - 50 cm**<br>19 - 19¾ in | | | **2.86**<br>6¼ | **3.15**<br>7 | **3.50**<br>7¾ | | | | | **3.02**<br>6¾ | **3.29**<br>7¼ | **3.59**<br>8 | | |
| **50 - 52 cm**<br>19¾ - 20½ in | | | **3.16**<br>7 | **3.48**<br>7¾ | **3.86**<br>8½ | | | | | **3.25**<br>7¼ | **3.55**<br>7¾ | **3.89**<br>8½ | | |
| **52 - 54 cm**<br>20½ - 21¼ in | | | **3.52**<br>7¾ | **3.88**<br>8½ | **4.28**<br>9½ | | | | | **3.56**<br>7¾ | **3.89**<br>8½ | **4.26**<br>9½ | | |
| **54 - 56 cm**<br>21¼ - 22 in | **3.49**<br>7¾ | **3.65**<br>8 | **3.95**<br>8¾ | **4.34**<br>9½ | **4.76**<br>10½ | **5.13**<br>11¼ | **5.33**<br>11¾ | **3.54**<br>7¾ | **3.64**<br>8 | **3.93**<br>8¾ | **4.29**<br>9½ | **4.70**<br>10¼ | **5.02**<br>11 | **5.21**<br>11½ |
| **56 - 58 cm**<br>22 - 22¾ in | **3.90**<br>8½ | **4.09**<br>9 | **4.43**<br>9¾ | **4.84**<br>10¾ | **5.29**<br>11¾ | **5.69**<br>12½ | **5.88**<br>13 | **3.93**<br>8¾ | **4.05**<br>9 | **4.37**<br>9¾ | **4.76**<br>10½ | **5.20**<br>11½ | **5.55**<br>12¼ | **5.77**<br>12¾ |
| **58 - 60 cm**<br>22¾ - 23½ in | **4.37**<br>9¾ | **4.58**<br>10 | **4.94**<br>11 | **5.38**<br>11¾ | **5.84**<br>12¾ | **6.28**<br>13¾ | **6.47**<br>14¼ | **4.38**<br>9¾ | **4.50**<br>10 | **4.85**<br>10¾ | **5.27**<br>11½ | **5.73**<br>12¾ | **6.12**<br>13½ | **6.36**<br>14 |
| **60 - 62 cm**<br>23½ - 24½ in | **4.88**<br>10¾ | **5.10**<br>11¼ | **5.49**<br>12 | **5.94**<br>13 | **6.42**<br>14¼ | **6.88**<br>15¼ | **7.08**<br>15½ | **4.85**<br>10¾ | **4.99**<br>11 | **5.37**<br>11¾ | **5.82**<br>12¾ | **6.30**<br>14 | **6.70**<br>14¾ | **6.95**<br>15¼ |
| **62 - 64 cm**<br>24½ - 25¼ in | **5.43**<br>12 | **5.65**<br>12½ | **6.05**<br>13¼ | **6.52**<br>14¼ | **7.02**<br>15½ | **7.50**<br>16½ | **7.72**<br>17 | **5.35**<br>11¾ | **5.50**<br>12 | **5.91**<br>13 | **6.39**<br>14 | **6.89**<br>15¼ | **7.30**<br>16 | **7.55**<br>16¾ |
| **64 - 66 cm**<br>25¼ - 26 in | **5.99**<br>13¼ | **6.20**<br>13¾ | **6.62**<br>14½ | **7.11**<br>15¾ | **7.63**<br>16¾ | **8.13**<br>18 | **8.36**<br>18½ | **5.87**<br>13 | **6.03**<br>13¼ | **6.47**<br>14¼ | **6.97**<br>15¼ | **7.48**<br>16½ | **7.90**<br>17½ | **8.15**<br>18 |
| **66 - 68 cm**<br>26 - 26¾ in | **6.55**<br>14½ | **6.76**<br>15 | **7.19**<br>15¾ | **7.70**<br>17 | **8.23**<br>18¼ | **8.75**<br>19¼ | **8.99**<br>19¾ | **6.38**<br>14 | **6.56**<br>14½ | **7.02**<br>15½ | **7.55**<br>16¾ | **8.07**<br>17¾ | **8.50**<br>18¾ | **8.75**<br>19¼ |
| **68 - 70 cm**<br>26¾ - 27½ in | **7.10**<br>15¾ | **7.31**<br>16 | **7.75**<br>17 | **8.27**<br>18¼ | **8.82**<br>19½ | **9.35**<br>20½ | **9.62**<br>21¼ | **6.89**<br>15¼ | **7.08**<br>15½ | **7.56**<br>16¾ | **8.11**<br>17¾ | **8.64**<br>19 | **9.08**<br>20 | **9.33**<br>20½ |
| **70 - 72 cm**<br>27½ - 28¼ in | **7.63**<br>16¾ | **7.84**<br>17¼ | **8.28**<br>18¼ | **8.82**<br>19½ | **9.39**<br>20¾ | **9.93**<br>22 | **10.21**<br>22½ | **7.37**<br>16¼ | **7.58**<br>16¾ | **8.08**<br>17¾ | **8.64**<br>19 | **9.18**<br>20¼ | **9.63**<br>21¼ | **9.88**<br>21¾ |
| **72 - 74 cm**<br>28¼ - 29¼ in | **8.13**<br>18 | **8.33**<br>18¼ | **8.78**<br>19¼ | **9.33**<br>20½ | **9.92**<br>21¾ | **10.48**<br>23 | **10.77**<br>23¾ | **7.82**<br>17¼ | **8.05**<br>17¾ | **8.56**<br>18¾ | **9.14**<br>20¼ | **9.68**<br>21¼ | **10.15**<br>22½ | **10.41**<br>23 |
| **74 - 76 cm**<br>29¼ - 30 in | **8.58**<br>19 | **8.78**<br>19¼ | **9.24**<br>20¼ | **9.81**<br>21¾ | **10.43**<br>23 | **10.99**<br>24¼ | **11.29**<br>25 | **8.24**<br>18¼ | **8.49**<br>18¾ | **9.00**<br>19¾ | **9.59**<br>21¼ | **10.14**<br>22¼ | **10.63**<br>23½ | **10.91**<br>24 |
| **76 - 78 cm**<br>30 - 30¾ in | **9.00**<br>19¾ | **9.21**<br>20¼ | **9.68**<br>21¼ | **10.27**<br>22¾ | **10.91**<br>24 | **11.48**<br>25¼ | **11.78**<br>26 | **8.62**<br>19 | **8.90**<br>19½ | **9.42**<br>20¾ | **10.02**<br>22 | **10.57**<br>23¼ | **11.08**<br>24½ | **11.39**<br>25 |
| **78 - 80 cm**<br>30¾ - 31½ in | **9.40**<br>20¾ | **9.62**<br>21¼ | **10.09**<br>22¼ | **10.70**<br>23½ | **11.36**<br>25 | **11.94**<br>26¼ | **12.25**<br>27 | **8.99**<br>19¾ | **9.29**<br>20½ | **9.81**<br>21¾ | **10.41**<br>23 | **10.97**<br>24¼ | **11.51**<br>25¼ | **11.85**<br>26 |
| **80 - 82 cm**<br>31½ - 32¼ in | **9.77**<br>21½ | **10.01**<br>22 | **10.49**<br>23¼ | **11.12**<br>24½ | **11.80**<br>26 | **12.39**<br>27¼ | **12.69**<br>28 | **9.34**<br>20½ | **9.67**<br>21¼ | **10.19**<br>22½ | **10.80**<br>23¾ | **11.37**<br>25 | **11.93**<br>26¼ | **12.29**<br>27 |
| **82 - 84 cm**<br>32¼ - 33 in | **10.14**<br>22¼ | **10.39**<br>23 | **10.88**<br>24 | **11.53**<br>25½ | **12.23**<br>27 | **12.83**<br>28¼ | **13.13**<br>29 | **9.68**<br>21¼ | **10.04**<br>22¼ | **10.57**<br>23¼ | **11.18**<br>24¾ | **11.75**<br>26 | **12.35**<br>27¼ | **12.72**<br>28 |
| **84 - 86 cm**<br>33 - 33¾ in | **10.49**<br>23¼ | **10.76**<br>23¾ | **11.27**<br>24¾ | **11.93**<br>26¼ | **12.65**<br>28 | **13.26**<br>29¼ | **13.56**<br>30 | **10.03**<br>22 | **10.41**<br>23 | **10.94**<br>24 | **11.56**<br>25½ | **12.15**<br>26¾ | **12.76**<br>28¼ | **13.15**<br>29 |
| **86 - 88 cm**<br>33¾ - 34¾ in | **10.85**<br>24 | **11.14**<br>24½ | **11.67**<br>25¾ | **12.34**<br>27¼ | **13.07**<br>28¾ | **13.69**<br>30¼ | **14.00**<br>30¾ | **10.39**<br>23 | **10.78**<br>23¾ | **11.33**<br>25 | **11.95**<br>26¼ | **12.55**<br>27¾ | **13.19**<br>29 | **13.57**<br>30 |
| **88 - 90 cm**<br>34¾ - 35½ in | **11.22**<br>24¾ | **11.53**<br>25½ | **12.08**<br>26¾ | **12.76**<br>28¼ | **13.50**<br>29¾ | **14.13**<br>31¼ | **14.44**<br>31¾ | **10.76**<br>23¾ | **11.17**<br>24½ | **11.74**<br>26 | **12.36**<br>27¼ | **12.98**<br>28½ | **13.63**<br>30 | **14.01**<br>31 |
| **90 - 92 cm**<br>35½ - 36¼ in | **11.60**<br>25½ | **11.94**<br>26¼ | **12.52**<br>27½ | **13.20**<br>29 | **13.94**<br>30¾ | **14.58**<br>32¼ | **14.90**<br>32¾ | **11.16**<br>24½ | **11.58**<br>25½ | **12.17**<br>26¾ | **12.80**<br>28¼ | **13.45**<br>29¾ | **14.10**<br>31 | **14.45**<br>31¾ |
| **92 - 94 cm**<br>36¼ - 37 in | **12.00**<br>26½ | **12.37**<br>27¼ | **12.97**<br>28½ | **13.65**<br>30 | **14.40**<br>31¾ | **15.05**<br>33¼ | **15.39**<br>34 | **11.59**<br>25½ | **12.02**<br>26½ | **12.63**<br>27¾ | **13.27**<br>29¼ | **13.95**<br>30¾ | **14.61**<br>32¼ | **14.92**<br>33 |
| **94 - 96 cm**<br>37 - 37¾ in | **12.42**<br>27½ | **12.81**<br>28¼ | **13.45**<br>29¾ | **14.14**<br>31¼ | **14.88**<br>32¾ | **15.54**<br>34¼ | **15.90**<br>35 | **12.05**<br>26½ | **12.48**<br>27½ | **13.12**<br>29 | **13.77**<br>30¼ | **14.48**<br>32 | **15.14**<br>33½ | **15.42**<br>34 |
| **96 - 98 cm**<br>37¾ - 38½ in | **12.88**<br>28½ | **13.28**<br>29¼ | **13.96**<br>30¾ | **14.66**<br>32¼ | **15.39**<br>34 | **16.06**<br>35½ | **16.43**<br>36¼ | **12.55**<br>27¾ | **12.98**<br>28½ | **13.64**<br>30 | **14.31**<br>31½ | **15.04**<br>33¼ | **15.71**<br>34¾ | **15.99**<br>35¼ |
| **98 - 100 cm**<br>38½ - 39¼ in | **13.37**<br>29½ | **13.78**<br>30½ | **14.50**<br>32 | **15.21**<br>33½ | **15.94**<br>35¼ | **16.62**<br>36¾ | **17.00**<br>37½ | **13.10**<br>29 | **13.51**<br>29¾ | **14.19**<br>31¼ | **14.87**<br>32¾ | **15.63**<br>34½ | **16.32**<br>36 | **16.64**<br>36¾ |
| **100 - 102 cm**<br>39¼ - 40¼ in | **13.90**<br>30¾ | **14.30**<br>31½ | **15.06**<br>33¼ | **15.81**<br>34¾ | **16.54**<br>36½ | **17.22**<br>38 | **17.60**<br>38¾ | **13.68**<br>30¼ | **14.08**<br>31 | **14.77**<br>32½ | **15.46**<br>34 | **16.25**<br>35¾ | **16.96**<br>37½ | **17.39**<br>38¼ |
| **102 - 104 cm**<br>40¼ - 41 in | **14.48**<br>32 | **14.85**<br>32¾ | **15.65**<br>34½ | **16.45**<br>36¼ | **17.18**<br>37¾ | **17.87**<br>39½ | **18.24**<br>40¼ | | | | | | | |

*National Center for Health Statistics, Health Resources Administration, DHEW, Hyattsville, Maryland 20782. Data from The Fels Research Institute, Yellow Springs, Ohio; smoothed by least-squares-cubic-spline technique.

Values correspond with NCHS percentile curves displayed in Ross NCHS Percentile Growth Charts. Conversion of metric data to inches and pounds by Ross Laboratories.

# NCHS PERCENTILES*–WEIGHT FOR STATURE
# BOYS AND GIRLS: PREPUBESCENCE

| STATURE | WEIGHT PERCENTILES, BOYS—kg and lb | | | | | | | WEIGHT PERCENTILES, GIRLS—kg and lb | | | | | | |
|---|---|---|---|---|---|---|---|---|---|---|---|---|---|---|
| | 5th | 10th | 25th | 50th | 75th | 90th | 95th | 5th | 10th | 25th | 50th | 75th | 90th | 95th |
| **90-92 cm**<br>35½-36¼ in | **11.70**<br>25¾ | **11.97**<br>26½ | **12.59**<br>27¾ | **13.41**<br>29½ | **14.35**<br>31¾ | **15.25**<br>33½ | **15.72**<br>34¾ | **11.45**<br>25¼ | **11.67**<br>25¾ | **12.28**<br>27 | **13.14**<br>29 | **14.11**<br>31 | **14.98**<br>33 | **15.74**<br>34¾ |
| **92-94 cm**<br>36¼-37 in | **12.07**<br>26½ | **12.36**<br>27¼ | **13.03**<br>28¾ | **13.89**<br>30½ | **14.84**<br>32¾ | **15.87**<br>35 | **16.41**<br>36¼ | **11.86**<br>26¼ | **12.10**<br>26¾ | **12.74**<br>28 | **13.63**<br>30 | **14.63**<br>32¼ | **15.57**<br>34¼ | **16.42**<br>36¼ |
| **94-96 cm**<br>37-37¾ in | **12.46**<br>27½ | **12.77**<br>28¼ | **13.49**<br>29¾ | **14.38**<br>31¾ | **15.34**<br>33¾ | **16.45**<br>36¼ | **17.06**<br>37½ | **12.26**<br>27 | **12.53**<br>27½ | **13.21**<br>29 | **14.12**<br>31¼ | **15.14**<br>33½ | **16.13**<br>35½ | **17.05**<br>37½ |
| **96-98 cm**<br>37¾-38½ in | **12.87**<br>28¼ | **13.21**<br>29 | **13.98**<br>30¾ | **14.89**<br>32¾ | **15.87**<br>35 | **17.01**<br>37½ | **17.69**<br>39 | **12.66**<br>28 | **12.97**<br>28½ | **13.70**<br>30¼ | **14.62**<br>32¼ | **15.66**<br>34½ | **16.69**<br>36¾ | **17.65**<br>39 |
| **98-100 cm**<br>38½-39¼ in | **13.31**<br>29¼ | **13.67**<br>30¼ | **14.48**<br>32 | **15.43**<br>34 | **16.41**<br>36¼ | **17.56**<br>38¾ | **18.29**<br>40¼ | **13.06**<br>28¾ | **13.42**<br>29½ | **14.19**<br>31¼ | **15.13**<br>33¼ | **16.19**<br>35¾ | **17.24**<br>38 | **18.23**<br>40¼ |
| **100-102 cm**<br>39¼-40¼ in | **13.77**<br>30¼ | **14.15**<br>31¼ | **15.00**<br>33 | **15.98**<br>35¼ | **16.98**<br>37½ | **18.11**<br>40 | **18.89**<br>41¾ | **13.48**<br>29¾ | **13.88**<br>30½ | **14.69**<br>32½ | **15.65**<br>34½ | **16.73**<br>37 | **17.80**<br>39¼ | **18.80**<br>41½ |
| **102-104 cm**<br>40¼-41 in | **14.25**<br>31½ | **14.65**<br>32¼ | **15.54**<br>34¼ | **16.55**<br>36½ | **17.57**<br>38¾ | **18.67**<br>41¼ | **19.50**<br>43 | **13.91**<br>30¾ | **14.36**<br>31¾ | **15.21**<br>33½ | **16.20**<br>35¾ | **17.28**<br>38 | **18.38**<br>40½ | **19.38**<br>42¾ |
| **104-106 cm**<br>41-41¾ in | **14.76**<br>32½ | **15.18**<br>33½ | **16.10**<br>35½ | **17.13**<br>37¾ | **18.18**<br>40 | **19.25**<br>42½ | **20.12**<br>44¼ | **14.36**<br>31¾ | **14.85**<br>32¾ | **15.75**<br>34¾ | **16.75**<br>37 | **17.86**<br>39¼ | **18.98**<br>41¾ | **19.98**<br>44 |
| **106-108 cm**<br>**41¾-42½ in** | **15.30**<br>33¾ | **15.73**<br>34¾ | **16.68**<br>36¾ | **17.74**<br>39 | **18.82**<br>41½ | **19.86**<br>43¾ | **20.76**<br>45¾ | **14.84**<br>32¾ | **15.37**<br>34 | **16.30**<br>36 | **17.33**<br>38¼ | **18.46**<br>40¾ | **19.62**<br>43¼ | **20.61**<br>45½ |
| **108-110 cm**<br>42½-43¼ in | **15.85**<br>35 | **16.31**<br>36 | **17.28**<br>38 | **18.37**<br>40½ | **19.49**<br>43 | **20.51**<br>45¼ | **21.45**<br>47¼ | **15.35**<br>33¾ | **15.91**<br>35 | **16.87**<br>37¼ | **17.94**<br>39½ | **19.09**<br>42 | **20.30**<br>44¾ | **21.29**<br>47 |
| **110-112 cm**<br>43¼-44 in | **16.43**<br>36¼ | **16.91**<br>37¼ | **17.90**<br>39½ | **19.02**<br>42 | **20.18**<br>44½ | **21.22**<br>46¾ | **22.18**<br>49 | **15.90**<br>35 | **16.48**<br>36¼ | **17.47**<br>38½ | **18.56**<br>41 | **19.76**<br>43½ | **21.03**<br>46¼ | **22.03**<br>48½ |
| **112-114 cm**<br>44-45 in | **17.04**<br>37½ | **17.53**<br>38¾ | **18.54**<br>40¾ | **19.70**<br>43½ | **20.91**<br>46 | **21.98**<br>48½ | **22.98**<br>50¾ | **16.48**<br>36¼ | **17.09**<br>37¾ | **18.08**<br>39¾ | **19.22**<br>42¼ | **20.47**<br>45¼ | **21.81**<br>48 | **22.84**<br>50¼ |
| **114-116 cm**<br>45-45¾ in | **17.66**<br>39 | **18.18**<br>40 | **19.20**<br>42¼ | **20.39**<br>45 | **21.66**<br>47¾ | **22.82**<br>50¼ | **23.85**<br>52½ | **17.11**<br>37¾ | **17.72**<br>39 | **18.72**<br>41¼ | **19.91**<br>44 | **21.23**<br>46¾ | **22.67**<br>50 | **23.73**<br>52¼ |
| **116-118 cm**<br>45¾-46½ in | **18.32**<br>40½ | **18.85**<br>41½ | **19.89**<br>43¾ | **21.11**<br>46½ | **22.45**<br>49½ | **23.73**<br>52¼ | **24.80**<br>54¾ | **17.77**<br>39¼ | **18.40**<br>40½ | **19.40**<br>42¾ | **20.64**<br>45½ | **22.04**<br>48½ | **23.60**<br>52 | **24.71**<br>54½ |
| **118-120 cm**<br>46½-47¼ in | **18.99**<br>41¾ | **19.55**<br>43 | **20.60**<br>45½ | **21.85**<br>48¼ | **23.28**<br>51¼ | **24.73**<br>54½ | **25.83**<br>57 | **18.48**<br>40¾ | **19.11**<br>42¼ | **20.11**<br>44¼ | **21.42**<br>47¼ | **22.92**<br>50½ | **24.62**<br>54¼ | **25.81**<br>57 |
| **120-122 cm**<br>47¼-48 in | **19.70**<br>43½ | **20.28**<br>44¾ | **21.34**<br>47 | **22.63**<br>50 | **24.15**<br>53¼ | **25.80**<br>57 | **26.96**<br>59½ | **19.22**<br>42¼ | **19.85**<br>43¾ | **20.87**<br>46 | **22.25**<br>49 | **23.88**<br>52¾ | **25.73**<br>56¾ | **27.03**<br>59½ |
| **122-124 cm**<br>48-48¾ in | **20.43**<br>45 | **21.03**<br>46¼ | **22.11**<br>48¾ | **23.45**<br>51¾ | **25.07**<br>55¼ | **26.96**<br>59½ | **28.18**<br>62¼ | **19.99**<br>44 | **20.64**<br>45½ | **21.68**<br>47¾ | **23.13**<br>51 | **24.91**<br>55 | **26.95**<br>59½ | **28.37**<br>62½ |
| **124-126 cm**<br>48¾-49½ in | **21.20**<br>46¾ | **21.82**<br>48 | **22.92**<br>50½ | **24.32**<br>53½ | **26.05**<br>57½ | **28.18**<br>62¼ | **29.50**<br>65 | **20.80**<br>45¾ | **21.47**<br>47¼ | **22.54**<br>49¾ | **24.09**<br>53 | **26.05**<br>57½ | **28.27**<br>62¼ | **29.87**<br>65¾ |
| **126-128 cm**<br>49½-50½ in | **21.99**<br>48½ | **22.64**<br>50 | **23.77**<br>52½ | **25.24**<br>55¾ | **27.10**<br>59¾ | **29.48**<br>65 | **30.92**<br>68¼ | **21.65**<br>47¾ | **22.34**<br>49¼ | **23.47**<br>51¾ | **25.11**<br>55¼ | **27.28**<br>60¼ | **29.71**<br>65½ | **31.51**<br>69½ |
| **128-130 cm**<br>50½-51¼ in | **22.82**<br>50¼ | **23.50**<br>51¾ | **24.67**<br>54½ | **26.22**<br>57¾ | **28.21**<br>62¼ | **30.86**<br>68 | **32.44**<br>71½ | **22.53**<br>49¾ | **23.25**<br>51¼ | **24.46**<br>54 | **26.22**<br>57¾ | **28.63**<br>63 | **31.28**<br>69 | **33.33**<br>73½ |
| **130-132 cm**<br>51¼-52 in | **23.69**<br>52¼ | **24.39**<br>53¾ | **25.62**<br>56½ | **27.26**<br>60 | **29.41**<br>64¾ | **32.31**<br>71¼ | **34.07**<br>75 | **23.44**<br>51¾ | **24.22**<br>53½ | **25.52**<br>56¼ | **27.40**<br>60½ | **30.09**<br>66¼ | **32.99**<br>72¾ | **35.33**<br>78 |
| **132-134 cm**<br>52-52¾ in | **24.59**<br>54¼ | **25.32**<br>55¾ | **26.62**<br>58¾ | **28.38**<br>62½ | **30.68**<br>67¾ | **33.82**<br>74½ | **35.81**<br>79 | **24.38**<br>53¾ | **25.22**<br>55½ | **26.66**<br>58¾ | **28.68**<br>63¼ | **31.68**<br>69¾ | **34.84**<br>76¾ | **37.53**<br>82¾ |
| **134-136 cm**<br>52¾-53½ in | **25.53**<br>56¼ | **26.30**<br>58 | **27.68**<br>61 | **29.58**<br>65¼ | **32.05**<br>70¾ | **35.40**<br>78 | **37.67**<br>83 | **25.35**<br>56 | **26.28**<br>58 | **27.88**<br>61½ | **30.06**<br>66¼ | **33.41**<br>73¾ | **36.84**<br>81¼ | **39.93**<br>88 |
| **136-138 cm**<br>53½-54¼ in | **26.51**<br>58½ | **27.32**<br>60¼ | **28.80**<br>63½ | **30.86**<br>68 | **33.51**<br>74 | **37.05**<br>81¾ | **39.65**<br>87½ | **26.34**<br>58 | **27.39**<br>60½ | **29.19**<br>64¼ | **31.54**<br>69½ | **35.29**<br>77¾ | **39.01**<br>86 | **42.54**<br>93¾ |
| **138-140 cm**<br>54¼-55 in | **27.53**<br>60¾ | **28.38**<br>62½ | **29.99**<br>66 | **32.23**<br>71 | **35.08**<br>77¼ | **38.77**<br>85½ | **41.74**<br>92 | | | | | | | |
| **140-142 cm**<br>55-56 in | **28.59**<br>63 | **29.48**<br>65 | **31.25**<br>69 | **33.70**<br>74¼ | **36.75**<br>81 | **40.55**<br>89½ | **43.97**<br>97 | | | | | | | |
| **142-144 cm**<br>56-56¾ in | **29.70**<br>65½ | **30.64**<br>67½ | **32.58**<br>71¾ | **35.27**<br>77¾ | **38.54**<br>85 | **42.39**<br>93½ | **46.32**<br>102 | | | | | | | |
| **144-146 cm**<br>56¾-57½ in | **30.86**<br>68 | **31.85**<br>70¼ | **34.00**<br>75 | **36.95**<br>81½ | **40.45**<br>89¼ | **44.29**<br>97¾ | **48.80**<br>107½ | | | | | | | |

*National Center for Health Statistics, Health Resources Administration, DHEW, Hyattsville, Maryland 20782. Data smoothed by least-squares-cubic-spline technique.

Values correspond with NCHS percentile curves displayed in Ross NCHS Percentile Growth Charts. Conversion of metric data to inches and pounds by Ross Laboratories.

# NCHS PERCENTILES*–STATURE AND WEIGHT
# BOYS AND GIRLS: 2 TO 18 YEARS

| AGE years | PERCENTILES, BOYS | | | | | | |
|---|---|---|---|---|---|---|---|
| | 5th | 10th | 25th | 50th | 75th | 90th | 9 |
| 2.0** | **82.5** 32½<br>**10.49** 23¼ | **83.5** 32¾<br>**10.96** 24¼ | **85.3** 33½<br>**11.55** 25½ | **86.8** 34¼<br>**12.34** 27¼ | **89.2** 35<br>**13.36** 29½ | **92.0** 36¼<br>**14.38** 31¾ | **94.4**<br>**15.50** |
| 2.5** | **85.4** 33½<br>**11.27** 24¾ | **86.5** 34<br>**11.77** 26 | **88.5** 34¾<br>**12.55** 27¾ | **90.4** 35½<br>**13.52** 29¾ | **92.9** 36½<br>**14.61** 32¼ | **95.6** 37¾<br>**15.71** 34¾ | **97.8**<br>**16.61** |
| 3.0 | **89.0** 35<br>**12.05** 26½ | **90.3** 35½<br>**12.58** 27¾ | **92.6** 36½<br>**13.52** 29¾ | **94.9** 37¼<br>**14.62** 32¼ | **97.5** 38½<br>**15.78** 34¾ | **100.1** 39½<br>**16.95** 37¼ | **102.0**<br>**17.77** |
| 3.5 | **92.5** 36½<br>**12.84** 28¼ | **93.9** 37<br>**13.41** 29½ | **96.4** 38<br>**14.46** 32 | **99.1** 39<br>**15.68** 34½ | **101.7** 40<br>**16.90** 37¼ | **104.3** 41¼<br>**18.15** 40 | **106.1**<br>**18.98** |
| 4.0 | **95.8** 37¾<br>**13.64** 30 | **97.3** 38¼<br>**14.24** 31½ | **100.0** 39¼<br>**15.39** 34 | **102.9** 40½<br>**16.69** 36¾ | **105.7** 41½<br>**17.99** 39¾ | **108.2** 42½<br>**19.32** 42½ | **109.9**<br>**20.27** |
| 4.5 | **98.9** 39<br>**14.45** 31¾ | **100.6** 39½<br>**15.10** 33¼ | **103.4** 40¾<br>**16.30** 36 | **106.6** 42<br>**17.69** 39 | **109.4** 43<br>**19.06** 42 | **111.9** 44<br>**20.50** 45¼ | **113.5**<br>**21.63** |
| 5.0 | **102.0** 40¼<br>**15.27** 33¾ | **103.7** 40¾<br>**15.96** 35¼ | **106.5** 42<br>**17.22** 38 | **109.9** 43¼<br>**18.67** 41¼ | **112.8** 44½<br>**20.14** 44½ | **115.4** 45½<br>**21.70** 47¾ | **117.0**<br>**23.09** |
| 5.5 | **104.9** 41¼<br>**16.09** 35½ | **106.7** 42<br>**16.83** 37 | **109.6** 43¼<br>**18.14** 40 | **113.1** 44½<br>**19.67** 43¼ | **116.1** 45¾<br>**21.25** 46¾ | **118.7** 46¾<br>**22.96** 50½ | **120.3**<br>**24.66** |
| 6.0 | **107.7** 42½<br>**16.93** 37¼ | **109.6** 43¼<br>**17.72** 39 | **112.5** 44¼<br>**19.07** 42 | **116.1** 45¾<br>**20.69** 45½ | **119.2** 47<br>**22.40** 49½ | **121.9** 48<br>**24.31** 53½ | **123.5**<br>**26.34** |
| 6.5 | **110.4** 43½<br>**17.78** 39¼ | **112.3** 44¼<br>**18.62** 41 | **115.3** 45½<br>**20.02** 44¼ | **119.0** 46¾<br>**21.74** 48 | **122.2** 48<br>**23.62** 52 | **124.9** 49¼<br>**25.76** 56¾ | **126.6**<br>**28.16** |
| 7.0 | **113.0** 44½<br>**18.64** 41 | **115.0** 45¼<br>**19.53** 43 | **118.0** 46½<br>**21.00** 46¼ | **121.7** 48<br>**22.85** 50¼ | **125.0** 49¼<br>**24.94** 55 | **127.9** 50¼<br>**27.36** 60¼ | **129.7**<br>**30.12** |
| 7.5 | **115.6** 45½<br>**19.52** 43 | **117.6** 46¼<br>**20.45** 45 | **120.6** 47½<br>**22.02** 48½ | **124.4** 49<br>**24.03** 53 | **127.8** 50¼<br>**26.36** 58 | **130.8** 51½<br>**29.11** 64¼ | **132.7**<br>**32.73** |
| 8.0 | **118.1** 46½<br>**20.40** 45 | **120.2** 47¼<br>**21.39** 47¼ | **123.2** 48½<br>**23.09** 51 | **127.0** 50<br>**25.30** 55¾ | **130.5** 51½<br>**27.91** 61½ | **133.6** 52½<br>**31.06** 68½ | **135.7**<br>**34.51** |
| 8.5 | **120.5** 47½<br>**21.31** 47 | **122.7** 48¼<br>**22.34** 49¼ | **125.7** 49½<br>**24.21** 53¼ | **129.6** 51<br>**26.66** 58¾ | **133.2** 52½<br>**29.61** 65¼ | **136.5** 53¾<br>**33.22** 73¼ | **138.8**<br>**36.96** |
| 9.0 | **122.9** 48½<br>**22.25** 49 | **125.2** 49¼<br>**23.33** 51½ | **128.2** 50½<br>**25.40** 56 | **132.2** 52<br>**28.13** 62 | **136.0** 53½<br>**31.46** 69¼ | **139.4** 55<br>**35.57** 78½ | **141.8**<br>**39.5** |
| 9.5 | **125.3** 49¼<br>**23.25** 51¼ | **127.6** 50¼<br>**24.38** 53¾ | **130.8** 51½<br>**26.68** 58¾ | **134.8** 53<br>**29.73** 65½ | **138.8** 54¾<br>**33.46** 73¾ | **142.4** 56<br>**38.11** 84 | **144.9**<br>**42.3** |
| 10.0 | **127.7** 50¼<br>**24.33** 53¾ | **130.1** 51¼<br>**25.52** 56¼ | **133.4** 52½<br>**28.07** 62 | **137.5** 54¼<br>**31.44** 69¼ | **141.6** 55¾<br>**35.61** 78½ | **145.5** 57¼<br>**40.80** 90 | **148.1**<br>**45.2** |
| 10.5 | **130.1** 51¼<br>**25.51** 56¼ | **132.6** 52¼<br>**26.78** 59 | **136.0** 53½<br>**29.59** 65¼ | **140.3** 55¼<br>**33.30** 73½ | **144.6** 57<br>**37.92** 83½ | **148.7** 58½<br>**43.63** 96¼ | **151.5**<br>**48.3** |
| 11.0 | **132.6** 52¼<br>**26.80** 59 | **135.1** 53¼<br>**28.17** 62 | **138.7** 54½<br>**31.25** 69 | **143.3** 56½<br>**35.30** 77¾ | **147.8** 58¼<br>**40.38** 89 | **152.1** 60<br>**46.57** 102¾ | **154.9**<br>**51.4** |
| 11.5 | **135.0** 53¼<br>**28.24** 62¼ | **137.7** 54¼<br>**29.72** 65½ | **141.5** 55¾<br>**33.08** 73 | **146.4** 57¾<br>**37.46** 82½ | **151.1** 59½<br>**43.00** 94¾ | **155.6** 61¼<br>**49.61** 109¼ | **158.5**<br>**54.7** |
| 12.0 | **137.6** 54¼<br>**29.85** 65¾ | **140.3** 55¼<br>**31.46** 69¼ | **144.4** 56¾<br>**35.09** 77¼ | **149.7** 59<br>**39.78** 87¾ | **154.6** 60¾<br>**45.77** 101 | **159.4** 62¾<br>**52.73** 116¼ | **162.3**<br>**58.0** |
| 12.5 | **140.2** 55¼<br>**31.64** 69¾ | **143.0** 56¼<br>**33.41** 73¾ | **147.4** 58<br>**37.31** 82¼ | **153.0** 60¼<br>**42.27** 93¼ | **158.2** 62¼<br>**48.70** 107¼ | **163.2** 64¼<br>**55.91** 123¼ | **166.1**<br>**61.5** |
| 13.0 | **142.9** 56¼<br>**33.64** 74¼ | **145.8** 57½<br>**35.60** 78½ | **150.5** 59¼<br>**39.74** 87½ | **156.5** 61½<br>**44.95** 99 | **161.8** 63¾<br>**51.79** 114¼ | **167.0** 65¾<br>**59.12** 130¼ | **169.8**<br>**65.0** |
| 13.5 | **145.7** 57¼<br>**35.85** 79 | **148.7** 58½<br>**38.03** 83¾ | **153.6** 60½<br>**42.40** 93½ | **159.9** 63<br>**47.81** 105½ | **165.3** 65<br>**55.02** 121¼ | **170.5** 67¼<br>**62.35** 137½ | **173.4**<br>**68.5** |
| 14.0 | **148.8** 58½<br>**38.22** 84¼ | **151.8** 59¾<br>**40.64** 89½ | **156.9** 61¾<br>**45.21** 99¾ | **163.1** 64¼<br>**50.77** 112 | **168.5** 66¼<br>**58.31** 128½ | **173.8** 68½<br>**65.57** 144½ | **176.7**<br>**72.1** |
| 14.5 | **152.0** 59¾<br>**40.66** 89¾ | **155.0** 61<br>**43.34** 95½ | **160.1** 63<br>**48.08** 106 | **166.2** 65½<br>**53.76** 118½ | **171.5** 67½<br>**61.58** 135¾ | **176.6** 69½<br>**68.76** 151½ | **179.5**<br>**75.6** |
| 15.0 | **155.2** 61<br>**43.11** 95 | **158.2** 62¼<br>**46.06** 101½ | **163.3** 64¼<br>**50.92** 112¼ | **169.0** 66½<br>**56.71** 125 | **174.1** 68½<br>**64.72** 142¾ | **178.9** 70½<br>**71.91** 158½ | **181.9**<br>**79.1** |
| 15.5 | **158.3** 62¼<br>**45.50** 100¼ | **161.2** 63½<br>**48.69** 107¼ | **166.2** 65½<br>**53.64** 118¼ | **171.5** 67½<br>**59.51** 131¼ | **176.3** 69½<br>**67.64** 149 | **180.8** 71¼<br>**74.98** 165¼ | **183.9**<br>**82.4** |
| 16.0 | **161.1** 63½<br>**47.74** 105¼ | **163.9** 64½<br>**51.16** 112¾ | **168.7** 66½<br>**56.16** 123¾ | **173.5** 68¼<br>**62.10** 137 | **178.1** 70<br>**70.26** 155 | **182.4** 71¾<br>**77.97** 172 | **185.4**<br>**85.6** |
| 16.5 | **163.4** 64¼<br>**49.76** 109¾ | **166.1** 65½<br>**53.39** 117¾ | **170.6** 67¼<br>**58.38** 128¾ | **175.2** 69<br>**64.39** 142 | **179.5** 70¾<br>**72.46** 159¾ | **183.6** 72¼<br>**80.84** 178¼ | **186.6**<br>**88.5** |
| 17.0 | **164.9** 65<br>**51.50** 113½ | **167.7** 66<br>**55.28** 121¾ | **171.9** 67¾<br>**60.22** 132¾ | **176.2** 69¼<br>**66.31** 146¼ | **180.5** 71<br>**74.17** 163½ | **184.4** 72½<br>**83.58** 184¼ | **187.3**<br>**91.3** |
| 17.5 | **165.6** 65¼<br>**52.89** 116½ | **168.5** 66¼<br>**56.78** 125¼ | **172.4** 67¾<br>**61.61** 135¾ | **176.7** 69½<br>**67.78** 149½ | **181.0** 71¼<br>**75.32** 166 | **185.0** 72¾<br>**86.14** 190 | **187.6**<br>**93.7** |
| 18.0 | **165.7** 65¼<br>**53.97** 119 | **168.7** 66½<br>**57.89** 127½ | **172.3** 67¾<br>**62.61** 138 | **176.8** 69½<br>**68.88** 151¾ | **181.2** 71¼<br>**76.04** 167¾ | **185.3** 73<br>**88.41** 195 | **187.6**<br>**95.7** |

*National Center for Health Statistics, Health Resources Administration, DHEW, Hyattsville, Maryland 20782. Data smoothed by least-squares-cubic spline technique. Values correspond with NCHS percentile curves displayed in Ross NCHS Percentile Growth Charts. Conversion of metric data to inches and pounds by Ross Lab

## PERCENTILES, GIRLS

| MEASUREMENT | 5th | 10th | 25th | 50th | 75th | 90th | 95th |
|---|---|---|---|---|---|---|---|
| Stature–cm and in | 81.6  32¼ | 82.1  32¼ | 84.0  33 | 86.8  34¼ | 89.3  35¼ | 92.0  36¼ | 93.6  36¾ |
| Weight–kg and lb | 9.95  22 | 10.32  22¾ | 10.96  24¼ | 11.80  26 | 12.73  28 | 13.58  30 | 14.15  31¼ |
| Stature–cm and in | 84.6  33¼ | 85.3  33½ | 87.3  34½ | 90.0  35½ | 92.5  36½ | 95.0  37½ | 96.6  38 |
| Weight–kg and lb | 10.80  23¾ | 11.35  25 | 12.11  26¾ | 13.03  28¾ | 14.23  31¼ | 15.16  33¼ | 15.76  34¾ |
| Stature–cm and in | 88.3  34¾ | 89.3  35¼ | 91.4  36 | 94.1  37 | 96.6  38 | 99.0  39 | 100.6  39½ |
| Weight–kg and lb | 11.61  25½ | 12.26  27 | 13.11  29 | 14.10  31 | 15.50  34¼ | 16.54  36½ | 17.22  38 |
| Stature–cm and in | 91.7  36 | 93.0  36½ | 95.2  37½ | 97.9  38½ | 100.5  39½ | 102.8  40½ | 104.5  41¼ |
| Weight–kg and lb | 12.37  27¼ | 13.08  28¾ | 14.00  30¾ | 15.07  33¼ | 16.59  36½ | 17.77  39¼ | 18.59  41 |
| Stature–cm and in | 95.0  37½ | 96.4  38 | 98.8  39 | 101.6  40 | 104.3  41 | 106.6  42 | 108.3  42¾ |
| Weight–kg and lb | 13.11  29 | 13.84  30½ | 14.80  32¾ | 15.96  35¼ | 17.56  38¾ | 18.93  41¾ | 19.91  44 |
| Stature–cm and in | 98.1  38½ | 99.7  39¼ | 102.2  40¼ | 105.0  41¼ | 107.9  42½ | 110.2  43½ | 112.0  44 |
| Weight–kg and lb | 13.83  30½ | 14.56  32 | 15.55  34¼ | 16.81  37 | 18.48  40¾ | 20.06  44¼ | 21.24  46¾ |
| Stature–cm and in | 101.1  39¾ | 102.7  40½ | 105.4  41½ | 108.4  42¾ | 111.4  43¾ | 113.8  44¾ | 115.6  45½ |
| Weight–kg and lb | 14.55  32 | 15.26  33¾ | 16.29  36 | 17.66  39 | 19.39  42¾ | 21.23  46¾ | 22.62  49¾ |
| Stature–cm and in | 103.9  41 | 105.6  41½ | 108.4  42¾ | 111.6  44 | 114.8  45¼ | 117.4  46¼ | 119.2  47 |
| Weight–kg and lb | 15.29  33¾ | 15.97  35¼ | 17.05  37½ | 18.56  41 | 20.36  45 | 22.48  49½ | 24.11  53¼ |
| Stature–cm and in | 106.6  42 | 108.4  42¾ | 111.3  43¾ | 114.6  45 | 118.1  46½ | 120.8  47½ | 122.7  48¼ |
| Weight–kg and lb | 16.05  35½ | 16.72  36¾ | 17.86  39¼ | 19.52  43 | 21.44  47¼ | 23.89  52¾ | 25.75  56¾ |
| Stature–cm and in | 109.2  43 | 111.0  43¾ | 114.1  45 | 117.6  46¼ | 121.3  47¾ | 124.2  49 | 126.1  49¾ |
| Weight–kg and lb | 16.85  37¼ | 17.51  38½ | 18.76  41¼ | 20.61  45½ | 22.68  50 | 25.50  56¼ | 27.59  60¾ |
| Stature–cm and in | 111.8  44 | 113.6  44¾ | 116.8  46 | 120.6  47½ | 124.4  49 | 127.6  50¼ | 129.5  51 |
| Weight–kg and lb | 17.71  39 | 18.39  40½ | 19.78  43½ | 21.84  48¼ | 24.16  53¼ | 27.39  60½ | 29.68  65½ |
| Stature–cm and in | 114.4  45 | 116.2  45¾ | 119.5  47 | 123.5  48½ | 127.5  50¼ | 130.9  51½ | 132.9  52¼ |
| Weight–kg and lb | 18.62  41 | 19.37  42¾ | 20.95  46¼ | 23.26  51¼ | 25.90  57 | 29.57  65¼ | 32.07  70¾ |
| Stature–cm and in | 116.9  46 | 118.7  46¾ | 122.2  48 | 126.4  49¾ | 130.6  51½ | 134.2  52¾ | 136.2  53½ |
| Weight–kg and lb | 19.62  43¼ | 20.45  45 | 22.26  49 | 24.84  54¾ | 27.88  61½ | 32.04  70¾ | 34.71  76½ |
| Stature–cm and in | 119.5  47 | 121.3  47¾ | 124.9  49¼ | 129.3  51 | 133.6  52½ | 137.4  54 | 139.6  55 |
| Weight–kg and lb | 20.68  45½ | 21.64  47¾ | 23.70  52¼ | 26.58  58½ | 30.08  66¼ | 34.73  76½ | 37.58  82¾ |
| Stature–cm and in | 122.1  48 | 123.9  48¾ | 127.7  50¼ | 132.2  52 | 136.7  53¾ | 140.7  55½ | 142.9  56¼ |
| Weight–kg and lb | 21.82  48 | 22.92  50½ | 25.27  55¾ | 28.46  62¾ | 32.44  71½ | 37.60  83 | 40.64  89½ |
| Stature–cm and in | 124.8  49¼ | 126.6  49¾ | 130.6  51½ | 135.2  53¼ | 139.8  55 | 143.9  56¾ | 146.2  57½ |
| Weight–kg and lb | 23.05  50¾ | 24.29  53½ | 26.94  59½ | 30.45  67¼ | 34.94  77 | 40.61  89½ | 43.85  96¾ |
| Stature–cm and in | 127.5  50¼ | 129.5  51 | 133.6  52½ | 138.3  54½ | 142.9  56¼ | 147.2  58 | 149.5  58¾ |
| Weight–kg and lb | 24.36  53¾ | 25.76  56¾ | 28.71  63¼ | 32.55  71¾ | 37.53  82¾ | 43.70  96¼ | 47.17  104 |
| Stature–cm and in | 130.4  51¼ | 132.5  52¼ | 136.7  53¾ | 141.5  55¾ | 146.1  57½ | 150.4  59¼ | 152.8  60¼ |
| Weight–kg and lb | 25.75  56¾ | 27.32  60¼ | 30.57  67½ | 34.72  76½ | 40.17  88½ | 46.84  103¼ | 50.57  111½ |
| Stature–cm and in | 133.5  52½ | 135.6  53½ | 140.0  55 | 144.8  57 | 149.3  58¾ | 153.7  60½ | 156.2  61½ |
| Weight–kg and lb | 27.24  60 | 28.97  63¾ | 32.49  71¾ | 36.95  81½ | 42.84  94½ | 49.96  110¼ | 54.00  119 |
| Stature–cm and in | 136.6  53¾ | 139.0  54¾ | 143.5  56½ | 148.2  58¼ | 152.6  60 | 156.9  61¾ | 159.5  62¾ |
| Weight–kg and lb | 28.83  63½ | 30.71  67¾ | 34.48  76 | 39.23  86½ | 45.48  100¼ | 53.03  117 | 57.42  126½ |
| Stature–cm and in | 139.8  55 | 142.3  56 | 147.0  57¾ | 151.5  59¾ | 155.8  61¼ | 160.0  63 | 162.7  64 |
| Weight–kg and lb | 30.52  67¼ | 32.53  71¾ | 36.52  80½ | 41.53  91½ | 48.07  106 | 55.99  123½ | 60.81  134 |
| Stature–cm and in | 142.7  56¼ | 145.4  57¼ | 150.1  59 | 154.6  60¾ | 158.8  62½ | 162.9  64¼ | 165.6  65¼ |
| Weight–kg and lb | 32.30  71¼ | 34.42  76 | 38.59  85 | 43.84  96¾ | 50.56  111½ | 58.81  129¾ | 64.12  141¼ |
| Stature–cm and in | 145.2  57¼ | 148.0  58¼ | 152.8  60¼ | 157.1  61¾ | 161.3  63½ | 165.3  65 | 168.1  66¼ |
| Weight–kg and lb | 34.14  75¼ | 36.35  80¼ | 40.65  89½ | 46.10  101¾ | 52.91  116¾ | 61.45  135½ | 67.30  148¼ |
| Stature–cm and in | 147.2  58 | 150.0  59 | 154.7  61 | 159.0  62½ | 163.2  64¼ | 167.3  65¾ | 170.0  67 |
| Weight–kg and lb | 35.98  79¼ | 38.26  84¼ | 42.65  94 | 48.26  106½ | 55.11  121½ | 63.87  140¾ | 70.30  155 |
| Stature–cm and in | 148.7  58½ | 151.5  59¾ | 155.9  61½ | 160.4  63¼ | 164.6  64¾ | 168.7  66½ | 171.3  67½ |
| Weight–kg and lb | 37.76  83¼ | 40.11  88½ | 44.54  98¼ | 50.28  110¾ | 57.09  125¾ | 66.04  145½ | 73.08  161 |
| Stature–cm and in | 149.7  59 | 152.5  60 | 156.8  61¾ | 161.2  63½ | 165.6  65¼ | 169.8  66¾ | 172.2  67¾ |
| Weight–kg and lb | 39.45  87 | 41.83  92¼ | 46.28  102 | 52.10  114¾ | 58.84  129¾ | 67.95  149¾ | 75.59  166¾ |
| Stature–cm and in | 150.5  59¼ | 153.2  60¼ | 157.2  62 | 161.8  63¾ | 166.3  65½ | 170.5  67¼ | 172.8  68 |
| Weight–kg and lb | 40.99  90¼ | 43.38  95¾ | 47.82  105½ | 53.68  118¼ | 60.32  133 | 69.54  153¼ | 77.78  171½ |
| Stature–cm and in | 151.1  59½ | 153.6  60½ | 157.5  62 | 162.1  63¾ | 166.7  65¾ | 170.9  67¼ | 173.1  68¼ |
| Weight–kg and lb | 42.32  93¼ | 44.72  98½ | 49.10  108¼ | 54.96  121¼ | 61.48  135½ | 70.79  156 | 79.59  175½ |
| Stature–cm and in | 151.6  59¾ | 154.1  60¾ | 157.8  62¼ | 162.4  64 | 166.9  65¾ | 171.1  67¼ | 173.3  68¼ |
| Weight–kg and lb | 43.41  95¾ | 45.78  101 | 50.09  110½ | 55.89  123¼ | 62.29  137¼ | 71.68  158 | 80.99  178½ |
| Stature–cm and in | 152.2  60 | 154.6  60¾ | 158.2  62¼ | 162.7  64 | 167.1  65¾ | 171.2  67½ | 173.4  68¼ |
| Weight–kg and lb | 44.20  97½ | 46.54  102½ | 50.75  112 | 56.44  124½ | 62.75  138¼ | 72.18  159¼ | 81.93  180½ |
| Stature–cm and in | 152.7  60 | 155.1  61 | 158.7  62½ | 163.1  64¼ | 167.3  65¾ | 171.2  67¼ | 173.5  68¼ |
| Weight–kg and lb | 44.74  98¾ | 47.04  103¾ | 51.14  112¾ | 56.69  125 | 62.91  138¾ | 72.38  159½ | 82.46  181¾ |
| Stature–cm and in | 153.2  60¼ | 155.6  61¼ | 159.1  62¾ | 163.4  64¼ | 167.5  66 | 171.1  67¼ | 173.5  68¼ |
| Weight–kg and lb | 45.08  99¼ | 47.33  104¼ | 51.33  113¼ | 56.71  125 | 62.89  138¾ | 72.37  159¼ | 82.62  182¼ |
| Stature–cm and in | 153.6  60½ | 156.0  61½ | 159.6  62¾ | 163.7  64½ | 167.6  66 | 171.0  67¼ | 173.6  68¼ |
| Weight–kg and lb | 45.26  99¾ | 47.47  104¾ | 51.39  113¼ | 56.62  124¾ | 62.78  138½ | 72.25  159¼ | 82.47  181¾ |

**Stature data for 2.0 to 3.0 years include some recumbent length measurements, which make values slightly higher than if all measurements had been of stature.

# Table of Weights and Measures

| | |
|---|---|
| 1 ounce | = 30 grams (actual weight 28.35 g) |
| 1 fluid ounce | = 30 millilitres (actual amount 28.35 ml) |
| 1 cup | = ½ pint = 240 ml = 8 fl ounces |
| 2 cups | = 1 pint = 480 ml = 16 fl ounces |
| 2 pints | = 1 quart = 960 ml = 32 fl ounces |
| 4 quarts | = 1 gallon |
| 2 gallons | = 1 peck |
| 4 pecks | = 1 bushel |
| | |
| 1 teaspoon fluid | = 5 ml or ⅙ oz or 1 dram |
| 1 tablespoon fluid | = 15 ml or ½ oz |
| 1 cup (standard) | = 16 tablespoons |
| | |
| 1 inch | = 2.54 cm |
| | |
| 1 milliequivalent | = one thousandth of an equivalent |
| 1 microgram | = one thousandth of a milligram |
| 1 milligram | = one thousandth of a gram |
| 1 gram | = one thousandth of a kilogram |
| | |
| 1 kilogram | = 2.2045 pounds (2.2 lb) |
| 1 litre | = 1.0567 quarts |
| 1 pound | = 453.6 grams |

To change pounds to kilograms multiply by 0.45

To change inches to centimetres multiply by 2.54

*Source*: Reprinted from Manual of Diets, Departments of Dietetics, Hospital of St. Raphael, New Haven, CT; Veterans Administration Hospital, West Haven, CT; and Yale-New Haven Hospital, Yale-New Haven Medical Center, New Haven, CT, 1972.

# Milliequivalents Conversion Table

To convert milligrams (mg) to milliequivalents (meq), the following formula is used:

$$\frac{\text{milligrams}}{\text{atomic weight}} \times \text{valence} = \text{milliequivalents}$$

Example: Convert 2,000 mg sodium to milliequivalents of sodium:

$$\frac{2,000}{23} \times 1 = 87 \text{ meq sodium}$$

To change milliequivalents back to milligrams, multiply the milliequivalents by the atomic weight and divide by the valence.

Example: Convert 20 meq sodium to milligrams of sodium:

$$\frac{20 \times 23}{1} = 460 \text{ mg sodium}$$

| Minerals | Atomic weights | Valences |
|---|---|---|
| Calcium | 40.00 | 2 |
| Chlorine | 35.40 | 1 |
| Magnesium | 24.30 | 2 |
| Phosphorus | 31.00 | 2 |
| Potassium | 39.00 | 1 |
| Sodium | 23.00 | 1 |
| Sulfur | 32.00 | 2 |
| Zinc | 65.37 | 2 |

# Osmolality of Common Foods

*Osmolality* refers to the number of osmoles of the particles (solutes) in a kilogram of solvent. It is generally expressed as milliosmoles (mOsm), a measure of osmotically active particles per kilogram of water. *Osmolarity*, a term often confused with osmolality, refers to the number of osmoles per litre of solution (solvent plus solute). In body fluids there is a minor and unimportant difference between osmolality and osmolarity. In liquid diets and certain other foods, however, the value for osmolarity is always less than the value of osmolality, usually about 80% as much. Osmolarity is influenced by the values of all solutes contained in a solution and by the temperature, while osmolality is not.

In comparing potential hypertonic effects of various tube feedings or liquid diets, osmolality is the preferred term. The osmolality of blood serum and other body fluids should normally be no greater than 300 mOsm/kg of water. The body attempts to keep the osmolality of the contents of the stomach and intestine at this level. Adverse effects of hyperosmolar tube feedings and synthetic fiber free liquid diets have been discussed elsewhere.

At a given concentration, the smaller the particle size the greater the number of particles present and therefore the higher the osmolality. Simple sugars or low molecular weight carbohydrates increase osmolality of solutions much more than complex carbohydrates with higher molecular weights and large particle size.

Fats, which are complex and water insoluble, do not increase the osmolality of solutions. Electrolytes, such as sodium and potassium, and amino acids, all contribute significantly to the osmolality of a solution or liquid feeding.

## Approximate Osmolality of Some Common Foods

| Food | mOsm/kg water |
|---|---|
| Ginger ale | 510 |
| Gelatin dessert | 535 |
| Tomato juice | 595 |
| 7-Up | 640 |
| Coca-Cola | 680 |
| Eggnog | 695 |
| Apple juice | 870 |
| Orange juice | 935 |
| Malted milk | 940 |
| Ice cream | 1,150 |
| Grape juice | 1,170 |
| Sherbet | 1,225 |

# Caffeine Content of Beverages

| Beverage | Caffeine (mg/100 ml) |
|---|---|
| *Carbonated* | |
| Coca Cola* | 17.97 |
| Dr. Pepper* | 16.92 |
| Mountain Dew* | 15.19 |
| Diet Dr. Pepper* | 15.06 |
| Tab* | 13.72 |
| Pepsi-Cola* | 11.98 |
| RC Cola* | 9.36 |
| Diet RC* | 9.17 |
| Diet Rite* | 8.81 |
| Fanta Root Beer† | 0 |
| *Coffee* | |
| Instant* | 44.00 |
| Percolated* | 73.00 |
| Dripolated* | 97.00 |
| *Coffee: decaffeinated* | |
| Infused‡ | 1.00–3.00 |
| Instant‡ | 0.50–1.50 |
| Decaf† | 0.90 |
| Nescafe† | 3.30–5.60 |
| Sanka† | 1.80 |
| *Tea, bagged* | |
| Black, 5 min brew* | 33.00 |
| Black, 1 min brew* | 20.00 |
| *Tea, loose* | |
| Black, 5 min brew* | 29.00 |
| Green, 5 min brew* | 25.00 |
| Green, Japan, 5 min brew* | 15.00 |
| *Cocoa; chocolate** | 6.00 |
| *Ovaltine‡* | 0.00 |

* Bunker, M. L., and McWilliams, M.: Caffeine content of common beverages. J. Am. Diet. Assoc. 74: 28, 1979.
† Nutritional analysis data supplied by the manufacturer.
‡ Nagy, M.: Caffeine content of beverages and chocolate. JAMA 229: 337, 1974.

# Zinc Content of Foods

| Food | Zinc (mg/100 g) |
| --- | --- |
| Applesauce | |
|    Unsweetened | 0.1* |
|    Canned | 0.013‡ |
| Apples | |
|    Raw | 0.05* |
|    Cider, bottled, pasteurized | 0.03† |
|    Juice, canned | 0.043‡ |
| Apricots, canned, drained | 0.085‡ |
| Artichokes, cooked, whole | 0.35† |
| Asparagus spears, frozen, uncooked | 0.76‡ |
| Avocados, peeled | 0.43† |
| Bagel | 0.96† |
| Bananas, raw | 0.2* |
| Barbecue sauce, tomato base | 0.13† |
| Beans, common, mature, dry | |
|    Raw | 2.8* |
|    Boiled, drained | 1.0* |
|    Baked with pork | 1.7‡ |
| Beans, lima, mature, dry | |
|    Raw | 2.8* |
|    Boiled, drained | 0.9* |
|    Baby, frozen, uncooked | 0.77‡ |
| Beans, snap, green | |
|    Raw | 0.4* |
|    Boiled, drained | 0.3* |
|    Canned, solids and liquid | 0.2* |
|    Canned, drained solids | 0.3* |
|    Frozen, uncooked | 0.31‡ |
| Beans, wax, canned, drained, salt free | 0.23‡ |
| Beef, corned, cooked | 1.94† |
| Beef, fresh, uncooked | |
|    Flank (U.S. Good) | 3.6‡ |
|    Ground (U.S. Cutter) | 3.4‡ |
|    Liver (U.S. Good) | 4.2‡ |
|    Round (U.S. Good) | 3.0‡ |
|    Rump (U.S. Good) | 3.3‡ |
|    Sirloin (U.S. Good Medium fat) | 3.1‡ |
|    Tenderloin (U.S. Prime) | 2.5‡ |
| Beef, ground (77% lean) | |
|    Raw | 3.4* |
|    Cooked | 4.4* |
| Beef, separable fat, raw | 0.5* |
| Beef, separable lean | |
|    Raw | 4.2* |
|    Cooked, dry heat | 5.8* |
|    Cooked, moist heat | 6.2* |
| Beef stew, canned | 1.60† |
| Beets, canned, no added salt, drained | 0.3‡ |
| Beverages, alcoholic | |
|    Domestic beer | 0.03† |
|    Domestic brandy | 0.07† |
|    Domestic red wine | 0.10† |
| Beverages, carbonated | |
|    Cola | 0.02† |
|    Diet cola | <0.01† |
|    Root beer | <0.01† |
|    Canned | 0.08* |

| Food | Zinc (mg/100 g) |
|---|---|
| Beverages, noncarbonated | |
|   Fruit punch drink | 0.02† |
|   Orange drink | 0.04† |
| Blueberries, water pack, drained | 0.085‡ |
| Bran, crude | 14.3* |
| Branflakes, 40% | 3.6* |
| Bread | |
|   Corn, molasses | 0.85† |
|   Italian | 0.05† |
|   Oatmeal | 1.04† |
|   Pumpernickel | 1.14† |
|   Rye | 1.6* |
|   Stone ground wheat | 2.03† |
|   White | 0.6* |
|   Whole wheat | 1.8* |
|   Crumbs, prepared | 0.38† |
|   Stuffing, prepared | 0.39† |
| Breakfast, complete, in liquid form, | |
|     milk added | 2.09† |
| Broccoli | |
|   Cooked | 0.15† |
|   Frozen, uncooked | 0.27‡ |
| Brussels sprouts | |
|   Boiled | 0.36† |
|   Frozen, uncooked | 0.37‡ |
| Butter | 0.1* |
| Cabbage, common | |
|   Raw | 0.4* |
|   Boiled, drained | 0.4* |
| Cake | |
|   Cheese, frozen, prepared | 0.51† |
|   Chocolate, chocolate icing | 1.26† |
|   Coffee | 0.86† |
|   Datenut, commercial | 0.15† |
|   White, no icing | 0.2* |
|   Frosting, buttercream | 0.16† |
| Candy bar | |
|   Almond | 0.40† |
|   Caramel filled | 0.41† |
|   Chocolate | 0.46† |
|   Mocha-type filled | 0.21† |
| Candy | |
|   Chocolate covered mint | 0.38† |
|   Marshmallow | 0.03† |
| Cantaloupe | 0.14‡ |
| Carrots, raw | 0.12‡ |
| | 0.4* |
|   Cooked, canned, drained solid | 0.03* |
| Cauliflower, frozen, uncooked | 0.46‡ |
| Celery, fresh | 0.065‡ |
| Cheerios | 3.0‡ |
| Cherries, Royal Anne, canned, drained | 0.11‡ |
| Cheese | |
|   Cheddar type | 4.0* |
|   American, processed | 3.00† |
|   Camembert, imported | 2.40† |
|   Cottage | 0.4‡ |
|   Cream | 0.26† |
|   Farmer | 0.46† |
|   Gouda, domestic | 3.86† |
|   Mozzarella, domestic | 3.88† |
|   Muenster, domestic | 3.36† |
|     99% fat free | 2.34† |
|   Parmesan, domestic | 5.50† |
|   Swiss | 4.6‡ |

| Food | Zinc (mg/100 g) |
|---|---|
| Chicken, broiler, fryer | |
| Breast, meat only | |
| Raw | 0.7* |
| Cooked, dry heat | 0.9* |
| Breast | |
| Raw (81% meat, 12% skin, 7% fat) | 0.7* |
| Cooked, dry heat | |
| (81% meat, 11% skin) | 0.9* |
| Drumstick, thigh, back, meat only | |
| Raw | 1.8* |
| Cooked, dry heat | 2.8* |
| Drumstick | |
| Raw (85% meat, 13% skin, 2% fat) | 1.7* |
| Cooked, dry heat | |
| (84% meat, 16% skin) | 2.5* |
| Neck, meat only | |
| Raw | 2.7* |
| Cooked, moist heat | 3.0* |
| Skin | |
| Raw | 1.0* |
| Cooked, dry heat | 1.2* |
| Wing, meat only | |
| Raw | 1.6* |
| Cooked | 2.4* |
| Chicken, roaster, uncooked | |
| Dark meat | 1.5‡ |
| White meat | 0.59‡ |
| Chickpeas or garbanzos, | |
| mature seeds, dry | |
| Raw | 2.7* |
| Boiled, drained | 1.4* |
| Chili con carne, canned | 1.63† |
| Chocolate | |
| Granular mix for milk | 0.82† |
| Hot | 0.96† |
| Hot, powder mix | 1.46† |
| Syrup | 0.9* |
| Clams, hard shell | |
| Raw | 1.5* |
| Cooked | 1.7* |
| Clams, soft shell | |
| Raw | 1.5* |
| Cooked | 1.7* |
| Clams, surf, canned, solid and liquid | 1.2* |
| Cocoa, dry powder | 5.6* |
| Coffee | |
| Dry, instant | 0.6* |
| Fluid beverage | 0.03* |
| Ground, dry | 0.36‡ |
| Instant, decaffeinated | <0.01† |
| Coleslaw, homemade | 0.24† |
| Cookies | |
| Chocolate chip | 0.96† |
| Chocolate fudge | 0.96† |
| Chocolate mint | 1.03† |
| Oatmeal | 1.31† |
| Shortbread | 0.42† |
| Vanilla wafers | 0.3* |
| Corn | |
| Canned, whole kernel, yellow | |
| Brine pack, solid and liquid | 0.3* |
| Brine pack, drained solids | 0.4* |
| Vacuum pack, solid and liquid | 0.4* |
| Creamed | 0.43† |
| Corn, field, whole grain, white, yellow | 2.1* |

| Food | Zinc (mg/100 g) |
|---|---|
| Corn, sweet yellow | |
|    Raw | 0.5* |
|    Boiled, drained | 0.4* |
| Corn chips | 1.5* |
| Cornflakes | 0.3* |
| Corn grits, white degermed, dry form | 0.4* |
| Cornmeal, white or yellow | |
|    Bolted (nearly whole grain) | 1.8* |
|    Degermed | |
|       Dry form | 0.8* |
|       Cooked | 0.1* |
| Cornstarch | 0.03* |
| Cowpeas (black eye), dry | |
|    Raw | 2.9* |
|    Boiled, drained | 1.2* |
| Crabs, blue and Dungeness | |
|    Raw | 4.0* |
|    Steamed | 4.3* |
|    Deviled, frozen | 1.71† |
| Crackers | |
|    Graham | 1.1* |
|    Round thin | 0.62† |
|    Saltines | 0.5* |
|    Sesame seed | 1.04† |
| Cranberry sauce | 0.01† |
| Cream | |
|    Artificial nondairy | 0.04† |
|    Table | 0.27† |
| Creamer, nondairy, coffee | 0.51† |
| Cucumber | 0.1‡ |
| Doughnuts, cake type | 0.5* |
| Drinking water | 0.015‡ |
| Eggs, fresh | |
|    White | 0.02* |
|    Yolk | 3.0* |
|    Whole | 1.0* |
| Egg noodles, uncooked | 2.2‡ |
| Farina, regular | |
|    Dry form | 0.5* |
|    Cooked | 0.006* |
| Fish, white varieties, flesh only | |
|    Raw | 0.7* |
|    Cooked, fillet | 1.0* |
|    Cooked, steak | 0.8* |
|    Gefilte | 0.45† |
|    Haddock, frozen, uncooked | 0.32‡ |
|    Salmon, canned, salt-free | 1.1‡ |
|    Sole, uncooked, frozen | 0.31‡ |
|    Tuna, canned, salt-free, water pack | 0.44‡ |
|    White, smoked | 0.36† |
| Flour | 0.93‡ |
| Garlic, raw | 1.25† |
| Gelatin dessert, cherry | 0.02† |
| Gizzard | |
|    Chicken, raw | 2.9* |
|          cooked, drained | 4.3* |
|    Turkey, raw | 2.8* |
|          cooked, drained | 4.1* |
| Granola | 2.1* |
| Gravy | |
|    Beef, canned | 1.80† |
|    Chicken, packaged | 0.12† |
| Grapes | |
|    Fresh with peel | 0.035‡ |
|    Juice, canned | 0.04‡ |

| Food | Zinc (mg/100 g) |
|---|---|
| Grapefruit | |
| Juice, canned | 0.03‡ |
| Fresh, skinless | 0.10‡ |
| Canned, drained | 0.04‡ |
| Heart, chicken | |
| Raw | 2.9* |
| Cooked, drained | 4.8* |
| Heart, turkey | |
| Raw | 2.8* |
| Cooked, drained | 4.8* |
| Honey | 0.08† |
| Horseradish, prepared | 1.07† |
| Ice cream | 0.5* |
| Ice cream cone | |
| Cake | 0.90† |
| Sugar | 1.03† |
| Ice milk | |
| Chocolate | 0.75† |
| Strawberry | 0.25† |
| Vanilla | 0.21† |
| Jam | |
| Peach | 0.06† |
| Strawberry | 0.01† |
| Lamb | |
| Chop, medium fat | 2.4‡ |
| Cooked, dry heat | 4.3* |
| Cooked, moist heat | 5.0* |
| Leg, medium fat | 3.2‡ |
| Raw | 3.0* |
| Separable fat, raw | 0.2* |
| Separable lean, raw | 3.0* |
| Lard | 0.2* |
| Lasagna, frozen | 0.61† |
| Lemonade, frozen, diluted | 0.01† |
| Lemon juice | 0.01† |
| Lentils, mature, dry | |
| Raw | 3.1* |
| Cooked, drained | 1.0* |
| Lettuce, head or leaf | 0.4* |
| Liver | |
| Beef, raw | 3.8* |
| cooked | 5.1* |
| Calf, raw | 3.8* |
| cooked | 6.1* |
| Chicken, raw | 2.4* |
| cooked | 3.4* |
| Turkey, raw | 2.7* |
| cooked | 3.4* |
| Lobster, steamed | 7.95† |
| Lobster, crayfish | |
| Raw | 1.8* |
| Cooked or canned | 2.2* |
| Luncheon meat, bologna | 1.5‡ |
| Macaroni | |
| Uncooked | 1.5* |
| Cooked, tender stage | 0.5* |
| Baked in frozen cheese | 0.67† |
| Baked in tomato sauce | 0.57† |
| Mangoes | 0.47† |
| Margarine | 0.2* |
| Meat loaf, homemade | 2.86† |
| Meriten, plain flavor, dry | 3.3‡ |
| Milk | |
| Fluid, whole or skim | 0.4* |
| Canned, evaporated | 0.8* |

| Food | Zinc (mg/100 g) |
|---|---|
| Chocolate drink | 0.32† |
| Dry, nonfat | 4.5* |
| Buttermilk | 0.37‡ |
| Mushroom, stems and pieces, canned | 1.1‡ |
| Mustard | |
| Brown | 0.21† |
| Yellow | 0.63† |
| Nuts | |
| Almonds, roasted | 2.56† |
| Brazil | 5.07† |
| Cashews | 4.38† |
| Filberts | 3.05† |
| Oatmeal or rolled oats | |
| Dry form | 3.4* |
| Cooked | 0.5* |
| Oat cereal, puffed, ready to eat | 3.0* |
| Oils, salad or cooking | 0.2* |
| Olives | |
| Black | 0.30† |
| Green, pimiento | 0.07† |
| Onions, mature or green, raw | 0.3* |
| Onion rings, frozen | 0.35† |
| Oranges | |
| Raw | 0.2* |
| Juice, canned, unsweetened | 0.07* |
| Juice, fresh or frozen | 0.02* |
| Sections, skinless | 0.02‡ |
| Oysters, raw or frozen | |
| Atlantic | 74.7* |
| Pacific | 9.0* |
| Pancakes, plain | 0.82† |
| Parsley, dry | 2.46† |
| Pastry, Danish | 0.84† |
| Peaches | |
| Raw | 0.2* |
| Canned, drained solid | 0.1* |
| Peanuts | |
| Raw | 2.9* |
| Roasted | 3.0* |
| Peanut butter | 2.9* |
| Peapods, snow, frozen | 0.41† |
| Pear, canned, drained | 0.055‡ |
| Peas, green, immature | |
| Raw | 0.9* |
| Boiled, drained | 0.7* |
| Canned, drained solids | 0.8* |
| Peas, green, mature seeds, dry | |
| Raw | 3.2* |
| Boiled, drained | 1.1* |
| Canned, salt free, drained | 1.3‡ |
| Pecans, unsalted | 4.1‡ |
| Pepper, green | 0.06† |
| Pineapple | |
| Crushed, canned, drained | 0.08‡ |
| Juice, canned | 0.07‡ |
| Pickle | |
| Dill | 0.27† |
| Pepper | 0.13† |
| Relish | 0.06† |
| Sweet | 0.14† |
| Tomato | 0.02† |
| Pie | |
| Apple | 0.09† |
| Blueberry | 0.01† |
| Cherry | 0.04† |

| Food | Zinc (mg/100 g) |
|---|---|
| Peach | 0.09† |
| Piecrust, homemade | 0.53† |
| Pizza, frozen | 1.22† |
| Popcorn | |
|   Unpopped | 3.9* |
|   Popped, plain | 4.1* |
|     oil and salt added | 3.0* |
| Pork | |
|   Bacon (medium fat) | 1.4‡ |
|   Boston butt, lean | |
|     Raw | 3.2* |
|     Cooked | 4.5* |
|   Ham or picnic lean | |
|     Raw | 2.8* |
|     Cooked | 4.0* |
|   Liver | 6.7‡ |
|   Loin, lean | |
|     Raw | 2.2* |
|     Cooked | 3.1* |
|   Separable fat, raw | 0.5* |
|   Trimmed lean cuts, lean | |
|     Raw | 2.7* |
|     Cooked | 3.8* |
| Pork roll sandwich meat | 2.67† |
| Pork sausage | 3.24† |
| Potato | |
|   Raw | 0.3* |
|   Boiled, drained | 0.3* |
|   Instant, mashed | 0.38† |
|   Chips | 0.81† |
|   French fries | 0.28† |
|   Knishes | 0.84† |
|   Salad | 0.24† |
|   Sticks, canned | 0.85† |
| Pretzels | 1.08† |
| Prunes | |
|   Cooked | 0.33‡ |
|   Juice, bottled | <0.01† |
|   Juice, canned | 0.12‡ |
| Pumpkin, canned | 0.19‡ |
| Puffed rice | 1.3‡ |
| Quick Cream of Wheat | |
|   Enriched, uncooked | 2.2‡ |
|   Regular, uncooked | 1.1‡ |
| Radishes | 0.27† |
| Raisins | 0.18† |
| Ravioli | |
|   Cheese, frozen | 0.76† |
|   Beef, canned | 0.48† |
| Rhubarb | |
|   Cooked, added sugar | 0.11† |
|   Raw | 0.37† |
| Rice | |
|   Brown, dry | 1.8* |
|   Cooked | 0.6* |
|   White, regular, dry | 1.3* |
|     cooked | 0.4* |
|   White, parboiled, dry | 1.1* |
|     cooked | 0.3* |
|   White, precooked, dry | 0.7* |
|     cooked | 0.2* |
|   Fried, mix | 0.69† |
|   White and wild, frozen, prepared | 0.47† |
| Rice pudding, homemade | 0.31† |
| Rice Krispies | 1.4‡ |

| Food | Zinc (mg/100 g) |
|---|---|
| Roll | |
|    Dinner | 1.22† |
|    Hamburger | 0.6* |
|    Hard | 1.13† |
| Salad dressing | |
|    Imitation mayonnaise | 0.11† |
|    Italian | 0.11† |
|    Mayonnaise | 0.16† |
|    Roquefort | 0.25† |
|    Russian | 0.43† |
|    Thousand Island | 0.14† |
|    Tomato—French | 0.08† |
| Salmon, canned (77% solid, 23% liquid) | 0.9* |
| Sauerkraut, canned | 0.81† |
| Sausages and cold cuts | |
|    Beef bologna | 1.8* |
|    Braunschweiger | 2.8* |
|    Frankfurter with beef | 2.0* |
|               with beef and pork | 1.6* |
| Sherbet | 0.24‡ |
| Shredded wheat | 3.2‡ |
| Shrimps | |
|    Raw | 1.5* |
|    Boiled, peeled, deveined | 2.1* |
|    Canned, drained solid | 2.1* |
| Soup, canned | |
|    Beef noodle | 1.41† |
|    Clam chowder | 0.58† |
|    Mushroom, cream of | 0.51† |
|    Shrimp, cream of | 0.60† |
|    Tomato | 0.07† |
|    Tomato, cream of | 0.43† |
|    Vegetable | 0.74† |
|    Vegetable beef | 1.58† |
| Soup, dry packaged | |
|    Chicken broth | 0.09† |
|    Onion | 0.03† |
|    Cup-sized, chicken noodle | 0.06† |
|             lobster bisque | 0.06† |
|             split pea | 0.24† |
| Sour cream | 0.27† |
| Spaghetti, uncooked | 1.7‡ |
| Spinach | |
|    Raw | 0.8* |
|    Boiled, drained | 0.7* |
|    Canned, solid and liquid | 0.6* |
|    Canned, solid | 0.8* |
|    Creamed | 0.61† |
|    Frozen, cooked | 0.37‡ |
| Squash, zucchini | |
|    Cooked | 0.18† |
|    Uncooked, frozen | 0.3‡ |
| Strawberry | 0.08* |
| Sugar | |
|    White, granulated | 0.06* |
|    Brown | 0.029‡ |
|    Powder | <0.02‡ |
| Sweet potatoes | |
|    Raw | 0.08† |
|    Canned | 0.16‡ |
| Sustagen, imitation vanilla flavor, dry | 2.9‡ |
| Syrup, pancake | 0.04* |
| Tea | |
|    Dry leaves | 3.3* |
|    Fluid beverage | 0.02* |
|    Instant beverage | 0.06† |

| Food | Zinc (mg/100 g) |
|---|---|
| Tomato, ripe | |
|   Raw | 0.2* |
|   Boiled, solids and liquids | 0.2* |
|   Canned, solids and liquids | 0.2* |
| Tomato catsup | 0.26† |
| Tomato sauce | |
|   Meat | 0.58† |
|   Mushroom | 0.53† |
| Tomato juice, salt free | 0.065‡ |
| Topping | |
|   Nondairy, whipped | 0.05† |
|   Sundae | 0.02† |
| Tuna fish, canned in oil | |
|   85% solid, 15% liquid | 1.0* |
|   Drained solids | 1.1* |
|   Casserole, dehydrated | 0.41† |
|   Salad | 0.32† |
| Turkey | |
|   Dark meat | |
|     Raw | 3.1* |
|     Cooked, dry heat | 4.4* |
|   Light meat | |
|     Raw | 1.6* |
|     Cooked, dry heat | 2.1* |
|   Neck meat | |
|     Raw | 5.0* |
|     Cooked | 6.4* |
|   Skin | |
|     Raw | 1.3* |
|     Cooked | 2.1* |
| Veal, separable lean | |
|   Raw | 2.8* |
|   Cooked, dry heat | 4.1* |
|   Cooked, moist heat | 4.2* |
| Veal, separable fat, raw | 0.05* |
| Vegetables | |
|   Bavarian style, frozen | 0.34† |
|   Mixed, frozen | 0.32† |
| Vinegar | 0.10† |
| Watermelon | 0.085‡ |
| Walnut, unsalted | 3.2‡ |
| Wheat, whole grain | |
|   Hard | 3.4* |
|   Soft | 2.7* |
|   White | 2.2* |
|   Durum | 2.7* |
| Wheat, flours | |
|   Whole | 2.4* |
|   80% extraction | 1.5* |
|   All-purpose | 0.7* |
|   Bread flour | 0.8* |
|   Cake or pastry flour | 0.3* |
| Wheat germ, crude | 14.3* |
| Wheat germ | 16.7† |
| Wheat cereal, whole meal | |
|   Dry form | 3.6* |
|   Cooked | 0.5* |
| Wheat, cereals ready to eat | |
|   Flakes | 2.3* |
|   Germ, toasted | 15.4* |
|   Puffed | 2.6* |
|   Shredded | 2.8* |
|   Wheaties | 2.4‡ |

* Murphy, E. W.; Willis, B. W.; and Watt, B. K.: Provisional tables on the zinc content of foods. J. Am. Diet. Assoc. 66: 345, 1975.
† Freeland, J. H., and Cousins, R. J.: Zinc content of selected foods. J. Am. Diet. Assoc. 68: 526, 1976.
‡ Gormican, A.: Inorganic elements in foods used in hospital menus. J. Am. Diet. Assoc. 56: 398, 1970.

# Cholesterol and Fatty Acid Composition of Foods

**Per 100 g Edible Portion**

| Food | Total fat (g) | Total saturated fatty acid (g) | Total unsaturated fatty acid | Oleic acid | Linoleic | Linolenic | Arachidonic | Cholesterol (mg) |
|---|---|---|---|---|---|---|---|---|
| | | | | | | | | |

Where the header spans are: "Unsaturated fatty acid (g)" spans Total unsaturated fatty acid / Oleic acid / Linoleic / Linolenic / Arachidonic; and "Polyunsaturated fatty acids" spans Linoleic / Linolenic / Arachidonic.

| Food | Total fat (g) | Total saturated fatty acid (g) | Total unsaturated fatty acid | Oleic acid | Linoleic | Linolenic | Arachidonic | Cholesterol (mg) |
|---|---|---|---|---|---|---|---|---|
| *Beef* | | | | | | | | |
| Composite of retail cut | | | | | | | | |
|   Total edible, | | | | | | | | |
|     cooked, bone removed | | | | | | | | 94 |
|   Lean, trimmed of separable | | | | | | | | |
|     fat, cooked | | | | | | | | 91 |
| Trimmed to retail level | | | | | | | | |
|   Brisket, cooked | | | | | | | | |
|     Total edible (69% lean) | | | | | | | | |
|       (31% fat) | 34.80 | 14.60 | 18.30 | 14.10 | 0.80 | 0.50 | 0.10 | |
|     Separable lean | 10.50 | 4.50 | 5.10 | 3.90 | 0.40 | 0.10 | 0.10 | |
|   Chuck, 5th rib, cooked | | | | | | | | |
|     Total edible (69% lean) | | | | | | | | |
|       (31% fat) | 36.70 | 15.30 | 19.30 | 14.80 | 0.90 | 0.50 | 0.10 | |
|     Separable lean | 13.90 | 6.00 | 6.70 | 5.10 | 0.50 | 0.10 | 0.10 | |
|   Flank steak, | | | | | | | | |
|     cooked (100% lean) | 7.30 | 3.10 | 3.60 | 2.67 | 0.28 | 0.06 | 0.07 | |
|   Porterhouse steak, cooked | | | | | | | | |
|     Total edible (57% lean) | | | | | | | | |
|       (43% fat) | 42.20 | 17.60 | 22.40 | 17.30 | 0.90 | 0.60 | 0.10 | |
|   T-bone steak, cooked | | | | | | | | |
|     Separable lean | 10.30 | 4.40 | 5.00 | 3.80 | 0.40 | 0.10 | 0.10 | |
|   Sirloin steak, cooked | | | | | | | | |
|     Separable lean | 7.70 | 3.30 | 3.80 | 2.82 | 0.30 | 0.06 | 0.08 | |
|   Short plate, total edible, | | | | | | | | |
|     simmered (58% lean) | | | | | | | | |
|       (42% fat) | 42.80 | 17.80 | 22.80 | 17.50 | 0.90 | 0.60 | 0.10 | |
|   Short plate, separable lean | | | | | | | | |
|     simmered | 10.50 | 4.50 | 5.10 | 3.80 | 0.40 | 0.10 | 0.10 | |
|   Entire rib, cooked | | | | | | | | |
|     Total edible (64% lean) | | | | | | | | |
|       (36% fat) | 39.40 | 16.50 | 20.70 | 16.00 | 0.90 | 0.50 | 0.10 | |
|     Separable lean | 13.40 | 5.90 | 6.40 | 4.90 | 0.50 | 0.10 | 0.10 | |
|   Round steak, separable lean, | | | | | | | | |
|     cooked, broiled | 6.40 | 2.70 | 3.20 | 2.34 | 0.25 | 0.05 | 0.06 | |
|   Rump, separable lean, | | | | | | | | |
|     cooked, roasted, not | | | | | | | | |
|     less than 77% lean | 9.30 | 3.90 | 4.60 | 3.40 | 0.36 | 0.07 | 0.09 | |
|   Ground beef, | | | | | | | | |
|     cooked, pan broiled | 22.70 | 9.50 | 11.90 | 9.10 | 0.60 | 0.30 | 0.10 | |
|   Heart, cooked, braised | 5.70 | 1.80 | 2.60 | 1.32 | 0.74 | 0.01 | 0.39 | 274 |
|   Liver, cooked, fried in | | | | | | | | |
|     margarine | 10.60 | 2.90 | 6.10 | 4.10 | 1.10 | 0.10 | 0.30 | 438 |
|   Kidney, cooked | | | | | | | | 804 |
|   Beef sausages | | | | | | | | |
|     Bologna | 29.20 | 11.90 | 15.30 | 12.40 | 0.70 | 0.20 | — | 65 |
|     Frankfurters | 29.10 | 11.20 | 15.80 | 12.30 | 0.90 | 0.30 | — | |
|     Cervelat | 27.20 | 11.00 | 14.40 | 11.20 | 0.80 | 0.20 | — | |
|     Salami (cooked) | 20.60 | 8.70 | 10.60 | 8.40 | 0.60 | 0.20 | — | |
|   Beef and vegetable stew, | | | | | | | | |
|     canned | 3.10 | | | | | | | 14 |
|   Beef, dried, chipped, creamed | 10.30 | | | | | | | 27 |
|   Beef pot pie, | | | | | | | | |
|     commercial, frozen, | | | | | | | | |
|       unheated | 9.90 | | | | | | | 18 |
|   Brains, raw | 8.60 | | | | | | | >2,000 |

| Food | Total fat (g) | Total saturated fatty acid (g) | Unsaturated fatty acid (g) | | | | | Cholesterol (mg) |
|---|---|---|---|---|---|---|---|---|
| | | | Total unsaturated fatty acid | Oleic acid | Polyunsaturated fatty acids | | | |
| | | | | | Linoleic | Linolenic | Arachidonic | |

| Food | Total fat (g) | Total saturated fatty acid (g) | Total unsaturated fatty acid | Oleic acid | Linoleic | Linolenic | Arachidonic | Cholesterol (mg) |
|---|---|---|---|---|---|---|---|---|
| *Cereals* | | | | | | | | |
| Barley, whole grain | 2.80 | 0.48 | 1.52 | 0.24 | 1.14 | 0.13 | | |
| Corn bread, baked from mix made with egg, milk | 8.40 | | | | | | | 69 |
| Corn grits, degermed, cooked | 0.10 | 0.01 | 0.07 | 0.02 | 0.05 | — | | |
| Cornmeal, degermed, cooked | 0.20 | 0.02 | 0.14 | 0.04 | 0.10 | | | |
| Corn pudding | 4.70 | | | | | | | 42 |
| Cornstarch | 0.60 | 0.07 | 0.44 | 0.13 | 0.31 | — | | |
| Farina, enriched, cooked | 0.20 | 0.03 | 0.10 | 0.01 | 0.09 | | | |
| Millet, whole grain | 4.10 | 0.86 | 2.67 | 0.83 | 1.69 | 0.13 | | |
| Muffins, plain, home recipe | 10.10 | 2.50 | | 5.00 | 2.50 | | | 53 |
| Noodles | | | | | | | | |
|   Whole egg, cooked | 1.50 | 0.70 | | 0.70 | tr. | | | 31 |
|   Chow mein, canned | 23.50 | | | | | | | 12 |
| Oats, puffed | | | | | | | | |
|   Without added ingredient | 5.50 | 1.02 | 4.18 | 1.93 | 2.13 | 0.11 | | |
|   With added nutrients, sugar covered | 3.40 | 0.63 | 2.60 | 1.20 | 1.32 | 0.07 | | |
| Oatmeal, cooked | 1.00 | 0.17 | 0.76 | 0.35 | 0.39 | 0.02 | | |
| Pancake from mix made with eggs and milk | 7.30 | 3.60 | | 3.60 | tr. | | | 74 |
| Rice, white, enriched, cooked | 0.20 | 0.05 | 0.12 | 0.05 | 0.07 | — | | |
| Rye flour | 1.40 | 0.16 | 0.77 | 0.13 | 0.56 | 0.07 | | |
| Sorghum, whole grain | 3.30 | 0.48 | 2.74 | 1.15 | 1.46 | 0.09 | | |
| Waffles, baked from mix made with eggs and milk | 10.60 | 4.00 | | 4.00 | 1.30 | | | 60 |
| Wheat, whole grain | | | | | | | | |
|   Hard, red spring | 2.70 | 0.37 | 1.56 | 0.25 | 1.20 | 0.10 | | |
|   Hard, red winter | 2.50 | 0.35 | 1.47 | 0.28 | 1.08 | 0.10 | | |
|   White | 2.00 | 0.30 | 1.14 | 0.18 | 0.88 | 0.07 | | |
| Wheat flours | | | | | | | | |
|   All-purpose | 1.40 | 0.23 | 0.72 | 0.11 | 0.58 | 0.03 | | |
| Wheat bran | 4.60 | 0.74 | 3.09 | 0.71 | 2.20 | 0.16 | | |
| Wheat germ | 10.90 | 1.88 | 8.18 | 1.54 | 5.86 | 0.74 | | |
| Wheat products | | | | | | | | |
|   Breakfast cereals | | | | | | | | |
|     Shredded wheat | 2.50 | 0.42 | 1.73 | 0.40 | 1.22 | 0.11 | | |
|     Wheat flakes | 2.40 | 0.36 | 1.55 | 0.34 | 1.12 | 0.09 | | |
|     Wheat meal | 1.40 | 0.26 | 0.75 | 0.10 | 0.65 | | | |
| Wheat, durum, semolina | 1.80 | 0.33 | 0.90 | 0.17 | 0.68 | 0.04 | | |
| *Dairy products* | | | | | | | | |
| Butter | 80.10 | 49.80 | 26.10 | 20.10 | 1.80 | 1.20 | | 250 |
| Buttermilk, fluid, cultured, made from nonfat milk | 0.10 | | | | | | | 2 |
| *Cheeses* | | | | | | | | |
| Natural cheeses | | | | | | | | |
|   Bel Paese | 25.10 | 15.70 | 8.00 | 6.56 | 0.22 | 0.26 | | |
|   Blue | 29.60 | 19.10 | 9.10 | 7.04 | 0.54 | 0.26 | | 87 |
|   Brick | 29.40 | 18.00 | 10.00 | 7.80 | 0.46 | 0.37 | | 90 |
|   Camembert | 26.10 | 16.40 | 8.50 | 6.44 | 0.43 | 0.34 | | 92 |
|   Cheddar | 32.80 | 20.20 | 10.70 | 8.24 | 0.51 | 0.42 | | 99 |
|   Colby | 30.80 | 19.40 | 9.80 | 7.50 | 0.65 | 0.27 | | 96 |
|   Cottage, creamed | 4.00 | 2.60 | 1.20 | 0.91 | 0.09 | 0.03 | | 19 |
|   Cottage, uncreamed | 0.40 | 0.20 | 0.10 | 0.08 | 0.01 | — | | 7 |
|   Cream cheese | 33.80 | 21.20 | 10.60 | 8.08 | 0.79 | 0.45 | | 111 |
|   Edam | 27.90 | 18.10 | 8.30 | 6.68 | 0.36 | 0.21 | | 102 |

| Food | Total fat (g) | Total saturated fatty acid (g) | Total unsaturated fatty acid | Oleic acid | Linoleic | Linolenic | Arachidonic | Cholesterol (mg) |
|---|---|---|---|---|---|---|---|---|
| | | | | | **Unsaturated fatty acid (g)** | | | |
| | | | | | | **Polyunsaturated fatty acids** | | |
| Farmer's whole milk | 18.10 | 10.90 | 6.20 | 4.80 | 0.38 | 0.26 | | |
| Feta | 24.80 | 17.30 | 6.10 | 4.63 | 0.38 | 0.31 | | 89 |
| Fontina | 30.20 | 18.60 | 10.00 | 6.89 | 0.84 | 0.77 | | 118 |
| Gzetost | 29.60 | 19.20 | 8.90 | 6.99 | 0.51 | 0.43 | | |
| Gouda | 27.40 | 17.60 | 8.40 | 6.39 | 0.26 | 0.39 | | 114 |
| Gruyère | 32.00 | 18.70 | 11.70 | 8.49 | 1.29 | 0.43 | | 111 |
| Leyden | 24.10 | 15.10 | 7.90 | 6.03 | 0.16 | 0.46 | | |
| Limburger | 26.80 | 16.50 | 9.00 | 7.06 | 0.33 | 0.15 | | 98 |
| Mozzarella low moisture, part skim | 16.40 | 10.20 | 5.10 | 3.98 | 0.34 | 0.14 | | 66 |
| Mozzarella low moisture, whole | 26.50 | 16.70 | 8.40 | 6.37 | 0.61 | 0.23 | | 97 |
| Muenster | 29.80 | 19.00 | 9.30 | 7.29 | 0.43 | 0.23 | | 91 |
| Neufchâtel | 24.20 | 15.40 | 7.70 | 5.85 | 0.46 | 0.21 | | 76 |
| Parmesan | 26.50 | 16.80 | 8.30 | 6.83 | 0.28 | 0.30 | | 95 |
| Port | 29.80 | 17.60 | 10.60 | 8.51 | 0.40 | 0.37 | | 125 |
| Provolone | 26.00 | 16.50 | 8.10 | 6.26 | 0.51 | 0.27 | | 101 |
| Ricotta whole milk | 14.60 | 9.30 | 4.50 | 3.22 | 0.31 | 0.13 | | 51 |
| part skim | 8.60 | 5.20 | 2.70 | 2.09 | 0.19 | 0.07 | | 32 |
| Roquefort | 33.80 | 21.20 | 10.80 | 8.22 | 0.68 | 0.78 | | 118 |
| Samsae | 21.40 | 13.40 | 6.90 | 5.41 | 0.31 | 0.33 | | |
| Swiss | 27.60 | 17.60 | 8.70 | 6.53 | 0.49 | 0.55 | | 100 |
| Tilsit | 28.80 | 18.60 | 8.70 | 6.73 | 0.44 | 0.36 | | 104 |
| Pasteurized process cheese American | 28.90 | 18.00 | 9.50 | 7.21 | 0.64 | 0.33 | | 90 |
| Cheddar | 29.60 | 18.30 | 9.80 | 7.55 | 0.74 | 0.37 | | |
| Swiss | 24.50 | 15.60 | 7.60 | 5.91 | 0.30 | 0.32 | | 93 |
| Pasteurized process cheese spread, plain | 20.80 | 13.10 | 6.70 | 5.13 | 0.39 | 0.22 | | 64 |
| Cheese sauce | 13.60 | | | | | | | 18 |
| Cheese soufflé, home recipe | 17.10 | | | | | | | 167 |
| Creams Half and half | 11.70 | 7.30 | 3.80 | 2.94 | 0.26 | 0.17 | | 43 |
| Light cream | 20.60 | 12.80 | 6.70 | 5.18 | 0.47 | 0.30 | | 66 |
| Light whipping cream | 32.40 | 20.20 | 10.60 | 8.13 | 0.65 | 0.28 | | 113 |
| Heavy cream | 37.80 | 23.50 | 12.30 | 9.50 | 0.85 | 0.55 | | 133 |
| Powdered cream | 29.10 | 17.90 | 9.70 | 7.26 | 0.40 | 0.32 | | |
| Sour cream | 18.40 | 11.50 | 6.00 | 4.63 | 0.42 | 0.27 | | 66 |
| Whipped topping (pressurized) | 23.30 | | | | | | | 85 |
| Custards, baked | 5.00 | 2.50 | 2.00 | 1.50 | 0.29 | 0.05 | | 105 |
| Ice cream Chocolate chip | 11.00 | 6.30 | 4.10 | 2.40 | 0.29 | 0.10 | | 40 |
| Vanilla | 12.30 | 7.70 | 4.00 | 3.09 | 0.28 | 0.18 | | 50 |
| Sandwich | 8.20 | 4.70 | 3.10 | 2.39 | 0.36 | 0.16 | | |
| Ice milk | 5.10 | 3.20 | 1.70 | 1.28 | 0.12 | 0.07 | | 20 |
| Milk Fluid Whole | 3.50 | 2.20 | 1.10 | 0.88 | 0.08 | 0.05 | | 14 |
| Low fat—1% fat | 1.00 | 0.60 | 0.30 | 0.25 | 0.02 | 0.01 | | 6 |
| 2% fat | 2.00 | 1.20 | 0.70 | 0.50 | 0.05 | 0.03 | | 9 |
| Canned, concentrated undiluted Evaporated, unsweetened | 8.00 | 4.90 | 2.70 | 2.21 | 0.18 | 0.08 | | 31 |
| Condensed, sweetened | 8.70 | 5.50 | 2.80 | 2.19 | 0.22 | 0.12 | | 34 |
| Dried Buttermilk, sweet cream | 5.30 | 3.30 | 1.70 | 1.33 | 0.12 | 0.08 | | 69 |
| Skim | 0.80 | 0.50 | 0.30 | 0.22 | 0.02 | 0.01 | | 22 |
| Whole | 26.80 | 16.50 | 8.60 | 6.22 | 0.46 | 0.21 | | 109 |

| Food | Total fat (g) | Total saturated fatty acid (g) | Total unsaturated fatty acid | Oleic acid | Linoleic | Linolenic | Arachidonic | Cholesterol (mg) |
|---|---|---|---|---|---|---|---|---|
| Flavored | | | | | | | | |
| Chocolate milk with whole milk | 3.40 | 2.10 | 1.10 | 0.88 | 0.08 | 0.05 | | 13 |
| Chocolate milkshake | 4.40 | 3.10 | 1.10 | 0.87 | 0.07 | 0.04 | | |
| Hot chocolate with whole milk | 5.00 | 3.10 | 1.70 | 1.38 | 0.12 | 0.05 | | 12 |
| Hot cocoa with whole milk | 4.60 | 2.80 | 1.50 | 1.21 | 0.11 | 0.06 | | 14 |
| Welsh rarebit | 13.60 | | | | | | | 31 |
| Whey, dried | | | | | | | | |
| Sweet | 1.00 | 0.60 | 0.30 | 0.20 | 0.02 | 0.01 | | |
| Cottage cheese | 0.50 | 0.30 | 0.20 | 0.11 | 0.02 | — | | |
| White sauce | | | | | | | | |
| Thin | 8.70 | | | | | | | 14 |
| Medium | 12.50 | 4.00 | | 4.00 | 0.25 | | | 13 |
| Thick | 15.60 | | | | | | | 13 |
| Yogurt, natural | | | | | | | | |
| Made from whole milk | 3.40 | 2.20 | 1.00 | 0.78 | 0.07 | 0.03 | | 14 |
| Made from skim milk | | | | | | | | |
| Plain or vanilla | 1.50 | 1.00 | 0.40 | 0.34 | 0.03 | 0.01 | | 8 |
| Fruit flavored (all kinds) | 1.20 | | | | | | | 7 |

*Desserts*

| Food | Total fat (g) | Total saturated fatty acid (g) | Total unsaturated fatty acid | Oleic acid | Linoleic | Linolenic | Arachidonic | Cholesterol (mg) |
|---|---|---|---|---|---|---|---|---|
| Cakes from home recipe | | | | | | | | |
| Fruit cake, dark | 15.30 | tr. | | 6.70 | tr. | | | 45 |
| Cakes, baked from mix | | | | | | | | |
| Angel food, made with water and flavorings | 0.20 | | | | | | | 0 |
| Chocolate (devil's food), 2 layer, made with egg, water, chocolate frosting | 13.00 | 4.35 | | 5.80 | 1.50 | | | 47 |
| Gingerbread made with water | 6.80 | 1.60 | | 3.20 | 1.60 | | | 1 |
| White, 2 layer, made with egg white, water, chocolate frosting | 10.70 | 4.20 | | 4.20 | 1.40 | | | 2 |
| Yellow, 2 layer, made with egg, water, chocolate frosting | 11.30 | | | | | | | 48 |
| Cookies | | | | | | | | |
| Lady fingers | 7.80 | | | | | | | 356 |
| Cream puffs with custard filling | 13.90 | | | | | | | 144 |
| Pies, baked | | | | | | | | |
| Apple | 11.10 | 2.90 | | 5.30 | 2.20 | | | 0 |
| Custard | 11.10 | 3.80 | | 4.60 | 1.50 | | | 105 |
| Lemon chiffon | 12.60 | | | | | | | 169 |
| Lemon meringue | 10.20 | 3.30 | | 5.10 | 1.70 | | | 93 |
| Peach | 10.70 | | | | | | | 0 |
| Pumpkin | 11.20 | 3.80 | | 4.60 | 1.50 | | | 61 |
| Popovers, home recipe | 9.20 | | | | | | | 147 |
| Puddings | | | | | | | | |
| Chocolate, home recipe | 4.20 | 2.60 | 1.40 | 1.12 | 0.10 | 0.05 | | |
| Chocolate, made from mix | 3.00 | | | | | | | 12 |
| Vanilla, home recipe | 3.50 | 2.20 | 1.10 | 0.88 | 0.08 | 0.05 | | 14 |
| Tapioca cream | 4.70 | 2.30 | 1.90 | 1.40 | 0.28 | 0.05 | | 97 |

*Chicken*

| Food | Total fat (g) | Total saturated fatty acid (g) | Total unsaturated fatty acid | Oleic acid | Linoleic | Linolenic | Arachidonic | Cholesterol (mg) |
|---|---|---|---|---|---|---|---|---|
| Broiler-fryer | | | | | | | | |
| Dark meat, roasted | 10.80 | 3.05 | 6.55 | 3.25 | 2.30 | 0.13 | 0.21 | 91 |
| Light meat, roasted | 6.38 | 1.86 | 3.66 | 1.77 | 1.27 | 0.07 | 0.16 | 80 |
| Flesh and skin only, roasted | 10.30 | 3.07 | 6.28 | 3.09 | 2.21 | 0.12 | 0.21 | 87 |

| Food | Total fat (g) | Total saturated fatty acid (g) | Unsaturated fatty acid (g) | | | | | Cholesterol (mg) |
|---|---|---|---|---|---|---|---|---|
| | | | Total unsaturated fatty acid | Oleic acid | Polyunsaturated fatty acids | | | |
| | | | | | Linoleic | Linolenic | Arachidonic | |
| Flesh only, roasted | 6.35 | 1.93 | 3.62 | 1.71 | 1.22 | 0.05 | 0.22 | 85 |
| Skin only, roasted | 29.70 | 8.62 | 19.30 | 9.84 | 7.05 | 0.48 | 0.17 | |
| Heart, cooked | 7.20 | | | | | | | 231 |
| Liver, raw | 4.50 | 1.66 | 2.08 | 0.96 | 0.56 | 0.09 | 0.22 | 555 |
| Hen, stewing | | | | | | | | |
| Dark meat, stewed | 9.50 | 2.61 | 5.45 | 2.65 | 1.85 | 0.08 | 0.28 | |
| Light meat, stewed | 4.70 | 1.37 | 2.32 | 1.03 | 0.74 | 0.03 | 0.21 | |
| Chicken à la king, home recipe | 14.00 | | | | | | | 76 |
| Chicken pot pie, commercial, frozen, unheated | 11.50 | | | | | | | 13 |
| Chop suey, with meat, canned | 3.20 | | | | | | | 12 |
| Chow mein, chix, no noodles, canned | 0.10 | | | | | | | 3 |
| Duck, raw, flesh plus skin | 28.60 | 6.86 | 17.70 | 13.00 | 3.09 | 0.22 | 0 | |
| *Eggs*, chicken, whole | | | | | | | | |
| Fresh or frozen | 11.30 | 3.40 | 6.00 | 4.16 | 1.26 | 0.03 | 0.09 | 504 |
| Cooked in shell | 11.30 | 3.40 | 6.00 | 4.16 | 1.26 | 0.03 | 0.09 | |
| Poached | 11.20 | 3.40 | 5.90 | 4.12 | 1.25 | 0.03 | 0.09 | |
| Scrambled in margarine | 12.60 | 3.70 | 7.20 | 5.20 | 1.28 | 0.07 | 0.08 | 411 |
| Whites, fresh, frozen, dried | tr. | | | | | | | 0 |
| Yolks | | | | | | | | |
| Fresh | 33.50 | 10.10 | 17.70 | 12.30 | 3.74 | 0.09 | 0.28 | 1,480 |
| Frozen, commercial | 29.40 | 8.90 | 15.50 | 10.80 | 3.28 | 0.08 | 0.25 | 1,270 |
| Frozen, sugared | 26.30 | 7.90 | 13.90 | 9.67 | 2.93 | 0.07 | 0.22 | |
| Dried, standard or stabilized | 58.40 | 17.60 | 30.90 | 21.50 | 6.51 | 0.16 | 0.49 | 2,630 |
| Eggs, duck, whole, fresh | 14.50 | 4.00 | 8.10 | 6.44 | 0.54 | 0.04 | 0.34 | |
| Eggs, goose, whole, fresh | 13.30 | 3.60 | 7.70 | 5.46 | 0.70 | 0.78 | 0.23 | |
| Eggs, turkey, whole, fresh | 11.80 | 3.70 | 6.30 | 3.94 | 1.22 | 0.07 | 0.12 | |
| *Fish and shellfish* | | | | | | | | |
| Anchovy, raw fillet | 6.40 | 1.66 | 4.28 | 0.80 | 0.12 | 0.08 | 0.02 | |
| Caviar, sturgeon, granular | 15.00 | | | | | | | >300 |
| Cod, raw, fillet | 0.69 | 0.11 | 0.16 | 0.06 | — | — | 0.02 | 50 |
| Cod, dried, salted | 0.70 | | | | | | | 82 |
| Flounder, raw, fillet | 1.20 | 0.28 | 0.56 | 0.11 | 0.01 | 0.01 | 0.04 | 50 |
| Haddock, raw, fillet | 0.66 | 0.11 | 0.27 | 0.06 | 0.01 | — | 0.01 | 60 |
| Halibut, raw, fillet | 1.10 | 0.20 | 0.60 | 0.10 | — | — | 0.02 | 50 |
| Herring, raw, fillet | 11.10 | 2.64 | 7.38 | 2.10 | 0.12 | 0.03 | 0.02 | 85 |
| Mackerel, raw, fillet | 9.80 | 2.42 | 6.88 | 1.60 | 0.14 | 0.10 | 0.12 | |
| Ocean perch, raw, fillet | 2.50 | 0.41 | 1.81 | 0.44 | 0.03 | 0.04 | 0.18 | |
| Pike, raw, fillet | 0.90 | 0.16 | 0.53 | 0.08 | 0.05 | 0.05 | 0.05 | |
| Roe, salmon, raw | 10.40 | | | | | | | 360 |
| Salmon, pink, raw, fillet | 5.20 | 0.85 | 3.89 | 0.83 | 0.08 | 0.05 | 0.03 | 35 |
| Salmon, sockeye, raw, fillet | 8.90 | 1.82 | 6.21 | 0.94 | 1.40 | 0.31 | — | 35 |
| Salmon, canned | 6.70 | 0.75 | 4.52 | 0.75 | 0.15 | 0.41 | 0.81 | 35 |
| Sardines, canned in oil | | | | | | | | |
| Solid and liquid | 24.40 | | | | | | | 120 |
| Drained, solid | 11.10 | | | | | | | 140 |
| Sturgeon, raw, fillet | 3.30 | 0.76 | 2.14 | 1.40 | 0.04 | 0.03 | 0.04 | |
| Trout, raw, fillet | 4.50 | 0.99 | 3.01 | 1.00 | 0.21 | 0.10 | 0.09 | 55 |
| Tuna, raw, white meat | 8.00 | 3.14 | 5.20 | 1.40 | 0.15 | 0.19 | 0.14 | 65 |
| Tuna, canned in water | 0.60 | 0.16 | 2.24 | 0.08 | — | — | 0.01 | 63 |
| Whitefish, raw, fillet | 5.20 | 0.86 | 3.88 | 1.30 | 0.26 | 0.17 | 0.18 | |
| Clams | | | | | | | | |
| Meat only, raw | 1.60 | | | | | | | 50 |
| Canned, drained solids | 2.50 | | | | | | | 63 |
| Crab, all kinds | | | | | | | | |
| Steam in shell, meat only | 1.90 | | | | | | | 100 |
| Canned, meat only | 2.50 | | | | | | | 101 |

| Food | Total fat (g) | Total saturated fatty acid (g) | Unsaturated fatty acid (g) | | | | | Cholesterol (mg) |
|---|---|---|---|---|---|---|---|---|
| | | | Total unsaturated fatty acid | Oleic acid | Polyunsaturated fatty acids | | | |
| | | | | | Linoleic | Linolenic | Arachidonic | |
| Crab, deviled | 9.40 | | | | | | | 102 |
| Crab, imperial | 7.60 | | | | | | | 140 |
| Lobster, cooked, meat only | 1.50 | | | | | | | 85 |
| Lobster Newburg | 10.60 | | | | | | | 182 |
| Oysters, raw | | | | | | | | |
|   Meat only, | | | | | | | | |
|     Eastern and Pacific | 2.00 | | | | | | | 50 |
|   Canned, solids and liquid | 2.20 | | | | | | | 45 |
| Scallops, muscle only | | | | | | | | |
|   Raw | 0.20 | | | | | | | 35 |
|   Steamed | 1.40 | | | | | | | 53 |
| Shrimp, raw | | | | | | | | |
|   Flesh only | 0.80 | | | | | | | 150 |
|   Canned, drained, solid | 1.10 | | | | | | | 150 |
| *Frog legs*, raw | 0.20 | | | | | | | 50 |
| *Goose*, raw, | | | | | | | | |
|   flesh and skin | 33.60 | 8.98 | 19.30 | 15.50 | 2.67 | 0 | 0 | |
| *Lamb* | | | | | | | | |
| Composite of retail cut | | | | | | | | |
|   Total edible, cooked | | | | | | | | 98 |
|   Separable lean, cooked | | | | | | | | 100 |
| Leg, cooked, roasted | | | | | | | | |
|   Total edible (83% lean) | | | | | | | | |
|     (17% fat) | 21.20 | 9.57 | 9.70 | 7.92 | 0.79 | 0.34 | 0.11 | |
|   Separable lean | 9.60 | 4.03 | 4.24 | 3.40 | 0.36 | 0.09 | 0.13 | |
| Loin, cooked, broiled | | | | | | | | |
|   Total edible (66% lean) | | | | | | | | |
|     (34% fat) | 32.40 | 15.10 | 15.10 | 12.40 | 1.23 | 0.61 | 0.05 | |
|   Separable lean | 6.13 | 2.57 | 2.71 | 2.17 | 0.23 | 0.06 | 0.08 | |
| Rib, cooked, broiled | | | | | | | | |
|   Total edible (68% lean) | | | | | | | | |
|     (32% fat) | 36.00 | 16.80 | 16.80 | 13.80 | 1.36 | 0.68 | 0.06 | |
|   Separable lean | 7.06 | 2.95 | 3.11 | 2.50 | 0.26 | 0.07 | 0.09 | |
| Shoulder, cooked, roasted | | | | | | | | |
|   Total edible (74% lean) | | | | | | | | |
|     (26% fat) | 26.90 | 12.60 | 12.50 | 10.30 | 1.01 | 0.50 | 0.05 | |
|   Separable lean | 5.60 | 2.33 | 2.45 | 1.98 | 0.21 | 0.05 | 0.07 | |
| Heart, lean, | | | | | | | | |
|   cooked, braised | 7.95 | 2.28 | 3.33 | 1.76 | 0.97 | 0.10 | 0.33 | |
| Kidney, raw | 3.85 | 1.41 | 1.51 | 0.90 | 0.27 | 0.04 | 0.22 | 375 |
| Liver, raw | 4.32 | 1.52 | 1.46 | 0.79 | 0.29 | 0.06 | 0.24 | 300 |
| Liver, cooked, broiled | | | | | | | | |
|   with margarine | 12.50 | 3.40 | 7.47 | 4.90 | 1.51 | 0.15 | 0.36 | 438 |
| *Macaroni and cheese* | | | | | | | | |
|   Baked, home recipe | 11.10 | | | | | | | 21 |
| *Fats* | | | | | | | | |
| Lard | 100 | 39.60 | 56.10 | 40.90 | 9.96 | 1.44 | 0.37 | 95 |
| Margarine | | | | | | | | |
|   All vegetable fat | 81.00 | | | | | | | 0 |
|   ⅔ animal fat, | | | | | | | | |
|   ⅓ vegetable fat | 81.00 | | | | | | | 50 |
| Nuts | | | | | | | | |
|   Acorn | 2.80 | 0.51 | 2.13 | 1.58 | 0.50 | 0.04 | | |
|   Almond | 53.90 | 4.31 | 47.00 | 36.50 | 9.86 | 0.26 | | |
|   Almond, bitter | 53.90 | 4.19 | 47.20 | 36.90 | 10.10 | 0 | | |
|   Apricot seed | 47.40 | 4.04 | 40.80 | 26.30 | 14.00 | 0.14 | | |

| Food | Total fat (g) | Total saturated fatty acid (g) | Unsaturated fatty acid (g) | | | | | Cholesterol (mg) |
|---|---|---|---|---|---|---|---|---|
| | | | Total unsaturated fatty acid | Oleic acid | Polyunsaturated fatty acids | | | |
| | | | | | Linoleic | Linolenic | Arachidonic | |
| Beechnut | 50.30 | 6.28 | 39.90 | 19.70 | 20.20 | 0 | | |
| Betel nut palm | 17.70 | 13.10 | 2.33 | 1.25 | 1.08 | 0 | | |
| Brazil nut | 68.20 | 17.40 | 47.90 | 22.20 | 25.40 | 0 | | |
| Cashew | 45.60 | 9.20 | 33.90 | 26.20 | 7.25 | 0.17 | | |
| Chestnut, European | 2.70 | 9.44 | 2.04 | 0.97 | 0.94 | 0.11 | | |
| Coconut | 35.50 | 31.20 | 2.82 | 2.03 | 0.66 | 0 | | |
| Filbert | 64.70 | 4.61 | 56.70 | 49.80 | 6.60 | 0.16 | | |
| Horsechestnut | 8.30 | 0.58 | 6.79 | 4.31 | 2.39 | 0.08 | | |
| Macadamia | 75.70 | 10.95 | 59.50 | 43.20 | 1.15 | 1.06 | | |
| Peanut | 49.70 | 9.43 | 37.80 | 22.90 | 14.40 | 0.55 | | |
| Pecan | 71.40 | 6.09 | 61.20 | 42.90 | 17.00 | 0.86 | | |
| Pili nut | 63.00 | 24.80 | 35.50 | 29.50 | 6.02 | 0 | | |
| Pine nut | 51.00 | 6.15 | 41.80 | 19.00 | 22.20 | 0.38 | | |
| Pistachio | 53.60 | 7.41 | 43.30 | 36.00 | 6.75 | 0.28 | | |
| Shea nut | 46.00 | 19.00 | 22.40 | 15.80 | 5.70 | 0.88 | | |
| Walnut, black | 59.60 | 5.08 | 51.60 | 10.70 | 36.80 | 3.99 | | |
| Walnut, English | 63.40 | 6.94 | 51.70 | 9.70 | 34.90 | 6.91 | | |
| *Oils* | | | | | | | | |
| Corn oil | 100 | 12.70 | 83.00 | 24.60 | 57.40 | 0.82 | | |
| Cottonseed oil | 100 | 26.10 | 69.60 | 18.10 | 50.30 | 0.40 | | |
| Olive oil | 100 | 14.20 | 81.40 | 71.50 | 8.23 | 0.72 | | |
| Palm oil | 100 | 47.90 | 47.70 | 37.90 | 8.96 | 0.33 | | |
| Safflower seed oil | | | | | | | | |
|   High linoleic | 100 | 9.40 | 86.20 | 11.90 | 73.30 | 0.46 | | |
|   High oleic | 100 | 6.39 | 89.20 | 76.90 | 12.30 | | | |
| Sesame seed oil | 100 | 15.20 | 80.40 | 39.10 | 40.00 | 0.46 | | |
| Soybean oil | 100 | 15.00 | 80.60 | 22.80 | 50.80 | 6.76 | | |
| Sunflower seed oil | 100 | 10.30 | 84.70 | 20.70 | 63.50 | 0.32 | | |
| Wheat germ oil | 100 | 17.50 | 76.90 | 15.00 | 54.40 | 6.69 | | |
| Salad dressings | | | | | | | | |
|   Mayonnaise, commercial | 79.90 | | | | | | | 70 |
|   Mayonnaise-type, commercial | 42.30 | 7.00 | | 7.00 | 21.10 | | | 50 |
| Tartar sauce, regular | 57.80 | 7.20 | | 7.20 | 28.90 | | | 51 |
| *Peppers*, sweet, stuffed with beef and crumb | 5.50 | | | | | | | 30 |
| *Pheasant*, raw, flesh plus skin | 11.40 | 3.58 | 6.82 | 4.24 | 0.64 | 0.70 | 0 | |
| *Pork*, fresh | | | | | | | | |
| Composite of retail cut | | | | | | | | |
|   Total edible, cooked | | | | | | | | 405 |
|   Separable lean, cooked | | | | | | | | 88 |
| Leg, cooked, roasted | | | | | | | | |
|   Total edible (82% lean) (18% fat) | 20.20 | 7.09 | 11.88 | 8.73 | 1.90 | 0.17 | 0.13 | |
|   Separable lean | 9.00 | 3.05 | 5.14 | 3.75 | 0.74 | 0.08 | 0.12 | |
| Loin, cooked, roasted | | | | | | | | |
|   Separable lean | 13.90 | 4.71 | 7.94 | 5.79 | 1.15 | 0.12 | 0.19 | |
| Shoulder | | | | | | | | |
|   Boston blade, total edible, roasted | 32.70 | 11.68 | 19.09 | 14.02 | 3.02 | 0.27 | 0.24 | |
|   Spareribs, cooked | 38.70 | 13.46 | 22.60 | 16.57 | 3.49 | 0.33 | 0.35 | |
| *Pork,* cured, smoked | | | | | | | | |
|   Leg, roasted | 22.10 | 7.75 | 12.98 | 9.95 | 2.09 | 0.19 | 0.14 | |
|   Leg (ham), canned | 11.30 | 3.97 | 6.66 | 4.90 | 1.08 | 0.09 | 0.06 | |
|   Loin (Canadian bacon), cooked, broiled, drained | 17.50 | 5.93 | 9.98 | 7.29 | 1.44 | 0.15 | 0.24 | |

| Food | Total fat (g) | Total saturated fatty acid (g) | Unsaturated fatty acid (g) | | | | | Cholesterol (mg) |
|---|---|---|---|---|---|---|---|---|
| | | | Total unsaturated fatty acid | Oleic acid | Polyunsaturated fatty acids | | | |
| | | | | | Linoleic | Linolenic | Arachidonic | |
| Shoulder, | | | | | | | | |
| Boston blade, roasted, | | | | | | | | |
| total edible (83% lean) | | | | | | | | |
| (17% fat) | 25.70 | 8.96 | 15.04 | 11.04 | 2.38 | 0.22 | 0.19 | |
| Pork, variety, other meats | | | | | | | | |
| Brain, cooked, braised | 8.70 | 2.07 | 2.81 | 1.07 | 0.10 | 0.13 | 0.50 | |
| Heart, cooked, braised | 6.90 | 1.99 | 3.45 | 1.60 | 1.03 | 0.10 | 0.34 | |
| Liver, raw | 3.70 | 1.29 | 1.45 | 0.56 | 0.31 | 0.01 | 0.27 | 300 |
| Liver, fried in margarine | 11.50 | 2.87 | 6.84 | 4.45 | 1.33 | 0.06 | 0.44 | 438 |
| Pork sausages and luncheon meats | | | | | | | | |
| Boiled ham | 17.00 | 5.92 | 9.92 | 7.29 | 1.57 | 0.14 | 0.12 | |
| Capocollo | 45.80 | 16.20 | 27.31 | 20.06 | 4.50 | 0.39 | 0.19 | |
| Chopped ham | 17.40 | 5.70 | 10.49 | 7.69 | 1.72 | 0.23 | 0.24 | |
| Deviled ham, canned | 32.30 | 11.30 | 19.04 | 13.98 | 3.13 | 0.27 | 0.14 | |
| Headcheese | 14.60 | 4.45 | 9.13 | 6.71 | 1.36 | 0.16 | 0.13 | |
| Liver cheese | 24.00 | 8.01 | 14.50 | 10.24 | 2.78 | 0.27 | 0.23 | |
| Liverwurst | 32.50 | 10.96 | 19.62 | 14.27 | 3.45 | 0.39 | 0.22 | |
| Luncheon meat, canned | 30.10 | 10.65 | 17.91 | 13.19 | 3.05 | 0.42 | 0.10 | |
| Olive loaf | 16.60 | 5.78 | 9.97 | 7.28 | 1.77 | 0.14 | 0.06 | |
| Pickle and pimento loaf | 15.80 | 5.83 | 9.16 | 6.71 | 1.65 | 0.23 | 0.06 | |
| Sausage, links or bulk | | | | | | | | |
| Raw | 36.50 | 13.15 | 21.45 | 15.85 | 3.82 | 0.43 | 0.12 | 62 |
| Cooked | 32.50 | 11.74 | 19.10 | 14.11 | 3.40 | 0.39 | 0.11 | 65 |
| Sausage, canned | | | | | | | | |
| Solids and liquid | 38.40 | 13.52 | 22.79 | 16.74 | 3.75 | 0.33 | 0.16 | |
| Drained, solid | 32.80 | 11.54 | 19.45 | 14.28 | 3.18 | 0.28 | 0.16 | |
| *Quail*, raw, | | | | | | | | |
| flesh and skin | 7.00 | 1.67 | 4.70 | 2.58 | 1.00 | 0.62 | 0 | |
| *Rabbit*, domesticated, | | | | | | | | |
| flesh only, cooked | 10.10 | | | | | | | 91 |
| *Soups*: commercially canned soup diluted with water (1:1), unless otherwise noted | | | | | | | | 9 |
| Bean and bacon | 2.40 | 0.61 | 1.60 | 0.82 | 0.55 | 0.17 | | |
| Bean and franks | 2.80 | 0.84 | 1.73 | 1.00 | 0.49 | 0.14 | | |
| Beef with vegetables | 0.80 | 0.34 | 0.36 | 0.27 | 0.04 | — | | |
| Beef noodle | 1.30 | 0.48 | 0.71 | 0.45 | 0.17 | 0.02 | | |
| Celery, cream of | | | | | | | | |
| Diluted with water | 2.30 | 0.57 | 1.53 | 0.48 | 0.98 | 0.03 | | |
| Diluted with milk | 4.00 | 1.64 | 2.07 | 0.91 | 1.00 | 0.05 | | |
| Chicken with dumplings | 2.50 | 0.59 | 1.72 | 1.02 | 0.55 | 0.01 | | |
| Chicken, cream of | | | | | | | | |
| Diluted with water | 3.00 | 0.85 | 1.94 | 1.20 | 0.57 | 0.03 | | |
| Diluted with milk | 4.70 | 1.92 | 2.48 | 1.62 | 0.60 | 0.05 | | |
| Chicken gumbo | 0.60 | 0.13 | 0.41 | 0.24 | 0.13 | — | | |
| Chicken noodle | 1.00 | 0.25 | 0.63 | 0.40 | 0.19 | 0.01 | | |
| Chicken and rice | 0.80 | 0.19 | 0.56 | 0.35 | 0.17 | — | | |
| Clam chowder, Manhattan | 0.90 | 0.17 | 0.69 | 0.15 | 0.49 | 0.04 | | |
| Minestrone | 1.10 | 0.23 | 0.77 | 0.28 | 0.41 | 0.06 | | |
| Mushroom and beef stock | 1.60 | 0.64 | 0.90 | 0.52 | 0.28 | 0.04 | | |
| Mushroom, cream of | | | | | | | | |
| Diluted with water | 3.90 | 1.06 | 2.58 | 0.70 | 1.82 | 0.01 | | |
| Diluted with milk | 5.60 | 2.13 | 3.10 | 1.13 | 1.83 | 0.04 | | |
| Oyster stew | | | | | | | | |
| Diluted with water | 1.60 | 1.03 | 0.44 | 0.33 | 0.05 | 0.01 | | |
| Diluted with milk | 3.30 | 2.12 | 1.01 | 0.77 | 0.09 | 0.04 | | |

| Food | Total fat (g) | Total saturated fatty acid (g) | Unsaturated fatty acid (g) Total unsaturated fatty acid | Oleic acid | Polyunsaturated fatty acids Linoleic | Linolenic | Arachidonic | Cholesterol (mg) |
|---|---|---|---|---|---|---|---|---|
| Potato, cream of | | | | | | | | |
| Diluted with water | 1.00 | 0.50 | 0.40 | 0.20 | 0.15 | 0.01 | | |
| Diluted with milk | 2.70 | 1.58 | 0.95 | 0.63 | 0.19 | 0.04 | | |
| Scotch broth | 1.10 | 0.47 | 0.56 | 0.30 | 0.19 | 0.04 | | |
| Tomato | | | | | | | | |
| Diluted with water | 0.80 | 0.15 | 0.55 | 0.16 | 0.31 | 0.07 | | |
| Diluted with milk | 2.50 | 1.22 | 1.10 | 0.59 | 0.35 | 0.09 | | |
| Turkey noodle | 1.10 | 0.30 | 0.69 | 0.36 | 0.25 | 0.01 | | |
| Vegetable | 0.90 | 0.20 | 0.61 | 0.24 | 0.31 | 0.05 | | |
| Vegetable beef | 1.40 | 0.32 | 1.02 | 0.35 | 0.59 | 0.05 | | |
| *Spaghetti* with meat balls in tomato sauce, canned | 4.10 | 0.80 | | 1.20 | 1.60 | | | 9 |
| *Sweetbreads* (thymus) | | | | | | | | |
| Raw | | | | | | | | 250 |
| Cooked | | | | | | | | 466 |
| *Turkey*, all classes, whole | | | | | | | | |
| Flesh and skin, cooked | 10.40 | 2.87 | 6.30 | 2.86 | 2.34 | 0.17 | 0.16 | 93 |
| Skin only, cooked | 37.00 | 9.68 | 25.50 | 12.90 | 9.15 | 0.74 | 0 | 127 |
| Flesh only, cooked | 6.10 | 1.76 | 3.17 | 1.22 | 1.23 | 0.08 | 0.19 | |
| Dark meat, cooked | 5.33 | 1.57 | 2.89 | 1.13 | 1.11 | 0.07 | 0.12 | 101 |
| Light meat, cooked | 2.58 | 0.73 | 1.28 | 0.47 | 0.51 | 0.03 | 0.11 | 77 |
| Heart, cooked | 13.2 | | | | | | | 238 |
| Liver, cooked | 4.8 | | | | | | | 599 |
| Turkey pot pie, commercial, frozen, unheated | 10.4 | | | | | | | 9 |
| *Veal* | | | | | | | | |
| Carcass, braised or stewed | | | | | | | | |
| Total edible (83% lean) (17% fat) | 14.5 | 6.19 | 7.19 | 5.25 | 0.61 | 0.22 | 0.07 | 101 |
| Separable lean | 2.4 | 0.73 | 1.02 | 0.60 | 0.13 | 0.03 | 0.08 | 99 |
| Retail cuts, untrimmed | | | | | | | | |
| Breast, total edible, stewed (73% lean) (27% fat) | 21.2 | 9.21 | 10.59 | 7.82 | 0.87 | 0.33 | 0.06 | |
| Foreshank, total edible, stewed (86% lean) (14% fat) | 10.4 | 4.35 | 5.09 | 3.68 | 0.45 | 0.16 | 0.07 | |
| Leg, total edible, broiled (79% lean) (21% fat) | 11.1 | 4.68 | 5.46 | 3.97 | 0.47 | 0.17 | 0.06 | |
| Rib, total edible, roasted (82% lean) (18% fat) | 16.9 | 7.12 | 8.32 | 6.04 | 0.72 | 0.25 | 0.10 | |
| Shoulder, total edible, braised (85% lean) (15% fat) | 12.8 | 5.42 | 6.31 | 4.60 | 0.54 | 0.20 | 0.07 | |

*Sources:*

Anderson, B. A.: Comprehensive evaluation of fatty acids in foods. VII. Pork products. J. Am. Diet. Assoc. 69: 44, 1976.

Anderson, B. A.; Fristrom, G. A.; and Weihrauch, J. L.: Comprehensive evaluation of fatty acids in foods. X. Lamb and veal. J. Am. Diet. Assoc. 70: 53, 1977.

Anderson, B. A.; Kinsella, J. E.; and Watt, B. K.: Comprehensive evaluation of fatty acids in foods. II. Beef products. J. Am. Diet. Assoc. 67: 35, 1975.

Brignoli, C. A.; Kinsella, J. E.; and Weihrauch, J. L.: Comprehensive evaluation of fatty acids in foods. V. Unhydrogenated fats and oils. J. Am. Diet. Assoc. 68: 224, 1976.

Composition of Foods, Dairy and Egg Products, Raw, Processed, Prepared. Agricultural Handbook No. 8–1. Washington, DC: Agricultural Research Service, U.S. Department of Agriculture, 1976.

Exler, J., and Weihrauch, J. L.: Comprehensive evaluation of fatty acids in foods. VIII. Finfish. J. Am. Diet. Assoc. 69: 243, 1976.

Feely, R. M.; Criner, P. E.; and Watt, B. K.: Cholesterol content of foods. J. Am. Diet. Assoc. 61: 134, 1972.

Fristrom, G. A.; Stewart, B. C.; Weihrauch, J. L.; and Posati, L. P.: Comprehensive evaluation of fatty acids in foods. IV. Nuts, peanuts, and soups. J. Am. Diet. Assoc. 67: 351, 1975.

Fristrom, G. A., and Weihrauch, J. L.: Comprehensive evaluation of fatty acids in foods. IX. Fowl. J. Am. Diet. Assoc. 69: 517, 1976.

Posati, L. P.; Kinsella, J. E.; and Watt, B. K.: Comprehensive evaluation of fatty acids in foods. I. Dairy products. J. Am. Diet. Assoc. 66: 482, 1975.

Posati, L. P.; Kinsella, J. E.; and Watt, B. K.: Comprehensive evaluation of fatty acids in foods. III. Eggs and egg products. J. Am. Diet. Assoc. 67: 111, 1975.

Robinson, C. H., and Lawler, M. R.: Normal and Therapeutic Nutrition. 15th ed. New York: Macmillan, 1977.

Weihrauch, J. L.; Kinsella, J. E.; and Watt, B. K.: Comprehensive evaluation of fatty acids in foods. VI. Cereal products. J. Am. Diet. Assoc. 68: 335, 1976.

# Folacin Content of Foods

**Folacin Content in Terms of 100 g Edible Portion and of Specified Units***

| Item number | Food and description | Per 100 g edible protion | | Per specified unit | | | |
|---|---|---|---|---|---|---|---|
| | | Free folacin (µg) | Total folacin (µg) | Approximate measure | Weight (g) | Free folacin (µg) | Total folacin (µg) |
| | *Cereal grains and their products* | | | | | | |
| 1 | Barley, pot | 9 | 20 | 1 cup | 200 | 18 | 40 |
| 2 | Corn, whole grain | 15 | 19 | | | | |
| 3 | Cornmeal, degermed | 9 | 24 | 1 cup | 122 | 11 | 29 |
| 4 | Macaroni, dry form | 4 | 12 | 8-oz pkg. | 227 | 9 | 27 |
| | Rice | | | | | | |
| 5 | Brown | 12 | 16 | 1 cup | 185 | 22 | 30 |
| 6 | White | —† | 10 | 1 cup | 185 | — | 18 |
| 7 | Parboiled | 9 | 11 | 1 cup | 185 | 17 | 20 |
| 8 | Rice bran | — | 39 | | | | |
| 9 | Rice germ | — | 64 | | | | |
| 10 | Rye flour, sifted | 31 | 78 | 1 cup | 88 | 27 | 69 |
| 11 | Sorghum, grain | 18 | 27 | | | | |
| 12 | Spaghetti, dry form | 4 | 12 | 8- oz pkg. | 227 | 9 | 27 |
| 13 | Wheat, whole grain | 39 | 52 | | | | |
| | Wheat flour | | | | | | |
| 14 | Whole | 40 | 54 | 1 cup | 120 | 48 | 65 |
| 15 | Clear | 29 | 32 | | | | |
| | Patent | | | | | | |
| 16 | Bread, sifted | 19 | 25 | 1 cup | 115 | 22 | 29 |
| 17 | All-purpose, sifted | 18 | 21 | 1 cup | 115 | 21 | 24 |
| 18 | Wheat bran | 134 | 258 | | | | |
| 19 | Wheat germ | 257 | 328 | | | | |
| | Breakfast cereals, dry | | | | | | |
| 20 | Farina | — | 24 | 1 cup | 180 | — | 43 |
| 21 | Farina, wheat germ added | 17 | 34 | 1 cup | 180 | 31 | 61 |
| 22 | Oatmeal | 16 | 52 | 1 cup | 80 | 13 | 42 |
| | Breakfast cereals, ready-to-eat; not fortified with folacin | | | | | | |
| 23 | Cornflakes | 9 | 12 | 1 oz | 28 | 3 | 3 |
| 24 | Oats, with added wheat gluten | 8 | 22 | 1 oz | 28 | 2 | 6 |
| 25 | Rice, puffed | 8 | 23 | 1 oz | 28 | 2 | 6 |
| 26 | Rice, with added protein concentrate and wheat gluten | 14 | 31 | | 28 | 4 | 9 |
| 27 | Wheat germ, toasted | 125 | 420 | 1 oz | 28 | 35 | 118 |
| 28 | Wheat and malted barley granules | 15 | 54 | 1 oz | 28 | 4 | 15 |
| 29 | Wheat, shredded | 10 | 50 | 1 oz | 28 | 3 | 14 |
| | Bakery products | | | | | | |
| | Bread | | | | | | |
| 30 | Rye | 6 | 23 | 1 slice | 25 | 2 | 6 |
| 31 | White | 13 | 39 | 1 slice | 25 | 3 | 10 |
| 32 | Whole wheat | 27 | 58 | 1 slice | 28 | 8 | 16 |
| | Cakes | | | | | | |
| 33 | Chocolate with icing | 4 | 6 | 1 slice (3 in. high; 2⅜ in. arc) | 99 | 4 | 6 |
| 34 | Sponge | 3 | 7 | 1 slice (3 in. high; 2¼ in. arc) | 44 | 1 | 3 |
| | Cookies | | | | | | |
| 35 | Chocolate chip | 4 | 9 | 1 cookie | 10 | <0.5 | 1 |
| 36 | Shortbread | 4 | 9 | 1 cookie | 8 | <0.5 | 1 |
| | Doughnuts | | | | | | |
| 37 | Cake type | 5 | 8 | 1 doughnut | 32 | 2 | 3 |
| 38 | Yeast leavened | 5 | 22 | 1 doughnut | 35 | 2 | 8 |
| 39 | Pie, apple | 2 | 4 | ⅙ of pie | 158 | 3 | 6 |

* Measure and weight apply to edible part of food only.
† Dash denotes value not available.

## Folacin Content in Terms of 100 g Edible Portion and of Specified Units*

| Item number | Food and description | Per 100 g edible protion | | Per specified unit | | | |
| --- | --- | --- | --- | --- | --- | --- | --- |
| | | Free folacin (μg) | Total folacin (μg) | Approximate measure | Weight (g) | Free folacin (μg) | Total folacin (μg) |
| | **Leguminous seeds and their products** | | | | | | |
| | Beans, common, mature seeds | | | | | | |
| | White | | | | | | |
| 40 | Raw, dry | 25 | 129 | 1 cup | 205 | 51 | 264 |
| 41 | Canned, baked with tomato sauce | 8 | 24 | 1 cup | 255 | 20 | 61 |
| | Red | | | | | | |
| 42 | Raw, dry | 24 | 133 | 1 cup | 185 | 44 | 246 |
| 43 | Cooked | — | 37 | 1 cup | 185 | — | 68 |
| | Pinto, mature seeds, dry | | | | | | |
| 44 | Raw, dry | 57 | 216 | 1 cup | 190 | 108 | 410 |
| 45 | Cooked | — | 59 | 1 cup | 190 | — | 112 |
| 46 | Canned, drained | — | 51 | 1 cup | 190 | — | 97 |
| | Beans, lima, mature seeds | | | | | | |
| 47 | Raw, dry | 25 | 113 | 1 cup | 190 | 48 | 215 |
| 48 | Cooked | — | 43 | 1 cup | 190 | — | 82 |
| 49 | Beans, mung, mature seeds, dry | 26 | 133 | 1 cup | 210 | 55 | 279 |
| 50 | Beans, mungo, mature seeds, dry | 28 | 108 | | | | |
| | Chickpeas or garbanzos, mature seeds | | | | | | |
| 51 | Raw, dry | 32 | 199 | 1 cup | 200 | 64 | 398 |
| 52 | Roasted | 22 | 139 | | | | |
| 53 | Canned, drained | — | 102 | | | | |
| | Cowpeas, mature seeds | | | | | | |
| 54 | Raw, dry | 69 | 133 | 1 cup | 170 | 117 | 226 |
| 55 | Canned, drained | — | 80 | 1 cup | 165 | — | 132 |
| 56 | Lentils, mature seeds, dry | 19 | 36 | 1 cup | 190 | 36 | 68 |
| 57 | Peanuts, roasted | 24 | 106 | 1 cup | 144 | 35 | 153 |
| 58 | Peanut butter | 20 | 79 | 1 tbsp | 16 | 3 | 13 |
| 59 | Pigeon peas, mature seeds, dry | 20 | 110 | | | | |
| 60 | Soybeans, mature seeds, dry | 75 | 171 | 1 cup | 210 | 158 | 359 |
| | Soybean products, fermented | | | | | | |
| 61 | Natto | 95 | 126 | | | | |
| 62 | Tempeh | 12 | 156 | | | | |
| 63 | Soy sauce | 8 | 28 | 1 tbsp | 18 | 1 | 5 |
| | **Nuts and seeds (other than leguminous seeds)** | | | | | | |
| 64 | Almonds | 33 | 96 | 1 cup | 142 | 47 | 136 |
| 65 | Brazil nuts, shelled | 1 | 4 | 1 cup | 140 | 1 | 6 |
| 66 | Cashew nuts, roasted | 8 | 68 | 1 cup | 140 | 11 | 95 |
| 67 | Coconut, shredded | 10 | 24 | 1 cup | 130 | 13 | 31 |
| 68 | Filberts (hazelnuts), shelled | 23 | 72 | 1 cup | 135 | 31 | 97 |
| 69 | Pecans, shelled | 13 | 24 | 1 cup | 108 | 14 | 26 |
| 70 | Pistachio nuts | 10 | 58 | | | | |
| 71 | Sesame seeds | 49 | 96 | | | | |
| 71a | Sesame seeds | | | 1 tbsp | 8 | 4 | 8 |
| 71b | Sesame seeds | | | 1 cup | 150 | 74 | 144 |
| 72 | Walnuts, English, shelled | 52 | 66 | 1 cup | 100 | 52 | 66 |
| | **Vegetables** | | | | | | |
| 73 | Asparagus, raw | 58 | 64 | 1 cup | 135 | 78 | 86 |
| 74 | Bean sprouts, canned | 7 | 10 | 1 cup | 125 | 9 | 12 |
| | Beans, snap | | | | | | |
| | Green | | | | | | |
| 75 | Raw | 33 | 44 | 1 cup | 110 | 36 | 48 |
| 76 | Cooked, drained | — | 40 | 1 cup | 125 | — | 50 |
| 77 | Frozen | 8 | 33 | 1 cup | 125 | 10 | 41 |
| | Yellow or wax | | | | | | |
| 78 | Frozen | 8 | 34 | 1 cup | 125 | 10 | 42 |
| 79 | Raw | 32 | 40 | 1 cup | 110 | 35 | 44 |

| Item number | Food and description | Per 100 g edible protion | | Per specified unit | | | |
|---|---|---|---|---|---|---|---|
| | | Free folacin (µg) | Total folacin (µg) | Approximate measure | Weight (g) | Free folacin (µg) | Total folacin (µg) |
| 80 | Beans, lima, frozen | 9 | 31 | 1 cup | 160 | 14 | 50 |
| | Beets, common, red | | | | | | |
| 81 | Raw | 69 | 93 | 1 cup | 135 | 93 | 126 |
| 82 | Cooked | 38 | 78 | 1 cup | 170 | 65 | 133 |
| | Broccoli | | | | | | |
| | Spears | | | | | | |
| 83 | Raw | 51 | 69 | 3 medium | 354 | 181 | 244 |
| 84 | Cooked | 27 | 56 | 1 medium | 180 | 49 | 101 |
| 85 | Flower, raw | 102 | 105 | | | | |
| 86 | Stem, raw | 35 | 59 | | | | |
| | Brussels sprouts | | | | | | |
| 87 | Raw | 55 | 78 | 6 medium | 114 | 63 | 89 |
| 88 | Cooked | 6 | 36 | 1 cup (7–8 sprouts) | 155 | 9 | 56 |
| | Cabbage | | | | | | |
| | Common varieties | | | | | | |
| 89 | Raw | 33 | 66 | 1 cup | 90 | 30 | 59 |
| 90 | Cooked | 2 | 18 | 1 cup | 145 | 3 | 26 |
| 91 | Red, raw | 23 | 34 | 1 cup | 90 | 21 | 31 |
| | Cabbage, Chinese (also called celery cabbage or petsai) | | | | | | |
| 92 | Raw | 42 | 83 | 1 cup | 75 | 32 | 62 |
| 93 | Cooked | 5 | 19 | | | | |
| | Carrots | | | | | | |
| 94 | Raw | 14 | 32 | 1 medium | 59 | 8 | 19 |
| 95 | Cooked | 2 | 24 | 1 cup | 155 | 3 | 37 |
| | Cauliflower | | | | | | |
| 96 | Raw | 31 | 55 | 1 cup | 100 | 31 | 55 |
| 97 | Cooked | 2 | 34 | 1 cup | 125 | 2 | 42 |
| 98 | Celery, raw | 6 | 12 | 1 cup | 100 | 6 | 12 |
| 99 | Chicory greens, raw | 33 | 52 | | | | |
| 100 | Collards, raw | — | 102 | 1 cup | 55 | — | 56 |
| | Corn, sweet | | | | | | |
| 101 | Raw, whole kernel | 27 | 33 | 1 cup | 165 | 45 | 54 |
| 102 | Frozen | 2 | 21 | 1 cup | 162 | 3 | 35 |
| 103 | Cucumber, raw, pared | 12 | 15 | 1 small | 128 | 15 | 19 |
| | Eggplant | | | | | | |
| 104 | Raw | 9 | 31 | | | | |
| 105 | Cooked | 2 | 16 | 1 cup | 200 | 4 | 32 |
| 106 | Endive, raw | — | 49 | 1 cup | 50 | — | 24 |
| 107 | Kale, raw | 44 | 60 | 1 cup | 110 | 48 | 66 |
| | Lettuce, raw | | | | | | |
| 108 | Leaf or head | 34 | 37 | 1 cup | 55 | 19 | 20 |
| 109 | Romaine | 60 | 179 | 1 cup | 55 | 33 | 98 |
| 110 | Mushrooms, raw | 20 | 23 | 1 cup | 68 | 14 | 16 |
| 111 | Okra, raw | 10 | 24 | 1 cup | 100 | 10 | 24 |
| 112 | Onion, mature, dry | 10 | 25 | | | | |
| 112a | Onion, mature, chopped | | | 1 cup | 170 | 17 | 42 |
| 112b | Onion, mature, chopped | | | 1 tbsp | 10 | 1 | 2 |
| | Onion, young green, raw | | | | | | |
| 113 | Bulbs and white portion of top | 40 | 36 | | | | |
| 113a | Bulbs and white portion of top | | | 1 cup | 100 | 40 | 36 |
| 113b | Bulbs and white portion of top | | | 1 tbsp | 6 | 2 | 2 |
| 114 | Tops only (green portion) | 52 | 80 | | | | |

| Item number | Food and description | Per 100 g edible protion | | Per specified unit | | | |
|---|---|---|---|---|---|---|---|
| | | Free folacin (µg) | Total folacin (µg) | Approximate measure | Weight (g) | Free folacin (µg) | Total folacin (µg) |
| 114a | Tops only (green portion), chopped | | | 1 cup | 100 | 52 | 80 |
| 114b | Tops only (green portion), chopped | | | 1 tbsp | 6 | 3 | 5 |
| | Onion, Welsh, raw | | | | | | |
| 115 | Bulbs and white portion of top | 16 | 66 | | | | |
| 116 | Tops only (green portion) | 49 | 105 | | | | |
| 117 | Parsnips, raw | 57 | 67 | 1 cup | 130 | 74 | 87 |
| 118 | Parsley, raw | 41 | 116 | 1 tbsp | 4 | 2 | 5 |
| 119 | Peas, green, frozen | 17 | 53 | 1 cup | 145 | 25 | 77 |
| 120 | Peppers, hot, mature, red, raw | 23 | 52 | | | | |
| 121 | Peppers, sweet, immature, green, raw | 8 | 19 | 1 medium | 164 | 13 | 31 |
| | Potatoes | | | | | | |
| 122 | Raw | 11 | 19 | 1 medium | 122 | 13 | 23 |
| | Cooked | | | | | | |
| 123 | French fried | 8 | 22 | 10 pieces | 50 | 4 | 11 |
| 124 | Hashed brown | 3 | 17 | 1 cup | 155 | 5 | 26 |
| 125 | Mashed | 5 | 10 | 1 cup | 210 | 10 | 21 |
| | Pumpkin | | | | | | |
| 126 | Raw | 5 | 36 | | | | |
| 127 | Cooked | 2 | 19 | 1 cup | 245 | 5 | 47 |
| 128 | Radishes, common, raw | 18 | 24 | 4 small | 36 | 6 | 9 |
| | Rutabagas | | | | | | |
| 129 | Raw | 23 | 27 | 1 cup | 140 | 32 | 38 |
| 130 | Cooked | 9 | 21 | | | | |
| 130a | Cooked, cubed | | | 1 cup | 170 | 15 | 36 |
| 130b | Cooked, mashed | | | 1 cup | 210 | 22 | 50 |
| | Spinach | | | | | | |
| 131 | Raw | 119 | 193 | 1 cup | 55 | 65 | 106 |
| 132 | Cooked | 60 | 91 | 1 cup | 180 | 108 | 164 |
| | Squash, summer | | | | | | |
| 133 | Raw | 23 | 31 | 1 cup | 130 | 30 | 40 |
| 134 | Frozen, cooked | 2 | 10 | 1 cup | 210 | 4 | 21 |
| | Sweet potatoes | | | | | | |
| 135 | Raw | 33 | 50 | 1 medium | 146 | 48 | 73 |
| 136 | Cooked | 7 | 18 | 1 medium | 146 | 10 | 26 |
| 137 | Tomatoes, raw | 21 | 39 | 1 medium | 135 | 28 | 53 |
| 138 | Tomato juice, canned | 10 | 26 | | | | |
| 138a | Tomato juice, canned | | | 1 cup | 243 | 24 | 63 |
| 138b | Tomato juice, canned | | | 6-oz glass | 182 | 18 | 47 |
| 139 | Turnips, raw | 17 | 20 | 1 cup | 130 | 22 | 26 |
| 140 | Turnip greens, raw | — | 95 | 1 cup | 55 | — | 52 |
| **Fruits** | | | | | | | |
| 141 | Apples, raw | 3 | 8 | 1 medium | 166 | 5 | 13 |
| 142 | Applesauce, sweetened | 1 | 1 | 1 cup | 255 | 3 | 3 |
| 143 | Apricots, dried | 10 | 14 | | | | |
| 143a | Apricots, dried | | | 10 halves | 35 | 4 | 5 |
| 143b | Apricots, dried | | | 1 cup | 130 | 13 | 18 |
| 144 | Avocados, raw | 31 | 51 | ½ medium | 115 | 36 | 59 |
| 145 | Bananas, raw | 22 | 28 | 1 medium | 119 | 26 | 33 |
| 146 | Blueberries, raw | 2 | 6 | 1 cup | 145 | 3 | 9 |
| | Cantaloupe, see muskmelon | | | | | | |
| 147 | Cherries, raw | 6 | 8 | | | | |
| 147a | Cherries, raw | | | 1 cup | 117 | 7 | 9 |
| 147b | Cherries, raw | | | 10 cherries | 68 | 4 | 5 |
| 148 | Cranberries, raw | 1 | 2 | 1 cup | 91 | 1 | 2 |
| 149 | Currants, dried | 4 | 11 | | | | |

| Item number | Food and description | Per 100 g edible protion | | Per specified unit | | | |
|---|---|---|---|---|---|---|---|
| | | Free folacin (µg) | Total folacin (µg) | Approximate measure | Weight (g) | Free folacin (µg) | Total folacin (µg) |
| 150 | Dates, dried | 14 | 21 | | | | |
| 150a | Dates, dried | | | 1 cup | 178 | 25 | 37 |
| 150b | Dates, dried | | | 10 dates | 80 | 11 | 17 |
| 151 | Figs, dried | 3 | 9 | 1 large | 21 | 1 | 2 |
| 152 | Grapefruit, raw | 8 | 11 | ½ medium | 98 | 8 | 11 |
| 153 | Grapefruit juice, fresh or frozen reconstituted | 8 | 21 | | | | |
| 153a | Grapefruit juice, fresh or frozen reconstituted | | | 1 cup | 247 | 20 | 52 |
| 153b | Grapefruit juice, fresh or frozen reconsituted | | | 6 oz glass | 185 | 15 | 39 |
| 154 | Grapes, red or white, raw | 4 | 7 | 1 cup | 152 | 6 | 11 |
| 155 | Grape juice, canned or frozen reconstituted | 2 | 2 | 1 cup | 253 | 5 | 5 |
| 156 | Lemon, raw | 12 | 12 | 1 medium | 74 | 9 | 9 |
| 157 | Lemonade | 2 | 5 | | | | |
| 157a | Lemonade | | | 1 cup | 248 | 5 | 12 |
| 157b | Lemonade | | | 6-oz glass | 185 | 4 | 9 |
| 158 | Limes, raw | 6 | 4 | 1 lime | 67 | 4 | 3 |
| 159 | Muskmelon or cantaloupe | 30 | 30 | ½ medium | 272 | 82 | 82 |
| 160 | Nectarines, raw | 7 | 5 | 1 medium | 138 | 10 | 7 |
| 161 | Oranges, raw | 32 | 46 | 1 medium | 141 | 45 | 65 |
| 162 | Orange juice, fresh or frozen reconstituted | 34 | 55 | | | | |
| 162a | Orange juice, fresh or frozen reconstituted | | | 1 cup | 248 | 84 | 136 |
| 162b | Orange juice, fresh or frozen reconstituted | | | 6-oz glass | 185 | 63 | 102 |
| 163 | Peaches, raw | 2 | 8 | 1 medium | 100 | 2 | 8 |
| 164 | Pears, raw | 5 | 14 | 1 medium | 164 | 8 | 23 |
| 165 | Pineapple, raw | 9 | 11 | 1 cup | 155 | 14 | 17 |
| 166 | Plantain (baking banana), raw | 2 | 16 | 1 medium | 263 | 5 | 42 |
| 167 | Plums, raw | 4 | 6 | 1 medium | 55 | 2 | 3 |
| 168 | Prunes, dried, softenized, raw | 1 | 4 | 1 medium | 26 | <0.5 | 1 |
| 169 | Raisins, natural (unbleached), raw | 3 | 4 | 1 cup | 145 | 4 | 6 |
| 170 | Rhubarb, raw | 9 | 7 | 1 cup | 122 | 11 | 9 |
| 171 | Stawberries, raw | 15 | 16 | 1 cup | 149 | 22 | 24 |
| 172 | Tangerines, raw | 19 | 21 | 1 medium | 86 | 16 | 18 |
| 173 | Watermelon, raw | 2 | 8 | 1 wedge, 4″ × 8″ | 426 | 9 | 34 |

## Meat

| Item number | Food and description | Per 100 g edible protion | | Per specified unit | | | |
|---|---|---|---|---|---|---|---|
| | Beef, separable lean | | | | | | |
| 174 | Raw | 4 | 7 | | | | |
| 175 | Cooked | — | 4 | 3 oz | 85 | — | 3 |
| | Beef, ground | | | | | | |
| 176 | Raw | 3 | 7 | | | | |
| 177 | Cooked | — | 4 | 3 oz | 85 | — | 3 |
| | Kidney | | | | | | |
| 178 | Beef, raw | 63 | 80 | | | | |
| | Lamb | | | | | | |
| 179 | Raw | 24 | 42 | | | | |
| 180 | Cooked | — | 32 | 3 oz | 85 | — | 27 |
| | Lamb | | | | | | |
| 181 | Raw | 1 | 4 | | | | |
| 182 | Cooked | — | 3 | 3 oz | 85 | — | 3 |

## Folacin Content in Terms of 100 g Edible Portion and of Specified Units*

| Item number | Food and description | Per 100 g edible protion | | Per specified unit | | | |
| --- | --- | --- | --- | --- | --- | --- | --- |
| | | Free folacin (µg) | Total folacin (µg) | Approximate measure | Weight (g) | Free folacin (µg) | Total folacin (µg) |
| | Liver | | | | | | |
| | Beef, lamb, or pork | | | | | | |
| 183 | Raw | 80 | 219 | | | | |
| 184 | Cooked | — | 145 | 3 oz | 85 | — | 123 |
| | Pork | | | | | | |
| | Separable lean | | | | | | |
| 185 | Raw | 3 | 8 | | | | |
| 186 | Cooked | — | 5 | 3 oz | 85 | — | 4 |
| 187 | Ham, smoked | — | 11 | 3 oz | 85 | — | 9 |
| | Veal | | | | | | |
| 188 | Raw | 4 | 5 | | | | |
| 189 | Cooked | — | 3 | 3 oz | 85 | — | 3 |
| | Sausages, cold cuts, and luncheon meats | | | | | | |
| 190 | Beerwurst | 1 | 3 | 1 slice (1 oz) | 28 | <0.5 | 1 |
| 191 | Bologna | 2 | 5 | 1 slice (1 oz) | 28 | 1 | 1 |
| 192 | Frankfurters, unheated | 2 | 4 | 1 (5″ long, ¾″ diam.) | 45 | 1 | 2 |
| 193 | Head cheese | 1 | 2 | 1 slice (1 oz) | 28 | <0.5 | 1 |
| 194 | Liverwurst | 20 | 30 | 1 slice (1 oz) | 28 | 6 | 8 |
| | Luncheon meats | | | | | | |
| 195 | Boiled ham | 1 | 4 | 1 slice (1 oz) | 28 | <0.5 | 1 |
| 196 | Pork, spiced | 1 | 3 | 1 slice (1 oz) | 28 | <0.5 | 1 |
| 197 | Sausage, pork, raw | — | 14 | 3 oz | 85 | — | 12 |
| **Poultry** | | | | | | | |
| | Chicken, without skin | | | | | | |
| | Dark meat | | | | | | |
| 198 | Raw | 5 | 11 | | | | |
| 199 | Cooked | — | 7 | 3 oz | 85 | — | 6 |
| | Light meat | | | | | | |
| 200 | Raw | 3 | 6 | | | | |
| 201 | Cooked | — | 4 | 3 oz | 85 | — | 3 |
| | Liver, chicken | | | | | | |
| 202 | Raw | — | 364 | | | | |
| 203 | Cooked | — | 240 | 3 oz | 85 | — | 204 |
| | Turkey, without skin | | | | | | |
| | Dark meat | | | | | | |
| 204 | Raw | 8 | 11 | | | | |
| 205 | Cooked | — | 7 | 3 oz | 85 | — | 6 |
| | Light meat | | | | | | |
| 206 | Raw | 4 | 9 | | | | |
| 207 | Cooked | — | 5 | 3 oz | 85 | — | 4 |
| **Fish and shellfish** | | | | | | | |
| 208 | Cod, frozen | 6 | 18 | 3 oz | 85 | 5 | 15 |
| 209 | Crab, frozen | 2 | 20 | 3 oz | 85 | 2 | 17 |
| 210 | Haddock, frozen | 4 | 10 | 3 oz | 85 | 3 | 8 |
| 211 | Halibut, frozen | 4 | 12 | 3 oz | 85 | 3 | 10 |
| 212 | Lobster, canned | 8 | 17 | 3 oz | 85 | 7 | 14 |
| 213 | Ocean perch, frozen | 5 | 9 | 3 oz | 85 | 4 | 8 |
| | Salmon | | | | | | |
| 214 | Canned | 10 | 20 | 3 oz | 85 | 8 | 17 |
| 215 | Frozen | 4 | 26 | 3 oz | 85 | 3 | 22 |
| 216 | Sardines, canned | 13 | 16 | 1 fish | 12 | 2 | 2 |
| 217 | Scallops, frozen | 18 | 16 | 3 oz | 85 | 15 | 14 |
| | Shrimp | | | | | | |
| 218 | Canned | 8 | 15 | 3 oz | 85 | 7 | 13 |
| 219 | Frozen | 8 | 11 | 3 oz | 85 | 7 | 9 |

| Item number | Food and description | Per 100 g edible protion | | Per specified unit | | | |
| | | Free folacin (µg) | Total folacin (µg) | Approximate measure | Weight (g) | Free folacin (µg) | Total folacin (µg) |
|---|---|---|---|---|---|---|---|
| 220 | Smelt, frozen | 6 | 16 | 3 oz | 85 | 5 | 14 |
| 221 | Sole, frozen | 5 | 11 | 3 oz | 85 | 4 | 9 |
| 222 | Tuna, canned | 8 | 15 | 3 oz | 85 | 7 | 13 |
| **Eggs and egg products** | | | | | | | |
| | Eggs | | | | | | |
| | Whole | | | | | | |
| 223 | Raw | 46 | 65 | 1 medium | 44 | 20 | 29 |
| 224 | Hard-cooked | — | 49 | 1 medium | 44 | — | 22 |
| 225 | White, raw | 3 | 16 | 1 medium | 29 | 1 | 5 |
| 226 | Yolk, raw | 121 | 152 | 1 medium | 15 | 18 | 23 |
| 227 | Eggnog | <0.5 | 1 | ½ cup | 128 | — | 1 |
| **Dairy products** | | | | | | | |
| 228 | Butter | 1 | 3 | | | | |
| 228a | Butter | | | 1 tbsp | 14 | <0.5 | <0.5 |
| 228b | Butter | | | 1 cup | 227 | 2 | 7 |
| | Cheeses, natural | | | | | | |
| 229 | Cheddar | 1 | 18 | | | | |
| 229a | Cheddar | | | 1 cup, shredded | 113 | 1 | 20 |
| 229b | Cheddar | | | 1 oz | 28 | <0.5 | 5 |
| 230 | Cottage | — | 12 | 1 cup, packed | 245 | — | 29 |
| 231 | Cream | — | 13 | | | | |
| 231a | Cream | | | 8-oz pkg. | 227 | — | 30 |
| 231b | Cream | | | 3-oz pkg. | 85 | — | 11 |
| 231c | Cream | | | 1 in.³ | 16 | — | 2 |
| 232 | Cheese spread, pasteurized process | 3 | 7 | 1 oz | 28 | 1 | 2 |
| | Cream, fluid | | | | | | |
| 233 | Half and half | 2 | 2 | | | | |
| 233a | Half and half | | | 1 cup | 242 | 5 | 5 |
| 233b | Half and half | | | 1 tbsp | 15 | <0.5 | <0.5 |
| 234 | Light coffee or table | 1 | 2 | | | | |
| 234a | Light coffee or table | | | 1 cup | 240 | 2 | 5 |
| 234b | Light coffee or table | | | 1 tbsp | 15 | <0.5 | <0.5 |
| 235 | Sour, cultured | — | 11 | | | | |
| 235a | Sour, cultured | | | 1 cup | 230 | — | 25 |
| 235b | Sour, cultured | | | 1 tbsp | 12 | — | 1 |
| 236 | Whipping, light | 2 | 4 | | | | |
| 236a | Whipping, light | | | 1 cup | 239 | 5 | 10 |
| 236b | Whipping, light | | | 1 tbsp | 15 | <0.5 | 1 |
| 237 | Ice cream, vanilla | 2 | 2 | 1 cup | 133 | 3 | 3 |
| | Milk, cow, fluid | | | | | | |
| 238 | Whole, pasteurized | 5 | 5 | 1 cup | 244 | 12 | 12 |
| 239 | Skim, raw | 3 | — | 1 cup | 245 | 7 | — |
| 240 | Evaporated | 4 | 8 | 1 cup | 252 | 10 | 20 |
| 241 | Milk, goat | 1 | 1 | 1 cup | 244 | 2 | 2 |
| 242 | Milk, human | 3 | 5 | 1 fl oz | 31 | 1 | 2 |
| 243 | Yogurt | <0.5 | 11 | 1 cup | 245 | — | 27 |
| **Mixed dishes, frozen** | | | | | | | |
| 244 | Beef with one vegetable | 2 | 5 | 1 pkg. | 254 | 5 | 13 |
| 245 | Beef with two vegetables, soup, dessert | 5 | 12 | 1 pkg. | 456 | 23 | 55 |
| 246 | Beef with three vegetables | 8 | 24 | 1 pkg. | 327 | 26 | 78 |
| 247 | Chicken, fried, with one vegetable | 6 | 12 | 1 pkg. | 205 | 12 | 25 |
| 248 | Chicken, fried, with two vegetables, dessert | 6 | 18 | 1 pkg. | 315 | 19 | 57 |

| Item number | Food and description | Per 100 g edible protion | | Per specified unit | | | |
| | | Free folacin (µg) | Total folacin (µg) | Approximate measure | Weight (g) | Free folacin (µg) | Total folacin (µg) |
| --- | --- | --- | --- | --- | --- | --- | --- |
| 249 | Haddock with one vegetable | 6 | 18 | 1 pkg. | 273 | 16 | 49 |
| 250 | Ham with two vegetables, dessert | 5 | 15 | 1 pkg. | 314 | 16 | 47 |
| 251 | Lasagna | — | 22 | 10 oz portion | 280 | — | 62 |
| | Pizza | | | | | | |
| 252 | Cheese | — | 37 | ⅛ pie, 13¾ in. diam. | 65 | — | 24 |
| 253 | Pepperoni | — | 38 | ⅛ pie, 13¾ in. diam. | 67 | — | 25 |
| 254 | Sausage | — | 35 | ⅛ pie, 13¾ in. diam. | 67 | — | 23 |
| 255 | Pork with one vegetable, one fruit, dessert | 2 | 7 | 1 pkg. | 303 | 6 | 21 |
| 256 | Poultry, Oriental style with rice, vegetables | 2 | 4 | 1 pkg. | 415 | 8 | 17 |
| 257 | Shrimp, Oriental style with rice, vegetables | 4 | 13 | 1 pkg. | 388 | 16 | 50 |
| 258 | Shrimp with one vegetable | 8 | 14 | 1 pkg. | 264 | 21 | 37 |
| 259 | Shrimp with two vegetables | 9 | 22 | 1 pkg. | 234 | 21 | 51 |
| 260 | Spaghetti with meatballs, one vegetable, dessert | 6 | 18 | 1 pkg. | 354 | 21 | 64 |
| 261 | Turkey with one vegetable | 4 | 11 | 1 pkg. | 264 | 11 | 29 |
| 262 | Turkey with two vegetables, dessert | 6 | 14 | 1 pkg. | 346 | 21 | 48 |
| *Baby foods—strained, canned* | | | | | | | |
| 263 | Applesauce | <0.5 | 1 | | | | |
| 263a | Applesauce | | | 1 jar | 134 | — | 1 |
| 263b | Applesauce | | | 1 oz | 28 | — | <0.5 |
| 264 | Apricots | <0.5 | 1 | | | | |
| 264a | Apricots | | | 1 jar | 134 | — | 1 |
| 264b | Apricots | | | 1 oz | 28 | — | <0.5 |
| 265 | Bananas | 1 | 2 | | | | |
| 265a | Bananas | | | 1 jar | 134 | 1 | 3 |
| 265b | Bananas | | | 1 oz | 28 | <0.5 | 1 |
| 266 | Beans, green or wax | 1 | 6 | | | | |
| 266a | Beans, green or wax | | | 1 jar | 128 | 1 | 8 |
| 266b | Beans, green or wax | | | 1 oz | 28 | <0.5 | 2 |
| 267 | Beef with broth | 1 | 6 | | | | |
| 267a | Beef with broth | | | 1 jar | 99 | 1 | 6 |
| 267b | Beef with broth | | | 1 oz | 28 | <0.5 | 2 |
| 268 | Beets | 2 | 10 | | | | |
| 268a | Beets | | | 1 jar | 128 | 3 | 13 |
| 268b | Beets | | | 1 oz | 28 | 1 | 3 |
| 269 | Carrots | 1 | 2 | | | | |
| 269a | Carrots | | | 1 jar | 128 | 1 | 3 |
| 269b | Carrots | | | 1 oz | 28 | <0.5 | 1 |
| 270 | Chicken with broth | 1 | 2 | | | | |
| 270a | Chicken with broth | | | 1 jar | 99 | 1 | 2 |
| 270b | Chicken with broth | | | 1 oz | 28 | <0.5 | 1 |
| 271 | Corn, creamed | 1 | 3 | | | | |
| 271a | Corn, creamed | | | 1 jar | 128 | 1 | 4 |
| 271b | Corn, creamed | | | 1 oz | 28 | <0.5 | 1 |
| 272 | Egg yolk | 8 | 20 | | | | |
| 272a | Egg yolk | | | 1 jar | 94 | 8 | 19 |
| 272b | Egg yolk | | | 1 oz | 28 | 2 | 6 |
| 273 | Fruit, mixed | 1 | 1 | | | | |
| 273a | Fruit, mixed | | | 1 jar | 134 | 1 | 1 |
| 273b | Fruit, mixed | | | 1 oz | 28 | <0.5 | <0.5 |
| 274 | Ham with broth | <0.5 | 6 | | | | |
| 274a | Ham with broth | | | 1 jar | 99 | <0.5 | 6 |

| Item number | Food and description | Per 100 g edible protion | | Per specified unit | | | |
|---|---|---|---|---|---|---|---|
| | | Free folacin (μg) | Total folacin (μg) | Approximate measure | Weight (g) | Free folacin (μg) | Total folacin (μg) |
| 274b | Ham with broth | | | 1 oz | 28 | <0.5 | 2 |
| 275 | Lamb with vegetables | 1 | 8 | | | | |
| 275a | Lamb with vegetables | | | 1 jar | 99 | 1 | 8 |
| 275b | Lamb with vegetables | | | 1 oz | 28 | <0.5 | 2 |
| 276 | Oatmeal | — | 4 | | | | |
| 276a | Oatmeal | | | 1 jar | 135 | — | 5 |
| 276b | Oatmeal | | | 1 oz | 28 | — | 1 |
| 277 | Peas | 1 | 7 | | | | |
| 277a | Peas | | | 1 jar | 128 | 1 | 9 |
| 277b | Peas | | | 1 oz | 28 | <0.5 | 2 |
| 278 | Spinach, creamed | 2 | 4 | | | | |
| 278a | Spinach, creamed | | | 1 jar | 128 | 3 | 5 |
| 278b | Spinach, creamed | | | 1 oz | 28 | 1 | 1 |
| 279 | Squash | 1 | 6 | | | | |
| 279a | Squash | | | 1 jar | 128 | 1 | 8 |
| 279b | Squash | | | 1 oz | 28 | <0.5 | 2 |
| 280 | Sweet potatoes | 1 | 3 | | | | |
| 280a | Sweet potatoes | | | 1 jar | 128 | 1 | 4 |
| 280b | Sweet potatoes | | | 1 oz | 28 | <0.5 | 1 |
| 281 | Turkey with broth | 2 | 4 | | | | |
| 281a | Turkey with broth | | | 1 jar | 99 | 2 | 4 |
| 281b | Turkey with broth | | | 1 oz | 28 | 1 | 1 |
| 282 | Veal with broth | 2 | 7 | | | | |
| 282a | Veal with broth | | | 1 jar | 99 | 2 | 7 |
| 282b | Veal with broth | | | 1 oz | 28 | 1 | 2 |
| 283 | Vegetables, mixed | 1 | 4 | | | | |
| 283a | Vegetables, mixed | | | 1 jar | 128 | 1 | 5 |
| 283b | Vegetables, mixed | | | 1 oz | 28 | <0.5 | 1 |

**Miscellaneous**

| Item number | Food and description | Free folacin (μg) | Total folacin (μg) | Approximate measure | Weight (g) | Free folacin (μg) | Total folacin (μg) |
|---|---|---|---|---|---|---|---|
| 284 | Barbecue sauce | 3 | 4 | | | | |
| 284a | Barbecue sauce | | | 1 cup | 250 | 8 | 10 |
| 284b | Barbecue sauce | | | 1 tbsp | 16 | <0.5 | 1 |
| 285 | Candy, milk chocolate, plain | 4 | 7 | 1 oz | 28 | 1 | 2 |
| 286 | Margarine | 2 | 2 | | | | |
| 286a | Margarine | | | 1 cup | 227 | 5 | 5 |
| 286b | Margarine | | | 1 tbsp | 14 | <0.5 | <0.5 |
| 287 | Mayonnaise | 1 | 3 | 1 tbsp | 14 | <0.5 | <0.5 |
| 288 | Rice pudding | 5 | — | | | | |
| 288a | Rice pudding | | | 1 cup | 255 | 13 | — |
| 288b | Rice pudding | | | ½ cup | 128 | 6 | — |
| | Soups, commercial, canned | | | | | | |
| 289 | Asparagus, cream of | 5 | 19 | 1 cup | 245 | 12 | 47 |
| 290 | Beef broth | 1 | 4 | 1 cup | 240 | 2 | 10 |
| 291 | Clam chowder | 3 | 7 | 1 cup | 250 | 8 | 18 |
| 292 | Mushroom, cream of | 1 | 3 | 1 cup | 245 | 2 | 7 |
| 293 | Vegetable beef | 2 | 6 | 1 cup | 250 | 5 | 15 |
| 294 | Strawberry jam | 7 | 8 | 1 tbsp | 20 | 1 | 2 |
| 295 | Tapioca, dry | 2 | 8 | | | | |
| 295a | Tapioca, dry | | | 1 cup | 152 | 3 | 12 |
| 295b | Tapioca, dry | | | 1 tbsp | 8 | <0.5 | 1 |
| 296 | Tapioca pudding | 2 | — | 1 cup | 255 | 5 | — |
| 297 | Tomato catsup | 2 | 5 | | | | |
| 297a | Tomato catsup | | | 1 cup | 273 | 5 | 14 |
| 297b | Tomato catsup | | | 1 tbsp | 15 | <0.5 | 1 |

**Folacin Content in Terms of 100 g Edible Portion and of Specified Units\***

| Item number | Food and description | Per 100 g edible protion | | Per specified unit | | | |
|---|---|---|---|---|---|---|---|
| | | Free folacin (μg) | Total folacin (μg) | Approximate measure | Weight (g) | Free folacin (μg) | Total folacin (μg) |
| | Yeast | | | | | | |
| 298 | Baker's dry, active | 140 | 4,090 | 1 pkg. | 7 | 10 | 286 |
| 299 | Brewer's, debittered | 175 | 3,909 | 1 tbsp | 8 | 14 | 313 |

Source: Reprinted from Perloff, B. P., and Butrum, R. R.: Folacin in selected foods. J. Am. Diet. Assoc. 70: 161, 1977.

# Classification of Infant Formulas

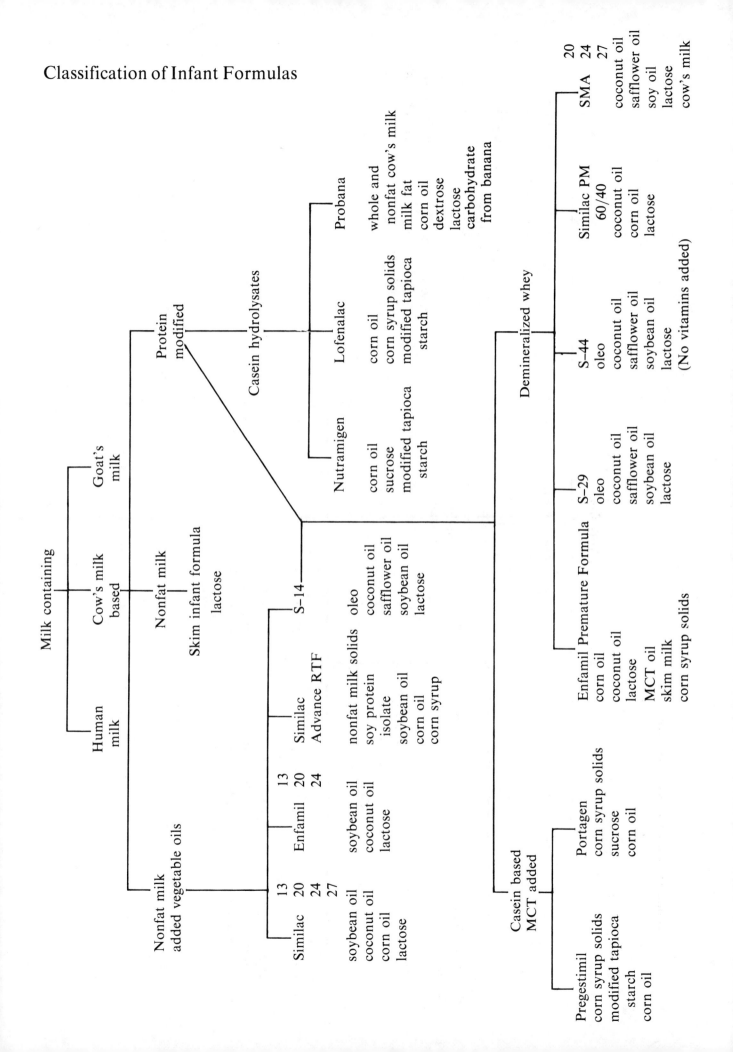

**Classification of Infant Formulas (*Continued*)**

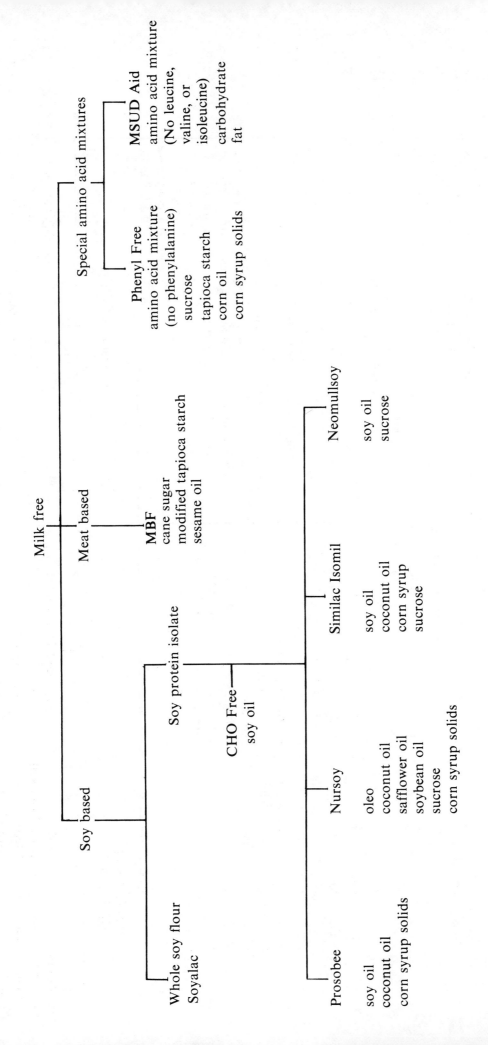

**Approximate Composition of Commonly Used Infant Formulas**

| | Protein (g) | Fat (g) | Carbohydrate (g) | Calcium (mg) | Phosphorus (mg) | Sodium (mg) | Potassium (mg) | Iron (mg) | Vitamin A (IU) | Vitamin D (IU) | Vitamin E (IU) | Vitamin C (mg) | Osmolality | Manufacturer |
|---|---|---|---|---|---|---|---|---|---|---|---|---|---|---|
| Skim infant formula | 3.55 | 0.10 | 4.89 | 130.0 | 95 | 52 | 171 | tr | 170 | 40.0 | 0.5 | 5.5 | 298 | Ross Laboratories* |
| Similac | 1.55 | 3.61 | 7.23 | 57.0 | 43 | 22 | 68 | tr | 250 | 40.0 | 1.5 | 5.5 | 290 | Ross |
| Enfamil 13 | 1.00 | 2.40 | 4.50 | 36.0 | 30 | 18 | 48 | 0.10 | 110 | 27.5 | 0.8 | 3.5 | 170 | Mead Johnson and Co.† |
| Enfamil 20 | 1.50 | 3.70 | 7.00 | 55.0 | 46 | 28 | 70 | 0.15 | 168 | 41.9 | 1.3 | 5.4 | 262 | Mead Johnson |
| Enfamil 24 | 1.80 | 4.50 | 8.30 | 66.0 | 56 | 34 | 83 | 1.52 | 203 | 50.6 | 1.5 | 6.5 | 314 | Mead Johnson |
| Advance RFT | 2.80 | 2.00 | 6.20 | 80.0 | 60 | 45 | 110 | 1.80 | 240 | 40.0 | 1.2 | 5.0 | 251 | Ross |
| S-14 | 1.10 | 3.70 | 7.10 | 40.0 | 30 | 15 | 45 | 0.04 | 250 | 40.0 | 0.9 | 5.5 | — | Wyeth Laboratories‡ |
| Enfamil Premature Formula | 2.40 | 4.10 | 8.90 | 95.0 | 47 | 31 | 89 | 0.13 | 250 | 50.0 | 1.6 | 6.8 | 300 | Mead Johnson |
| Similac PM 60/40 | 1.58 | 3.76 | 6.88 | 40.0 | 20 | 16 | 58 | 0.26 | 250 | 40.0 | 1.5 | 5.5 | 281 | Ross |
| SMA 20 | 1.50 | 3.60 | 7.20 | 44.0 | 33 | 15 | 56 | 1.27 | 261 | 42.0 | 0.9 | 5.7 | 300 | Wyeth |
| SMA 24 | 1.80 | 4.30 | 8.64 | 53.0 | 39 | 18 | 67 | 1.52 | 317 | 51.0 | 1.1 | 6.9 | 364 | Wyeth |
| SMA 27 | 2.47 | 4.81 | 9.55 | 60.0 | 45 | 20 | 76 | 1.71 | 357 | 57.0 | 1.3 | 7.8 | — | Wyeth |
| Pregestimil | 1.40 | 2.70 | 9.10 | 63.0 | 42 | 32 | 73 | 1.27 | 208 | 42.0 | 1.5 | 5.4 | 338 | Mead Johnson |
| Portagen | 2.40 | 3.20 | 7.80 | 63.0 | 47 | 32 | 84 | 1.27 | 523 | 52.0 | 2.1 | 5.4 | 211 | Mead Johnson |
| Nutramigen | 2.20 | 2.60 | 8.80 | 63.0 | 47 | 32 | 68 | 1.27 | 168 | 42.0 | 1.1 | 5.4 | 397 | Mead Johnson |
| Lofenalac | 2.20 | 2.70 | 8.80 | 63.0 | 47 | 32 | 68 | 1.27 | 168 | 42.0 | 1.1 | 5.4 | 407 | Mead Johnson |
| Probana | 4.20 | 2.20 | 7.90 | 116.0 | 89 | 61 | 121 | 0.15 | 523 | 105.0 | 1.1 | 5.4 | 531 | Mead Johnson |
| Prosobee | 2.00 | 3.60 | 6.90 | 65.0 | 50 | 28 | 68 | 1.27 | 208 | 42.0 | 1.1 | 5.4 | 160 | Mead Johnson |
| Isomil 20 | 2.00 | 3.60 | 6.80 | 70.0 | 50 | 30 | 71 | 1.20 | 250 | 40.0 | 1.5 | 5.5 | 253 | Ross |
| Neomullsoy 20 | 1.86 | 3.60 | 6.60 | 84.5 | 63 | 36 | 90 | 1.04 | 212 | 42.0 | 1.1 | 5.5 | 273 | Syntex Laboratories§ |
| CHO Free (diluted with equal volume of 12.8% CHO solution) | 1.80 | 3.50 | 12.8% CHO solution added | 85.0 | 65 | 35 | 85 | 0.80 | 200 | 40.0 | 1.0 | 5.2 | — | Syntex |
| MBF (dilution of 1:1½) | 2.90 | 3.30 | 4.20 | 253.5 | 169 | 45 | 96 | 3.90 | 390 | — | 1.3 | 13.0 | — | Gerber Products Co.⊥ |
| Phenyl Free | 2.10 | 0.70 | 6.80 | 63.0 | 47 | 26 | 73 | 1.25 | 208 | 42.0 | 1.0 | 5.4 | — | Mead Johnson |
| MSUD Aid | 1.20 | 2.90 | 8.90 | 69.0 | 38 | 31 | 47 | 1.25 | 167 | 42.0 | 1.0 | 4.3 | 300 | |
| Breast milk | 1.10 | 4.50 | 6.80 | 34.0 | 14 | 15 | 56 | 0.02 | 190 | 2.2 | 0.2 | 1.0 | 288 | |
| Cow's milk | 3.60 | 3.60 | 5.00 | 122.0 | 96 | 52 | 149 | tr | 145 | 42.0 | 0.1 | 5.4 | — | Mead Johnson |

*Note:* Values are per 100 ml of ready to use formula.
* Columbus, OH 43216.
† Evansville, IN 47721.
‡ Philadelphia, PA 19101.
§ Palo Alto, CA 94304.
⊥ Fremont, MI 49412.

## Composition and Indications for Use

| Product | Composition | Indications for use |
|---|---|---|
| *Nonfat milk formulas* | | |
| Skim infant formula (10 kcal/oz) | Skimmed milk, lactose, carrageen, ascorbic acid, vitamin A palmitate, niacin, vitamin $D_3$ concentrate, cupric sulfate, alpha tocopheryl acetate, pyridoxine, thiamine, calcium pantothenate, folic acid, cyanocobalamin | In instances when a more dilute formula is indicated, e.g., as initial formula feedings in infants in the recovery stage of acute diarrhea, as a transition between clear liquids and a more concentrated formula; when a low fat, low kilocalorie formula is indicated |
| *Nonfat milk formulas with added vegetable oils* | | |
| Similac (13 kcal/oz) | Water, nonfat milk, lactose, soy, coconut and corn oils, mono- and diglycerides, soy lecithin, carrageen, ascorbic acid, zinc sulfate, niacinamide, alpha tocopheryl acetate, cupric sulfate, vitamin A palmitate, calcium pantothenate, thiamine chloride hydrochloride, pyridoxine hydrochloride, riboflavin, manganese chloride, vitamin $D_3$ concentrate, cyanocobalamin, folic acid | In instances when a more dilute formula is indicated, e.g., as initial formula feedings in the recovery stage of acute diarrhea, as a transition between clear liquids and a more concentrated formula |
| Similac (20 kcal/oz) | Same as Similac (13 kcal/oz) | Routine infant feeding |
| Similac (24 kcal/oz) | Same as Similac (13 kcal/oz) | In premature, small for dates or underweight young infants; whenever a formula with increased kilocalories is indicated |
| Similac (27 kcal/oz) | Same as Similac (13 kcal/oz) | In premature, small for dates or underweight infants; whenever a high kilocalorie formula is indicated and a higher than normal renal solute load is not contraindicated (e.g., contraindicated in renal or heart disease) |
| Enfamil (13 kcal/oz) | Water, nonfat milk, lactose, coconut oil, soy and corn oils, mono- and diglycerides, soy lecithin, carrageen, ascorbic acid, ferrous sulfate, potassium citrate, niacin, vitamin A palmitate, vitamin $D_3$ concentrate, thiamine chloride hydrochloride, calcium pantothenate, pyridoxine hydrochloride, riboflavin, alpha tocopherol acetate, cupric sulfate, cyanocobalamin, folic acid | Same indications for use as Similac (13 kcal/oz) |
| Enfamil (20 kcal/oz) | Same as Enfamil (13 kcal/oz) | Same indications for use as Similac (20 kcal/oz) |
| Enfamil (24 kcal/oz) | Same as Enfamil (13 kcal/oz) | Same indications for use as Similac (24 kcal/oz) |
| Similac Advance RTF (16 kcal/oz) | Water, nonfat milk solids, corn syrup, soybean oil, isomerized corn syrup, soy protein isolate, corn oil, mono- and diglycerides, lecithin, carrageen, ascorbic acid, ferrous sulfate, magnesium chloride, zinc sulfate, vitamin A palmitate, vitamin $D_3$ concentrate, niacinamide, potassium citrate, calcium pantothenate, copper sulfate, alpha tocopherol acetate, riboflavin, pyridoxine hydrochloride, thiamine chloride hydrochloride, folic acid, cyanocobalamin, artificial flavorings | For the older infant, e.g., 4–12 months; an alternative to cow's milk for the infant in whom an iron fortified formula higher in polyunsaturated fat than cow's milk is indicated; contains some soy protein as well as cow's milk protein |

| Product | Composition | Indications for use |
| --- | --- | --- |
| *Nonfat milk formulas with MCT added* | | |
| Enfamil Premature Formula (24 kcal/oz) | Concentrated sweet skim milk, corn syrup solids, demineralized whey, MCT oil, corn oil, coconut oil, lactose, vitamins, and minerals | For the premature or underweight infant in whom an increased caloric intake and MCT oil are indicated, whenever a low renal solute load or low phosphate formula is indicated or a Ca:P ratio of 2:1 is indicated |
| *Nonfat milk based, leucine restricted* | | |
| SMA S–14 (20 kcal/oz) | Lactose, nonfat milk, oleo, coconut oil, safflower oil, soybean oil, soy lecithin, vitamins and minerals | For leucine sensitive hypoglycemia; as part of overall dietary management of branched chain ketoaciduria |
| *Protein modified (demineralized whey) formulas* | | |
| SMA–S–29 (20 kcal/oz) | Electrodialyzed whey (protein and lactose), oleo, coconut oil, soybean oil, vitamins and minerals | In the dietary management of infants who can tolerate only an exceptionally low renal solute load, e.g., infants with renal disease, diabetes insipidus, severe cardiac malfunction |
| SMA–S–44 (20 kcal/oz) | Same as SMA–S–29 except no vitamins and minerals | In the dietary management of infants who can tolerate only an exceptionally low renal solute load or who have severe hypercalcemia, e.g., congenital idiopathic hypercalcemia |
| Similac PM 60/40 (20 kcal/oz) Protein = 60% whey, 40% casein | Demineralized whey solids, coconut oil, lactose, corn oil, calcium citrate, potassium chloride, mono- and diglycerides, lecithin, potassium phosphate, sodium chloride, magnesium chloride, ascorbic acid, zinc sulfate, niacinamide, vitamin A palmitate, vitamin $D_3$ concentrate, ferrous sulfate, alpha tocopherol acetate, potassium citrate, cupric sulfate, calcium pantothenate, thiamine chloride hydrochloride, riboflavin, pyridoxine hydrochloride, potassium iodide, phytonadione (vitamin $K_1$), folic acid, manganese chloride, cyanocobalamin | In renal or heart disease, whenever a low renal solute load or low phosphate formula is indicated or a Ca:P ratio of 2:1 is indicated |
| SMA 20 (20 kcal/oz) Protein = 60% whey, 40% casein | Water; nonfat milk; electrodialyzed whey; lactose; oleo, coconut, oleic (safflower), and soybean oils; soy lecithin; calcium carrageen; vitamins and minerals | Routine infant feeding |
| SMA 24 (24 kcal/oz) Protein = 60% whey, 40% casein | Same as SMA 20 | In premature, underweight, low birth weight infants or whenever a high kilocalorie formula with a more normal percentage of whey to casein is indicated |
| SMA 27 (27 kcal/oz) Protein = 60% whey, 40% casein | Same as SMA 20 | In premature, underweight, low birth weight infants or whenever a high kilocalorie, electrodialyzed whey formula is indicated and a higher than normal renal solute load is not contraindicated |
| *Casein based, MCT added formulas* | | |
| Pregestimil (20 kcal/oz) | Corn syrup solids, casein enzymatically hydrolyzed and charcoal treated to reduce allergenicity, tapioca starch, MCT, corn oil, vitamins and minerals | When MCT oil is indicated or in instances where the digestion, absorption, transport, or utilization of long chain fats is impaired, e.g., in chylous ascites, Hirschsprung's disease, massive ileal resections, type I hyperlipidemia, pancreatitis; when monosaccharides as opposed to large amounts of disaccharides are indicated, e.g., in disaccharidase deficiencies |

| Product | Composition | Indications for use |
|---------|-------------|---------------------|
| Portagen (20 kcal/oz) | Sodium caseinate, MCT oil, corn oil, corn syrup solids, sucrose and other carbohydrates, vitamins and minerals | When MCT oil is indicated and disaccharide absorption is not also impaired |
| *Casein hydrolysate formulas* | | |
| Nutramigen (20 kcal/oz) | Sucrose, casein enzymatically hydrolyzed and charcoal treated to reduce allergenicity, tapioca starch, corn oil, vitamins and minerals | In galactosemia, lactose intolerance, lactalbumin and/or lactoglobulin milk protein allergy |
| Probana (20 kcal/oz) | Protein milk powder (whole milk curd and skim milk curd with added lactic acid and calcium chloride), banana powder, dextrose, an enzymatic casein hydrolysate, corn oil, vitamins and minerals | In the older child when a high protein formula is indicated and a high renal solute load is not contraindicated, e.g., in cystic fibrosis |
| *Casein based, amino acid modified formulas* | | |
| Lofenalac (20 kcal/oz) | Specially processed casein hydrolysate, corn oil, corn syrup solids, modified tapioca starch, vitamins and minerals | In phenylketonuria, where a low phenylalanine, high tyrosine formula is indicated |
| *Soy protein isolate formulas* | | |
| Prosobee (20 kcal/oz) | Corn syrup solids, soy oil, soy protein, vitamins and minerals | In milk protein allergy, allergy to both casein and whey fractions of milk protein, lactose and/or sucrose intolerance |
| Nursoy (20 kcal/oz) | Water, corn syrup solids, sucrose, soy protein isolate, oleo, coconut oil, safflower oil, soy lecithin, methionine, calcium carrageen, vitamins and minerals | Same as Prosobee |
| Similac Isomil (20 kcal/oz) | Water, sucrose, corn syrup solids, soy protein isolate, corn oil, coconut oil, corn starch, dibasic calcium phosphate, potassium citrate, potassium chloride, calcium carbonate, magnesium chloride, soy phospholipids, mono- and diglycerides, calcium carrageen, vitamins and minerals | Same as Prosobee |
| Neomullsoy (20 kcal/oz) | Sucrose, soy oil, soy protein isolate, vitamins and minerals | Same as Prosobee |
| Soyalac (20 kcal/oz) | Soy flour, soy oil, vitamins and minerals | Same as Prosobee |
| CHO Free (20 kcal/oz when reconstituted according to directions with 56 g sugar) | Water, soy oil, soy protein isolate, potassium citrate, tricalcium phosphate, dibasic magnesium phosphate, lecithin, methionine, choline chloride salt, calcium carrageen, ascorbic acid, ferrous sulfate, zinc sulfate, niacinamide, dl-alpha tocopheryl acetate, manganese sulfate, calcium pantathonate, vitamin A palmitate, cupric sulfate, riboflavin, thiamine hydrochloride, pyridoxine hydrochloride, vitamin $D_3$, biotin, potassium iodide, folic acid, vitamin $B_{12}$ | A carbohydrate free formula to which a carbohydrate source of choice is added—an aid to the diagnosis and treatment of inborn errors of carbohydrate metabolism, e.g., fructose, sucrose, isomaltose, or lactose intolerance |
| *Meat based formulas* | | |
| Meat Base Formula (20 kcal/oz) | Beef hearts, water, cane sugar, sesame oil, modified tapioca starch, tricalcium phosphate, calcium citrate, sodium ascorbate, ferrous sulfate, thiamine hydrochloride, tocopherol acetate, vitamin A palmitate, pyridoxine hydrochloride, vitamin D, phytonadione (vitamin $K_1$), folic acid, potassium iodide | In lactose intolerance, galactosemia, milk allergy, soy allergy |

| Product | Composition | Indications for use |
|---|---|---|
| *Selective amino acid restricted formulas* | | |
| Lofenalac (Listed under casein based, amino acid modified formulas) | | |
| SMA S–14 (Listed under nonfat milk based, leucine restricted formulas) | | |
| PKU-Aid | A hydrolysate of beef serum from which phenylalanine has been removed | In phenylketonuria, in which additional supplementation with carbohydrate, fat and vitamins and minerals is necessary to provide nutritional requirements |
| MSUD Aid | A mixture of crystalline L-amino acids devoid of the branched chain amino acids | In branched chain ketoaciduria, in which fat soluble vitamins and additional kilocalories from carbohydrate and fat are needed to meet nutritional requirements, and additional protein as a minimal source of branched chain amino acids is needed to meet daily nutrient requirements |
| Methionaid | A methionine free mixture of L-amino acids, water soluble vitamins and minerals, fortified with cystine | In homocystinuria due to diet responsive form of cystathionine syntetase deficiency; not indicated in pyridoxine responsive form of homocystinuria |
| Low Methionine Isomil | A low methionine, low cystine soy based product containing carbohydrate, fat, protein, vitamins and minerals | Whenever it is desirable to reduce the intake of sulfur containing amino acids |
| Histinaid | An L-amino acid mixture devoid of histidine and containing water soluble vitamins and minerals | Whenever selective restriction of histidine is indicated—other foods must be utilized in order to provide kilocalories, fat soluble vitamins, and essential fatty acids |
| Phenyl Free | An amino acid mixture devoid of phenylalanine, contains vitamins, minerals, carbohydrate and fat; fewer calories than Lofenalac | For the older child with phenylketonuria |

# Product Information: Composition of Nutritional Supplements

I. HIGH PROTEIN SUPPLEMENTS

| Product | Manufacturer | Nutrient analysis | Composition | Remarks |
|---|---|---|---|---|
| Casec (powder) 3⅓-oz cans | Mead Johnson and Co., Evansville, IN 47721 | Per 100 g powder: protein 88 g, fat 0 g, CHO 2 g, Na 51 mg | Calcium caseinate derived from dried skim skim milk curd and lime water (calcium carbonate) | No vitamins |
| Gevral Protein (powder) 8-oz pkg. 5-lb pkg. | Lederle Laboratories, Division American Cyanamid Co., Pearl River, NY 10965 | Per ⅓ cup powder mixed with approx. 8 oz water: protein 15.60 g, fat 0.52 g, Na 20.70 mg | Calcium caseinate, lactose, artificial flavors, malt extract, sucrose, yeast, vitamins and minerals | Recommended dilution 1:3 with water |
| Citrotein (powder) | Doyle Pharmaceutical Co., Minneapolis, MN 55416 | Per 1 pkg. reconstituted to provide approx. 8 fl oz: protein 6.70 g, fat 0.33 g, CHO 23.30 g, Na 130.00 mg | Sugar, egg white solids, maltodextrin, natural and artificial flavors, vegetable oil, emulsifiers, vitamins and minerals | Dilute with water Lactose free, low fat, low residue |
| Dietene (powder) 1-lb cans 4½-lb cans | Doyle Pharmaceutical Co. | Caloric distribution (%): protein 35, fat 2, CHO 63, 0.8 kcal/ml | Nonfat dry milk, sugar, milk protein, carrageen, artificial flavor, lecithin, vitamins | Dilute with skim milk, 1 oz powder to 8 oz milk |
| Instant Breakfast (powder) | Carnation Co., Los Angeles, CA 90036 | Per 1 envelope powder mixed with 8 oz milk: protein 17.5 g, fat 9.0 g, CHO 35.0 g, Na 234.0 mg | Nonfat dry milk, sucrose, lactose, sodium caseinate, corn syrup solids, lecithin, salts, stabilizers, artificial flavors, vitamins and minerals | Dilute with whole milk Flavors: chocolate, chocolate malt, eggnog, plain, strawberry |
| Liquid Predigested Protein | Hospital Diet Products Corp., Buena Park, CA 90621 | Per 30 ml: 15 g protein, 2 kcal/ml | Hydrolyzed animal collagen with added tryptophan | |
| Delmark Milkshake (powder) | Delmark Food Service Co., Minneapolis, MN 55416 | Caloric distribution (%): protein 14.4, fat 34.6, CHO 51.0, 0.95 kcal/ml (when mixed with whole milk) | *Strawberry and vanilla flavors:* sugar, maltodextrin, ice cream mix, carrageen, natural and artificial flavors, vegetable oil, mono- and diglycerides, salt, xanthan gum, artificial flavors | Also comes in chocolate malt flavor, which contains cocoa. Salmonella free. May be mixed with whole or skim milk |
| Delmark Eggnog (powder) | Delmark Food Service Co. | Per 1 envelope when mixed with 8 oz whole milk: protein 15.2 g, fat 8.8 g, CHO 37.5 g, Cholesterol 30.0 mg, Na 220.0 mg, K 590.0 mg | Nonfat dry milk, maltodextrin, sugar, egg white and egg yolk solids, vegetable oil, artificial vanilla, artificial color, vitamins | May be diluted with whole or skim milk. Salmonella free |
| Lolactene 2-oz packets | Doyle Pharmaceutical Co. | Per 1 pkg. mixed with 8 oz water: protein 15.0 g, fat 5.3 g, CHO 30.0 g, Na 250.0 mg, K 700.0 mg | Low lactose nonfat dry milk, corn syrup solids, vegetable oil, sucrose, sodium caseinate, natural and artificial flavors, mono- and diglycerides, hydroxylated lecithin, polyglycerol esters, artificial color, vitamins and minerals | Milk based feeding, 99.6% lactose free |

## II. CARBOHYDRATE SUPPLEMENTS

| Product | Manufacturer | Nutrient analysis | Composition | Remarks |
|---------|--------------|-------------------|-------------|---------|
| Cal-Power (liquid) 8-oz cartons 12 cartons per case | Henkel Corp., Minneapolis, MN 55435 | Caloric distribution (%): protein 0.1 fat 0.0 CHO 99.9 2.25 kcal/ml | Deionized water, deionized corn syrup, natural and/or artificial flavors, natural and/or artificial color, preservatives | High kilocalorie, low electrolye product  Flavors: lemon cherry grape apple fruit punch |
| Controlyte (powder) 14-oz cans 7-oz cans | Doyle Pharmaceutical Co. | Caloric distribution (%): protein trace fat 43 CHO 57 5.04 kcal/g of powder | Polysaccharides obtained by deionization of a partial enzymatic hydrolysate of corn starch, vegetable oil, emulsifier | High kilocalorie, low electrolyte product  Powder can be added to liquids or foods |
| Hycal 4-oz glass bottles | Beecham-Massengill Pharmaceuticals, Melrose, MA 02176 | Caloric distribution (%): protein trace fat trace CHO 97.6 295 kcal/4-oz bottle | Liquid glucose that has been specially demineralized, deionized water, natural flavorings, artificial color, citric acid, sodium benzoate 0.06% as a preservative | High osmolality  Ready to use flavors: lemon lime orange black walnut |
| Polycose (powder) 14-oz cans 6 cans per case  (liquid) 4-fl oz bottles 48 bottles per case | Ross Laboratories, Columbus, OH 43216 | Powder contains 94% CHO; liquid contains 100% CHO. Minerals do not exceed the following values per 100 g powder: Na 122 mg K 8 mg Cl 234 mg Ca 14 mg P 9 mg 4 kcal/g of powder 2 kcal/g of liquid Minerals do not exceed the following values per 100 ml liquid: Na 70 mg K 4 mg Cl 110 mg Ca 16 mg P 3 mg | Glucose polymers derived from controlled hydrolysis of corn starch | Dissolved powder or opened liquid should be discarded if not used within 24 hours  Low electrolyte content, low osmolality, less sweet than ordinary sugar |
| Dextro-Maltose | Mead Johnson and Co. | CHO equals 99.5% of product Minerals per 100 g powder: Na 10.0 mg Ca 10.0 mg P 30.0 mg K 120.0 mg Mg 10.0 mg Fe 0.8 mg | Cornstarch hydrolysate: 56% maltose 42% dextrins | Powder equals 150 g/cup  Used in infant feeding |

III. FAT SUPPLEMENTS

| Product | Manufacturer | Nutrient analysis | Composition | Remarks |
|---------|--------------|-------------------|-------------|---------|
| MCT Oil<br>1-qt bottles<br>1-gallon bottles | Mead Johnson and Co. | 14 g fat/tbsp and 8.3 kcal/g of fat or approx. 115 kcal | Lipid fraction of coconut oil consisting primarily of triglycerides of medium length carbon chains, i.e.,<br>decanoic acid ($C_{10}$) 24%<br>octanoic acid ($C_8$) 68%<br>fatty acids longer than decanoic 5%<br>fatty acids with carbon chains shorter than octanoic 3% | To be used only in instances when long chain fats are poorly tolerated or in cases of diseases interfering with digestion, absorption, or utilization of ordinary fats<br><br>Must be mixed with other foods and consumed slowly; should be served chilled when used in beverages |
| Lipomul<br>16-fl oz bottles | Upjohn Co., Needham Heights, MA 02194 | Fat equals 100% of kilocalories | Corn oil in a liquid formula containing Polysorbate 80, glyceride phosphate, sodium saccharin, artificial flavoring, preservatives | Indicated when a concentrated source of kilocalories is necessary |
| Microlipid | Hospital Diet Product Corp. | Fat equals 100% of kilocalories<br><br>Per 5 fl oz: 75 g fat or 675 kcal | Fat emulsion containing the following fatty acids: lauric, myristic, palmitic, stearic, oleic, linoleic, linolenic | May be purchased in solutions with different P/S ratios as a soy oil emulsion, corn oil emulsion, or safflower oil emulsion |

## Composition of Selected Special Dietary Products

| Product | Manufacturer | Nutrient analysis | Composition | Remarks |
|---------|--------------|-------------------|-------------|---------|
| Aproten Macaroni Products<br><br>Anellini—imitation ring macaroni<br>200 g boxes | Henkel Corp. | Per 100 g cooked weight:<br>protein 0.14 g<br>fat 0.01 g<br>CHO 21.80 g<br>Na 8.00 mg<br>K 2.00 mg<br>phenylalanine 4.00 mg | Cornstarch, tapioca starch, microcrystalline cellulose, artificial color | Indicated for low protein, low phenylalanine diets |

| Product | Manufacturer | Nutrient analysis | Composition | Remarks |
|---|---|---|---|---|
| Rigatini—imitation elbow macaroni 250 g boxes | | | | |
| Tagliatelle—imitation spaghetti 250 g boxes | | | | |
| Aproten Rusks 1 box or 24/box or 240 g boxes | Henkel Corp. | Per 100 g:<br>protein 1.0 g<br>fat 8.5 g<br>CHO 86.2 g<br>Na 30.0 mg<br>K 40.0 mg<br>(One slice or 1 rusk equals approximately 10 g) | Wheat starch, rice starch, honey, butter, locust bean gum, sorbitol, sucrose, monoglycerides, yeast | Indicated for low protein, low phenylalanine diets<br><br>Low protein, yeast leavened bread, diced and toasted |
| Prono | Henkel Corp. | Per ⅓ cup serving:<br>protein 0.02 g<br>fat 0.0 g<br>CHO 14.0 g<br>phenylalanine 0 mg<br>Na <8 mg<br>K <97 mg | Sugar, carrageen, adipic acid, potassium citrate, locust bean gum, natural and imitation flavors, calcium sulfate, artificial colors | A gelatin dessert indicated for use on low protein, low phenylalanine diets |
| Cellu Wheat Starch | Chicago Dietetic Supply, Lagrange, IL 60525 | Per 100 g starch:<br>protein 0.5%<br>CHO 89.2% | Wheat starch | Indicated for baking breads, cakes, cookies, etc. for use in protein restricted diets<br><br>Gluten content reduced to approximately 0.2% of protein content |
| Low Pro Bread | Henkel Corp. | Per serving (one ½-in. slice, 32 g):<br>protein 0.3 g<br>fat 1.8 g<br>CHO 15.8 g<br>phenylalanine 11 mg<br>Na 13 mg<br>K 13 mg | Dietetic Paygel wheat starch, sugar, vegetable shortening, yeast, egg albumen, tapioca starch methylcellulose, citric acid | Indicated for use in low protein diets or low phenylalanine diets |
| Low Pro Cookies 12 cookies per pkg. | Henkel Corp. | Per cookie:<br>protein 0.1 g<br>fat 10.0 g<br>CHO 4.0 g<br>Na 30 mg<br>K 12 mg<br>P 5 mg<br>phenylalanine 2 mg<br>gluten 0.1 g | Wheat starch, vegetable shortening, brown sugar, corn syrup, cocoa processed with alkali, monoglyceride, lecithin, methylcellulose, artificial flavors, baking soda, salt | Contains chocolate flavored chips<br><br>Indicated for use in low protein, low phenylalanine or gluten restricted diets |
| Fleischmann's Egg Beaters | Standard Brands New York, NY 10022 | Serving size equals ¼ cup or 2 fl oz, which is a substitute for 1 egg | Egg white, corn oil, nonfat dry milk, emulsifiers, (vegetable lecithin, mono- and diglycerides and PGM), cellulose and xanthan gums, trisodium and triethyl citrate, artificial flavor, artificial color, vitamins and minerals | Pasteurized, homogenized, cholesterol free egg substitute, salmonella free<br><br>Indicated on low cholesterol diets |

| Product | Manufacturer | Nutrient analysis | Composition | Remarks |
|---|---|---|---|---|
| Coffee Rich Non-Dairy Creamer | Rich Products Corp., Buffalo, NY 14212 | Per 100 g liquid:<br>protein 0.8 g<br>fat 12.2 g<br>CHO 12.2 g<br>Na 129 mg<br>K 27 mg | Water, corn syrup, vegetable fat, mono- and diglycerides, soy protein, sodium stearoyl-2 lactylate, polysorbate 60, dipotassium phosphate, sodium acid pyrophosphate, artificial color | Indicated in protein restricted diets as a concentrated source of kilocalories |
| Poly Perx Cream substitute | Mitchell Foods, Inc., Fredonia, NY 14063 | Per 100 g:<br>protein<br>(sodium caseinate) 0.75 g<br>fat (soy bean oil) 10 g<br>CHO<br>(corn syrup solids) 11.8 g<br>Ca 0<br>P 91.0 mg<br>Na 6.0 mg<br>K 17.0 mg | Vegetable oil composition (%):<br><br>Total polyunsaturated 38.8<br>Cis-cis polyunsaturated 28.7<br>Monounsaturated 45.9<br>Saturates 15.3<br>P/S ratio = 2<br>The polyunsaturated oil consists of linoleic and linolenic fatty acids. The monounsaturated oil is an oleic triglyceride | Indicated on low cholesterol, high polyunsaturated fat diets<br>Contains no coconut oil |

# Index

intestinal lymphangiectasia, E66
iodine: deficiency signs, A25; number, E51
iodized salt, A4
Isocal, B33, B36
Isomil, I81, I83, I86; low methionine, I87

Jaretsky diet, H24

K, vitamin. *See* vitamins
Karrell diet, H24
Kempner rice-fruit diet, H24
keratomalacia, F11
ketoacidosis, F11
ketogenic diet, MCT, E71–75. *See also* medium chain triglyceride (MCT)
ketogenic diet, traditional, E77–80; equivalent food groups list, E78–79; nutritional value, E77; nutritional inadequacy, E77; meal patterns, E78; sample menus, E80; use, E77
kidney: disease, A87; reabsorption and drugs, H8–9
kilocalorie:nitrogen ratio, TPN, B56; anabolic prescription, A29
kilocalorie, protein, fat, and carbohydrate controlled diet, F11–29; adverse reactions, F13; American Diabetes Association statement, F3–9; calculations, F17–20; characteristics, F11; check list for prescription, F14–15; contraindications, F13; defined, F11; diet for insulin dependent, F6–7; diet for non-insulin dependent, F7; dietary strategies, F15; effects, F12; exchange lists, F20–25; fiber, F5; hemoglobin variant A1C, F12; high carbohydrate diet effect, F12; hyperlipidemia, F12; hypoglycemic agents, F12; individualization, F8; meal spacing, F13; nutritional analysis (1800 kcal), A14; nutrient distribution, F16; planning, F13–15; purpose, F11–12; regularity of meals, F6; sample menu (1800 kcal), F26; use, F12–13
kilocalorie restricted diet, F31–34; adverse reactions, F32; behavioral modification and weight reduction, F32; characteristics, F31; contraindications, F32; deficiencies, F32; defined, F31; drugs and weight reduction, F32; nutritional analysis, A14; Pickwickian syndrome, F31; planning, F32; purpose, F31; protein intake, F31, F32; use, F31–32
kilocalories in pregnancy and lactation, A8, A48
kwashiorkor, C4

laboratory evaluations, nutritional assessment, A21, A25–26
laboratory tests, nutritional assessment, A16–17
laboratory values, I19–26; abbreviations, I26

lactase, D14
lactation, A52; kilocalories, A8, A52; sample menu, A8; nutritional analysis, A14; nutritional needs, A52
lactose free diet, D13–17; adverse reactions, D13–14; characteristics, D13; contraindications, D14; defined, D13; effects, D13; foods allowed and excluded, D15–16; nutritional analysis, A14; planning, D14; purpose, D13; sample menu, D16; use, D13
lactose intolerance, D21–29; congenital, D27; defined, D21; milk in diet, D24; primary, D21–24; secondary, D25–27; treatment, D27
lactose restricted diet, D19–20; characteristics, D19; defined, D19; duration, D19; purpose, D19; use, D19
lactoovovegetarian: defined, A31; nutritional analysis, A14
lactovegetarian: defined, A31; nutritional analysis, A14
laxatives, H3–4
LCT restricted, MCT diet, E65–68; adverse reactions, E66; characteristics, E65; contraindications, E66; daily food plan, E69; defined, E65; effect, E65; foods allowed and excluded, E67–68; nutritional analysis, A14; planning, E66–67; purpose, E65; uses, E32, E65–66
LDL: fat controlled diet effect, E9; levels, E27; nomogram, E28; vegetarian, A33
lean body mass–creatinine index, A19
leavening agents, G4
legume equivalent list, vegetarian diet, A35
Lenhartz diet, H24
lente insulin, F16
Levodopa and vitamin B$_6$, H9
lignin, B11–12
linoleic acid, E11, E13; food composition, I61–69
linolenic acid, food composition, I61–69
lipase, pancreatic, deficiency, E65–66
lipid cholesterol, E27
lipid lowering diets, E53–55; American Heart Association, E53; diets A, B, C, D, E54; differences, American Heart Association—National Institutes of Health, E55; National Institutes of Health, E53–55; selection, E53–55; types, E53
Lipomul, I91
lipoproteins: compsition, E26; defined, E23; cholesterol, E27; nomogram, E28
liquid diets, B3–7
—clear, adverse reactions, B3; characteristics, B3; contraindications, B3; defined, B3; nutritional analysis, A14; planning, B3; purpose, B3; sample menu, B3; use, B3
—fiber free semisynthetic, B43–53; administration, B47–48; adverse reac-

tions, B45–46; composition, B49; contraindications, B46; characteristics, B43; defined, B43; effect, B43–45; for infants, B48; kilocalorie:nitrogen ratios, B52; nutritional analysis, B50–51; proper storage, B48; purpose, B43; selection guidelines, B46–47, use, B45
—full: adverse reactions, B5; characteristics, B5; contraindications, B5; defined, B5; daily food plan, B6; low sodium, B5; nutritional analysis, A14; planning, B5; purpose, B5; sample menus, B6–7; use, B5
liver disease, A87, G3
liver function test, I24
Lofenolac, C29, C31, C32, I81, I83, I86, I87
Lolactine, I89
long chain triglyceride, defined, E65
long chain triglyceride restricted, medium chain triglyceride diet. *See* LCT restricted, MCT diet
low protein bread, I90
low protein cookies, I90
lymphocyte count, A18–19

malabsorption disorders, E65; fat, E3; 100 g fat diet, H15–16
malnutrition: food and drug interactions, H11; indications, A17–18; protein-kilocalorie, C3; phenylketonuria, C31
mannitol, F5
MAO. *See* monoamine oxidase
MCT. *See* medium chain triglyceride
MCT, LCT restricted diet. *See* LCT restricted, MCT diet
meat base infant formulas, I82, I83, I86
meat exchange lists: basic, F23–24; controlled protein, potassium, sodium, C17; high potassium, G19; low sodium, G10
medical combining forms, I9–11
medical records, I13–18; criteria for assessment of nutritional care, I14; educational plan, example, I17; how to record, I14–15; method of recording, I16; problem oriented medical record (POMR), I13, I16–17; Professional Standards Review Organization (PSRO) I14; SOAP format, I17; what to record, I15–16; who to record, I15; treatment plan, example, I17
medication, oral timing, H7
medium chain triglycerides (MCT): defined, E65; infant formulas, I85; oil, I91; type I hyperlipoproteinemia, E31, E35
—ketogenic diet, E71–75; adverse reactions, E72; calculation, E72–73; characteristics, E71; contraindications, E72; defined, E71; diet for 1–3 year old, E73; effects, E72; essential fatty acid deficiency, E72; meal plan and sample menu, E74; nutritional analy-

sis, A14; planning, E72; purpose, E71; side effects, E72; use in epileptic seizures, E72

megavitamins: therapy in childhood psychoses and learning disabilities, A89–91; orthomolecular approach, A89

—claims, vitamin, A42; vitamin C, A42; vitamin D, A43; vitamin E, A43

men: Recommended Dietary Allowances, (RDA), I3, I4, I5

Meritene, B33, B36, C5

metabolic complications in TPN, B58

metabolic disturbances in obesity, F32

Methionaid, I87

Meulengracht diet, H24

microlipid, I91

mild fat restricted diet, E3

milk: human, nutrient composition, A63–67; nonfat infant formulas, I83; with MCT, I84; skim infant formula, I81, I83, I84; use, in bland diet, B23, B27; in lactose free diet, D13

—exchange lists: basic, F20, controlled protein, potassium, sodium diet, C17; high potassium, G19, low sodium, G9

Milkshake, I89

milliequivalant conversion table, I45

minerals: in controlled protein, potassium, sodium diet, C14; in pregnancy, A48; recommended intake (RDA), I3, I5; in TPN, B57

modified diets, xi, xii

moderate fat restricted diet, E3

monoamine oxidase (MAO): and food interactions, H6–7; inhibitors, C49, C50

MSUD Aid, I82, I83, I87

multivitamin preparations, parenteral: adult, B60; children, B60

myocardial infarct, E10

myoclonic seizures, E71

myxedema, G7

National Academy of Science, Food and Nutrition Board, A37, A85, A87, E21–22; Recommended Dietary Allowances (RDA), I3, I4, I5

National Institutes of Health, E23, E25, E32, E35, E53–55

natural foods: defined, A43

Neomulsoy, I82, I83, I86

nervous system and drugs, H4

Newburgh diet, H24

niacin deficiency signs, A25

nitrogen metabolism, A20

N′methyl nicotinamide, urinary, A27

nonfat milk infant formulas, with vegetable oil, I83; leucine restricted, I85

norepinephrine, C50

normal diet, A3–10

NPH insulin, F16

Nursoy, I82, I83, I86

nut and seed equivalent list for vegetarians, A35

Nutri 1000, B34, B36

Nutri 1000 LF, B34, B36, D15

Nutramigen, I81, I83, I86

nutrients and drugs, availability, H5–6

nutritional analysis of diets, A11–15

nutritional assessment, A17–31; albumin, serum, A26; anemia, A18, A22; ascorbic acid, serum, A26; basal energy expenditure (BEE) calculation, A20; carotene, plasma, A26; clinical data included, A18; physical exam, clinical signs, A25; creatinine urinary values, A30; dental examination, A19; EGOT, A27; EGPT, A27; folacin, serum, A26; glutathione reductase-FAD effect, A29; hematocrit, A26; hemoglobin, A26; immune function, A19–20; iron, serum, A26; kilocalorie intake, A20; lean body mass–creatinine index, A20; nitrogen metabolism, A19; N′methyl nicotinamide, A27; pantothenic acid, A27; protein, serum, A26; pyridoxine, A27; RBC transketolase-TPP effect, A27; riboflavin, urinary, A27; thiamine, urinary, A26; transaminase index, A27; transferrin saturation, A19, A26; tryptophan load index, A27; visceral protein status, A19; vitamin A, plasma, A26; vitamin B$_{12}$, serum, A26; vitamin E, plasma, A26; weight changes evaluation, A19, A27

—anthropometry: arm, nomogram, adult, A29, children, A28; measurement procedures, A19; muscle mass and fat stores, A19

—nutrition care planning: algorithm, A17, A21; areas of investigation, A17; diet history, A17; dietary intake information, A22; form, A23–24; malnutrition indications, A18–19; methodology, A17; nutrition problems identified, A17; patient interview, A18; screening patients, A21; screening tests, A18, A21

nutritional care therapy, I15

nutritional deficiency, B3; in vegetarians, A37, A41

nutritional status, A17; and drugs, H11; in vegetarians, A38, A40

nutritional inadequacy, tube feedings, B36

nutritional therapy, anabolic prescriptions, A30

oatmeal cure, H14

obesity: in coronary heart disease, E57; in diabetes, F12; endocrine or metabolic disturbances, F32; fat cell size, F31; hypertension, F31; in infant overfeeding, A67; non-insulin dependent diabetics, F7; respiratory difficulties, F31

obsolete diets, H23–25

oil, MCT, I91

olecranon, A19

oleic acid, E65; food composition, I61–69

oral hyperalimentation: protein, A29; infant formula, I83

oral medications, timing, H7

organic foods, defined, A43

orthomolecular therapy, A90

osmolality, B47, B50–51; common foods, I47; infant foods, I83; vs osmolarity, I47

osteoarthritis, F32

pancreatic function test, I24

pancreatic lipase deficiency, E65–66

pancreatitis, E3

pantothenate, urinary, A27

peritoneal dialysis, C16

petechiae, A25

phenylalanine restricted diet, C29–44; adverse reactions, C31, calculations, C42; characteristics, C29; defined, C29; deficiency, C31; effects, C30; food lists, C34–41; hyperphenylalaninemia, C32; meal guide, C41; menu, C42–43; planning, C31–32; prescription, C33; purpose, C29–30; use, C30–31

Phenyl Free, C32, I82, I83, I87

phosphorus: in controlled protein, potassium, sodium diet, C13–14

physical exam: clinical signs, A25

phytate, B19

PKU aid, C32, I87

plant fiber, nonnutritive, B9

plasma levels, laboratory values, I20–21

Polycose, C9, I90

Poly Perx, I93

polysaccharides; noncellulose, B11–12; starch, F16

POMR, I13, I16–17

Portagen, I81, I83, I86

postoperative diet, B3, B5

potassium: hypertension, G8, G17; renal failure, C12–13, C15

potassium chloride, G17

potassium diet, controlled. See controlled protein, potassium, sodium diet

potassium diet, high, G17–23; adverse reactions, G18; characteristics, G17; contraindications, G18; daily food plan, G19; defined, G17; diuretics, use, G17; effects of depletion, G17; food lists, G19–23; insulin, G17; nutritional analysis, A14; planning, G18; purpose, G17; salt substitute use, G18; use, G17

Precision LR, B49, B50, B52; moderate nitrogen, B49, B52; HN, B49, B50, B52; isotonic, B49, B51, B52; Gelatin LR, B49, B51, B52

predigested protein, I89

Pregestimil, E67, I81, I83, I85

pregnancy: diet, A51–52; diabetes in, F11; kilocalorie content, A8, A51; fluid intake, A52; folic acid, A51; iron, A51; menu pattern, A8; nutritional analysis, A14; protein content, A8, A51; sodium intake, A52; sodium